Respiratory Disease

A Case Study Approach
to Patient Care

Respiratory Disease

A Case Study Approach to Patient Care

Second Edition

Robert L. Wilkins, PhD, RRT
Professor and Chair
Department of Cardiopulmonary Sciences
School of Allied Health Professions
Loma Linda University
Loma Linda, California

James R. Dexter, MD, FACP, FCCP
Associate Clinical Professor
School of Medicine
Loma Linda University
Loma Linda, California

F. A. DAVIS COMPANY • Philadelphia

F. A. Davis Company
1915 Arch Street
Philadelphia, PA 19103

Printed in the United States of America

Last digit indicates print number: 10 9 8 7 6 5 4 3 2 1

Publisher: Jean-François Vilain
Senior Editor: Lynn Borders Caldwell
Production Editor: Devorah W. Zuckerman
Cover Designer: Louis J. Forgione

As new scientific information becomes available through basic and clinical research, recommended treatments and drug therapies undergo changes. The authors and publisher have done everything possible to make this book accurate, up to date, and in accord with accepted standards at the time of publication. The authors, editors, and publisher are not responsible for errors or omissions or for consequences from application of the book, and make no warranty, expressed or implied, in regard to the contents of the book. Any practice described in this book should be applied by the reader in accordance with professional standards of care used in regard to the unique circumstances that may apply in each situation. The reader is advised always to check product information (package inserts) for changes and new information regarding dose and contraindications before administering any drug. Caution is especially urged when using new or infrequently ordered drugs.

Library of Congress Cataloging-in-Publication Data

Respiratory disease: a case study approach to patient care / [edited
  by] Robert L. Wilkins, James R. Dexter. — 2nd ed.
      p.   cm.
    Includes bibliographical references and index.
    ISBN 0-8036-0155-7 (cloth : alk. paper)
    1. Respiratory organs—Diseases. 2. Respiratory organs—Diseases—
  Case studies.   I. Wilkins, Robert L.   II. Dexter, James R., 1948-   .
    [DNLM: 1. Respiration Disorders.   2. Respiration Disorders—case
  studies. WF 140 R4341022 1998]
RC731.R466 1998
616.2—dc21
DNLM/DLC   97-9419
for Library of Congress

This book is dedicated to our wives,
Kris and Kathy,
and our children,
Tyler, Nicholas, Kimberly,
and Scott.

Foreword to the Second Edition

In the current era of outcome-based assessment, respiratory care faces the same challenge posed to all health-care providers—to demonstrate that respiratory care practitioners (RCPs) enhance the clinical well-being of the patients we serve. Thankfully, a maturing body of literature demonstrates that RCPs do, in fact, strengthen clinical outcomes by:

- Implementing therapist-driven protocols for adult non-ICU inpatient care
- Accelerating patients' weaning from mechanical ventilation
- Overseeing the use of diagnostic tests, such as arterial blood gases and pulmonary function tests

However gratifying these study conclusions may be, they bring along with them the requirement for a high level of competence on the part of RCPs. The "value added" by RCPs in these studies refers to therapists' roles in correct assessment of patients' clinical needs and competent application of respiratory care protocols, care plans, and algorithms to address and treat these clinical needs. Thus, in the current era of cost-conscious and quality-attentive health care, RCPs must be highly skilled, with a solid foundation in clinical practice, including:

- Understanding the pathophysiology of pulmonary disease
- Knowing the scientific underpinnings of respiratory care treatments
- Developing and projecting a sense of professionalism and craftsmanship in the care we provide
- Valuing attention to detail and thoroughness
- Maintaining the caring attributes that led us initially to a career in health care

These clinical "reflexes," particularly the attribute of caring, must develop early in the clinician's career and be cultivated through careful instruction by committed and capable teachers.

As RCPs face the challenge of becoming astute clinicians, respiratory care educators face a similar challenge: how to develop these important clinical skills by clearly explaining pathophysiology, therapeutic principles, and physical diagnosis, while preserving enthusiasm for learning in a field in which knowledge is continually evolving. Respiratory care educators must empower their students with information that will allow them to understand and treat patients' illnesses as well as to communicate with physicians with whom they interact and collaborate. More and more, clinical teaching has adopted an interactive, case-based approach, using clinical vignettes to engage trainees' attention and to foster critical thinking. Indeed, interactive, case-based learning has become a keystone of current health-care education.

How fortunate then, that this book, *Respiratory Disease: A Case Study Approach to Patient Care,* is available. The second edition revises and updates a very solid first edition by Drs. Wilkins and Dexter. The authors and their contributors present a case-study-based text addressing 25 common clinical conditions that RCPs face, both in adult and in pediatric/neonatal care. Each chapter is meticulously organized around discussions of etiology, pathophysiology, and clinical features, including aspects of the physical examination, and laboratory evaluation. Treatment is described with an emphasis on the scientific foundations of respiratory care. Following these succinct discussions, each chapter presents several case studies with focused questions that challenge the respiratory care student to apply the information to clinical situations. The questions are accompanied by clear answers, which are nicely annotated with explanatory illustrations in the format of line drawings, chest radiographs, pulmonary function test results, and electrocardiograms.

In addition to the new title, *Respiratory Disease: A Case Study Approach to Patient Care,* which aptly calls attention to the case-based nature of the book, new chapters in the second edition include an introduction to patient assessment and chapters that address ethics in respiratory care, tuberculosis, and pneumonia in the immuno-compromised host. An expanded glossary of terms and a list of key terms at the beginning of each chapter are also welcome features that enhance the usefulness of the book to the respiratory care student.

The authors, Robert L. Wilkins, PhD, RRT, and James R. Dexter, MD, FACP, FCCP, have a longstanding interest and expertise in both respiratory care and respiratory care education at Loma Linda University, an institution with an outstanding reputation in the field. To complement their own chapters, the authors have assembled a talented group of physicians, respiratory care practitioners, and educators who have translated their longstanding involvement in respiratory care into a clear, relevant, case-based book that will be an asset to every respiratory care curriculum. This book will help all of us, educators and clinicians alike, to meet the ongoing challenges of providing superb respiratory care to the patients we serve.

James K. Stoller, MD
Head, Section of Respiratory Therapy
Department of Pulmonary and
Critical Care Medicine
Cleveland Clinic Foundation
Cleveland, Ohio

Foreword to the First Edition

The treatment of respiratory disease requires a breadth and depth of knowledge that challenges even the most dedicated respiratory therapist. Analyses of respiratory disturbances require an understanding of the etiology, pathophysiology, and clinical signs of the disease, thus leading to a plan for treatment, establishment of therapeutic goals, and a schedule for ongoing assessment. Today, microprocessor-controlled ventilators, because they have so many possible modes of operation, demand an even greater understanding of the underlying causes of respiratory failure.

Many respiratory care books focus on equipment, respiratory therapy, or pathophysiology, but unlike *Respiratory Disease: Principles of Patient Care,* few organize this information by specific medical and surgical problems. Wilkins and Dexter have assembled a text written specifically for respiratory therapists that addresses the most crucial aspects of twenty-two commonly encountered respiratory diseases.

Once you review this text, I'm sure you'll agree that a great deal of thought went into what to include, or perhaps more importantly, what *not* to include. The writing style is clear without being boring; the material in each chapter is comprehensive with just the right depth of coverage; and the medical terminology is appropriate for health professionals with treatment and assessment responsibilities.

Educators will better prepare their students if this book is assigned as required reading since it will help them understand a lecture on the pathophysiology of a particular respiratory disease and will prompt thought about assessment and a therapeutic plan. Having this understanding will help new therapists begin their practice at a high level. The text should be used during the student's second clinical rotation and before studying advanced critical care topics. Individual chapters should be assigned prior to lectures on each disease entity with lectures focusing on the pathophysiology and etiology of the disease as found in the book. Discussion of each chapter's case study(ies) will enhance class time and reinforce the concepts presented in each chapter, especially since questions accompanying each case will trigger a discussion of the treatment plan and the assessment of therapeutic goals.

In addition to being of great value to students, this book is also a good reference for the beginning therapist. Its format summarizes pertinent information and makes it easy to locate quickly.

Candidates for the National Board of Respiratory Care registry written and clinical simulation examinations will find this to be an excellent review text. It covers important information about each disease and offers case studies so that readers can verify their knowledge of clinical application.

Loma Linda University has a reputation for having an excellent respiratory therapy program, and the Medical Center Respiratory Care Department has been a role model for others. Students at Loma Linda University have been fortunate to benefit from this great resource. Now, with this text, Loma Linda educators have made it possible for *all* students to benefit from their experience in treating respiratory disease.

I plan to make this a required text for a course I teach called "Respiratory Care for Medical and Surgical Patients."

Thomas A. Barnes, EdD, RRT
Associate Professor of Cardiopulmonary Sciences
Northeastern University
Boston, Massachusetts

Preface

The goal of this second edition remains to provide students in respiratory care, nursing, medicine, and other health-care programs with the critical information needed to treat patients with cardiopulmonary ailments. Clinicians who care for patients with cardiopulmonary disease will benefit from reviewing the topics most applicable to their work. A background in pulmonary anatomy and physiology, pharmacology, and medical terminology is needed to fully benefit from the information contained in this book.

The format is the same as that of the first edition. Each chapter begins with a description of the etiology, pathophysiology, clinical findings, and treatment for each disorder. This is followed by the detailed presentation of a related case study. Questions and answers highlighting key points are interspersed throughout the case study to stimulate better understanding of the topic.

All chapters have been updated; presented here are key changes in the book:

- The addition of a chapter on patient assessment. This provides the reader with a strong background in patient evaluation, which is essential for understanding the clinical assessment portion of the case studies.
- The addition of a chapter on tuberculosis. This was prompted by the recent resurgence of TB in the United States.
- The addition of a chapter on pneumonia in the immunocompromised patient. Caring for patients with defects in their immune system has become a common problem confronting all health-care providers.
- The addition of a chapter on ethics in respiratory care. We believe that respiratory care practitioners need to be familiar with the current code of conduct for their profession and must understand how this code applies to patient care. The case study approach and discussion in this new chapter are designed to help the reader better understand and apply the Code of Conduct of the American Association for Respiratory Care.

Also new to this edition is a list of key terms provided at the beginning of each chapter. These terms appear in bold within their respective chapters, and they are defined in the glossary at the end of the text. Lists of normal values for the more common laboratory tests are also provided in the Appendix to help the reader interpret the findings in the case studies.

We hope you find this book helpful in caring for your patients.

Robert L. Wilkins
James R. Dexter

Acknowledgments

Major projects are often the product of teamwork; this book is no exception. First, we would like to thank the contributors who wrote many of the chapters. They are busy professionals willing to share their expertise to help students and clinicians learn. They did an excellent job and their support is appreciated.

Once a chapter was written, it was sent to reviewers for a critique. The feedback provided by these experts was critical in making the final product complete and accurate. Reviewers for this edition included:

David W. Chang, EdD, RRT
Professor/Program Director
Respiratory Therapy Program
Columbus State University
Columbus, Georgia

Charles S. Cornfield, MS, RRT
Program Director and Assistant
  Professor
Respiratory Care Program
Gannon University
Erie, Pennsylvania

William F. Galvin, MSEd, RRT, CPFT
Program Director/Assistant Professor
Respiratory Care Program
Gwynedd Mercy College
Gwynedd Valley, Pennsylvania

Philip Geronimo, BA, RRT
Assistant Professor
Department of Respiratory Therapy
University of Toledo
Toledo, Ohio

S. Lee King, MS, RRT
Chair
Respiratory Care Department
Pearl River Community College
Hattiesburg, Mississippi

Robert McGee, MS, RRT
Program Director
Respiratory Care Technology
Walters State Community College
Greenville, Tennessee

Mimi Yee Norwood, MA, MS, RRT
Program Director/Department Chair
Department of Respiratory Therapy
Washtenaw Community College
Ann Arbor, Michigan

Sam Gregory Marshall, PhD, RRT
Associate Professor/Director of Clinical
  Education
Respiratory Care Program
Southwest Texas State University
San Marcos, Texas

In addition, we thank Wayne Harlow for providing many of the illustrations in this second edition.

Finally, we would like to mention the reviewers of the first edition—Thomas Barnes, Dean Hess, Allen Marangoni, Anna Parkman, Yvonne Robbins, John Riggs, and Lee Robinson—who played a key role in making the initial version of the text a success.

RLW and JRD

Contributors

Gregory A. B. Cheek, MD, MSPH
Clinical Instructor
Department of Internal Medicine
Pulmonary/Critical Care Fellow
Loma Linda University
Loma Linda, California

James R. Dexter, MD, FACP, FCCP
Associate Clinical Professor
School of Medicine
Loma Linda University
Loma Linda, California
and
Medical Director
Department of Respiratory Care
Redlands Community Hospital
Redlands, California

Enrique Gil, MD, FCCP
Pulmonary and Critical Care Specialist
Beaver Medical Clinic
Redlands, California

George H. Hicks, MS, RRT
Instructor and Clinical Coordinator
Respiratory Care Program
Mt. Hood Community College
Gresham, Oregon

Patrice A. Johnson, BS, RRT
Respiratory Care Manager
The Children's Mercy Hospital
Kansas City, Missouri

David Lopez, MA, RRT
Assistant Professor
Department of Cardiopulmonary
  Sciences
School of Allied Health Professions
Loma Linda University
Loma Linda, California

Cynthia Malinowski, MA, RRT
Assistant Professor
Department of Cardiopulmonary
  Sciences
School of Allied Health Professions
Loma Linda University
Loma Linda, California

**Thomas P. Malinowski, BS, RRT,
  RCP**
Clinical Director
Respiratory Care Services
Loma Linda University Children's
  Hospital and Medical Center
Loma Linda, California

Arthur B. Marshak, BS, RRT
Instructor/Clinical Coordinator
Department of Cardiopulmonary
  Sciences
School of Allied Health Professions
Loma Linda University
Loma Linda, California

Kenneth D. McCarty, MS, RRT, RCP
Former Assistant Professor
Department of Cardiopulmonary Sciences
School of Allied Health Professions
Loma Linda University
Loma Linda, California

Victoria C. Sciacqua, BS, RRT
Respiratory Care Practitioner II
San Bernardino County Medical Center
San Bernardino, California

N. Lennard Specht, MD, FACP
Medical Director
Department of Cardiopulmonary Sciences
School of Allied Health Professions
Loma Linda University
Loma Linda, California

David M. Stanton, MS, RRT, CPFT, RCP
Assistant Professor
Program Director, Respiratory Therapy
Associate Program
Department of Cardiopulmonary Sciences
School of Allied Health Professions
Loma Linda University
Loma Linda, California

Hoi N. Tran, RCP, CRTT
Staff Therapist
Loma Linda University Medical Center
Loma Linda, California

Robert L. Wilkins, PhD, RRT
Professor and Chair
Department of Cardiopulmonary
    Sciences
School of Allied Health Professions
Loma Linda University
Loma Linda, California

Gerald R. Winslow, PhD
Dean and Professor
Faculty of Religion
Loma Linda University
Loma Linda, California

Contents

CHAPTER **4**

Asthma 59

Robert L. Wilkins, PhD, RRT
James R. Dexter, MD, FACP, FCCP

CHAPTER **5**

Chronic Bronchitis 73

Robert L. Wilkins, PhD, RRT
James R. Dexter, MD, FACP, FCCP

CHAPTER **6**

Emphysema 88

Kenneth D. McCarty, MS, RRT, RCP

CHAPTER **11**
Smoke Inhalation and Burns 176
George H. Hicks, MS, RRT

CHAPTER **12**
Near Drowning 199
David M. Stanton, MS, RRT, CPFT, RCP

CHAPTER **13**
Adult Respiratory Distress Syndrome 222
Kenneth D. McCarty, MS, RRT, RCP

CHAPTER **14**

Chest Trauma..241

George H. Hicks, MS, RRT

CHAPTER **15**

Postoperative Atelectasis............................267

Thomas P. Malinowski, BS, RRT, RCP

CHAPTER **16**

Interstitial Lung Disease..............................280

N. Lennard Specht, MD, FACP

CHAPTER **17**

Neuromuscular Diseases...............................302

N. Lennard Specht, MD, FACP
Robert L. Wilkins, PhD, RRT

CHAPTER **18**

Bacterial Pneumonia 323

Robert L. Wilkins, PhD, RRT

James R. Dexter, MD, FACP, FCCP

CHAPTER **19**

Pneumonia in the Immunocompromised Patient 339

N. Lennard Specht, MD, FACP

CHAPTER **20**

Tuberculosis 357

David Lopez, MA, RRT

Arthur B. Marshak, BS, RRT

CHAPTER **21**

Lung Cancer.. 372
Gregory A. B. Cheek, MD, MSPH

CHAPTER **22**

Sleep Apnea 394
Enrique Gil, MD, FCCP

CHAPTER **23**

Croup and Epiglottitis.. 410
Robert L. Wilkins, PhD, RRT
James R. Dexter, MD, FACP, FCCP

Hoai N. Tran, RCP, CRTT

A Note to the Reader

In addition to giving you a working knowledge of the most commonly encountered respiratory diseases, this text has been specifically designed to help improve your clinical reasoning skills. Each chapter begins with background information about a certain disease, then a detailed case study is presented. The case study will help bring the information to life and give you the opportunity to test your knowledge.

To use this text most effectively, we recommend that you approach each chapter in the following manner:

- Study the background information at the beginning of each chapter. This information about etiology, pathophysiology, clinical features, and treatment will be very helpful to you as you review the related case study.
- If, during the study of any chapter, you see a term or abbreviation with which you are unfamiliar, take a moment to look it up in the glossary provided at the back of the book.
- Key questions appear throughout each case study; the questions are there to make you think about important issues related to the case. After reading each question, take a moment to write your answer either in the space provided in the text or on a separate sheet of paper. If you need to review normal values to interpret data presented in the cases, refer to the tables of normal values for clinical laboratory tests, pulmonary function tests, arterial blood gases, and hemodynamic monitoring values in the Appendix.
- Compare your answer with the one we provide.

We hope you enjoy reading each chapter with its accompanying case study and find the information helpful to your understanding and treatment of respiratory disease.

Robert L. Wilkins
James R. Dexter

CHAPTER **1**

Introduction to Patient Assessment

Robert L. Wilkins, PhD, RRT

Key Terms

abdominal paradox
acidosis
adventitious lung sounds
alkalosis
anemia
apnea
barrel chest
bradycardia
bradypnea
breath sounds
bronchial breath sounds
cardiomegaly
chest pain
chest percussion
copious
cough
crackles
cyanosis
digital clubbing

dyspnea
fetid
fever
heave
hemoptysis
history of present illness
hypercapnia
hypocapnia
hypotension
hypothermia
hypoxemia
ischemia
kyphoscoliosis
kyphosis
leukocytosis
leukopenia
monophonic wheeze
mucoid
orthopnea

pectus carinatum
pectus excavatum
platypnea
polycythemia
polyphonic wheeze
precordium
purulent
rhonchi
scoliosis
sensorium
sputum
stridor
tachycardia
tachypnea
tracheal breath sounds
vesicular breath sounds
vital capacity
wheeze

Introduction

Patient assessment is a vital part of patient care. Whether in the emergency room, intensive care unit (ICU), or home-care setting, patient assessment skills make the difference between inadequate and effective patient care. The purpose of this chapter is to provide the reader with an overview of how patient assessment is done, with an emphasis on assessment skills for the respiratory care practitioner (RCP). The therapist does not evaluate patients to make a diagnosis, but to assist the physician in determining the appropriate therapy and the effects of that therapy. In many cases, modifications in the treatment plan are based on observations by the RCP.

The clinicians who are best at patient assessment are the ones who are rigorous in their daily patient care. This entails asking all relevant questions, examining all sides of the patient's chest wall, and reviewing other data such as the chest x-ray. Clinicians who take a superficial approach to patient assessment are likely to miss important clues to changes in the patient's condition and render inappropriate care.

This chapter is divided into three parts. First, the patient interview and the medical history are reviewed, and then a brief case study is presented to show how the interview is applied in practice. Second, use of the physical examination is presented; this is followed by continuation of the case study to illustrate use of the examination. Finally, use of laboratory data is described, followed by continuation of the illustrative case study.

The Medical History and the Interview

Most patient evaluations begin with the interview. The interview is done to gather important information about what is currently wrong with the patient. It is also useful because it allows you to establish a rapport with the patient before other procedures are done, such as a physical examination. As an interviewer, you must be knowledgeable about diseases and typical patterns of diseases in order to ask the most appropriate questions. For this reason, the study of cardiopulmonary diseases, as presented in this text, will make you a better interviewer. Examples of basic questions to ask your patient, regardless of the symptoms, include the following:

1. When did the problem start?
2. Have you ever had this problem before?
3. How severe is the problem?
4. What seemed to provoke the problem, and does anything seem to make it better?
5. What region of the body is affected by the problem? If pain is the symptom, exactly where is the pain, and does it radiate to any other part of the body?

Answers to these questions will help determine a differential diagnosis, what further tests may be needed, and what initial therapy may be appropriate. The length of the interview is often determined by the severity of the patient's illness. Patients who are acutely ill may need immediate care (e.g., oxygen therapy or metered-dose inhaler treatment) before you can conduct a lengthy interview or examination.

Symptoms

The following are among the most common symptoms that patients with cardiopulmonary disease experience:

- Shortness of breath (dyspnea)
- Cough
- Sputum production
- Chest pain
- Coughing up bloody sputum (hemoptysis)
- Fever
- Wheeze

Each of these symptoms will be described in detail to give you a better background regarding each symptom, thus allowing you to ask the right questions when your patient mentions these problems during your interview.

Shortness of Breath. Shortness of breath, as perceived by the patient, is known as **dyspnea.** It is a common problem in patients with cardiopulmonary disease. Patients who experience dyspnea are also often anxious because of the fear associated with feeling short of breath. Dyspnea usually worsens with exertion (termed *exertional dyspnea*) and improves with rest. Patients with the least cardiopulmonary reserve will be dyspneic even at rest. If the dyspnea occurs only during exertion, you should identify the level of exertion at which the patient must stop to catch his breath. Is it after climbing one flight of stairs or after walking a certain distance on a flat surface? You also can ask the patient to rate his dyspnea on a scale from 1 to 10, 10 being the worst. This type of questioning helps identify the severity of the dyspnea and the urgency of therapy.

Dyspnea may be more severe in certain positions. Patients experiencing shortness of breath only in the reclining (supine) position are said to have **orthopnea.** Orthopnea is most commonly associated with heart failure, but it may also be present in patients with lung disease. **Platypnea** refers to dyspnea in the upright position. This may occur after lung surgery to remove a diseased segment or lobe. Dyspnea occurring with any change in position is abnormal and should be reported to the patient's attending physician.

The physiologic mechanisms causing dyspnea are not well understood. Most experts believe it occurs when the patient senses that his work of breathing is excessive for the level of activity in which he is engaged. Any pathologic lung change (e.g., bronchospasm or lung consolidation) that increases the work of breathing usually will lead to dyspnea, especially during exertion. Patients with severe disease, or with an acute problem superimposed on a chronic problem (e.g., pneumonia in a patient with chronic obstructive lung disease), tend to have dyspnea with very little activity or even at rest. Abnormalities that stimulate the drive to breathe (e.g., metabolic acidosis) also lead to dyspnea (Table 1-1).

Cough. **Cough** is one of the most frequent symptoms seen in patients with cardiopulmonary disease. It typically occurs when the cough receptors of the larger airways are stimulated. These receptors respond to stimulation from mechanical, chemical, inflammatory, and thermal sources. Mechanical stimulation occurs when foreign bodies touch the airway wall. Food, liquid, and suction catheters are examples of mechanical stimulators of the cough receptors. Chemical stimulation of the cough receptors occurs when the patient inhales an irritating gas, such as cigarette smoke. Infection and inflammation of the larger airways can irritate the cough receptors and is a common cause of coughing. Breathing extremely cold air can also stimulate the cough receptors. Cough receptors are also located in the pleural lining of the lung and may be stimulated when pleural inflammation is present.

A rule of thumb is that cough is usually associated with airway disease. Common

TABLE 1-1   **Physiologic Causes of Dyspnea**

INCREASES IN THE DRIVE TO BREATHE
- Significant hypoxemia
- Acidosis
- Fever
- Exercise

INCREASES IN AIRWAY'S RESISTANCE
- Asthma
- Acute bronchitis
- Croup and epiglottitis
- Chronic obstructive pulmonary disease

DECREASES IN LUNG OR CHEST WALL COMPLIANCE
- Severe pneumonia
- Severe pulmonary edema
- Adult respiratory distress syndrome
- Atelectasis
- Kyphoscoliosis
- Pneumothorax

causes of cough include acute upper respiratory infections, asthma, and bronchitis. Other causes include sinusitis or postnasal drip and reactive airway disease not severe enough to be classified as asthma.

You should identify the severity of the cough, when and how often it occurs, and whether it is productive. A productive cough can occur with infection of the airways or pneumonia. A weak cough may indicate abdominal pain or neuromuscular disease. Emphysema patients often have a weak cough because of poor respiratory muscle mechanics. Patients with chronic bronchitis often cough and produce sputum for the first hour or two after getting out of bed in the morning. Heart failure may be associated with a dry cough.

Sputum Production. **Sputum** refers to excessive production of secretions from the lung. Sputum is often contaminated with oral secretions and may not accurately reflect what is occurring in the lung. Sputum is normally produced in small amounts in the airways as part of the lungs' defense against invasion by germs. It is moved to the larynx by cilia (tiny waving fingers on the cells lining the airways). It is not normally noticed by healthy people.

Noticeable sputum production is a sign of disease of the airways. The most common cause of excessive mucus production is cigarette smoking. Cigarette smoke is irritating to the airways and causes them to produce excessive mucus as a reflex response. This in turn causes the smoker to cough and produce mucus every day, especially in the morning. Other causes of increased sputum production include inflammation associated with asthma and infection associated with pneumonia.

Sputum is described as **mucoid** when it is clear and thick, **fetid** when it is foul smelling, **purulent** when it contains pus, and **copious** when it is present in large amounts. Mucoid sputum is a common finding in airway disease without infection. Bacterial infections cause the sputum to become purulent and colored, often green or yellow. Some bacteria, especially anaerobes, will cause fetid sputum. Copious mucus production most often is seen in patients with bronchiectasis (see Chapter 7).

Ask questions to clarify any recent changes in the amount and color of the patient's sputum. Increases in the amount and changes in the color from clear to yellow or green often indicate acute infection. Stagnation of the mucus in the airways also will lead to discoloration of the sputum. Patients who have trouble coughing up their excessive mucus tend to retain it longer than normal and produce discolored sputum, even when infection is not present. Patients with asthma and extensive inflammation in the airways have so many eosinophils in their sputum that it appears purulent when no infection is present.

Chest Pain. **Chest pain** often is divided into two types: pleuritic and nonpleuritic. Pleuritic chest pain is made worse by breathing. It is usually sharp in nature and located laterally or posteriorly on the chest wall. Diseases that affect the lining of the lung (e.g., pneumothorax, pulmonary embolism, pneumonia) may cause pleuritic chest pain.

Nonpleuritic chest pain is more often located centrally in the chest and is usually not affected by respiratory efforts. It may radiate to the shoulder, arm, jaw, or back and is more often a dull pressure type of sensation. It is often associated with diseases such as ischemic heart disease.

Hemoptysis. **Hemoptysis** refers to the spitting up of blood from the tracheobronchial tree or lungs. When the hemoptysis is caused by an infectious disease, the blood is often mixed with sputum. The presence of blood-tinged sputum is strong evidence that the blood is coming from the respiratory tract, rather than the gastrointestinal tract. Pneumonia, trauma, bronchitis/bronchiectasis, bronchogenic carcinoma, tuberculosis, and pulmonary embolism are common causes of hemoptysis. Even after extensive evaluation, the cause of massive hemoptysis (more than 400 mL of blood in 24 hours) is undetermined 20 to 30 percent of the time. Chronic hemoptysis that has been occurring over many years is usually associated with a relatively benign condition, such as bronchiectasis. Acute hemoptysis also may be harmless when associated with acute bronchitis, but the potentially life-threatening causes of hemoptysis (e.g., carcinoma) must be ruled out before it is assumed that the problem is self-limited.

Fever. **Fever** is an abnormal increase in body temperature due to disease. It is a nonspecific response to many problems, but most often occurs in response to an infection. Pulmonary infections are a common cause of infection-related fever and should always be considered in the evaluation of fever. Fevers tend to increase in the afternoon and evening and decrease in the early morning.

Fever causes an increase in oxygen consumption and carbon dioxide production. Patients with high fever need to take deeper breaths at a faster rate in order to accommodate the fever-related increase in metabolism. Some patients report having a fever when they feel warm even though they have not measured their temperature. This subjective sensation of feeling warm may simply reflect the temperature of their environment. It is important to know whether the report of fever is based on actual temperature measurements.

Common respiratory problems associated with fever include viral infections, bacterial bronchitis, bacterial pneumonia, fungal infections, and tuberculosis. The degree of fever in any illness depends on the severity of the infection and the patient's ability to respond to the infection. A patient with a compromised immune system may not generate a significant fever despite having a severe infection.

Wheeze. **Wheeze** is a common complaint in patients with asthma, congestive heart failure, and bronchitis. It is often associated with shortness of breath and is caused by rapid airflow through one or more narrowed airways. Airway walls will vibrate between a partially open and closed position as air passes through at high speed.

Wheezing may be associated with cough, sputum, and dyspnea when airways disease is present. More information about wheezing is presented in the Physical Examination section of this chapter.

Outline for the Medical History

In addition to interviewing the patient to evaluate the onset and relief of symptoms, you will need to examine the patient's chart to identify the previously documented medical history. This requires familiarity with the outline used to document the patient's medical history. The typical outline and the common information listed in each category are presented in Table 1–2.

The most important category is the **history of present illness.** This section describes the crucial information that the physician obtains for each of the patient's complaints. All clinicians should be familiar with this section before caring for any patient. Each symptom is described as to when it started, what may have provoked it, how severe it is, and what seems to relieve it. The symptoms are usually put into chronological perspective, and the effect of the illness on the patient's life is often also described. Your responsibility is to read this section before seeing the patient so

TABLE 1–2   **Outline of the Medical History**

I. Patient Identification
    A. Name of patient
    B. Address of patient
    C. Age of patient
    D. Date and place of birth
    E. Marital status
    F. Current occupation
    G. Religious preference
II. Chief Complaint(s)
    A. List of patient complaints in the order of severity
III. History of Present Illness
    Chronological description of each symptom including:
    A. When it started and what seemed to provoke it
    B. Severity
    C. Location on the body
    D. Aggravating/alleviating factors
    E. Frequency (how often it occurs)
IV. Past Medical History
    A. Childhood illnesses and development
    B. Hospitalizations, surgeries, injuries, and major illnesses
    C. Allergies/immunizations
    D. Drugs and medications
    E. Smoking history and attempts at quitting
V. Family History
    A. List of living close relatives and their health condition
    B. List of close relatives who are deceased and the causes of death
    C. Marital history
VI. Social and Environmental History
    A. Education level
    B. Military experience
    C. Occupational history
    D. Hobbies and recreation activities
    E. Current life situation, including stresses from employment and
       relationship problems
    F. Recent travel that might have an impact on the patient's health
VII. Review of Systems

that you can be apprised of the initial symptoms and their severity. Changes in these symptoms may occur with the therapy you provide, and you will recognize this change more easily if you are familiar with the history of present illness.

In addition to finding out the details surrounding each of the patient's pertinent complaints, the interviewer should ask about the possible presence of other symptoms. This helps define the problem better, as well as clarifying a possible diagnosis. For example, if the patient comes to the doctor complaining of cough, the interviewer should ask about fever, sputum production, shortness of breath, hemoptysis, or recent exposure to tuberculosis. If the patient denies the existence of any of these other symptoms, they become a list of pertinent negatives. The list is presented in the history of present illness as "the patient denies fever, sputum production," and so on.

The history of present illness for a pulmonary patient should address the patient's smoking history. In this paragraph the physician describes at what age the patient started smoking, how many packs of cigarettes are smoked each day, and if any attempts have been made to stop smoking. The smoking history is important for patient assessment whenever cardiopulmonary disease is present. Occupational information, exposure to pets or animals, travel history, hobbies, sexual exposure, drug use, and family illnesses also provide important clues about possible causes of pulmonary disease.

CASE STUDY

History

William B. is a 49-year-old white man who came to the emergency room at 2 AM complaining of chest pain and shortness of breath. The chest pain started about 12 hours previously, when Mr. B was mowing the grass. The shortness of breath started while Mr. B was reclining, which was about 2 hours before he came to the emergency room.

QUESTIONS

1. What details about the chest pain need to be identified?
2. What details about the shortness of breath need to be identified?
3. What term is used to describe dyspnea in a reclining position?
4. What other possible symptoms need to be asked about in order to define the problem better?
5. What social habits need to be identified?

ANSWERS

1. Mr. B should be asked where his chest pain is located and to point to the spot. Constant chest pain under the sternum is consistent with cardiac **ischemia.** Pleuritic chest pain located laterally or posteriorly is more consistent with pleuritic involvement. Questions should be asked about the effect of breathing on the chest pain: Does the chest pain increase with a deep breath? Does the pain radiate to other parts of the body? How severe is the pain? Is it associated with nausea, diaphoresis, weakness, or faintness?
2. The shortness of breath needs to be clarified as to its severity. Does it occur at rest or only with exertion? Has Mr. B ever had this shortness of breath before? Did the dyspnea occur only when he was supine, or did it improve when he sat upright?
3. Dyspnea in the reclining position is known as orthopnea.

4. The interviewer should ask Mr. B if he has any other symptoms, such as fever, cough, sputum production, hemoptysis, recent exposure to tuberculosis, or swollen or sore calf muscles. His cholesterol level, family history of heart disease, stress levels, and personal history of heart disease should be evaluated.

5. Mr. B's cigarette smoking history must be identified. His symptoms could be consistent with a myocardial infarction, which occurs more often among patients with a significant smoking history.

CASE STUDY—continued

Mr. B explains that the chest pain is centrally located and radiates to his left shoulder and jaw. The chest pain started when he was pushing a lawn mower. The pain decreased with rest but did not subside totally. It is not affected by breathing. He has not taken any medication for the chest pain. On a scale from 1 to 10, Mr. B says that at its worst the pain was a 7. Currently he rates the chest pain as a 3.

The shortness of breath is described as severe; it awakened Mr. B from sleep about 2 hours after going to bed. It improved when he sat upright. He has never experienced shortness of breath before. He describes it as a feeling of suffocation.

Mr. B denies cough, sputum production, hemoptysis, fever, or exposure to tuberculosis. He does admit to having some diaphoresis, weakness, and nausea, but denies having vomited. He states that he smokes about two packs of cigarettes per day and has been smoking since the age of 16. He has tried to quit on several occasions, but was never successful for more than 6 weeks.

QUESTIONS

6. What pathology probably is responsible for the chest pain?
7. What pathology probably is responsible for the shortness of breath?
8. What problems are decreased in likelihood by the list of pertinent negatives?
9. If Mr. B had a dry, nonproductive cough, what pathology would probably explain it?
10. Should Mr. B be admitted to the hospital?

ANSWERS

6. Centrally located chest pain that worsens with exertion and radiates to the shoulder is the classic description of cardiac pain. Mr. B's coronary vessels are probably narrowed and preventing adequate blood flow to the heart muscle, resulting in an ischemic myocardium. Exertion increases the difference between the amount of oxygen needed by the heart and the amount that can be supplied by the narrowed coronary arteries. As a result, exertion causes the chest pain to worsen.

7. The shortness of breath is probably related to buildup of fluid in the lung. Left ventricular failure causes an increased hydrostatic pressure in the pulmonary capillaries, which leads to pulmonary edema. This makes it more difficult for the lung to expand and increases the work of breathing. In such cases, the patient often complains of labored breathing. Oxygenation of the arterial blood also will be reduced as a result of the pulmonary edema, which causes an increase in the drive to breathe via the carotid bodies and

adds to the sensation of dyspnea. The entire process is worsened when the patient lies flat in bed. Reclining causes the venous return to the heart to increase, which in turn increases the hydrostatic pressure in the pulmonary capillaries.

8. The lack of fever, cough, and sputum helps rule out pneumonia. The lack of leg tenderness, swelling, hemoptysis, or pleuritic chest pain helps rule out pulmonary embolism. The acute onset and lack of exposure help rule out tuberculosis.

9. A dry, nonproductive cough is common in heart failure patients with pleural effusion.

10. Yes, Mr. B should be admitted to the telemetry ward or ICU for close monitoring and treatment.

Physical Examination

Once you have established a rapport with the patient via the interview, you and the patient will usually find the physical examination a more comfortable experience. The physical examination is done to confirm or rule out certain illnesses suspected by the results of the interview. For example, in the case above, it is suspected that Mr. B has ischemic heart disease and pulmonary edema. The clinician should perform the physical examination with this tentative diagnosis in mind and seek evidence of heart failure and pulmonary edema. The physical examination is also done to identify all abnormalities, some of which may be very important but unrelated to the current problem. RCPs most often use the physical examination to evaluate the patient's response to therapy. This calls for a brief and well-focused examination, primarily centered around the cardiopulmonary system. For this reason, this section will emphasize examination of the cardiopulmonary system.

The physical examination is simple, quick, and inexpensive. In many cases, it also is sensitive, resulting in the identification of the initial evidence of disease. The examination may need to be brief when the patient is in serious distress and initial treatment is needed. A more thorough examination can be done when the patient is stable. A typical outline for documentation of a complete physical examination is listed in Table 1–3.

Vital Signs and Sensorium

In general, the vital signs provide an index of the patient's condition. Many medical problems will be reflected by abnormal vital signs as the problem increases in severity.

The four basic vital signs are heart rate, respiratory rate, blood pressure, and body temperature. A rapid increase in heart rate to greater than 100/minute is known as **tachycardia.** A decrease in the heart rate to less than 60/minute is known as **bradycardia.** Common causes of tachycardia and bradycardia are listed in Table 1–4. The heart rate is determined by counting the rate of the peripheral pulse or by using a cardiac monitor.

A respiratory rate higher than 18/minute in the adult is known as **tachypnea,** a common finding in patients with cardiopulmonary disease. Common causes of tachypnea are disorders of the lung that cause a reduction in lung volume (**restrictive**

TABLE 1-3 **Format for Documenting the Physical Examination**

INITIAL IMPRESSION
Age, height, weight, and general appearance

VITAL SIGNS
Heart rate, respiratory rate, temperature, and blood pressure

HEAD, EARS, EYES, NOSE, AND THROAT (HEENT)

NECK
Evidence of jugular venous distention; position of the trachea; any lymphadenopathy

THORAX
Heart: Evidence of heaves or lifts, heart sounds, and murmurs
Lungs: Lung sounds, breathing pattern, chest configuration, percussion findings, etc.

ABDOMEN
Evidence of distention and hepatomegaly
Degree of obesity

EXTREMITIES
Evidence of cyanosis, clubbing, and pedal edema

defect). A loss of lung volume forces the patient to breathe more rapidly in order to compensate for the shallow volume. Disorders such as atelectasis, pulmonary edema, pneumonia, pneumothorax, and pulmonary fibrosis cause loss of lung volume and result in a proportionate increase in respiratory rate. Other causes of tachypnea include hypoxemia, pain, anxiety, fever, and exertion.

Bradypnea, a respiratory rate in the adult of less than 10/minute, is not common but may be seen with hypothermia and central nervous system (CNS) disorders. Hypothermia causes a decrease in the amount of oxygen consumed and carbon dioxide produced by the body and results in a reduced need for breathing. CNS disorders may interfere with the brain activity responsible for breathing and cause bradypnea or even a complete lack of breathing, known as **apnea.**

Normal blood pressure is approximately 120/80 mm Hg in the adult patient. A blood pressure less than 90/60 mm Hg is known as **hypotension.** Mild levels of hypotension may be seen in normal persons or healthy athletes. Severe hypotension occurs when the heart fails as a pump, when peripheral vasculature dilates excessively, or when the circulating blood volume is severely reduced. Severe hypotension is to be avoided at all costs because it indicates that blood flow to important vascular beds is inadequate.

Normal body temperature is approximately 37°C plus or minus 0.5°C (98.6°F plus or minus 1°F). Elevation of body temperature due to disease is known as **fever.**

TABLE 1-4 **Common Causes of Abnormal Heart Rate**

TACHYCARDIA
- Anxiety
- Stress
- Response to medications, such as bronchodilators
- Hypoxemia
- Heart failure
- Fever

BRADYCARDIA
- Hypothermia
- Myocardial infarction with damaged SA node
- Stimulation of the vagus nerve

Fever is common in patients with infections, such as respiratory infections due to viral, fungal, or bacterial organisms. Fever causes the metabolic rate of the patient to increase slightly, and this requires an increase in the oxygen consumption and carbon dioxide production each minute. As a result, a febrile patient needs to breathe at a slightly faster rate to accommodate the increased metabolic rate.

A low body temperature is referred to as **hypothermia.** It is not common, but does occur in patients with head injuries that damage the hypothalamus and in those who have been exposed to cold temperatures for long periods of time. Near-drowning victims are frequently admitted to the hospital in a hypothermic condition. Some medications make patients more likely to become hypothermic. Although hypothermic patients need less oxygen to survive, the heart and some other body systems do not function well when body temperature is severely reduced. Blood flow is shunted to vital organs in hypothermic patients, which is why resuscitation of the hypothermic patient often requires special procedures and slow warming of the patient.

Sensorium assessment is done by evaluating the patient's level of consciousness. It is an important parameter in monitoring the patient with cardiopulmonary disease because it reflects the adequacy of blood flow and oxygenation of the brain as well as the net effect of acid-base imbalance, electrolyte imbalance, nutritional deficiency, and other signs of organ-system failure. The patient who is alert and oriented as to time, place, and person is said to be "oriented $\times 3$"; that is, the patient knows the correct date and time, where he is physically located, and who he is. Confusion with regard to any of these items indicates that the patient is disoriented. As cerebral function continues to deteriorate, the patient will become semiconscious and eventually comatose.

Pulse oximetry has recently become a very popular noninvasive technique for monitoring the patient with acute cardiopulmonary disease. The popularity of pulse oximetry has caused some clinicians to refer to it as the "fifth vital sign." It can be used intermittently or continuously to monitor the oxygenation status of the patient. The probe is attached to the patient's finger or ear lobe and shines an infrared light through the tissues. Red, oxygenated blood absorbs infrared light differently in comparison to bluish, deoxygenated blood. The oximeter reads the amount of light absorption and determines the degree of oxygenation.

Although pulse oximetry has proved very useful in a variety of settings, it does not evaluate the patient's ability to ventilate, fails when peripheral circulation is poor, and can read falsely high when the hemoglobin is saturated with carbon monoxide. For these reasons, pulse oximetry should not be the only parameter used to evaluate the respiratory status of the patient suspected of having circulatory problems, ventilatory problems, or carbon monoxide poisoning. Clinical examination and arterial blood gases (see later discussion) are needed in such cases.

Chest Inspection

An important parameter to evaluate during chest inspection is breathing pattern, because it can provide important clues regarding the underlying lung pathology. Patients who breathe with a prolonged expiratory phase usually have narrowed intrathoracic airways. Patients with acute asthma, bronchitis, or emphysema tend to breathe with a prolonged expiratory phase when airway obstruction is severe. Patients with a narrowed upper airway breathe with a prolonged inspiratory phase. The upper airway tends to narrow more during inspiratory efforts, making gas flow into the lung more difficult. Patients with restrictive lung disease (i.e., loss of lung volume) breathe with a rapid and shallow breathing pattern. The greater the loss of lung volume, the faster the respiratory rate.

Abdominal paradox is an abnormal breathing pattern seen in patients who have diaphragm fatigue. It is recognized by observing the abdomen sink inward with each inspiratory effort. Fatigue of the diaphragm, which is the major muscle for breathing, occurs when it has been overworked and underfed. These circumstances are common in patients with acute exacerbations of chronic obstructive pulmonary disease (COPD). The abdomen sinks inward with each breath because the negative intrathoracic pressure created by the accessory respiratory muscles causes the diaphragm and abdomen contents to be pulled upward into the chest during inspiration. This, in turn, causes the flaccid abdomen to sink inward during each respiratory inspiration.

Inspection of the chest includes notation of the degree of symmetrical chest expansion. Normally, both sides of the chest expand evenly with each inspiratory effort. Unilateral chest diseases, such as pneumonia or pneumothorax, may result in better expansion of the healthy side of the chest compared to the diseased side. The diseased side is said to "lag behind" the normal side.

Inspection of the chest wall for possible deformities is important. Abnormal curvature of the spine can cause poor lung expansion and significant restrictive lung disease. Lateral curvature of the spine is termed **scoliosis,** and anteroposterior curvature of the spine is termed **kyphosis.** The term **kyphoscoliosis** is used when both are present. Older patients with emphysema and osteoporosis will usually develop severe kyphosis. A premature anteroposterior increase in the diameter of the chest (referred to as **barrel chest**) often develops in the adult COPD patient (Fig. 1–1). Barrel chest occurs when the lung loses its elastic recoil and can no longer appropriately oppose the outward spring of the ribs. Other chest deformities to inspect for include **pectus excavatum** (abnormal permanent depression of the sternum) and **pectus carinatum** (abnormal prominence of the sternum).

Palpation and Percussion of the Chest

Palpation of the chest wall is done in certain circumstances to evaluate lung disorders. Palpation of the chest wall for tactile fremitus can be helpful in detecting significant changes in the pathology of the lung. The patient is asked to repeat the phrase "1-2-3" or "99" while the examiner palpates the chest wall comparing side to side. Diseases of the lung that cause it to become more dense (e.g., pneumonia) will cause an increase in tactile fremitus over the affected area. The vibrations created by the patient's larynx will travel more rapidly through consolidated lung tissue and result in a noticeable increase in fremitus. Diseases that cause the lung to become less dense (e.g., emphysema, pneumothorax) will cause a decrease in tactile fremitus.

The chest wall is also palpated to detect evidence of air leakage into the skin around the chest in certain circumstances. Air may leak into the surrounding tissues when chest trauma has occurred or when the patient has been mechanically ventilated with high pressure. Air leakage into the chest wall results in **subcutaneous emphysema;** this is detected by palpating the chest wall for areas that produce a distinctive crackling sound and sensation.

Tapping on the chest wall for the purpose of evaluating underlying lung pathology is known as **chest percussion.** Chest percussion is done when major changes in the density of the lung are suspected based on the history and previous physical examination findings. Normal lung tissue is air filled and produces a resonant sound in response to percussion. Diseases that produce increased lung density, such as

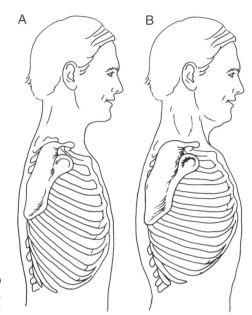

FIGURE 1–1 *(A)* Normal chest configuration vs. *(B)* increased AP diameter consistent with a barrel chest. Note the hypertrophy of the accessory muscles in B.

pneumonia, will result in decreased resonance upon percussion. Air trapped in the pleural space and emphysema cause increased resonance upon percussion. Chest percussion for evaluation of changes in lung pathology is not done routinely by health care providers, but can be very useful in some circumstances.

Chest Auscultation

The majority of health care providers routinely listen to the chest to evaluate the sounds of breathing. Chest auscultation provides immediate information about the patency of the airways and condition of the lung parenchyma. It is inexpensive and reliable and is done with a stethoscope (Fig. 1–2). To detect unilateral changes in lung pathology, the clinician compares the sounds of breathing on one side to those at the same location on the opposite side (Fig. 1–3).

Breath sounds are the normal sounds of breathing. There are three different types of breath sounds: tracheal, bronchovesicular, and vesicular. **Tracheal breath sounds** are heard directly over the trachea and are loud and high-pitched. It has a relatively equal inspiratory and expiratory phase and is produced by the turbulent flow in the trachea (Fig. 1–4).

Bronchovesicular breath sounds are heard around the sternum on the anterior chest wall and between the scapulae on the posterior chest wall. They are softer in intensity compared to tracheal breath sounds, but they also have equal inspiratory and expiratory components. These sounds are also produced by turbulent flow in the larger airways, but they are not as loud or high-pitched as tracheal breath sounds because they are filtered by healthy lung tissue, which lies between the area of sound production and the surface of the chest wall.

Vesicular breath sounds are heard over the areas of the chest wall overlying lung parenchyma. This sound is very soft and primarily heard on inspiration. The expiratory component is normally minimal and heard only during the initial one-fourth

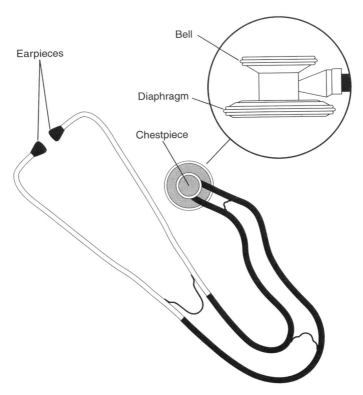

FIGURE 1-2   Diagram of a stethoscope used to auscultate the heart and lungs.

of the expiratory phase. Vesicular breath sounds are lower pitched than tracheal breath sounds and are also produced by turbulent flow in the larger airways. Vesicular breath sounds are significantly softer and lower pitched because they represent the turbulent flow sounds heard after they have passed through normal lung tissue. Normal lung tissue acts as a low-pass filter to sound traveling through it and changes normal tracheal breath sounds to normal vesicular breath sounds. Changes in lung-tissue density due to disease (e.g., pneumonia) will cause normal vesicular breath sounds to be altered.

Lung diseases that cause the parenchyma to become denser will result in less filtering of the turbulent flow sounds of the larger airways. This causes the normal vesicular breath sounds to be replaced with a harsher version that is louder and more bronchovesicular or tracheal in character. Atelectasis, pulmonary fibrosis, and pneumonia are examples of lung disorders that can cause harsh breath sounds over the affected region, which are termed **bronchial breath sounds.**

Disorders of the lung that result in a loss of lung tissue density, such as emphysema, result in excessive filtration of the turbulent flow sounds of the larger airways. This causes the normal breath sounds to be replaced by diminished sounds that are much harder to hear. Diseases of the chest wall can also cause diminished or absent breath sounds when excessive fluid or air build up in the pleural space, resulting in an acoustical sound barrier that prevents the transmission of normal breath sounds through the chest wall. Finally, diminished breath sound can be present when the

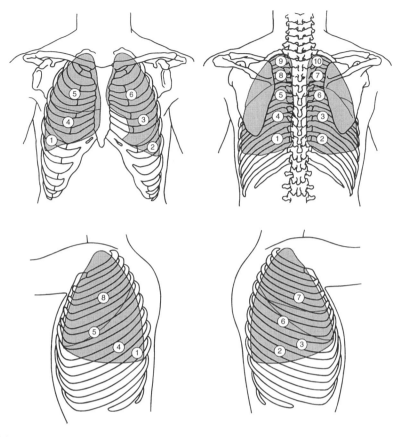

FIGURE 1-3   Sequence for chest auscultation. Note that examiner begins in the bases and compares side to side.

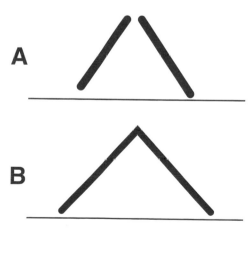

A

B

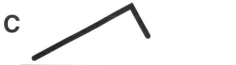

C

FIGURE 1-4   Diagram of *(A)* tracheobronchial, *(B)* bronchovesicular, and *(C)* vesicular breath sounds. The upstroke represents inspiration and the downstroke expiration. The thickness of the line represents the intensity of the sound.

patient is breathing excessively shallowly. This is common in cases of drug overdose, which suppresses the patient's drive to breathe.

Chest auscultation may reveal **adventitious lung sounds,** which are abnormal noises superimposed on the breath sounds. There are two basic types of adventitious lung sounds: continuous and discontinuous (Fig. 1–5). This categorization is based on acoustical recordings of the sounds. Study of these recordings reveals that the continuous type has a consistent sound pattern for at least one tenth of a second, whereas the discontinuous type has no such pattern.

The continuous type of adventitious lung sounds often has a musical quality and is associated with narrowed intrathoracic airways. Rapid airflow through a site of obstruction is believed to cause the airway wall to flutter rapidly between a partially open and closed position. This rapid fluttering causes a continuous type of whistling sound, known as a wheeze. Wheezes are most often heard during exhalation because this is when the intrathoracic airways naturally narrow.

Wheezing produced by multiple airways fluttering, which produces numerous musical notes that begin and end simultaneously, is known as **polyphonic wheezing.** Wheezing resulting from one airway's becoming partially obstructed produces a single note, and is known as a **monophonic wheeze.** Some clinicians refer to low-pitched wheezes as **rhonchi.**

Partial upper airway obstruction can cause a wheezing type of sound to come from the neck. This sound is most often heard during inspiration and is referred to as **stridor.** Stridor is a serious abnormality, since it signifies that the major airway into the lung is compromised; patients with stridor must be carefully monitored and treated. Not all patients with upper airway compromise present with stridor. In patients with partial upper airway obstruction, fatigue or the use of sedatives, or both, will reduce the degree of air movement past the site of obstruction and cause the absence of stridor. Clinicians should never assume the upper airway is patent simply because the patient lacks noisy breathing.

Discontinuous adventitious lung sounds are termed **crackles.** Clinicians used to use the term *rales* to describe several abnormal lung sounds, but more recently this term has been used to describe only discontinuous adventitious lung sounds, and therefore it is an imprecise term.

Crackles are believed to be produced by two different mechanisms: (1) sudden

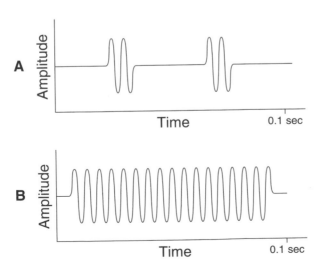

FIGURE 1–5   Time-expanded wave-form anaylsis of *(A)* continuous adventitious lung sound (wheeze) *(B)* discontinuous adventitious lung sound (crackles).

TABLE 1–5   **Interpreting Abnormal Lung Sounds**

Name of Sound	Mechanism	Characteristics
Bronchial BS	Increased sound transmission	Equal inspiratory and expiratory components
Diminished BS	Decreased sound transmission	Soft and low-pitched
Wheezes	Airflow through narrowed airway	Musical, with a continuous pattern
Crackles	Sudden opening of closed airways or movement of airway secretions	Fine, late-inspiratory Coarse, inspiratory and expiratory
Stridor	Upper airway narrowing	Often high-pitched

BS = breath sounds

opening of small airways and (2) movement of excessive airway secretions with breathing. Sudden opening of small airways occurs when a patient with collapsed small airways inhales deeply enough to overcome the surface tension of fluid, causing the airways to stay collapsed. Such crackles are typically heard late in inspiration and occur most often in patients with congestive heart failure and in the lower lung fields of bedridden patients. Crackles from the movement of excessive airway secretions are lower pitched (coarse) and occur during inhalation and exhalation. They may clear with a strong cough or if the airway is aspirated with a suction catheter (Table 1–5).

Examination of Other Parts of the Body

You should inspect the neck for evidence of jugular venous distention (JVD) when you suspect right heart failure. Failure of the right ventricle can occur with chronic lung disease or when chronic left heart failure is severe enough to affect the right heart. Failure of the right ventricle leads to backup of blood into the jugular vein, causing it to distend. Before examining the patient for JVD, you should ensure that the head of the patient's bed is slightly elevated so that the distention reaches the mid neck. The level of elevation should be recorded to provide an index of pressure.

The area of the chest overlying the heart is known as the **precordium.** You should inspect and palpate this area for abnormal pulsations. Enlargement of the right ventricle usually results in an abnormal pulsation around the sternum, known as a right ventricular **heave,** which occurs with each systolic heart beat. Left ventricular enlargement causes an abnormal heave in the left anterior axillary region and is associated with left ventricular failure.

To identify the heart sounds, you should perform auscultation over the precordium. Normally the heart sounds are soft and maintain a consistent "lub-dub" rhythm. The first heart sound is produced by closure of the mitral and tricuspid valves during systole, whereas the second heart sound is produced by closure of the aortic and pulmonary valves during diastole. The heart sounds may take on a "galloping" rhythm when added sounds are produced by abnormal cardiac pathology. For example, when the left ventricle becomes stiff after a myocardial infarction, an additional sound may be produced by the sudden filling of the ventricle with blood from the atrium during diastole. This added sound causes an additional heart sound, known as an S_3 gallop.

Murmurs are adventitious heart sounds that may also be heard during auscultation over the heart. They are caused by turbulent blood flow through a narrow opening. For example, when one of the heart valves becomes stenotic, rapid blood flow through the constriction causes an abnormal sound similar to a low-pitched blowing sound. Murmurs are typically rated on a scale from 1 to 6, according to their location and loudness.

You should examine the extremities for possible **digital clubbing** and for their color and temperature. Digital clubbing is a nonspecific sign that occurs in a variety of chronic cardiopulmonary diseases. You will recognize it by inspecting the fingers and toes for enlargement of soft tissue at the base of the nails and by examining the nails for abnormal lateral and longitudinal curvature. A bluish discoloration of the skin due to poorly oxygenated blood is known as **cyanosis.** Peripheral cyanosis indicates suboptimal circulation or oxygenation, or both. Extremities that are cyanotic as a result of poor circulation are usually also cool to the touch.

You should inspect and palpate the abdomen for evidence of distention. Abdominal distention can limit function of the diaphragm and further increase the severity of respiratory failure in the patient with a compromised respiratory condition. An enlarged liver, known as *hepatomegaly,* is often present in the patient with right ventricular failure. Right heart failure occurs as a result of chronic left heart failure or when cor pulmonale is present as a result of chronic lung disease.

You should inspect the mouth for evidence of cyanosis. A cyanotic oral mucosa indicates the presence of *central cyanosis.* This is a sign of severe hypoxemia and indicates that the respiratory system is not fulfilling its obligations to the body. The presence of central cyanosis strongly suggests that the patient needs oxygen therapy and that you should investigate the respiratory system further.

Examination of the mouth may also reveal pursed-lip breathing. This breathing technique is naturally adopted by COPD patients as they attempt to maintain patency of distal airways during exhalation. COPD patients often have difficulty exhaling fully because of premature collapse of distal airways. Pursed-lip breathing helps these patients exhale more fully and maintain better gas exchange.

Physical Examination

Vital Signs (in the Emergency Room): heart rate 112/minute, respiratory rate 28/minute, blood pressure 105/66 mm Hg, and temperature 36.7°C (98.0°F); alert but disoriented

HEENT: Normal

Neck: JVD noted at mid neck with the head of the bed at 45°

Chest: A heave is noted at the left anterior axillary line; S_3 gallop rhythm noted on auscultation; no murmurs heard

Lungs: Fine, late-inspiratory crackles are noted in the bases bilaterally; respiratory rate rapid and shallow

Extremities: Digits mildly cyanotic and cool to the touch

QUESTIONS

11. How would you interpret the vital signs and sensorium? What could be the cause of the blood pressure finding?

12. What pathophysiology explains the JVD?

13. What pathophysiology explains the heave at the left anterior axillary line and the gallop rhythm?

14. Why does this patient have fine, late-inspiratory crackles in the bases?

15. What probably explains Mr. B's cool and cyanotic extremities?

ANSWERS

11. The heart rate and respiratory rate are increased. Blood pressure is reduced, while body temperature is essentially normal. The reduced sensorium suggests that the brain may not be getting adequate blood flow and may not be well oxygenated. The low blood pressure is probably the result of poor pumping ability of the heart due to acute ischemia.

12. The JVD is probably related to left heart failure. As the left ventricle fails to pump blood forward into the aorta, the blood backs up into the lungs. This puts a heavy load on the right heart, which also fails and causes the blood to back up and distend the jugular veins.

13. The heave at the left anterior axillary line is caused by left ventricular distention. The gallop rhythm is the result of a stiffened left ventricular wall following the myocardial injury. This stiff left ventricle causes turbulence and an added heart sound as blood from the left atrium fills the ventricle. The sudden deceleration of blood entering the right ventricle produces a third heard sound in a rhythm similar to a horse's gallop.

14. The fine, late-inspiratory crackles in the lung bases are due to the accumulation of pulmonary edema fluid in the small airways. Left heart failure increases the blood pressure in the capillaries, causing fluid to leak into the interstitial space and from there into the small airways. The airways collapse on exhalation and are stuck shut by the surface tension of the fluid within them. Subsequent inspiration will cause these collapsed units to pop open, making characteristic crackling sounds.

15. Mr. B's cool and cyanotic extremities are probably related to poor cardiac output. Poor perfusion of the extremities causes them to become cool to the touch, and the cyanosis is related to the presence of deoxygenated hemoglobin.

Laboratory Data

Laboratory data are used for continuous evaluation of the patient in order to diagnose the problem as well as determine the effectiveness of therapy. This section focuses on those tests that are more frequently ordered for patients with cardiopulmonary disease.

The most common laboratory test is the complete blood count (CBC). The CBC measures the number and type of circulating white blood cells (WBCs) and the number and size of red blood cells (RBCs). The WBCs primarily fight invading organisms, such as bacteria. Elevation of the WBC count is known as **leukocytosis** and is a common finding in patients with pneumonia. A decrease in the WBC count is termed **leukopenia** and is less common than leukocytosis. It is seen in cases of bone marrow disease and overwhelming infection.

The WBC count represents a total number of circulating WBCs per cubic mil-

TABLE 1-6   **Interpretation of the White Blood Cell Count Differential**

Cell Type	Normal Values	Cause of Increase	Description
Neutrophil	40–60%	Acute illness/stress	Neutrophilia
Lymphocyte	20–40%	Viral infections	Lymphocytosis
Eosinophil	0–6%	Allergic reaction	Eosinophilia
Monocyte	2–10%	Chronic infection, malignancies	Monocytosis
Basophil	0–1%	Bone marrow disease	Basophilia

limeter. Five different cells make up the WBCs (Table 1-6). *Neutrophils* are the most common type of WBC and are primarily responsible for fighting bacterial organisms. Two types of neutrophils are counted: the segmented neutrophils (segs) and the immature segs (bands). Segs are the first line of defense against infection, but when they cannot be produced rapidly enough, bands are called into action. Thus, the presence of a high number of bands usually means that a severe infection is present. *Lymphocytes,* another common type of WBC, are mostly responsible for fighting viral infections. *Eosinophils* help the body deal with allergic reactions; thus, an elevation in eosinophils often indicates the presence of an allergic stimulus. See Appendix for tables on normal values for laboratory tests.

The RBC count helps determine the ability of the blood to carry oxygen. A low RBC count is termed **anemia,** whereas a high RBC count is called **polycythemia.** Anemia is common after surgery or hemorrhage, and it decreases the oxygen-carrying capacity of the blood. Polycythemia is seen most often in cases of chronically low blood oxygen levels due either to lung disease or to living at high altitudes. Chronically low oxygen levels stimulate the bone marrow to produce more RBCs to compensate for low oxygen availability. This allows an adequate quantity of oxygen to be carried in the blood despite a reduced partial pressure of oxygen.

In addition to the total RBC count, the amount of hemoglobin per 100 mL of blood is reported. In cases of *microcytic, hypochromic anemia,* the total number of circulating RBCs is normal, but their size is small and the amount of hemoglobin is reduced. This disorder is common among patients with iron-deficient diets or chronic blood loss.

Serum electrolytes are also frequently measured as a routine test for patients with cardiopulmonary disease. Most often, the serum sodium (Na^+), potassium (K^+), chloride (Cl^-), and total (HCO_3^-) are evaluated. Normal values are listed for these tests in the Appendix. Electrolyte abnormalities are associated with a large number of diseases; they can also occur as a complication of certain medications. In most cases, electrolytes are measured not to confirm suspicion of a specific disease, but rather to evaluate the general health condition of the patient and potential side effects of therapy. For example, the patient with heart failure may have a reduced serum sodium (*hyponatremia*) as a result of retaining too much water and a reduced serum potassium (*hypokalemia*) as a side effect of diuretic therapy. If either abnormality is present, the heart may pump suboptimally until the problem is corrected.

The clinical laboratory department has a microbiology section to evaluate the type of organisms present in body fluids. An example would be the patient with pneumonia who produces a sputum sample for laboratory evaluation. The laboratory technician attempts to identify the type of organisms present in the lung sputum. This can be very helpful for starting the patient on a good course of antibiotics. The Gram stain is used to initially evaluate sputum, and it is usually followed by a bacterial culture.

The Gram stain will help identify whether the sample consists of sputum from the lung or just secretions from the mouth. True sputum from the infected airways has few epithelial cells and numerous pus cells. Once the sample has been found to represent lower airway secretions, a portion of the sample is placed in an appropriate nutrient container and warmed to promote growth. In about 48 to 72 hours, the sample will reveal the identity of the organisms present in the specimen and the antibiotics to which they are most sensitive.

Cardiac enzymes are measured in patients suspected of having a myocardial infarction. Acute injury to the myocardium causes the heart muscle cells to release excessive amounts of enzymes into the circulating blood. For example, CPK enzymes are usually elevated within hours of a heart attack. If the chest pain is not due to ischemia of the heart muscle, the enzymes will not be released into the blood. Other laboratory tests performed periodically in the patient with cardiopulmonary disease are listed in Table 1-7.

Another common test done to evaluate patients with cardiopulmonary disease is the arterial blood gas (ABG). This test measures the ability of the lungs to oxygenate the blood and remove carbon dioxide from it. When the lungs are working well, the arterial oxygen tension (PaO_2) will be 90 to 100 mm Hg. **Hypoxemia** is present when the blood oxygen level is below normal. Mild hypoxemia is present when the PaO_2 is below normal for the age of the patient but above 59 mm Hg. Moderate hypoxemia

TABLE 1-7   **Other Laboratory Tests**

Test Name	Purpose	Implications of Results
Platelet count	Assess blood clotting ability	Reduced with bone marrow dysfunction and chemotherapy
Sweat chloride	Assess excretory function of sweat glands	>60–80 mEq/liter consistent with cystic fibrosis
Blood glucose	Measure blood sugar	Increased with diabetes; decreased with inadequate food intake or excessive use of insulin
BUN	Measure BUN level	Increased with renal disease and heart failure severe enough to cause renal dysfunction
Creatinine	Assess renal function	Increased with renal failure; more specific test
Serum protein/ albumin	Assess protein synthesis	Decreased with liver disease and malnutrition; decreased serum albumin may contribute to pulmonary edema
PTT	Test blood clotting ability	Lengthened with heparin therapy, but not common
PT	Test blood clotting ability	Lengthened with warfarin, but not heparin therapy
INR	Test blood clotting ability	More accurate calculation of the PT
Urinalysis	Assess urine for:	
	WBCs	Many WBCs indicate infection
	RBCs	Many RBCs indicate kidney inflammation or infection
	Protein	Protein indicates renal disease
	Glucose	Presence of sugar may indicate diabetes

BUN = blood urea nitrogen; INR = international normalized ratio; PT = prothrombin time; PTT = partial thromboplastin time; RBCs = red blood cells; WBCs = white blood cells is present when the Pao_2 is 40 to 59 mm Hg, and severe hypoxemia is defined as a Pao_2 of less than 40 mm Hg.

The normal carbon dioxide level is about 35 to 45 mm Hg. Elevation of the Pao_2 above 45 mm Hg is termed **hypercapnia** (or hypercarbia). It indicates that the degree of ventilation is inadequate to keep up with the rate of carbon dioxide production. Hypercarbia is common with hypoventilation caused by drug overdose, severe airways obstruction and neuromuscular disease.

Hypocapnia (or hypocarbia) is present when the arterial tension of carbon dioxide ($Paco_2$) is less than 35 mm Hg. This indicates that the rate of ventilation is excessive for the rate of carbon dioxide production. It is common with acute pain, exercise, anxiety, and CNS disorders.

ABG measurements also evaluate the acid-base status of the patient. Normal arterial blood pH is 7.35 to 7.45. A pH of less than 7.35 is termed **acidosis** (or acidemia) and is caused by elevation of the arterial blood CO_2 (called *respiratory acidosis*) or by reduction in blood bicarbonate (called *metabolic acidosis*). Respiratory acidosis, also called ventilatory failure, is caused by failure of the lungs to provide adequate gas exchange between the blood and the environment. Disorders that break down the neuromuscular system or obstruct the airways commonly cause ventilatory failure (Table 1-8). Reduction in blood bicarbonate occurs in conditions such as diarrhea, toxicity by some poisons, diabetes, renal failure, and anaerobic metabolism.

An arterial blood pH of greater than 7.45 is termed **alkalosis** (or alkalemia) and occurs with hyperventilation, which causes a reduction of $Paco_2$ (termed *respiratory alkalosis*), and with elevation of arterial blood bicarbonate (called *metabolic alkalosis*). Respiratory alkalosis is frequently caused by anxiety, pain, acidosis, or hypoxemia. Metabolic alkalosis can occur with a loss of acid (e.g., nasogastric suctioning, vomiting).

Pulmonary function tests are done to evaluate lung volumes and airway patency. The **vital capacity** is a measure of all usable lung volume. The patient inhales maximally and then exhales maximally into the spirometer; the amount of gas fully exhaled after a maximum inhalation is the vital capacity. Reductions in the vital capacity can be due to low lung volumes (restrictive disease) or narrowed airways with air trapping (obstructive disease).

The most common measures of airway patency are the forced expiratory volume in 1 second (FEV_1) and the forced expiratory flow during the middle half of the forced vital capacity ($FEF_{25-75\%}$). These measures of flow help determine whether obstructive lung disease is present. An FEV_1 of less than 80 percent of predicted is abnormally low, and an $FEF_{25-75\%}$ of less than 60 percent of predicted is abnormally low. Low FEV_1 and $FEF_{25-75\%}$ in the presence of a normal forced vital capacity documents airway obstruction. Low FEV_1 and $FEF_{25-75\%}$ with a reduced vital capacity could be caused by either restrictive lung disease or by obstructive lung disease with air trapping. Further testing with a body box or helium dilution would be necessary to de-

TABLE 1-8   **Common Causes of Respiratory Acidosis**

Category of Problem	*Clinical Examples*
Decreased drive to breathe	Drug overdose; head trauma
Neuromuscular defect	Guillain-Barré syndrome, myasthenia gravis, muscular dystrophy, cervical neck injury
Thoracic cage defect	Kyphoscoliosis, chest trauma/flail chest
Airway obstruction	Asthma, chronic obstructive pulmonary disease, epiglottitis

termine the exact cause. A bronchodilator is usually given to the patient with reduced flow measurements to see if it has therapeutic effect. If the flow measurements increase significantly (i.e., by greater than 15 percent) after bronchodilator therapy, the patient is said to have improved with bronchodilation. Many patients benefit from a bronchodilator even if it does not produce a change in the above values: A positive response to a bronchodilator means that the therapy is definitely helpful and that the patient will also likely respond to steroid treatment.

Chest Radiographs

Chest radiographs (x-rays) provide a view of the patient's internal thoracic anatomy as shadows of different shades of gray cast upon the x-ray. Diseases of the chest that alter lung pathology are visible on chest x-rays as they change the density of unusual structures. The chest x-ray is also useful for identifying the position of tubes and catheters. For example, after intubation of the trachea, a chest x-ray is useful for determining whether the tube is in the correct position. The tip of the endotracheal tube is properly positioned if it is found to be 3 to 5 cm above the carina on the chest x-ray. Insertion of the endotracheal tube too far usually results in its passing into the right mainstem bronchus (Fig. 1–6). If the tube is not inserted into the trachea far

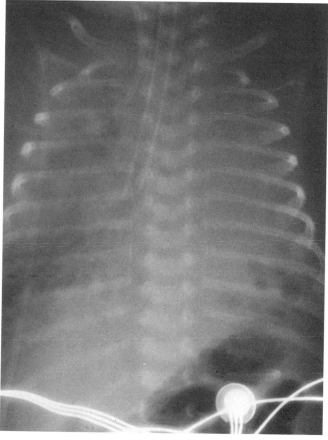

FIGURE 1–6   Chest radiograph showing endotracheal tube in the right mainstem bronchus.

enough, the tip will be seen near the larynx, where it is prone to accidental extubation (Fig. 1–7). After placement of a chest tube to drain fluid out of the pleural cavity, a chest x-ray is used to see if the tube is in good position and if the lung has re-expanded. A chest x-ray following placement of a nasogastric tube is sometimes needed if the clinician suspects that it has accidentally entered the lung (Fig. 1–8).

Reading chest x-rays requires many hours of supervised practice and cannot be taught in a book chapter. A few general guidelines, however, are presented in this section to help get you started. X-ray beams pass through the patient's chest and put different shades of gray shadows on the chest x-ray according to the density of the tissue through which the beam passes. Four different densities can be detected by examining the shadows on a chest x-ray: bone, water, fat, and air. For example, x-rays passing through bony structures are absorbed by the dense material and leave a whitish shadow on the corresponding portion of the chest x-ray. Conversely, x-rays that pass through lung tissue (air) are not blocked and burn the corresponding portion of the chest x-ray black. Inspection of the shadows seen on the chest x-ray allows identification of the changes in chest anatomy that may be present with disease. A normal chest x-ray with the more prominent anatomical structures labeled is presented in Figure 1–9.

Diseases of the chest that cause the lung tissue to become more dense, such as pneumonia, cause the affected region to absorb more than a normal amount of the chest x-rays and leave a white shadow on the x-ray. Lung tumors also cause the corresponding portion of the chest x-ray to have a white shadow instead of the expected dark shadow, as seen in normal lung tissue.

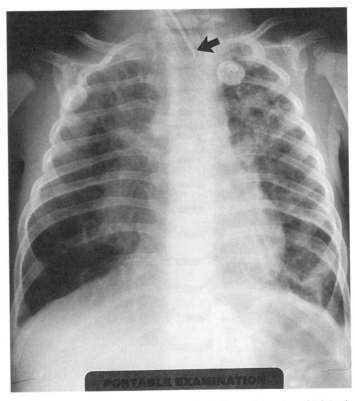

FIGURE 1–7   Chest radiograph showing endotracheal tube positioned too high in the trachea.

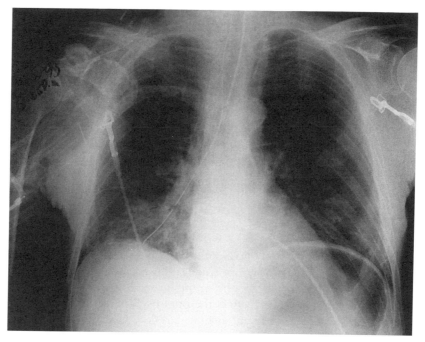

FIGURE 1-8   Chest radiograph showing the endotracheal tube in good position but the nasogastric tube accidentally placed in the right lung.

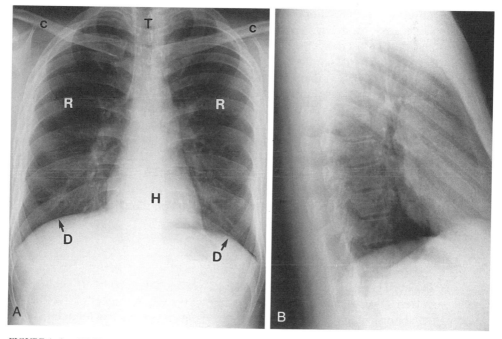

FIGURE 1-9   *(A)* Normal chest radiograph with normal structures labeled T = tracheal air shadow, R = ribs, C = clavicle, H = heart shadow, and D = diaphragm. *(B)* Normal lateral chest film.

Decreases in lung tissue density will cause the chest x-ray to be abnormally dark in the corresponding regions. Emphysema and pneumothorax are examples of lung conditions that cause darker shadows on the chest x-ray. Examples of abnormal chest x-rays are presented throughout this text to help you learn the skill of interpreting x-rays.

The size of the heart is evaluated by examining the width of the cardiac shadow on the chest x-ray. Normally the heart shadow is less than half the width of the entire chest. **Cardiomegaly** causes the heart shadow to enlarge to the point where it is larger than half the width of the chest on the chest x-ray. Cardiomegaly is most often seen in patients with left ventricular hypertrophy due to ischemic heart disease.

Electrocardiography

The electrocardiogram (ECG) is a recording of electrical activity in the heart. It clearly shows cardiac rate and rhythm and also gives some information about the status of the electrical conducting system in the heart, as well as the status of the heart muscle. It does not, however, reflect the pumping ability of the heart.

The SA node in the right atrium starts the heartbeat with an electrical impulse that causes the right and left atria to depolarize (P wave) and pump blood into the ventricles. Next, the impulse travels through the atrioventricular node to the ventricles, where it causes the ventricular muscles to depolarize (QRS wave), pumping blood into the arterial systems (Fig. 1–10). The muscle then returns to ready condition by repolarizing (T wave) in preparation for the next beat.

P waves are normally small, but may become larger when the atria hypertrophy. The QRS complex is divided into three waves. The Q wave is the first downward deflection of the QRS complex. It may not be present in some ECG recordings. The R wave is any upward movement following the Q wave, and the S wave is any subsequent downward deflection. The QRS complex is referred to as such even if not all three waves are present.

The normal ECG demonstrates an interval between the start of the P wave and the start of the QRS complex (known as the PR interval) of no longer than 0.20 seconds (five small boxes on the ECG grid), a QRS complex no wider than 0.12 seconds, and a flat (isoelectric) ST segment. A PR interval of longer than 0.20 seconds is known as heart block. A widened QRS interval is a sign of an internal conduction defect within the ventricles, and an elevated ST segment is consistent with myocardial ischemia.

The electrical activity can be observed from several angles to provide a three-dimensional view of the heart. The following are common observation sites (leads):

Lead I, aVL, V_1, V_4
Lead II, aVR, V_2, V_5
Lead III, aVF, V_3, V_6

Cardiac ischemia will cause tall, peaked T waves, followed by ST-segment elevation, inverted T waves, and eventually large Q waves when the cells have died. A lack of ECG abnormalities in the patient with chest pain provides evidence that the source of the discomfort may lie outside the heart. Please refer to the references at the end of this chapter for more detailed sources on ECG interpretation.

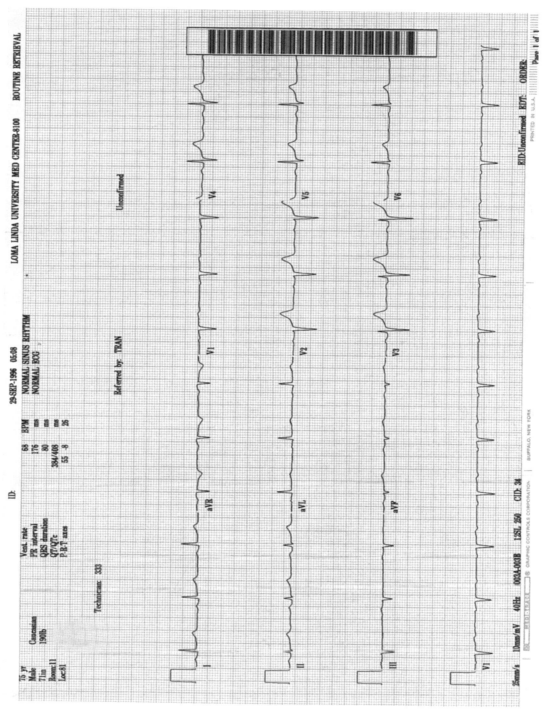

FIGURE 1-10   Normal ECG tracing demonstrating a normal P wave, normal PR interval, normal QRS complex, and normal T wave. Note that the ST segment is flat.

Mr. B is admitted to the coronary ICU. He is started on oxygen therapy with a nasal cannula at 4 liters/minute. Venous blood is drawn to measure a CBC, which reveals the following: WBCs 14,000/mm³, neutrophils 60 percent, bands 8 percent, lymphocytes 30 percent, and monocytes 2 percent.

Arterial blood is drawn for measuring ABGs. Results are as follows: pH 7.40, $PaCO_2$ 30 mm Hg, PaO_2 55 mm Hg, HCO_3^- 15 mEq/liter, base excess −3, FIO_2 4 liters/minute by nasal cannula. A portable chest x-ray is taken to evaluate the heart and lungs (Fig. 1–11), and a 12-lead ECG is taken (Fig. 1–12).

QUESTIONS

16. How would you interpret the CBC?

17. How would you interpret the ABGs?

18. What other test(s) should be done on the venous sample in this patient?

19. Do you see any significant abnormalities on the chest x-ray?

20. What does the ECG show?

ANSWERS

16. The WBC is elevated. This is common in response to stress and does not always indicate that infection is present.

17. The ABG results reveal respiratory alkalosis and metabolic acidosis with inadequate oxygenation despite administration of oxygen at a rate of 4 liters/minute.

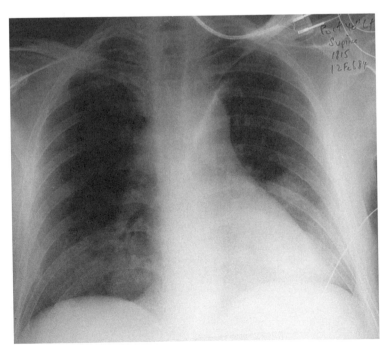

FIGURE 1–11   Mr. B's chest film demonstrating an enlarged heart.

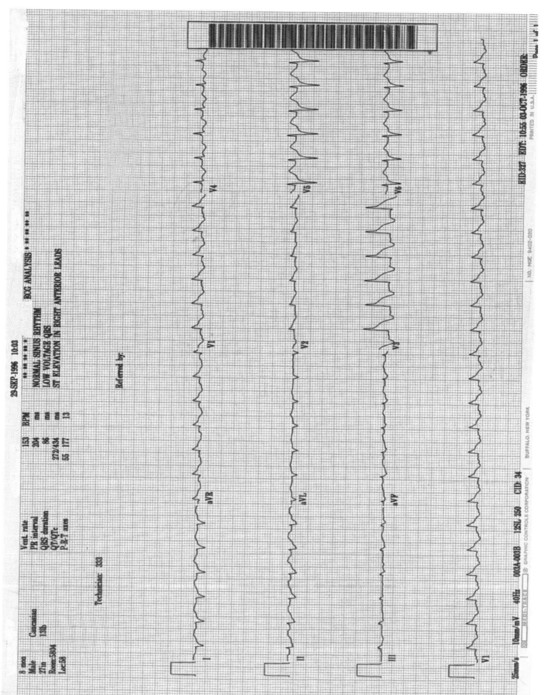

FIGURE 1–12   Mr. B's ECG showing elevated ST segments consistent with ischemia.

18. The venous blood should be analyzed for cardiac enzyme levels.

19. The chest x-ray demonstrates an enlarged heart. Notice that the width of the cardiac shadow is greater than one half the width of the chest. This is consistent with acute cardiac ischemia and heart failure. The chest x-ray also shows interstitial pulmonary edema, which is consistent with left ventricular failure.

20. There are elevated ST segments in V_1, aVL, and V_{2-5}.

CASE STUDY—continued

Over the next 24 hours, Mr. B gradually improved. He was treated with furosemide (Lasix) to reduce the pulmonary edema, which allowed better oxygenation on day 2. The cardiac enzymes were found to be elevated and confirmed the diagnosis of myocardial infarction. Mr. B remained hospitalized for 10 days and was sent home and enrolled in a cardiac rehabilitation program.

REFERENCES

Grauer, K: A Practical Guide to ECG Interpretation. Mosby–Year Book, St. Louis, 1992.

Malasanos, L, et al: Health Assessment, ed 4. CV Mosby, St. Louis, 1990.

Pierson, DJ, and Wilkins, RL: Clinical skills in respiratory care. In Pierson, DJ, and Kacmarek, RM (eds): Foundations of Respiratory Care. Churchill Livingstone, New York, 1992, pp 423–448.

Wilkins, RL, et al: Clinical Assessment in Respiratory Care, ed 3. Mosby–Year Book, St. Louis, 1995.

CHAPTER 2

Ethics in Respiratory Care

Gerald R. Winslow, PhD

Key Terms

active euthanasia
beneficence
common morality
competent
ethical principles
ethics

moral dilemma
moral virtues
principle of double effect
principle of fidelity
principle of justice

principle of
    nonmaleficence
principle of respect for
    personal autonomy
professional ethics

Introduction

The rapid pace of change and the power of new technology have combined to make the study of ethics in health care increasingly important. This chapter is devoted to a basic introduction to ethics for respiratory care professionals. Discussions of ethics are usually more fruitful when they occur within the context of specific cases. Cases are like prisms, allowing us to view more clearly the spectrum of issues that deserve ethical attention. The following case, which involves a patient who needs respiratory care, raises some ethical questions.

CASE STUDY

History

Mrs. W is a 64-year-old woman who was hospitalized because of progressive dyspnea and weakness in her extremities. At 14 years of age, she was diagnosed with poliomyelitis and was required to spend several weeks in an iron lung. She had made what appeared to be a complete neurologic recovery with minimal residual effects. Neurologic and pulmonary evaluations suggest that postpolio syndrome is the most likely cause of her respiratory deterioration. Her condition has recently deteriorated to the point of respiratory failure, and it was necessary for her to be endotracheally intubated and supported with continuous mechanical ventilation. After 3 days of mechanical ventilation, several unsuccessful attempts were made to wean Mrs. W from the ventilator. The patient asked if she would eventually be able to live without ventilatory support. Her pulmonary physician indicated that she would almost certainly continue to be ventilator dependent for the rest of her life. Other consultants agreed with this conclusion. After careful consideration, Mrs. W decided that she did not want to continue life on a ventilator. She insisted that all ventilatory support be discontinued, even though she knew that this was likely to lead to her death.

Over the next month, the patient continued to demand that the ventilator be removed. She also requested that she be heavily sedated when the ventilator was discontinued because she was afraid of feeling suffocation. At first, her husband and two children were reluctant to agree with Mrs. W's decision. Eventually, her husband and son accepted her wishes and offered their support. But the patient's daughter objected and pled with the caregivers to continue all measures needed to keep the patient alive. The daughter raised questions about her mother's mental ability to make a competent decision, given her depressing situation. A psychiatrist evaluated Mrs. W and concluded that, despite her discouragement, she was mentally able to make a competent decision.

The case of Mrs. W introduces a number of significant questions. Is it permissible to terminate life support for a mentally alert patient? Who should have the authority to decide? Is the patient's decision to refuse the ventilator evidence that depression has interfered with her mental competence? Must the patient's family agree with her decision? What if the family is divided? Is it necessary, under these circumstances, to involve other decision-making entities, such as an institutional ethics committee or the legal system? If the patient's decision to terminate the ventilator is accepted, should her wish to have heavy sedation also be accepted, even though such sedation will make survival without ventilation even less likely? Such questions are an invitation to think about ethics.

Ethics is the systematic study of the moral principles and virtues that should direct a person's decisions and actions. The goal of ethics is to provide guidance for living a virtuous life and for building a good society. When applied to a profession such as respiratory care, ethics is the endeavor to state clearly how members of the profession should conduct their professional lives. Thus, the study of ethics provides opportunities to think clearly about the central values that an individual, a professional group, or an entire society should embrace.

An individual's personal system of ethics consists of his or her moral convictions about how life ought to be lived. There are many traditional sources of these convictions, including family, religious community, and culture. Among the acknowledged goals of moral maturity are the assessment of the moral values that have been received from such conventional sources and the development of a personal system of ethics that has been carefully considered. Mrs. W arrived at a personal decision that we can assume fits with her considered values.

A society's ethics consists of the moral values held by people who share common territory and systems of meaning. These values are fundamental to the society's culture. In cases such as Mrs. W's, for example, it has become common in our society to accept termination of artificial life support, if we are convinced that a mentally competent patient has opted to discontinue the life support. But the practice of ac-

tive euthanasia, taking direct action to end a patient's life, is highly controversial and still condemned by most health care professional organizations and legal jurisdictions. Mrs. W's request to be heavily sedated at the time of withdrawal of ventilatory support illustrates the difficulty of deciding whether or not the line of active euthanasia would be crossed. Debates about the social acceptability of such sedation continue.[1] Sometimes referred to as the **common morality,** society's shared moral values are developed gradually, and often after periods of controversy. Society's common morality creates mutual expectations about what is acceptable and unacceptable within the society. It is usually assumed that new members of the society will learn these expectations.

Today, there is general awareness that moral values may differ from one culture to the next. As contemporary societies become increasingly multicultural, one of the major challenges of social life is to find sufficient agreement on basic moral values to sustain society's essential functions. Current debates in our society not only about active euthanasia, but also about termination of life support, allocation of medical resources, experimentation with human subjects, and many other issues in modern health care are illustrations of efforts either to build or to revise the common morality.

Professional ethics comprises the ethical convictions of a specific segment of society recognized as a profession. The members of a profession have received specialized training that enables them to provide needed services. One of the most important characteristics of a profession is the responsibility for stating the ethical standards that govern professional activities. Society generally places significant trust in the profession. This trust includes a high level of self-governance. In cases such as Mrs. W's, it is assumed that the professionals involved in her care will be governed by the relevant rules or principles in their professional association's code of ethics. The profession is expected to teach new members this code and to discipline those members who fail to comply with it. Respiratory care practitioners have followed the traditional pattern of professions by establishing an official code of ethics. Developed by the American Association for Respiratory Care (AARC), this code deserves the careful study of respiratory care professionals in this society (Table 2–1).

The Function of Codes of Ethics

The code of ethics for respiratory care professionals bears many similarities to the codes of other health care professions, both ancient and modern. For example, the code calls for the respiratory care professional to hold in strict confidence all privileged information concerning the patient. This commitment to confidentiality can be traced all the way back to the Oath of Hippocrates, an ancient Greek pledge of physicians to care honorably for their patients.[2] Patients such as Mrs. W rightly assume that information about them will be held in strict confidence by their caregivers. Virtually every code of ethics for health care professionals contains a similar rule for protecting the privacy of patient information.

Codes for health care professionals are not always the same. Such codes express the distinctive aspirations, prescriptions, and prohibitions of the various professions. In so doing, they often reveal interesting differences in the traditions of the professions. For example, the AARC's code of ethics calls for respiratory care professionals to provide care without discrimination on any basis. This statement is nearly identical to the American Nurses' Association's Code for Nurses.[3] But these two codes are in

TABLE 2-1   **AARC Statement of Ethics and Professional Conduct**

In the conduct of their professional activities the Respiratory Care Practitioner shall be bound by the following ethical and professional principles. Respiratory Practitioners shall:

- Demonstrate behavior that reflects integrity, supports objectivity, and fosters trust in the profession and its professionals.
- Actively maintain and continually improve their professional competence, and represent it accurately.
- Perform only those procedures or functions in which they are individually competent and which are within the scope of accepted and responsible practice.
- Respect and protect the legal and personal rights of patients they treat, including the right to informed consent and refusal of treatment.
- Divulge no confidential information regarding any patient or family unless disclosure is required for responsible performance of duty, or required by law.
- Provide care without discrimination on any basis, with respect for the rights and dignity of all individuals.
- Promote disease prevention and wellness.
- Refuse to participate in illegal or unethical acts, and shall refuse to conceal illegal, unethical, or incompetent acts of others.
- Follow sound scientific procedures and ethical principles in research.
- Comply with state or federal laws which govern and relate to their practice.
- Avoid any form of conduct that creates a conflict of interest, and shall follow the principles of ethical business behavior.
- Promote the positive evolution of the profession, and health care in general, through improvement of the access, efficacy, and cost of patient care.
- Refrain from indiscriminate and unnecessary use of resources, both economic and natural, in their practice.

Source: AARC and Respir Care 41(9):835, 1996.
Code revised, December 1994.

sharp contrast to the American Medical Association's Principles of Medical Ethics, which states that, except in emergencies, physicians shall "be free to choose whom to serve."[4] Such obvious differences in codes should not suggest that one profession is necessarily more virtuous than another. The differences do indicate, however, that the codes of health care professions, like those of all other professions, manifest distinctive differences that are linked to the professions' distinctive traditions.

A profession's ethical code accomplishes a number of important functions. First, it tells members of the profession what their fellow professionals expect of them. Although there are many additional expectations of a competent professional, the code establishes the fundamental norms that must be observed. For example, according to the AARC code, respiratory care professionals should refuse to conceal incompetence and illegal or unethical conduct of members of the profession. Thus, a member of the profession should neither be surprised nor feel mistreated if his or her incompetent, illegal, or unethical conduct is brought to light by a fellow member of the profession. The rule is, in part, an expression of the profession's commitment to **self-regulation.**

A second function of a code is the establishment of society's trust in the profession. If the members of society are to grant the privileges of self-governance to a profession, they need to be assured that the profession will not abuse the privileges. Patients, for example, need to be confident that their health care providers will place benefit to the patients' health ahead of other potentially conflicting considerations. Thus, the AARC code admonishes respiratory care professionals to guard against conflicts of interest. So Mrs. W and her family should not have to worry that their care-givers are likely to base treatment decisions on considerations that conflict with Mrs. W's interests. The commitment of health care professionals to avoid conflicts of interest takes on new significance in a time when cost containment is a major concern and when new arrangements for financing health care, such as managed care, are growing more prevalent.

A third function of an ethics code is the statement of the profession's aspirations. Beyond the "do's and don'ts," codes often state the ideals and hopes of the profession. Thus, the AARC Code commits respiratory care professionals to promote disease prevention and wellness and improve access to care. As a practical matter, it may never be possible to meet all of the health care needs of every citizen. Nevertheless, the statement means that the profession is bound to continue efforts to achieve the goal.

As valuable as codes may be in establishing professional identity, securing the public's trust, and stating the profession's aspirations, there are a number of ways in which codes are insufficient. Codes tend to fall short in at least four ways:

1. Codes of ethics usually omit important norms and virtues. No list of rules could be fully adequate to prescribe every feature of a virtuous life. Codes of ethics for health care professionals, including the AARC code, have generally emphasized the importance of benefiting rather than harming the patient, preserving confidentiality, and acting equitably. Such codes have not typically featured other important values, such as patient autonomy and truth-telling. So, for example, nothing in the AARC code indicates how much weight, if any, should be given to Mrs. W's personal decision to have her ventilator discontinued.

2. Codes of ethics are never extensive enough to cover all possible cases. Codes are like maps of the moral territory: They are always simpler and smaller than the territory they cover. Failure to anticipate the complexity of all possible cases is a problem inherent to any code, and it cannot be remedied merely by adding more rules. The case of Mrs. W illustrates the impossibility of developing a code that will prescribe specific solutions for every set of circumstances. Even the most careful reading of the AARC code will not lead to answers for all of the questions that her case raises.

3. Over time, codes no longer conform to the values of a changing society. Again, like maps, codes need to be updated as the territory they cover changes. Not only do new cases and new technical capabilities arise, but changing social attitudes also affect important values. For example, nursing codes of the past called for strict loyalty to the physicians.[5] The most recent code for nurses, however, does not mention physicians. Society has also been experiencing significant changes in moral attitudes toward practices as diverse as the use of human reproductive technology, abortion, assisted suicide, and euthanasia. Such changes challenge all health care professions to relate ethically to the new developments. For example, at the time of the Karen Ann Quinlan case, in the 1970s, there was widespread debate about the termination of any artificial life support, including mechanical ventilation.[6] Now, there is general agreement that such support can be ethically terminated. As Mrs. W's case illustrates, however, there is still disagreement about the line between withdrawing life support and actions aimed directly at ending a patient's life.

4. In some circumstances, codes may present conflicting rules. For example, the AARC code calls for compliance with the laws that govern the practice of res-

piratory care and also mandates that patient information be kept confidential. It is possible, however, to think of cases in which the law may require reporting information about a patient that would not be permitted by strict adherence to confidentiality. Most jurisdictions require that certain injuries, such as gunshot wounds or suspected child abuse, be reported to government authorities. It is not possible to include all of these exceptions in the code. Moreover, some health care professionals may be convinced that certain laws are misguided and ought to be challenged. For example, Dr. Jack Kevorkian, the Michigan physician who has assisted in the suicides of a number of patients, believes the laws forbidding doctors actively to aid the dying of their patients should be challenged.

Because codes of ethics are both valuable and limited, an important task for all professionals is to think critically about their code. Professionals should be prepared to join in the process of interpreting and updating their code. They should also understand how to relate their code not only to specific cases, but also to broad ethical principles.

Ethical Principles

It would, of course, be convenient if perfect harmony always existed among the values and principles of an individual's personal ethics, his or her professional code of ethics, and the norms of the society. But, as the case of Mrs. W shows, moral reality is more complex and often includes difficult moral dilemmas. A **moral dilemma** arises whenever circumstances are such that two or more moral values are in conflict. For example, in Mrs. W's case, the value we place on continued life is in conflict with the value we place on the personal choices of the competent patient. In such cases, no decision is possible without some residue of regret, because any decision will represent the loss of something considered morally valuable. Conflicts may develop because different individuals give priority to different values. This was apparently true in Mrs. W's case, when her daughter arrived at a different conclusion from that of the rest of the family. Conflicts also develop, at times, because different individuals may interpret or apply the same rules in different ways. For example, whether or not heavy sedation in Mrs. W's case is viewed as the equivalent of active euthanasia will depend on a number of complex interpretations of both the facts and concepts involved.

In the face of moral complexity, one way to preserve integrity is to adopt a set of basic **ethical principles,** which are broad statements of obligation that cover large sectors of the moral obligation. Such principles can help to unify various elements of an individual's personal moral convictions and his or her professional code. When confronted with moral dilemmas, a principled approach to decision making facilitates careful consideration of the main elements of a case. In a diverse society such as ours, where people are free to live by many different sets of moral convictions, we cannot expect uniformity even at the level of broad principles. In recent years, however, the presentation of four basic principles for biomedical ethics offered by Beauchamp and Childress has gained wide acceptance.[7] These four principles—respect for personal autonomy, nonmaleficence, **beneficence,** and justice—have helped to establish a beneficial measure of shared ethical language in health care. They can also form a useful basis for further discussion of ethics in respiratory care.

The **principle of respect for personal autonomy** is the first of these four principles. To be autonomous is to govern oneself rather than to be controlled by others. Respecting another's autonomy means permitting that person to live according to his or her own intentions. For persons to be autonomous, they must be able to formulate and understand plans and make decisions about alternatives. Many factors may interfere with a person's ability to make autonomous decisions. Someone may be able to function autonomously with regard to some areas of decision making, but not others. Thus, there is a wide range of possibilities from fully autonomous to completely dependent on the decisional capacity of others. Respecting the autonomy of individuals requires efforts to enable them, as much as possible, to live in accordance with their own expressed will. Such efforts include providing accurate information so that the person can make knowledgeable decisions.

In health care, the principle of respect for autonomy is often linked to the practice of seeking the informed consent of mentally competent adult patients. Except in rare instances, such as an emergency in which a patient's mental competence is uncertain, treating a competent patient against his or her will is both unethical and illegal.[8] Because of the importance attached to the concept of competence, much hinges on whether or not a person is deemed to be competent. There are numerous arguments about how to assess a person's competence. In health care, however, a person is generally considered **competent** if he or she can comprehend the basic elements of a proposed treatment, including its potential risks and benefits, and form a decision based on the information. It should be noted that competence is a legal concept and, in cases of dispute, it may be necessary to seek the decision of a court. Although psychiatrists are often asked to consult in disputed cases, as happened with Mrs. W, there is no legal requirement to seek such a consultation.[9]

The AARC code of ethics upholds the principle of autonomy when it states that patients' personal rights should be respected, including the right to informed consent and to refuse treatment. It is to be expected that respiratory care professionals would join other health care professionals in respecting patients' decisions. Even though the principle of patient autonomy has long been upheld in case law, the ethical significance of autonomy has been given major emphasis only in the last couple of decades, beginning with the patients' rights movement of the 1970s. The various codes of the health professions are still in the process of shifting toward greater attention to autonomy.

If the principle of autonomy is given priority in the case of Mrs. W, the conclusion seems clear: The patient's decision to terminate ventilation should be honored. The durable wishes of an informed and mentally competent patient should hold sway. However, questions remain:

- How much time is needed to assess the durability and competence of a patient's choices?
- Was the month that had elapsed in Mrs. W's case too long or too short?
- What weight, if any, should be given to the daughter's objections?
- What are the implications of Mrs. W's request for heavy sedation?

The second of the four principles elaborated by Beauchamp and Childress is the **principle of nonmaleficence.** This is the "no harm" principle. It forbids deliberately injuring or harming a person. This principle may seem all too obvious at first glance, but it requires careful amplification. Many health care interventions run the risk of harming patients. Termination of some interventions may also risk harm. A health care professional who is unwilling ever to risk harm to a patient will be able to help very few patients. Thus, it is necessary to understand the principle of non-maleficence as calling for a cautious weighing of risks and benefits. The principle mandates that we not subject patients to risks without the promise of proportionately greater benefits. Inevitably, such decisions include assessments of the quality of life that will likely result from proposed treatments.

The basic idea of nonmaleficence appears in a number of places in the AARC code. For example, the code forbids that respiratory care professionals extend their practice beyond their competence. Presumably, the commitment to stay within one's area of professional competence is intended, at least in part, to protect patients from incompetent care. Similarly, as mentioned earlier, the code mandates that incompetent, illegal, or unethical actions of one's colleagues should not be concealed. Again, this may be understood as protection of patients from harmful treatment.

Mrs. W concluded that life on a ventilator was not acceptable to her. From the perspective of some caregivers as well as Mrs. W's daughter, the desire to avoid the harm of death outweighs concerns about any harm caused by the ventilator. Mrs. W, however, saw it differently. She found the prospect of death more acceptable than long-term survival with ventilatory support. In the past, the decision to honor Mrs. W's wishes would have been complicated by the fact that many health care professionals drew a distinction between withholding potentially life-sustaining treatments and withdrawing them after they were in use. Clinicians often considered the decision to withhold artificial life support less ethically problematic than the decision to withdraw it; this distinction has now been widely discredited.[7] The withdrawal of life support from a patient may be potentially more emotionally traumatic for those involved. This is especially true if life support is being withdrawn from an alert patient. Clinicians and family members may feel as though they are abandoning the patient. Nevertheless, it is now generally acknowledged that it is as ethically permissible to withdraw treatments deemed harmful, or not in keeping with the patient's wishes, as it would have been to withhold such treatments in the first place.

The third principle described by Beauchamp and Childress is beneficence. The **principle of beneficence** prescribes actions that will be of benefit to others. Deeds that are intended to help another person flourish are in keeping with this principle. Thus, beneficence is the "do good" principle. The AARC code evidences a commitment to beneficence when it obligates respiratory care professionals to improve their professional competence and promote wellness.

Recent discussions of beneficence have often focused attention on the potential conflicts between doing good for patients and abiding by patients' decisions. In former times, it was often considered acceptable, or even advisable, for health care professionals to override the wishes of patients on the grounds that the professionals knew what was best for the patients. Such paternalism was considered part of the ordinary provision of health care. The current emphases on patients' rights and the importance of autonomy suggest a much more limited role for paternalism. Still, some health care decisions must be paternalistic. This is obvious in cases involving young children and individuals clearly lacking the mental capacity to decide for themselves. More difficult cases arise when caregivers are uncertain about a patient's ability to understand the medical alternatives or their likely consequences. In Mrs. W's case, for example, some paternalism was probably at work in the process of allowing time to elapse in order to be certain that her wishes were sufficiently deliberate and stable.

A further question regarding beneficence arises because of Mrs. W's request to have heavy sedation when her ventilator is discontinued. A large dose of morphine, for example, may be in keeping with beneficence by providing a more peaceful death in such cases,[10] but it could also suppress respiration and thus eliminate the chance, however small, that Mrs. W will have sufficient respiration without ventilatory support. The balance between the beneficent goal of alleviating air hunger and the goal of avoiding respiratory arrest is not always easy to achieve.[11] There is growing consensus that it is better to be certain that the patient will be kept comfortable. Such decisions have long been justified in terms of the **principle of double effect.** This principle permits the achievement of a beneficent and ethically proper goal, such as the alleviation of Mrs. W's air hunger, through the use of sedatives and narcotics, even if the necessary means might have unintended but foreseen secondary effects, such as suppressing respiration and thus possibly hastening the patient's death. New developments in health care and changing social attitudes will necessitate continued discussion about the full meaning of beneficence on the part of health care professionals.

The fourth principle is justice. The **principle of justice** forbids unfair discrimination and mandates that individuals be given what they have the right to receive. An important requirement of the concept of justice is that benefits and burdens be distributed fairly. This principle has achieved greater prominence in health care delivery as the health care system has become one of society's largest enterprises. When the capacity of health care to make a helpful difference in people's lives was extremely limited, few questions regarding social justice arose. Today, however, the health care systems of industrialized nations distribute enormous benefits and burdens. There is increasing awareness that difficult decisions must be made about the capacity of society to provide all the beneficial care that modern health care has generated. Greater emphasis is now placed on cost containment and even rationing of health care. In such circumstances, attention to the principle of justice is becoming increasingly significant.

The AARC code includes elements related to the principle of justice. For example, when the code prescribes that care be rendered without discrimination, justice is clearly the underlying principle. Similarly, justice is likely the main reason for forbidding conduct that involves a conflict of interest. All patients deserve competent, considerate care, regardless of their ability to provide special gratuities. To give less considerate care to those unable to grant such tips would be unfair. No patient should have to wonder if his or her care is being negatively affected because a health care professional harbors attitudes of unjust discrimination or has conflicts of interest.

The statement of these four principles—autonomy, beneficence, nonmaleficence, and justice—should not be taken to suggest that they exhaust the list of significant ethical principles. For example, some may want to add specific reference to the **principle of fidelity,** which prescribes that we maintain patients' trust by preserving confidentiality and practicing truthfulness. The AARC code bears witness to the importance of fidelity when it calls on respiratory care professionals to maintain integrity and foster trust. Thus, it is to be assumed that the now well-established ethical commitment of the health care professions to be honest with patients would be shared by respiratory care professionals. This commitment to the truth, which has both ethical and legal underpinnings, has grown stronger in recent decades.

Just as with codes of ethics, no set of ethical principles, however comprehensive they appear, will fully serve the complexity of the moral decisions that must be made. Recently, a number of commentators have also pointed to the importance of **moral virtues,** which are those inner traits of character such as courage. Others have suggested that more attention be given to the details of each person's and each community's narrative or story. Such emphases should be viewed as enhancing the possibilities for moral perception, rather than diminishing the importance of stating clear ethical principles. Knowledge of one's professional code of ethics and of basic ethical principles is central to the establishment of a framework for the professional's ethical decisions (Table 2–2).

TABLE 2-2   **Framework for Ethical Decisions in Respiratory Care**

CLARIFICATION OF THE CASE
- What facts are in question?
- What concepts need clarification?
- What values are in conflict?
- What authorities have power to act?
- What relationships will be affected?

EXPLORATION OF ALTERNATIVES
- What courses of action are possible?
- What are the likely results of such actions?

ELABORATION OF GOALS AND PRINCIPLES
- What guidance is available from the profession's code of ethics?
- What broad ethical principles should guide the decision?
- What goals are most appropriate under the circumstances of the case?

DECISION
- What decision best fits with professional responsibility and personal integrity?
- What challenges must be met in order to carry out the decision?

EVALUATION OF OUTCOMES
- What were the results of the decision?
- What is the assessment of the decision after the passage of time?

Applying a Framework

The primary value of a framework for ethical decisions is the order that it may lend to the consideration of cases that present moral dilemmas. No framework can provide a foolproof recipe for correct decisions, but an orderly approach to thinking about the moral dimensions of a case can ensure that areas of major significance are not ignored. It should be helpful to illustrate the value of such a framework by applying it to a specific case.

CASE STUDY

History

Mr. P is a 66-year-old white man admitted to the local emergency room for severe dyspnea at rest. He had been diagnosed with chronic obstructive pulmonary disease (COPD) more than 10 years ago. Mr. P currently does not smoke cigarettes, but he did smoke about two packs a day for 50 years. Recently Mr. P's dyspnea has progressed to the point of being severe after walking only a short distance on a flat surface. One year ago, his forced expiratory volume in one second (FEV_1) was measured at 0.8 L after bronchodilator treatment.

Mr. P is now depending on his accessory respiratory muscles to breathe. He is confused and somnolent. His vital signs show a heart rate of 124/minute, respiratory rate of 34/minute, and a normal blood pressure and body temperature. Mr. P's breath sounds are very diminished in all lung fields. There are no crackles or wheezes. Pulse oximetry reveals a saturation of 84 percent on 1 liter/minute via nasal cannula. A chest radiograph is taken immediately and shows clear lung fields but marked hyperinflation.

The hemidiaphragms are flat, and the heart is narrow and midline. The lateral projection shows a large retrosternal airspace consistent with severe emphysema. The current complete blood count shows slight polycythemia with normal white blood cell count and differential. Total CO_2 is increased on the electrolyte panel. Arterial blood gas results are pending on 2 liters/minute via nasal cannula.

Several hours after admission, Mr. P's clinical condition deteriorated. His respiratory rate increased to 56/minute, and his heart rate climbed to 152/minute. His blood pressure dropped to 70/40 mm Hg, and his sensorium deteriorated further. The attending physician consulted with the family members to determine if aggressive therapy was desired. Mr. P's wife and son indicated that they had anticipated the need for such a decision, but they still felt unprepared. They wanted Mr. P's life to be extended, if possible, so that his daughter, who lived abroad, would have time to make travel arrangements for a final visit with him. The physician offered a short-term solution: noninvasive positive pressure ventilation (NIPPV) via mask. The physician told the family that this low-risk therapy would allow Mr. P temporarily improved gas exchange, and this might enable him to regain consciousness and complete life-closure tasks. The family agreed.

Discussion

Initially, it may appear that the case of Mr. P does not raise obvious ethical issues. If the family and the caregivers agree that the use of NIPPV in this case is desirable, what is the dilemma? Some commentators have suggested that just such application of NIPPV is clinically and ethically appropriate.[12] Its use in this manner may provide some time for patients to complete important duties at the end of life. In opposition to this proposal, other observers have argued that such use of NIPPV may represent a breach of the principle of nonmaleficence because patients may be harmed by the painful extension of their lives in an unsuitable acute care setting and by the further risk that they could be subjected to inappropriate endotracheal intubation.[13] These opponents to such application of NIPPV also point to the social harm that may be caused if many thousands of terminally ill patients and their families are offered such treatment. The critics claim that providing NIPPV in the United States to 10% of dying lung cancer and COPD patients for just 2 days would result in added costs of more than $300 million per year.

These differences of perspective regarding NIPPV illustrate the need for careful reflection on cases such as that of Mr. P. The framework proposed in this chapter suggests that decision makers begin by clarifying the case. For example, is there evidence that Mr. P is suffering from an acute illness superimposed on his COPD? An answer to this question is obviously significant before alternatives for treatment can be considered. An acute problem, such as pneumonia, might be treated successfully, leading to significant improvement in Mr. P's clinical condition. Mechanical ventilation, under such circumstances, might be needed to allow the patient to recover and return to his baseline condition. Weaning from mechanical ventilation might be difficult, but it is not impossible. In Mr. P's case, however, there is no evidence of acute, reversible illness. It appears that he is suffering from end-stage COPD. This conclusion is based on the history, the clear chest radiograph, normal white cell count, and the lack of adventitious lung sounds.

Other questions that should be asked by decision makers seeking clarity about Mr. P's case include the following:

- Is Mr. P's condition considered "terminal"? (This is a conceptual question that requires clarity regarding the use of basic terms.)
- What values are Mr. P's family members attempting to preserve?
- Are there other important values that may be in conflict?
- If conflict about the use of NIPPV arises, who finally has decisional authority?
- Are the lines of authority affected by alternative reimbursement systems, such as managed care?
- If uncertainty or conflict is present, would the assistance of an institutional ethics committee be helpful?
- How much weight should be given to the family's desire for extra time so that Mr. P's daughter can travel to see him?
- Should concerns about society's allocation of health care resources have any bearing on this particular case?

Once decision makers have become as clear as possible about the dynamics of the case, it is important to attend carefully to treatment alternatives and their probable outcomes. For example, how likely is it that the use of NIPPV will accomplish what the family wants? If Mr. P receives NIPPV, how probable is it that he will then be given endotracheal intubation? Are there other treatment options that will better preserve both the family's and society's values?

After considering a range of options, decision makers should ponder the relevance of their professional codes of ethics and the application of broad ethical principles. For example, the AARC code gives primary weight to serving the health needs of patients in ways that are nondiscriminatory and respectful of their dignity. The code also calls for the respiratory care professional to seek improvement in "the access, efficacy, and cost of patient care" and to refrain from unnecessary use of resources. This would appear to prescribe that the respiratory care professional focus attention first on the patient's health care needs, while also being attentive to the social consequences of health care decisions for the public. The AARC code's commitment to fairness is also significant. The treatment options offered to Mr. P and his family should be similar to those offered others in similar circumstances. The principle of justice would challenge the decision to make a treatment option, such as NIPPV, available to some patients when it is apparent that it would generally be unwise or impossible to offer this option to other similarly situated patients. The principle of autonomy does not apply directly to Mr. P in his current condition, because he is unable to express his own wishes about treatment alternatives. It is usually reasonable to assume, however, that a patient's family can help to determine what he or she would want under the circumstances. The principles of beneficence and nonmaleficence call for the decision makers to give conscientious reflection to what would likely benefit or harm Mr. P.

After ethical norms are considered, a decision is in order. It is likely in Mr. P's case that no decision is without uncertainty. It is best to acknowledge from the beginning that equally well-motivated decision makers may differ. The goal of ethics is not absolute certainty: It is careful discernment, integrity, and accountability, often in the face of uncertainty. In Mr. P's case, it is not unreasonable to conclude that a limited use of NIPPV, in keeping with the family's decision, will preserve the greatest number of ethical values. If there is a residue of regret about the decision to use NIPPV, it is likely to result in added burdens for Mr. P, his family, and society. His family appears to be prepared to accept the burdens and to support this decision on his behalf. It may eventually happen that society, through appropriately accountable and representative mechanisms, will decide to limit some forms of expensive health care, including NIPPV for cases such as Mr. P's. Such a societal decision is not necessarily unfair, and it may be imperative given the fact that human beings can invent more technology, including health care technology, than they can afford financially. In the absence of such a societal decision about the use of NIPPV, however, it is ethically permissible to leave decisions about its use to patients, their families, and their caregivers.

Once a decision has been made and the case has progressed to its conclusion, it is useful to evaluate the decision. Mr. P's case raises a number of retrospective questions:

- Did the outcome in this case indicate the wisdom of limited use of NIPPV?
- Conversely, did any negative effects (e.g., added pain and suffering and eventual endotracheal intubation, as predicted by some) lead to reconsideration of the use of NIPPV?
- Were Mr. P's family members satisfied with the care that he received?
- Might the case have unfolded differently if Mr. P and his family had been informed earlier that his condition was terminal, so that more life-closure tasks, including a final visit with his daughter, could have been concluded before his final hospitalization?
- Might Mr. P's end-of-life treatment have been improved if it had occurred within the context of hospice care?

Such retrospective questions should not be addressed to second-guess what actually occurred. Rather, they represent an opportunity for us to learn systematically from our experience and to use what we learn to enhance ethical decision making in the future.

Conclusion

Respiratory care professionals have established a valuable ethical tradition. It is part of the professional responsibility of the respiratory care practitioner (RCP) to understand this tradition, know how to apply it to specific cases, and participate in its revision. The challenging ethical issues that continue to arise from the increased power of medical technology call for careful ethical reflection and practice on the part of all health care professionals. The distinctive perspectives of respiratory care professionals should help to ensure the future integrity of ethics in health care.

Questions for Reflection

1. What elements of the AARC code do you find most helpful? What elements of the code would you like to change? What features would you like to add to this code?

2. What changes currently taking place in health care are likely to affect the ethics of RCPs? What, for example, are the probable effects of changing patterns of health care financing and the emphasis on cost containment in terms of the ethics of the profession?

3. What role should RCPs have in the development of ethics in the facilities where they work? Should they be involved, for example, in their institution's ethics committee? If the facility does not have an ethics committee, should RCPs join in efforts to establish one? Should RCPs have the professional independence to bring difficult cases to their institution's ethics committee for discussion?

4. If a conflict arises about the ethics of a case, what resources, beyond the professional code of ethics, do RCPs have? If conflicts are unresolved, are there steps toward resolution that can be taken before there is judicial intervention?

5. What distinctive ethical issues, if any, do RCPs face? Are there ethical dilemmas that are more likely in the provision of respiratory care than in some other areas of health care?

Suggested Activities

1. Join a group of respiratory therapy students in writing a revised code of ethics for the profession.

2. Use the framework for ethical decisions to discuss current cases and arrive at conclusions that preserve the greatest number of ethical values.

3. Discuss the implications of the respiratory care profession's tradition of ethics when applied to recent developments in health care financing.

4. In the United States, there are more than 100 research centers that focus on ethics in health care. If possible, visit such a center in your region and discover what resources they make available for the study of ethics.

5. Explore the Internet using the keyword "bioethics," and find out what sites offer resources for health care ethics.

REFERENCES

1. Edwards, BS, and Ueno, WM: Sedation before ventilator withdrawal. J Clin Ethics 2:118–122, 1991.
2. Edelstein, L: The Hippocratic Oath: Text, translation, and interpretation. In Veatch, RM (ed): Cross Cultural Perspectives in Medical Ethics. Jones and Bartlett, Boston, 1989, pp 6–24.
3. American Nurses' Association: The Code for Nurses with Interpretive Statements. American Nurses' Association, Chicago, 1985.
4. American Medical Association: Principles of Medical Ethics, 1980.
5. Winslow, GR: From loyalty to advocacy. Hastings Center Report 14:32–40,1984.
6. In re Quinlan, 70 NJ 10, 355 A.2d 647 (1976), at 663–64.
7. Beauchamp, TL, and Childress, JF: Principles of Biomedical Ethics, ed. 4. Oxford University Press, New York, 1994.
8. Schloendorff, V: Society of New York Hospitals, 211 N.Y. 125, N.E. 90–93 (1917); Cruzan v. Director, Missouri Department of Health, 110 S.C. 2841 (1990).
9. Schneiderman, LJ: Is it morally justifiable not to sedate this patient before ventilator withdrawal? J Clin Ethics 2:129–130, 1991.
10. Schneiderman, LJ, and Spragg, RG: Ethical issues in discontinuing mechanical ventilation. N Engl J Med 318:987, 1988.
11. Edwards, MJ, and Tolle, SW: Disconnecting a ventilator at the request of a patient who knows he will then die: The doctor's anguish. Ann Intern Med 117:254–256, 1992.
12. Freichels, TA: Palliative ventilatory support: Use of noninvasive positive pressure ventilation in terminal respiratory insufficiency. Am J Crit Care 3:6–10, 1994.
13. Clarke, DE, et al: Noninvasive positive pressure ventilation for patients with terminal respiratory failure: The ethical and economic costs of delaying the inevitable are too great. Am J Crit Care 3:4–5, 1994.

CHAPTER 3

Introduction to Respiratory Failure

Robert L. Wilkins, PhD, RRT
James R. Dexter, MD, FCCP

Key Terms

abdominal paradox
anatomical shunt
continuous positive airway
 pressure
cor pulmonale
external respiration
hypoxemia

intermittent mandatory
 ventilation
internal respiration
mechanical
 ventilation
oxygenation failure
physiologic shunt

positive end-expiratory
 pressure (PEEP)
respiratory alternans
respiratory failure
ventilation-perfusion
 mismatching
ventilatory failure
weaning

Introduction

The production of energy in the body, which is necessary to maintain life, requires a constant supply of oxygen and nutrients to the tissues. Breathing provides a steady intake of oxygen to the lungs, where the oxygen diffuses through the alveolar capillary membrane into the blood (**external respiration**). The circulatory system distributes the oxygenated blood to the various vascular beds, where oxygen is given up to the tissues (**internal respiration**). In addition to oxygenation of the blood, the lungs also serve to rid the body of carbon dioxide (CO_2), a waste product of metabolism. The venous blood transports CO_2 to the lungs. The CO_2 diffuses into the alveoli and is subsequently exhaled into the atmosphere. This chapter is an introduction to the various medical problems that can lead to inadequate gas exchange. Subsequent chapters provide specific examples of diseases that affect the heart and lungs in adults, children, and neonates.

Respiratory failure is a general term that indicates failure of the lungs to provide adequate oxygenation or ventilation for the blood. **Oxygenation failure** is a more specific term indicating an arterial oxygen tension (Pao_2) of less than 60 mm Hg despite a fraction of inspired oxygen (FIO_2) of 0.50 or higher. **Ventilatory failure** refers to inadequate ventilation between the lungs and atmosphere that results in an inappropriate elevation of arterial carbon dioxide tension ($PaCO_2$) of greater than 45 mm Hg.

The term respiratory failure may be used in a more general fashion to describe failure of either external or internal respiration. For example, if the circulatory system fails to move the blood at a sufficient rate to meet metabolic demands, the transport of oxygen is inadequate and the tissues may become hypoxic. Although this is more accurately an example of circulatory failure, it does represent a breakdown in the system needed for respiration.

The amount of oxygen consumed and CO_2 produced each minute is dictated by the metabolic rate of the patient. Exercise and fever are examples of factors that increase the metabolic rate and place more demands on the cardiopulmonary system. When the cardiopulmonary reserve is limited by disease, fever may represent an added stress that precipitates respiratory failure and tissue hypoxia.

This chapter provides an overview of the concepts important for managing respiratory failure and applies these concepts to a specific case of drug overdose. Drug overdose can often cause neuromuscular deficiency leading to ventilatory failure. This chapter provides specific information about drug overdose in addition to information about respiratory failure.

Etiology

Oxygenation Failure

Hypoxemia is present when the PaO_2 is below the predicted normal value for a given patient. Hypoxemia is classified as mild (PaO_2 60 to 79 mm Hg), moderate (PaO_2 40 to 59 mm Hg), or severe (PaO_2 less than 40 mm Hg). This classification is based on predicted normal values for a patient who is less than 60 years old and breathing room air. For older patients, the practitioner should subtract 1 mm Hg for every year over 60 years of age from the limits of mild and moderate hypoxemia. A PaO_2 of less than 40 mm Hg represents severe hypoxemia at any age.

Hypoxemia has potentially serious consequences because it can lead to inadequate tissue oxygenation (*hypoxia*). When hypoxemia is present, tissue oxygenation may be preserved by an increase in cardiac output. Patients with severe hypoxemia or marginal cardiac function may not be able to compensate adequately for the hypoxemia, resulting in tissue hypoxia. Tissue hypoxia of the heart complicates the problem by causing dysrhythmias and poor contractility, which adds to the lack of oxygen delivery throughout the body.

The most common cause of hypoxemia is **ventilation-perfusion ($\dot{V}/\dot{Q}$) mismatching.** $\dot{V}/\dot{Q}$ mismatching occurs when some regions of the lung are poorly ventilated but remain perfused by pulmonary blood (low $\dot{V}/\dot{Q}$) (Fig. 3–1). Although regional vasoconstriction typically occurs in the pulmonary capillaries of the affected region, blood flow is not entirely stopped. As a result, some blood leaves the lungs without receiving adequate oxygenation and lowers the PaO_2. $\dot{V}/\dot{Q}$ mismatching also occurs when perfusion of a portion of the lung is reduced or absent despite adequate ventilation of the affected region (high $\dot{V}/\dot{Q}$).

Shunt is another cause of hypoxemia and refers to the movement of blood from the right side of the heart to the left side of the heart without its coming into contact with ventilated alveoli. Shunt can be caused by a congenital heart defect

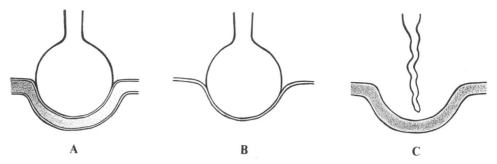

FIGURE 3-1   *(A)* Normal matching of ventilation to perfusion. *(B)* High V̇/Q̇, where ventilation is in excess of perfusion. *(C)* Low V̇/Q̇, where perfusion is in excess of ventilation (shunt).

(**anatomical shunt**), which allows the venous blood to bypass the pulmonary circulation through abnormal channels (e.g., ventricular septal defect). The most common cause of shunt, however, is pulmonary disease that results in collapsed or unventilated alveoli (**physiologic shunt**).[1] In this situation, blood flow through the affected lung regions does not participate in gas exchange and may result in severe hypoxemia (PaO_2 less than 40 mm Hg) that does not respond well to oxygen therapy (Fig. 3-1).

Hypoxemia can occur when an individual inhales a gas mixture that does not contain an adequate partial pressure of oxygen (PO_2). Breathing gas that lacks adequate oxygen results in a below-normal PaO_2 (arterial hypoxemia). This situation can occur at high altitude, during fires in an enclosed structure, and in cases of equipment failure while the patient is attached to a ventilator circuit.

Hypoventilation increases the alveolar PCO_2 ($PACO_2$) and decreases alveolar PO_2 (PAO_2). If the patient is breathing room air, hypoventilation can result in hypoxemia. Hypoxemia is less likely if the hypoventilating patient is breathing an elevated FIO_2. Causes of hypoventilation are described later in the chapter.

Ventilatory Failure

The ability to inhale requires a healthy neurological system that stimulates the respiratory muscles. Contraction of the diaphragm decreases the intrathoracic pressure and causes gas to flow into the lungs. Minimal effort is required if the chest cage is intact, airways are patent, and lungs are compliant. The ability to exhale requires patent airways and a lung parenchyma with sufficient elastic recoil to hold the bronchioles open until exhalation is complete.

Causes of ventilatory failure include depression of the respiratory center by drugs, diseases of the brain, spinal cord abnormalities, muscular diseases (see Chapter 17), thoracic cage abnormalities (see Chapter 14), and upper and lower airway obstruction (Table 3-1). Upper airway obstruction may occur with acute infection (see Chapter 23) and during sleep when muscle tone is reduced (see Chapter 22).

A number of factors can contribute to weakness of the inspiratory muscles and may tip the balance in favor of acute ventilatory failure. Malnutrition and electrolyte disturbances can weaken the ventilatory muscles, and pulmonary hyperinflation (e.g., emphysema) can make the diaphragm less efficient. Lung hyperinflation causes the diaphragm to assume an abnormally low position that results in a mechanical disadvantage (Fig. 3-2). These problems are common in patients with acute and chronic obstructive pulmonary disease (e.g., asthma, chronic bronchitis, emphysema; see Chapters 4, 5, and 6).

TABLE 3-1   **Causes of Ventilatory and Respiratory Failure**

VENTILATORY FAILURE
Dysfunction of the central nervous system
  Drug overdose
  Head trauma
  Infection
  Hemorrhage
  Sleep-related apnea
Neuromuscular dysfunction
  Myasthenia gravis
  Guillain-Barré syndrome
  Poliomyelitis
  Amyotrophic lateral sclerosis
  Spinal cord trauma
  Long-term use of aminoglycosides
Musculoskeletal dysfunction
  Chest trauma (flail chest)
  Kyphoscoliosis
  Malnutrition
Pulmonary dysfunction
  Emphysema
  Chronic bronchitis
  Asthma
  Cystic fibrosis

OXYGENATION FAILURE
Pneumonia
Adult respiratory distress syndrome
Congestive heart failure
Obstructive lung diseases (e.g., asthma, bronchitis)
Pulmonary embolism
Restrictive lung diseases (e.g., pulmonary fibrosis, kyphoscoliosis)

Pathophysiology

Oxygenation Failure

The severity of the hypoxemia and the patient's preexisting condition determine a patient's response to hypoxemia. A previously healthy patient will be unaffected by mild hypoxemia. A patient with severe cardiopulmonary disease, however, is likely to be in grave danger.

Patients usually respond to hypoxemia by increasing the rate of breathing (*tachypnea*). Tachypnea increases minute ventilation, decreases P_{ACO_2}, and to some extent increases P_{AO_2}. Since anatomical dead space (i.e., parts of the lung ventilated but not perfused) is fixed, the work of breathing increases. If the patient's respiratory system is unhealthy, as in obstructed airways, tachypnea may represent a serious increase in the work of breathing.

Hypoxemia stimulates the pulmonary capillaries to constrict in the affected regions. The pulmonary vasoconstriction will be widespread if the disease causing hypoxemia is prevalent throughout the lungs. Pulmonary vascular resistance (PVR) is markedly increased when widespread pulmonary vasoconstriction is present. This increases right heart workload and, if it continues for many months, can result in right

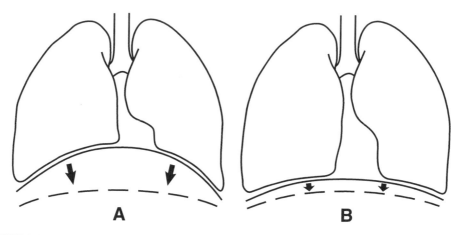

FIGURE 3-2 *(A)* Normal position of the diaphragm at end exhalation and end inhalation (dotted line). *(B)* Abnormal position of the diaphragm demonstrating the mechanical disadvantage associated with pulmonary hyperinflation.

heart failure. Right heart failure is characterized by increased pressure and dilatation of the right heart (as the heart pumps against the constricted capillaries). The combination of lung disease and right heart failure is known as **cor pulmonale.**

Cardiac rate and strength of contraction increase to compensate for hypoxemia. If coronary artery disease is present, the increased cardiac workload can lead to ischemia and irreversible damage (infarction). If the hypoxemia is severe or the heart cannot provide a sufficient increase in cardiac output to maintain adequate oxygen transport, the brain may be affected, resulting in a diminished sensorium and cognitive function. If the brain continues to be hypoxic, the patient will lose consciousness.

Ventilatory Failure

An acute increase in $PaCO_2$ decreases arterial blood pH. The combination of an elevated $PaCO_2$ and acidosis may have a profound effect on the body, especially when the ventilatory failure is acute. Ventilatory failure with rising PCO_2 affects the brain much like an anesthetic and results in somnolence and eventually coma.

Clinical Features

Oxygenation Failure

Inspection of the patient with severe hypoxemia typically reveals central cyanosis unless anemia is present and obscures the cyanosis. Central cyanosis is seen as a bluish discoloration of the tongue and mucous membranes. Anemia reduces the ability of clinicians to detect cyanosis because the bluish discoloration of tissues is due to desaturation of the hemoglobin. Vital signs are typically abnormal and demonstrate tachycardia, tachypnea, and hypertension. Severe hypoxemia may leave the patient confused, agitated, and slow to respond.

If the hypoxemia is chronic, right heart failure due to a persistent increase in PVR may develop and cause jugular venous distention. Right heart failure related to chronic pulmonary hypertension is known as cor pulmonale. Chronic hypoxemia also leads to other signs of right heart failure, including an enlarged liver (hepatomegaly), pedal edema, loud pulmonic valve closure,[2] and digital clubbing.

Laboratory abnormalities associated with hypoxemia include low Pao_2, Sao_2, and arterial oxygen content on ABG analysis. If the hypoxemia is chronic, bone marrow is stimulated to produce red blood cells, which results in polycythemia, increased hemoglobin, and hematocrit. When the hemoglobin increase is significant, the oxygen content of the arterial blood may be normal or near-normal despite the presence of hypoxemia.

Diseases of the lung that cause oxygenation failure usually also cause abnormalities on the chest radiograph. Typical abnormalities include infiltrates consistent with pulmonary edema, adult respiratory distress syndrome (ARDS), atelectasis, or pneumonia (see Chapters 10, 13, 15, and 18, respectively). When the primary cause of the hypoxemia is outside the lung (e.g., shunting from a congenital heart defect), the chest radiograph is often normal unless a complicating respiratory problem is present.

Ventilatory Failure

There are few clinical findings specifically suggestive of an elevated $Paco_2$. Clinical findings that suggest ventilatory failure include headache, diminished alertness, warm and flushed skin, and bounding peripheral pulses. These findings are very nonspecific, as they occur in a variety of conditions other than ventilatory failure. Since hypoxemia is often present in the patient with ventilatory failure, the clinical signs of inadequate oxygenation are often simultaneously present.

Hypothermia and loss of consciousness are common when the ventilatory failure is the result of an overdose of sedatives. Tricyclic antidepressants frequently increase heart rate and blood pressure. Breath sounds are often clear in the presence

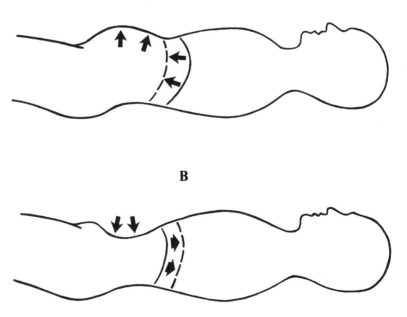

FIGURE 3-3   *(A)* Normal movement of the diaphragm and abdominal contents with breathing. *(B)* Abnormal, inward movement of the abdomen with each inspiratory effort as seen with diaphragm fatigue. This is known as abdominal paradox.

of drug overdose unless aspiration has occurred. Aspiration is more likely to occur when sedatives and alcohol are abused (due to a diminished gag reflex) and may result in crackles in the lower lobes with a predominance in the right lower lobe.

The clinical signs of diaphragm fatigue provide an early warning of respiratory failure in the patient with respiratory distress. It strongly suggests that the patient is in need of ventilatory assistance (see Treatment section). Fatigue of the diaphragm initially results in tachypnea. This is followed by periods of respiratory alternans or abdominal paradox.[3] The term **respiratory alternans** describes short-term alternation between using the diaphragm for breathing and using the accessory muscles. The term **abdominal paradox** describes the inward movement of the abdomen with each inspiratory effort (Fig. 3-3). This is due to the flaccid status of the diaphragm, which results in its being drawn upward when the accessory muscles create a negative intrathoracic pressure.

Arterial blood gases (ABGs) are very helpful for assessing the patient with ventilatory failure. The severity of ventilatory failure will be indicated by the degree to which the $Paco_2$ increases. Measurement of arterial pH identifies the degree of respiratory acidosis present and suggests the level of urgency at which treatment needs to be implemented. The patient needs immediate care when the pH drops below 7.2, as is discussed in the next section.

Treatment

Oxygenation Failure

Elevation of Fio_2 is the initial treatment for hypoxemia. Oxygen supplementation rapidly corrects hypoxemia associated with $\dot{V}/\dot{Q}$ mismatching or hypoventilation. Oxygen therapy in this situation can be given by nasal cannula, simple mask, or entrainment mask. The entrainment mask delivers a specific Fio_2 regardless of the patient's breathing pattern. This is in contrast to the nasal cannula and simple mask, which will allow the inhaled Fio_2 to vary as the patient's respiratory rate and tidal volume vary.

Hypoxemia due to either anatomical or physiologic shunting is usually not responsive to increases in Fio_2 because blood traversing the shunt does not come into contact with ventilated alveoli. Treatment of anatomical shunt requires closure of the defect, if possible. Treatment of physiologic shunt requires reopening of alveoli. Shunt caused by collapse of alveoli often responds to positive pressure ventilation (PPV). PPV can decrease the patient's work of breathing and open collapsed alveoli to allow better gas exchange.

PPV is generally used to treat hypoxemia when the patient has a Pao_2 of less than 60 mm Hg despite an increase in the Fio_2 to 0.50 or higher (Table 3-2). The application of **continuous positive airway pressure** (CPAP) by mask is an acceptable temporary measure as long as ventilation is adequate and the patient's problem is likely to resolve quickly (e.g., postoperative atelectasis). Intubation and **mechanical ventilation** are needed if mask CPAP is not successful in correcting the hypoxemia and reducing the patient's work of breathing or when the problem is not likely to resolve quickly (e.g., ARDS). The application of **positive end-expiratory pressure** (PEEP) in conjunction with mechanical ventilation is usually needed to treat patients with severe hypoxemia due to shunting. PEEP and CPAP allow adequate oxygenation at a lower Fio_2, thus reducing the risk of oxygen toxicity. The use of PEEP and its potential complications are described in more detail in Chapter 13.

TABLE 3-2   **Clinical Guidelines for Initiation of Mechanical Ventilation
(Adult Patients)**

Respiratory rate	> 35/minute
Vital capacity	< 15 mL/kg
Minute ventilation	> 10 liters/minute
Maximum inspiratory pressure	< -20 cm/H_2O
Pa_{CO_2}	> 50 mm Hg
Pa_{O_2}	< 60 mm Hg on O_2

Conventional modes of mechanical ventilation are adequate for most patients. These include assist/control or **intermittent mandatory ventilation** (IMV). A ventilator set to assist/control delivers a preset tidal volume at a specified rate. The ventilator will also deliver a full mechanical breath each time the patient initiates an inspiratory effort. A ventilator set to IMV delivers preset tidal volumes at the preset rate, but does not provide mechanical breaths when the patient takes spontaneous breaths in between the mechanical breaths. As a result, the patient may receive the preset number of mechanical breaths and as many spontaneous breaths each minute as desired. Although IMV was popularized initially as a mode of **weaning** patients from mechanical ventilation, it is now also popular as a form of ventilator support. See the following discussion on treatment of ventilatory failure to become familiarized with setting tidal volume and rate during mechanical ventilation.

Mechanical ventilation is almost always initiated with inspiratory times much shorter than expiratory times. A long expiratory time allows adequate time for exhalation and reduces the chance of inadvertent air trapping. Prolonged inspiratory times with short expiratory times (inverse I:E) may improve oxygenation in some patients with low lung compliance and poor gas exchange. Inverse ratio ventilation (IRV) was first applied in neonates but is now also used in adult patients with refractory hypoxemia.[1]

Ventilatory Failure

An acute elevation in Pa_{CO_2} indicates that the patient is unable to maintain adequate alveolar ventilation and may be in need of ventilatory assistance. The Pa_{CO_2} does not necessarily have to be above normal range to indicate the need for mechanical ventilation in all circumstances. For example, if an asthmatic patient is in acute respiratory distress and the Pa_{CO_2} increases from 30 to 40 mm Hg because of muscle fatigue, the patient would benefit from intubation and mechanical ventilation. This example illustrates how trends in the Pa_{CO_2} can be helpful in determining the need for mechanical ventilation.

Once the patient is intubated, the tidal volume selected should be based on the presenting pathophysiology.[4] Generally the tidal volume is set in the range of 8 to 12 mL/kg of ideal body weight (e.g., obese patients do not need enormous tidal volumes) Tidal volumes smaller than this tend to result in collapse of peripheral lung units, especially in the patient with healthy lungs. Tidal volumes larger than 12 mL/kg or large enough to produce peak airways pressure of greater than 40 to 50 cm H_2O tend to overinflate the lungs and may result in barotrauma (e.g., pneumothorax, pneumomediastinum). This is especially true for patients with stiff lungs, such as those with ARDS.

The respiratory rate needed by the patient depends on his or her metabolic rate, but adults typically require 8 to 15/minute. Rates as low as 6 to 8/minute may be needed in patients with obstructive lung disease to minimize air trapping by allowing long expiratory times. Ventilation is adjusted in most patients to keep the $Paco_2$ between 35 and 45 mm Hg. One exception is the patient with cerebral edema in whom a lower $Paco_2$ may be therapeutic by lowering intracranial pressure. Another exception is the patient with a chronically elevated $Paco_2$ in whom the goal of mechanical ventilation is to return the pH to the normal range and the $Paco_2$ to the patient's baseline, rather than to the normal range.[5] If patients with chronic hypoventilation and CO_2 retention are ventilated with enough vigor to achieve a normal $Paco_2$, respiratory alkalosis becomes a problem in the short term and weaning a problem in the long term.

Initially the Fio_2 is set at 1.0 to ensure adequate oxygenation during this stressful period. An exception might be in the patient in whom a recent ABG has demonstrated supranormal Pao_2 on an increased Fio_2. A Fio_2 of about 0.40 to 0.60 should be adequate in such cases. Once the patient stabilizes, the Fio_2 can be adjusted on the basis of pulse oximetry or ABGs.

Clinicians should determine the cause of the ventilatory failure while initiating symptomatic treatment. In the case of drug overdose, attempts should be made to identify the type of drug, the amount ingested, the length of time since ingestion, and whether trauma occurred. General goals in management of drug overdose are to prevent toxin absorption (e.g., stomach lavage, inducement of vomiting, use of charcoal), to enhance drug excretion (e.g., dialysis), or to prevent accumulation of toxic metabolic products (e.g., acetylcysteine as an antidote for acetaminophen overdose).

Weaning the patient from mechanical ventilation can begin as soon as the cause of the respiratory failure has been corrected and the patient's medical problems are stable. Weaning parameters help determine when weaning is likely to be successful (Table 3-3). Clinicians should use numerous parameters to decide when to begin weaning, since use of any single parameter can be misleading. A spontaneous tidal volume of greater than 325 mL combined with a spontaneous respiratory rate of less than 38/minute appear to be better than most predictors of weaning success in adults.[6]

Methods of weaning include IMV, pressure support (PS), and T-piece. Each method has advantages and disadvantages, but any one should effectively wean most patients when they are ready. Each method depends on decreasing the patient's ventilatory support under controlled circumstances while the patient is closely monitored. Extubation can occur when the patient's gag reflex is intact and the patient has demonstrated that the endotracheal tube is no longer needed.

TABLE 3-3 **Weaning Criteria**

Cause of respiratory or ventilatory failure is resolved
Patient condition is stable and improving
Vital capacity is > 10–15 mL/kg
Resting minute volume is < 10 liters/minute
Maximum inspiratory pressure is > −20 cm H_2O
Adequate oxygenation on an Fio_2 < 0.50
Spontaneous respiratory rate < 35/minute
Spontaneous tidal volume > 325 mL

IMV weaning is done by decreasing the number of mechanical breaths per minute every few hours until the patient no longer needs mechanical support or demonstrates poor tolerance of the weaning (e.g., 20 percent changes in pulse rate and blood pressure). The primary disadvantage of IMV is the potential increase in the work of breathing imposed on the patient by the ventilator circuit during spontaneous breaths.[7] This increased workload is primarily due to excessive resistance at the demand valve. Newer ventilators have improved this problem, but it remains a clinical issue in some patients.

PS helps overcome the workload imposed by the resistance of the artificial airway and ventilator circuitry and assists ventilation by providing a set amount of positive airway pressure during inspiration.[2] Weaning with PS is begun by setting it at a level that results in an acceptable tidal volume and rate without use of accessory muscles.[4] The practitioner gradually lowers the preset PS on a regular basis (over a period of hours to days) while the patient is monitored. Mechanical ventilation can be discontinued once the patient is tolerating a low PS level (e.g., less than 5 cm H_2O), as evidenced by the patient's maintaining a normal pattern of breathing.

T-piece weaning is done by discontinuing mechanical ventilation for short periods of time and placing the patient on "blow-by" at an appropriate FIO_2. The duration during which the patient is allowed to breathe spontaneously is gradually increased until the patient either shows signs of stress or no longer requires mechanical ventilation. This method of weaning has the advantage of giving patients periods of rest when they are reconnected to the ventilator.

CASE STUDY

History

Ms. N is a 47-year-old white woman who was found unconscious on the floor of her apartment by a relative. Empty bottles of diazepam (Valium), amitriptyline (antidepressant), and beer cans were nearby. The relative dialed 911, and the patient was transported to a local emergency room. During transportation, the patient had an adequate pulse rate but required ventilatory assistance with a bag-valve mask on oxygen. An ABG was obtained immediately, and a drug screen was ordered in the emergency room.

QUESTIONS

1. What complications are likely to occur in this patient?
2. What information should the attending physician attempt to identify from the relative or paramedics?
3. Is this patient most likely to be experiencing ventilatory or oxygenation failure?
4. Should the patient be intubated? If so, why?
5. What treatment should be provided?

ANSWERS

1. Common complications include respiratory depression, hypothermia or hyperthermia, cardiac irregularities, and vomiting and aspiration.

2. The physician should attempt to identify how much medication the patient swallowed and how much time has passed since ingestion. Some of the pertinent information could be obtained from the prescription labels on the bottles.

3. The patient is most likely to experience ventilatory failure due to depression of the central nervous system. Oxygenation failure would be expected only if gastric acid aspiration has occurred.

4. Yes, the patient should be intubated to ensure adequate ventilation and to protect the airway from aspiration. The need for bag-valve-mask assistance demonstrates the need for intubation and mechanical ventilation.

5. The most urgent treatment needed after establishing an airway and ensuring adequate ventilation is to prevent further absorption of the overdose medication. This is accomplished with the use of charcoal to absorb and bind with the toxins. If the patient is awake and alert, vomiting is induced with syrup of ipecac; however, if the patient is lethargic or if mental status is rapidly deteriorating, stomach lavage is preferable. To protect the lungs, it is important to place an endotracheal tube before performing stomach lavage.

Physical Examination

General: An unconscious, slightly obese female with a 8.0-mm transoral endotracheal tube in place being ventilated with a hand resuscitator; Ewald tube in left nostril; gastric lavage fluid containing a large number of pill fragments; strong smell of alcohol; patient approximately 5 foot, 8 inches and 155 pounds

Vital Signs: Pulse 124/minute, respiratory rate 12 to 16/minute with bag-valve mask, body temperature 35.3 C° (95.6°F), blood pressure 120/75 mm Hg

HEENT: No signs of trauma; pupils dilated with sluggish response to light

Heart: Normal heart sounds with no murmurs

Lungs: Breath sounds clear except in right lower lobe, where inspiratory crackles are heard

Abdomen: Soft, obese, with no organomegaly or tenderness; bowel sounds present, but hypoactive

Extremities: Warm to palpation with no edema, clubbing, or cyanosis

Initial ABG Findings (while patient is being ventilated with an FIO_2 of 1.0 via a bag-valve mask prior to intubation): pH 7.28, $PaCO_2$ 54 mm Hg, PaO_2 135 mm Hg, SaO_2 99 percent, HCO_3^- 26 mEq/liter

---

QUESTIONS

6. What accounts for the hypothermia?

7. What accounts for the dilated and sluggishly reactive pupils?

8. What could account for the crackles heard in the right lower lobe?

9. How would you interpret the ABG findings?

10. What is the significance of the pill fragments found in the contents of the stomach? Why was the charcoal given?

ANSWERS

6. Hypothermia is common in patients with an overdose of sedatives. Amitriptyline overdose especially disrupts temperature regulation.

7. Dilated and slowly reactive pupils are common in patients who overdose on sedatives and tricyclic antidepressants.

8. Crackles in the right lower lobe are most likely due to aspiration of stomach contents. Sedatives and alcohol cause decreased mental acuity and depressed pharyngeal muscle function, both of which contribute to a disturbed gag reflex and increase the chance of aspiration.

9. The ABG reveals an acute respiratory acidosis with adequate oxygenation. Respiratory acidosis is common in patients who overdose on sedatives, as sedatives depress the central nervous system and diminish the drive to breathe. Bag-valve-mask ventilation is often less effective than ventilation with a bag valve and a properly placed endotracheal tube because face masks can leak, causing some air to go down the esophagus (gastric inflation).

10. The presence of pill fragments in the stomach indicates that at least some of the pills were ingested somewhat recently. Gastric lavage and charcoal will probably prevent absorption of a large amount of the medication in the stomach.

CASE STUDY—continued

The patient was transferred from the emergency room to the intensive care unit (ICU). While in the ICU, she was placed on continuous mechanical ventilation with a volume ventilator, and cardiac monitoring was continued.

QUESTIONS

11. What laboratory tests would you suggest at this time?

12. What ventilator settings would you recommend? Specifically suggest the mode of ventilation, tidal volume, rate, FIO_2, and PEEP level.

ANSWERS

11. To ensure adequate ventilation, it would be helpful to order a repeat ABG after initiation of mechanical ventilation. A chest x-ray would be helpful to investigate the crackles in the right lower lobe.

12. The patient should be ventilated with the assist/control or IMV mode. The tidal volume should be in the range of 500 to 600 mL, since Ms. N's ideal body weight is approximately 60 kg. The mechanical rate should be about 10 to 14/minute. The presence of inspiratory crackles indicates that the patient may have lung pathology that could lead to $\dot{V}/\dot{Q}$ mismatch or shunt. This suggests that an elevated FIO_2 will be needed to maintain adequate oxygenation. An FIO_2 in the range of 0.40 to 0.60 is a reasonable place to start, since we know the patient has more than adequate oxygenation on an FIO_2 of 1.0. PEEP levels of greater than 5 cm H_2O should not be necessary unless the patient requires an FIO_2 of greater than 0.60 on mechanical ventilation.

CASE STUDY—continued

The ventilator was set to deliver a tidal volume of 600 mL at a rate of 12/minute with an FIO_2 of 0.45 in the assist/control mode. Twenty minutes after initiation of mechanical ventilation, an arterial blood sample was drawn and revealed the following: pH 7.51, $PaCO_2$ 32 mm Hg, PaO_2 88 mm Hg, and HCO_3^- 25 mEq. The chest x-ray showed patchy infiltrates in the right lower lobe, which is consistent with aspiration pneumonia (Fig. 3–4). The electrocardiogram monitor revealed a sinus rate of 115 to 130/minute. Breath sounds were clear in all areas except the right lower lobe.

A drug screening demonstrated that the patient had also taken acetaminophen. The patient's blood alcohol level was 0.155, and the presence of amitriptyline was confirmed via urinalysis.

QUESTIONS

13. How would you interpret the ABG results?

14. What changes in the ventilator settings would you suggest based on the ABG results?

15. What is the treatment for acetaminophen overdose?

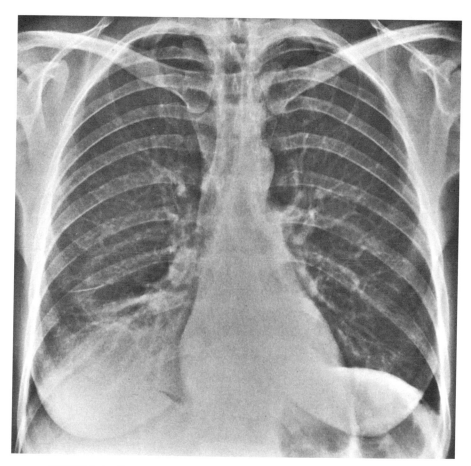

FIGURE 3–4   Chest radiograph demonstrating infiltrates in the right lower lobe.

ANSWERS

13. The ABG reveals an acute respiratory alkalosis with adequate oxygenation on an FIO_2 of 0.45. The respiratory alkalosis is the result of the mechanical ventilation with an excessive minute ventilation.

14. The ventilator should be adjusted to deliver a lower minute volume. A reduction in the tidal volume or rate would reduce alveolar ventilation and allow the $PaCO_2$ to increase to a more normal range.

15. The antidote for acetaminophen overdose is acetylcysteine (Mucomyst). The need for treatment with the antidote is determined by the use of a nomogram to compare the amount of time passed since ingestion versus the acetaminophen plasma blood level. If the acetaminophen plasma level is at or above the minimum "treatment" level, the patient should be given an oral loading dose of *N*-acetylcysteine (140 mg/kg) followed by 17 maintenance doses of 70 mg/kg at 4-hour intervals. The *N*-acetylcysteine should be diluted with water, juice, or soda. *N*-acetylcysteine is also given when an acetaminophen plasma level is not available and the history of ingestion is greater than 7.5 g or 140 mg/kg.

CASE STUDY—continued

The rate of the mechanical ventilator was reduced to 8/minute at the same tidal volume. Acetylcysteine was given to the patient to treat the acetaminophen overdose. Over the next 24 hours, the patient regained consciousness and was able to respond to commands and communicate by way of paper and pencil. She was weaned via T-piece and carefully observed. After 4 hours, her vital signs were normal and ABGs as follows: pH 7.43, $PaCO_2$ 36 mm Hg, and PaO_2 79 mm Hg on an FIO_2 of 0.40. Based on these findings, the patient was extubated and placed on oxygen by mask with aerosol at an FIO_2 of 0.45. Over the next 24 hours, her pneumonia and general condition improved, and she was transferred to the psychiatric ward on day 3. The remainder of her hospital stay was uneventful.

REFERENCES

1. Marini, JJ, and Wheeler, AP: Critical Care Medicine: The Essentials. Williams & Wilkins, Baltimore, 1989.
2. Butler, J: Cardiac evaluation. In Murray, JF and Nadel, JA (eds): Textbook of Respiratory Medicine. WB Saunders, Philadelphia, 1988.
3. Mier-Jedrzejowicz, A, et al: Assessment of diaphragm weakness. Am Rev Respir Dis 137:877, 1988.
4. Hess, DR, and Kacmarek, RM: Essentials of Mechanical Ventilation. McGraw-Hill, New York, 1996.
5. Dantzker, DR, et al: Comprehensive Respiratory Care. WB Saunders, Philadelphia, 1995.
6. Yang, KL, and Tobin MJ: A prospective study of indexes predicting the outcome of trials of weaning from mechanical ventilation. N Engl J Med 324:1445, 1991.
7. Beydon, L, et al: Inspiratory work of breathing during spontaneous ventilation using demand valves and continuous flow systems. Am Rev Respir Dis 138:300, 1988.
8. Fiastro, JF, et al: Pressure support compensation for inspiratory work due to endotracheal tubes and demand continuous positive airway pressure. Chest 93:499, 1988.

CHAPTER 4

Asthma

Robert L. Wilkins, PhD, RRT
James R. Dexter, MD, FCCP

Key Terms

abdominal paradox	cromolyn sodium	occupational asthma
anticholinergics	exercise-induced asthma	paradoxical pulse
asthma	extrinsic asthma	stable asthma
bronchial provocation	intrinsic asthma	status asthmaticus
bronchodilators	metered-dose inhaler	theophylline
corticosteroids	(MDI)	unstable asthma

Introduction

Asthma is a chronic obstructive pulmonary disease characterized by diffuse airway inflammation and bronchospasm that, in many cases, occurs in response to various stimuli. A key feature of asthma is that the airways obstruction is reversible. In fact, between episodes the patient often is without symptoms and pulmonary function may be normal. When the patient has an asthmatic attack that does not respond to conventional treatment, the condition is called **status asthmaticus.**

Although much overlap occurs, it is helpful to divide asthma into two categories: extrinsic and intrinsic. **Extrinsic asthma** is characterized by bronchospasm that occurs in an atopic patient (someone who has an allergic reaction in response to exposure to allergens) when exposed to environmental irritants. **Intrinsic asthma** is present when the patient suffers asthma attacks without evidence of atopy. Children most commonly exhibit extrinsic asthma, whereas intrinsic asthma often starts in adulthood.

Occupational asthma is the term used to describe bronchospasm that occurs in response to a provoking agent in the work place. Typically the individual with this type of asthma becomes asymptomatic during periods of time away from work, such as weekends and vacations.

Stable asthma is present when a period of 4 weeks has passed during which an asthma-prone patient has had no increase in symptoms or no need for an increase in medication. Conversely, **unstable asthma** is present when the patient has experienced increased symptoms sometime during the past 4 weeks.[1]

The highest incidence of asthma occurs within the first 10 years of life, but it can develop at any age. Asthma occurs more often in men during early adulthood, but more often in women when the onset of disease is beyond the age of 40 years.[2] Recent studies have demonstrated an increase in asthma morbidity and mortality during the past decade. The exact cause of this increase in morbidity and mortality is not known.

Etiology

In some cases of extrinsic asthma a specific provoking situation can be linked to the patient's asthma attacks, and thus terms such as **exercise-induced asthma** or pollen asthma are frequently used. Most patients with extrinsic asthma can have attacks provoked by many different allergens, such as house dust mites, animal danders, and certain foods or food additives (e.g., sulfites). In addition to allergens, asthma attacks can be provoked by pharmacological agents (e.g., β-adrenoceptor antagonists, aspirin), by air pollutants (e.g., sulfur dioxide, oxidants), exercise, cigarette smoke, and airway infections. Infection of the airways represents one of the most common causes of asthma attacks.

Pathophysiology

In addition to bronchospasm, asthmatics' airways may be obstructed by mucosal edema and excessive secretions (Fig 4–1). Frequently asthmatics have thick, tenacious mucus that causes plugging in the distal airways. The lack of uniform ventilation throughout the lung causes ventilation-perfusion ($\dot{V}/\dot{Q}$) mismatching, which results in hypoxemia. Pulmonary vascular resistance may increase as a result of hypoxemia.

Initially the airways obstruction primarily hinders exhalation. This results in air trapping and progressive hyperinflation of the lungs. With air trapping, the residual volume increases at the expense of the vital capacity. The combination of increased airway resistance and lung hyperinflation significantly elevates the work of breathing in asthmatics.

Clinical Features

Typically the patient suffering from an acute asthma attack will complain of one or more of the following: chest tightness, difficulty breathing, wheezing, and coughing. The onset of these symptoms may be rapid or relatively slow. When the symptoms have a rapid onset, they may disappear rapidly with appropriate treatment. Although some idea of the seriousness of an asthma attack can be determined from the history, the degree of dyspnea is not a reliable predictor of severity. The interviewer should ask the patient about recent exacerbations, their severity, and their response to therapy.

Although dyspnea and wheezing are suggestive of asthma, disorders such as con-

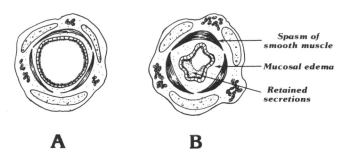

FIGURE 4-1   Cross-sectional view of a normal airway *(A)* and from a patient with asthma *(B)*. A combination of airway secretions, edema, and bronchospasm contribute to a reduction in the airway diameter.

gestive heart failure, bronchitis, pulmonary embolism, and upper airway obstruction can cause similar symptoms. In most cases the patient's age, medical history, physical findings, radiographic studies, and laboratory tests will confirm the diagnosis.

Physical examination of the asthmatic can provide important objective information that will assist in confirming the diagnosis and identifying the severity of the obstruction. Inadequate assessment of the patient's status can be a fatal mistake because it can result in insufficient treatment and monitoring.[1,3,4] Common findings associated with asthma include tachypnea, use of accessory muscles of breathing, a prolonged exhalation, increased anteroposterior diameter of the chest, expiratory polyphonic wheezing, diaphoresis, and intercostal retractions. Severe asthma is suggested by pronounced use of accessory muscles, abnormal sensorium, **paradoxical pulse,** tachypnea, inability to speak, and wheezing on inhalation and exhalation.[5-8]

Accessory muscles of breathing are used because of the pulmonary hyperinflation that causes the diaphragm to assume a flat position less capable of effective ventilation.[8] A prolonged expiratory phase occurs as the intrapulmonary airways become obstructed and slow the movement of gas out of the lungs. Increased anteroposterior diameter occurs when air trapping and pulmonary hyperinflation are present. *Wheezing* is produced as rapid airflow occurs through narrowed airways, resulting in vibration of the airway walls.[9] *Retractions* are seen as intermittent depressions of the skin around the rib cage with each inspiratory effort. Retractions result when a significant drop in intrapleural pressure causes the skin overlying the chest wall to sink inward. This suggests that the patient's work of breathing is markedly increased. The significant drop in intrapleural pressure is also responsible for the drop in pulse pressure during inspiration (*paradoxical pulse*).[10,11]

It is not uncommon to see patients lean forward and brace their hands or elbows on a nearby table during an acute asthma attack. This position may provide a better mechanical advantage for the accessory muscles to assist breathing. The reclining position is assumed only when the patient with a severe episode of asthma is exhausted.

The chest radiograph is most helpful for identifying the presence of complications such as pneumonia, atelectasis, or pneumothorax. The use of chest radiographs to evaluate routine asthma attacks is not recommended. In the absence of complications, the chest radiograph is often normal or may demonstrate hyperinflation of the lung fields.

Complete pulmonary function studies are not typically done when the patient is suffering from an acute asthma attack. Simple bedside spirometry, however, is appropriate and very useful in determining the severity of obstruction and the response to therapy. Measurement of peak flow and forced expiratory volume in one second

(FEV$_1$) is commonly used and easy to obtain unless the patient has severe dyspnea. A peak flow of less than 100 liters/minute or a FEV$_1$ of less than 1.0 liter suggests severe obstruction.[8]

Bronchial provocation testing is useful in identifying the degree of airway reactivity in patients whose symptoms are typical of asthma, but who have normal pulmonary function studies. Methacholine is most often used for bronchial provocation testing because it increases parasympathetic tone in the smooth muscles of the airways, resulting in bronchospasm. Asthmatics will have a greater than 20 percent decrease in FEV$_1$ in response to methacholine, whereas normal subjects have little or no response.

Arterial blood gases (ABGs) are extremely useful for assessing the severity of an asthma attack, especially when the bronchospasm is severe enough to prevent the patient from performing a forced expiratory maneuver. The degree of hypoxemia and hypercapnia present is a reliable indicator of the severity of the airway obstruction.[8] Typically the Paco$_2$ is decreased with the onset of an asthma attack.[4,5] A normal or increased Paco$_2$ indicates that a more severe degree of obstruction is present or that the patient has started to become fatigued. Additional signs of fatigue include tachypnea, diaphoresis, abdominal paradox, disturbed consciousness, and decreasing peak flow.[8] **Abdominal paradox** is seen as an inward movement of the abdominal wall during inspiration and is associated with fatigue of the diaphragm (see Chapter 1).

One important goal of assessment in acute asthma is an efficient evaluation. Most asthmatic patients need immediate care, and the experienced clinician will perform an efficient yet effective assessment without delaying the onset of treatment. Avoiding unnecessary evaluation tools is an essential part of any assessment, especially when the patient is acutely ill.

Treatment

Initially the clinician should direct treatment toward achieving adequate oxygenation, providing bronchodilators, and decreasing airway inflammation. The majority of patients suffering from an acute asthma attack will become hypoxemic as a result of V/Q mismatching. In some cases the hypoxemia will be severe enough to represent a serious threat to the patient's life, but it can almost always be corrected with appropriate oxygen therapy.

Numerous pharmacological agents are available to promote bronchodilation and reduce airway inflammation, such as β-adrenergics, xanthines, parasympatholytics, and steroids. In the majority of mild cases, the bronchospasm can be reversed by use of an aerosolized β$_2$-adrenergic. Inhaled β-agonist bronchodilators offer the following advantages over oral bronchodilators: a more rapid onset, lower dosage requirements, a lower incidence of systemic side effects, and better protection of the airways against provoking agents.[1,12] The **metered-dose inhaler** (MDI) is a popular route for administering bronchodilators because it is simple for patients to use.

Aerosolized bronchodilator treatments with a small volume nebulizer (SVN) are useful for the patient who is unable to use MDIs and during life-threatening episodes. The SVN treatments are most often given every 3 to 6 hours, but during severe bronchospasm they may be provided more often as long as the patient is monitored carefully. Continuous nebulization therapy for the administration of bronchodilator may prove useful when the asthmatic is not responding to conventional therapy and is on the verge of respiratory failure.[13,14] Continuous nebulization therapy is usually given in the intensive care unit (ICU) or emergency room.

During an acute, severe asthma attack, if the patient fails to respond adequately to inhaled β-agonists, intravenous (IV) **corticosteroids** can be added to the treatment plan. The anti-inflammatory effects of corticosteroids may take several hours to cause beneficial results and therefore should be started as soon as indicated. A large dose (500 mg) of methylprednisolone offers no advantage over a more conservative dose (100 mg) in the emergency room treatment of acute asthma.[15] Use of corticosteroids early in the treatment of an acute episode may reduce the need for hospitalization.[16] IV aminophylline is not recommended for treatment of acute asthma in the emergency room or outpatient clinic. Use of aminophylline in combination with repetitively administered β-agonist bronchodilators and corticosteroids has not proved beneficial in reversing acute, severe episodes.[17] Patients who respond minimally to initial therapy can be given inhaled β-agonists hourly and a subcutaneous injection of epinephrine. In such cases, patients must be monitored closely, especially those who are more than 45 years and at risk for myocardial ischemia.

Anticholinergics such as ipratropium (Atrovent) constitute a third therapeutic option after β-agonists and corticosteroids.[18] The combination of anticholinergic therapy and β-agonists is safe and may be more effective than either drug alone. Repeated doses of the two drugs may reduce the need for hospitalization in patients with very severe asthma.[19]

Magnesium sulfate has been shown to produce rapid reversal of bronchospasm in some patients with severe asthma.[17] Its exact mechanism of action is not known, and it is not considered standard care in the treatment of asthma.

Clinicians should avoid giving asthmatics certain medications during an acute asthma attack. Sedatives can induce ventilatory failure and should be given only if the patient is intubated and being mechanically ventilated. Inhaled corticosteroids, acetylcystcine (Mucomyst), **cromolyn sodium,** and dense aerosols may increase bronchospasm, since these agents tend to be irritating to the airways.[8]

Other goals of management include treatment of airway infections, mucolysis, and maintenance of adequate hydration. Hydration improves the patient's pulmonary condition by aiding in the expectoration of secretions.

Favorable prognostic signs include improvement in the vital signs, PaO_2, $PaCO_2$, breath sounds, sensorium, and breathing pattern. Since any one of these parameters can be misleading by itself, it is always best to assess numerous values to obtain a more accurate clinical picture of the patient's response to therapy.

If the patient becomes fatigued despite treatment, mechanical ventilation will be necessary. Although not every acute asthmatic patient with respiratory acidosis needs to be intubated and mechanically ventilated, a rising PCO_2 despite aggressive therapy is strong evidence that the patient is in serious respiratory distress and needs breathing assistance. The decision to intubate and mechanically ventilate the patient can be difficult, especially when the clinical findings are not convincing (Table 4–1). The physical findings, ABGs, and peak flow parameters (described earlier and in the following case study) provide the most reliable data for evaluating the need for mechanical ventilation.

Once the clinician decides to intubate the patient and begin mechanical ventilation, the patient must be sedated. Sedation improves patient comfort and reduces

TABLE 4-1   **Decision Making in Asthma**

Admit Patient? *Yes, if:*	*How to Recognize*
The attack is severe	Use of accessory muscles at rest Paradoxic pulse present Inspiratory and expiratory wheezing present Peak flow is <100 L/min FEV, <1.0 L Significant hyperinflation noted on chest radiograph
The patient does not respond to initial therapy	Vital signs not improving Continued use of accessory muscles PaO_2 responds minimally to O_2 therapy

Intubate and initiate CMV? *Yes, if:*	*How to Recognize?*
The patient fatigues	$PaCO_2$ rising Sensorium deteriorates Abdominal paradox present Peak flow decreasing
Respiratory failure present	Hypoxemia is present despite high FIO_2 Severe respiratory acidemia (pH <7.25) occurs Central cyanosis
Cardiopulmonary arrest occurs	Pulse and respiratory effort absent Pallor Patient becomes unconscious

oxygen consumption during mechanical ventilation. Ventilator management of the severe asthmatic can be challenging because of the high risk of air trapping and barotrauma. For this reason, the clinician should chose ventilator settings that result in a low minute ventilation to allow maximum time for exhalation and minimize air trapping.[17] This may cause $PaCO_2$ elevation, but the benefit of avoiding barotrauma outweighs the risk of mild acidosis. Most asthmatics who are mechanically ventilated are able to be weaned within a few days. Weaning can begin when airway resistance returns to near-normal.

The ultimate goal in the management of asthma is to prevent or at least minimize future attacks by decreasing the level of airway responsiveness. Consequently, once the episode is over and the patient has recovered, the clinician should assess the severity of the underlying asthma via the following: a careful history, pulmonary function testing, and in selected cases, investigations of provoking agents (e.g., in suspected occupational asthma). Clinicians should educate patients with regard to avoidance of provoking agents, use of medications, and medication side effects, thus enabling them to live an active, independent lifestyle. Cromolyn sodium is helpful in stabilizing the mast cells to prevent the release of mediators, such as histamine, that can cause bronchospasm.[20] The patient should be trained to use a peak flowmeter in order to monitor the degree of airway obstruction; such training allows patients to know when to increase their medication or when they need to seek medical attention. Low-dose **theophylline** may be beneficial in reducing the symptoms and number of hospitalizations of chronic asthmatics.[21]

History

Ms. B is a 19-year-old bareback-bronco rider seen in the emergency room because of shortness of breath. The dyspnea began during a particularly hard ride, which culminated in modest dust inhalation on the rodeo floor. She states that the tightness in her chest and shortness of breath were so severe that she had to eventually leave the rodeo and seek medical help. She is now very uncomfortable, even at rest. During the past week she has had a cough productive of greenish yellow sputum, mild fever, malaise, and fatigue, but she did not feel seriously ill until the onset of dyspnea at the rodeo earlier in the day. She denies previous lung problems except for mild "whistling" in her chest, which has occurred off and on during the past several years. She denies the use of any prescription medications, or any previous episodes of dyspnea, chest pain, leg pain, hemoptysis, sinusitis, or allergies. Her family history is negative for lung disease.

QUESTIONS

1. What is the key symptom to explore in greater detail?

2. What are the differential diagnoses of this patient's problem, and what is the most likely diagnosis?

3. Toward what details should the physical examination be specifically directed?

4. Why is Ms. B having trouble now rather than, say, 2 months ago?

ANSWERS

1. The key symptom is dyspnea. Ms. B should be questioned to evaluate the severity of the dyspnea because this determines the speed at which further evaluation and treatment should be pursued.

2. Asthma, acute bronchitis, congestive heart failure, flu syndrome, pneumothorax, pulmonary embolus, and psychogenic dyspnea are the differential diagnoses. Asthma exacerbated by acute bronchitis is the most likely diagnosis.

3. The physical examination should be directed toward identifying (1) signs that confirm or rule out the differential diagnoses and (2) the severity of the airway obstruction (see later in the chapter).

4. Ms. B is having trouble now because she has had a triple airway insult of respiratory tract infection, allergen (dust) inhalation, and recent severe exertion.

Physical Examination

General: Patient alert but restless and in moderate respiratory distress, mildly diaphoretic, sitting up on the edge of the bed leaning forward with her arms braced on her knees; cough frequent and productive of small amounts of greenish sputum

Vital Signs: Temperature 37.5°C (99.5°F), respiratory rate 38/minute, blood pressure 170/95 mm Hg, heart rate 140/minute, paradoxical pulse 25 mm Hg

HEENT: Sinuses not tender to palpation; alae nasii flare with inspiration

Neck: Trachea midline and mobile to palpation; no stridor; carotid pulsations ++ and symmetrical bilaterally with no bruit; no lymphadenopathy, thyroidomegaly, or jugular venous distention; sternocleidomastoid muscles tensed during inspiration

Chest: Increased anteroposterior diameter with decreased expansion during breathing; resonance to percussion moderately increased bilaterally; mild abdominal paradox with respiratory efforts

Lungs: Rapid respiratory rate with prolonged expiratory phase and polyphonic wheezing heard over entire chest during inhalation and exhalation (Fig. 4–2)

Heart: Regular rhythm at 140/minute; no murmurs, gallops, or rubs; point of maximum impulse in normal position

Abdomen: Soft, nontender; bowel sounds present; no masses or organomegaly

Extremities: No clubbing, cyanosis, or edema; pulses ++ and symmetrical in all areas

QUESTIONS

5. What is causing Ms. B's wheezing?

6. What is causing the paradoxical pulse, and what is the significance of this finding?

7. What is the cause and significance of the accessory muscle usage?

8. What is the cause and significance of the paradoxical breathing pattern?

9. Why do patients in respiratory distress lean forward and brace their hands or elbows?

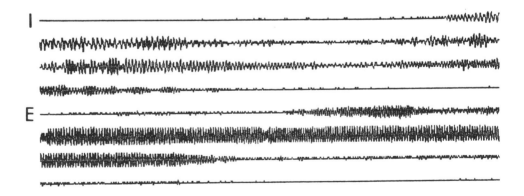

Wheeze/Stridor

FIGURE 4–2   Waveform analysis demonstrating an inspiratory and expiratory high-pitched wheeze. Time is represented on the horizontal axis and intensity (loudness) on the vertical axis. The pitch is indicated by the number of deflections per time period. Each horizontal line represents 0.34 second. (Reprinted from Respir Care 35:969, 1990, with permission.)

10. What pathophysiology accounts for Ms. B's increased anteroposterior diameter?

11. Does the physical examination provide evidence that hypoxemia is present, and if so what are the signs?

ANSWERS

5. Wheezing is caused by a decreased airway diameter, which is the result of bronchospasm, airway edema, and secretions. Rapid airflow through the partial obstruction causes the airway walls to "flutter," much like the reed in a musical instrument.[9] It is important to note that relatively rapid airflow is needed to cause the flutter effect, and wheezing stops when the patient fatigues to the point where airflow is no longer rapid enough to vibrate the airway wall.

6. Paradoxical pulse (variation of the systolic pressure by greater than 10 mm Hg due to breathing efforts) can be caused by wide swings in intrathoracic pressure or by cardiac tamponade.[10,11] In this case, the airway obstruction is requiring vigorous respiratory muscle effort, which causes large changes in intrathoracic pressure. Although this finding has been shown to occur in more severe cases of asthma,[22,23] its absence does not preclude severe airway obstruction.[8]

7. Accessory muscle usage occurs when the lung hyperinflation associated with asthma causes the diaphragm to become flattened and therefore less effective. Retraction of the sternocleidomastoid is a reliable sign of severe airway obstruction.[8]

8. The paradoxical breathing pattern is a sign of diaphragm fatigue.[24,25] It is recognized by noting inward movement of the abdomen during inspiration. Normally diaphragm contraction pushes the abdominal contents downward and the anterior abdominal wall out during inspiration. Fatigue of the diaphragm allows it to be "sucked" upward into the chest when the accessory muscles create a negative intrathoracic pressure during inspiration.

9. Patients in respiratory distress who have developed diaphragmatic fatigue lean forward and brace their arms or elbows to stabilize the shoulder girdle and to provide a better mechanical advantage for the accessory respiratory muscles.

10. The increased anteroposterior diameter is caused by air trapping, which occurs when partial airway obstruction is present in the medium to small bronchi.

11. Although cyanosis is not present, there are other clues that Ms. B is probably hypoxemic. The tachycardia, tachypnea, diaphoresis, restlessness, and wheezing suggest that oxygenation is not optimal.

Laboratory Evaluation

Chest Radiograph: Moderate hyperexpansion with no evidence of infiltrates (Fig 4–3)

ABGs: pH 7.38, $PaCO_2$ 43 mm Hg, PaO_2 49 mm Hg on room air

Spirometry:

FEV_1 = 1.5 liters (27 percent of predicted)

Peak flow = 140 liters/minute

FVC = 2.1 liters (40 percent of predicted)

Hematology: Results pending

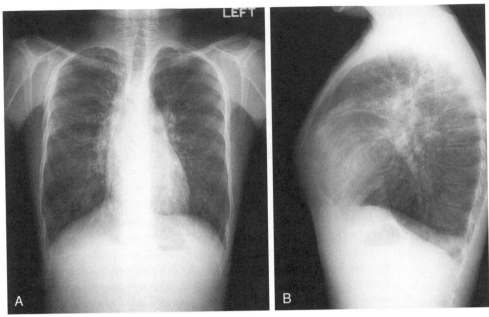

FIGURE 4-3   *(A)* Anteroposterior (AP) chest film of Ms. B. *(B)* Lateral view, showing increased AP diameter and low, flat diaphragm.

QUESTIONS

12. How would you interpret the ABGs and spirometry results?

13. What treatment should be planned?

14. What are the possible medication side effects?

15. Should you leave Ms. B to go take care of other patients while you are waiting for other test results?

16. Should you admit Ms. B to the hospital?

17. How would you evaluate Ms. B's response to therapy?

18. What therapies should be avoided in this patient?

19. If Ms. B fails to improve with conventional bronchodilator and corticosteroids, what other medication should be added to the treatment regimen?

20. When should mechanical ventilation be considered?

ANSWERS

12. The ABG results suggest that Ms. B is tiring, because the $Paco_2$ is now in the upper limits of normal. In most cases of asthma, the $Paco_2$ is reduced below normal until the patient becomes fatigued. The Pao_2 of 49 mm Hg indicates moderate hypoxemia on room air. These ABG results would strongly suggest the need for mechanical ventilation if Ms. B had been on maximum treatment before the arterial sample was obtained.

    The spirometry results are consistent with obstructive lung diseases such as asthma. The peak flow of 140 liters/minute and FEV_1 of 1.5 liters indicate moderate obstruction. The significant reduction in the forced vital capacity (FVC) indicates air trapping, which is most likely in this case (but could indicate restrictive lung disease).

13. Treatment should include oxygen, aerosolized and IV bronchodilators, antibiotics, and hydration. Oxygen should be started at 4 to 6 liters/minute via nasal cannula or at 40 percent by entrainment mask and should be adjusted to keep the arterial oxygen saturation (SaO_2) greater than 90 percent (or the PaO_2 in the 60 to 80 mm Hg range). A β-adrenergic bronchodilator should be administered. This is typically accomplished by administering aerosolized albuterol or other $β_2$-specific bronchodilators by an MDI or SVN. This may be supplemented by a subcutaneous injection of a β-agonist when a rapid peak effect is desired. High-dose parenteral corticosteroids should be started if the patient fails to respond adequately to β-adrenergic bronchodilators. IV fluids are given to establish optimum thinning of airway secretions. Antibiotics may be needed to treat an upper respiratory tract infection if there is evidence of a bacterial infection (e.g., purulent sputum with numerous pus cells).

14. The bronchodilator can cause tachycardia, tremor, nausea, and dysrhythmias. Oxygen therapy is not likely to cause any side effects, since most asthmatics are not CO_2 retainers and do not depend on their hypoxic drive.

15. This patient should not be left unattended for any reason. Ms. B needs close monitoring and evaluation, since respiratory failure could occur at any moment.

16. Unless Ms. B improves dramatically with treatment in the emergency room, she should be admitted to the ICU. If she improves significantly in the emergency room, she could be admitted to the pulmonary ward for treatment and observation (Table 4–1).

17. The same techniques used for the initial assessment should be used to evaluate Ms. B's response to therapy. Sensorium is an important parameter to monitor, because it will help evaluate the patient's condition and her ability to cooperate with treatment.[8] Other physical examination findings, such as the degree of accessory muscle usage and the vital signs, can be very useful. Simple spirometry tests such as the FEV_1 or peak flow, or both, can provide objective data regarding the course of recovery. ABGs should be used when the physical examination findings suggest a change in the patient's status.

18. In this patient, sedatives,[26] inhaled corticosteroids, cromolyn sodium, acetylcysteine, and dense aerosols should be avoided.[8] In the presence of airway obstruction, cromolyn sodium can be added to the treatment plan once bronchodilator therapy has stabilized lung function.[12,20] If this patient had presented with a history of hypertension, she might have been given a β-adrenergic antagonist (e.g., Inderal), which increases bronchospasm. In such a case, a trial of calcium channel blockers to treat the hypertension would be an appropriate choice, as they do not increase airway resistance.

19. Inhaled ipratropium bromide or atropine could be added to her treatment plan if the more conventional bronchodilators are not effective. The effects of atropine are additive to those of the adrenergic agonists.[1,27]

20. Mechanical ventilation should be considered if Ms. B's mental status deteriorates significantly, especially if this is associated with a rising $PaCO_2$ (Table 4–1) despite bronchodilator and oxygen therapy. Once mechanical ventilation is started, sedation can be used to make Ms. B more comfortable. Since the patient is alert and since treatment has not been initiated, mechanical ventilation is not yet mandatory.

CASE STUDY—continued

In the emergency room Ms. B was started on oxygen via nasal cannula at 4 liters/minute. This resulted in an improvement in oxygen saturation from 87 to 97 percent as obtained by pulse oximetry. An IV line was established to deliver steroids, fluids, and antibiotics. Additionally, an SVN treatment with 0.3 to 0.5 mL albuterol diluted in 3 mL saline was provided.

Although this treatment resulted in improvement in Ms. B's dyspnea, the peak flow improved only slightly (150 liters/minute), and Ms. B continued to use her accessory muscles heavily to breathe. Based on the minimal improvement 1 hour after the initiation of bronchodilator therapy, it was decided to admit the patient for further care and close observation.

Ms. B was admitted to the respiratory ICU, where oxygen therapy, steroids, and fluids were given. The nebulized albuterol treatment was repeated. Ninety minutes after admission to the ICU, ABGs revealed the following: pH = 7.43, $PaCO_2$ = 36 mm Hg, PaO_2 84 mm Hg, and HCO_3^- 25 mEq/liter. Peak flow measurement at this point was 145 liters/minute. The clinical examination revealed polyphonic wheezing throughout exhalation, normal sensorium, a respiratory rate of 32/minute, and a pulse rate of 126/minute. Because it was determined that Ms. B was responding minimally to the aerosolized bronchodilator and aminophylline, the attending physician started IV methylprednisolone with a bolus of 30 mg to be repeated every 4 to 6 hours. The Gram stain revealed numerous pus cells and gram-positive organisms.

QUESTIONS

21. Should the use of methylprednisolone result in rapid improvement in Ms. B's airway obstruction?

22. What are the potential side effects of steroids?

23. Is this patient a candidate for continuous nebulization of bronchodilator?

24. Are any favorable prognostic signs present at this point?

ANSWERS

21. The use of IV corticosteroids is not expected to result in rapid improvement in Ms. B's airway obstruction.[8] In most cases, 4 to 6 hours is needed before significant improvement in peak flow or FEV_1 can be expected with the use of corticosteroids.

22. The potential systemic side effects of high-dose oral corticosteroids taken for prolonged periods of time are significant, including depletion of bone calcium, impairment of immunologic response, increased fat cell production and deposition in the subcutaneous tissues of the neck and trunk, and hypertension. With the use of aerosolized corticosteroids, candidiasis (oral thrush) and dysphonia can occur.[1] Since the patient in this case is expected to need only a short course of IV steroids, these side effects are not of concern at this point.

23. This patient could be a candidate for continuous nebulization therapy for the administration of aerosolized bronchodilator. This therapy has been shown to be safe and effective for the treatment of acute asthma in children[13,14] and adults. Continuous bronchodilator nebulization has been suggested as a

treatment alternative to intermittent therapy, because the continuous administration could allow more optimal delivery of the nebulized medication. Prolonged inhalation should promote better distribution of the aerosolized drug and a more consistent topical administration of the bronchodilator to the bronchial smooth muscle. To avoid toxic side effects, a more dilute solution of the medication should be used such that the dose typically given in a 15-minute treatment is given over a 1-hour period. Bronchodilators that have more specific β_2 response, such as terbutaline and salbutamol, are recommended to avoid cardiac side effects (e.g., tachycardia, palpitations). Continuous nebulization therapy appears to be indicated in asthmatics with impending respiratory failure who are not responding optimally to conventional therapy. More studies need to be conducted to identify the role of this therapy in severe cases of asthma and the exact criteria for its use.

24. The improvement in Pao_2 and $Paco_2$ are favorable prognostic signs.[8]

CASE STUDY—continued

Over the next 24 hours, Ms. B steadily improved. Peak flow improved to 220 liters/minute the next day, and her vital signs returned to near-normal. The wheezing improved: it was heard only during the latter half of exhalation, and the use of accessory muscles was minimal at this point. Ms. B was transferred to the general floor for maintenance therapy and evaluation of prophylactic therapy.

The remainder of Ms. B's hospital stay was uneventful, and she was discharged 3 days later with a follow-up outpatient appointment in 2 weeks. Ms. B was discharged on oral antibiotics and an MDI (albuterol). She was counseled on how to avoid dust inhalation, how to recognize and what to do in response to respiratory infections, and how to use the MDI. She was advised to use the MDI before performing any heavy exercise.

REFERENCES

1. Woolcock, AJ: Asthma. In Murray, JF, and Nadel, JA (eds): Textbook of Respiratory Medicine. WB Saunders, Philadelphia, 1988.
2. Kussin, PS: Pathophysiology and management of life-threatening asthma. Respir Care Clin North Am 1:177–192, 1995.
3. Rebuck, AS, and Read, J: Assessment and management of severe asthma. Am J Med 51:788, 1971.
4. Kelsen, SG, et al: Emergency room assessment and treatment of patients with acute asthma: Adequacy of the conventional approach. Am J Med 64:622, 1978.
5. Shim, CS, and Williams, MH Jr: Relationship of wheezing to the severity of obstruction in asthma. Arch Intern Med 143:890, 1983.
6. McFadden, ER Jr, et al: Acute bronchial asthma: Relations between clinical and physiologic manifestations. N Engl J Med 288:221, 1973.
7. George, RB: Monitoring of patients during asthma attacks. In Lavietes, M, and Reichman, LB (eds): Diagnostic aspects and management of asthma. Purdue Frederick, Norwalk, CT, 1981.
8. George, RB: Management of the acute asthma attack. In Bone, RC, et al (eds): Acute Respiratory Failure. Churchill Livingstone, New York, 1987.
9. Forgacs, P: The functional basis of pulmonary sounds. Chest 73:399, 1978.
10. Henkind, SJ, et al: The paradox of pulsus paradoxus. Am Heart J 114:198, 1987.
11. Rebuck, AS, and Pengelly, LD: Development of pulsus paradoxus in the presence of airway obstruction. N Engl J Med 288:66, 1973.
12. Canny, GJ, and Levison, H: Aerosols: Therapeutic use and delivery in childhood asthma. Ann Allergy 60:11, 1988.
13. Moler, FW, et al: Improvement in clinical asthma score and $Paco_2$ in children with severe asthma treated with continuously nebulized terbutaline. J Allergy Clin Immunol 81:1101, 1988.
14. Portnow, J, and Aggarwal, J: Continuous terbutaline nebulization for the treatment of severe exacerbation of asthma in children. Ann Allergy 60:368, 1988.

15. Emerman, CL, and Cydulka, RK: A randomized comparison of 100mg vs 500mg dose of methylprednisolone in the treatment of acute asthma. Chest 107:1559, 1995.

16. Rowe, BH, et al: Effectiveness of steroid therapy in acute exacerbations of asthma: A meta-analysis. Am J Emerg Med 10:301–310, 1992

17. Luna, CM, et al: Acute, severe, life-threatening asthma. Clin Pulm Med 3:119–128, 1996.

18. International consensus report on diagnosis and treatment of asthma. Publication No. 92:3091. National Institutes of Health, National Heart, Lung, and Blood Institute, 1992.

19. Schuh, S, et al: Efficacy of frequent nebulized ipratropium bromide added to frequent high-dose albuterol therapy in severe childhood asthma. J Pediatr 126:639–645, 1995.

20. Blumenthal, MN, et al: A multicenter evaluation of the clinical benefits of cromolyn sodium aerosol by metered-dose inhaler in the treatment of asthma. J Allergy Clin Immunol 81:681–687, 1988.

21. Emad, A: Effectiveness of adding alternate-day theophylline to the treatment regimen of patients with moderate to severe asthma. Respir Care 41:520, 1996.

22. Shim, C, and Williams, MH Jr: Pulsus paradoxus in asthma. Lancet 1:530, 1978.

23. Knowles, GK, and Clark, TJH: Pulsus paradoxus as a valuable sign indicating severity of asthma. Lancet 2:1356, 1973.

24. Mier-Jedrezejawicz, A, et al: Assessment of diaphragm weakness. Am Rev Respir Dis 137:877, 1988.

25. Cohen, CA, et al: Clinical manifestations of inspiratory muscle fatigue. Am J Med 73:308, 1982.

26. Neder, GA, et al: Death in status asthmaticus: Role of sedation. Dis Chest 44:263, 1963.

27. Brady, RE, and Easton, JG: The value of atropine in the documentation of reversible airways obstruction. Ann Allergy 42:211, 1979.

CHAPTER 5

Chronic Bronchitis

Robert L. Wilkins, PhD, RRT
James R. Dexter, MD, FCCP

Key Terms

chronic obstructive
   pulmonary disease
   (COPD)
cor pulmonale
cyanosis
hepatojugular reflex

jugular venous distention
   (JVD)
loud pulmonary valve
   sound
mucoid sputum
mucus

pedal edema
pulmonary hypertension
right ventricular heave
sympathomimetics

Introduction

Chronic bronchitis is a pulmonary disease that causes a chronically productive cough due to bronchial inflammation. A disease is termed chronic when it lasts for at least 3 consecutive months of the year for 2 successive years. In a patient with a chronic productive cough, other potential causes of this problem (e.g., tuberculosis, lung cancer, congestive heart failure) must be excluded before the diagnosis of chronic bronchitis can be made.

This chapter on chronic bronchitis and the following one on emphysema present two commonly encountered problems known as **chronic obstructive pulmonary disease** (COPD). COPD occurs worldwide and is a common cause of death and disability in adults. Although many patients with COPD have a combination of emphysema and chronic bronchitis, for teaching purposes we are presenting each disease separately. A third condition that some experts include under the heading of COPD is asthma (Fig. 5-1). Chapter 4 provides background information and a case presentation on asthma.

Etiology

The most important factor contributing to the onset of chronic bronchitis is cigarette smoking.[1] Compared to nonsmokers, cigarette smokers have a more rapid decline in

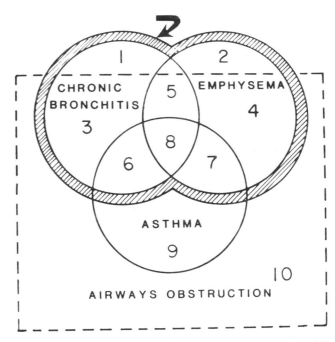

FIGURE 5-1   Schema of chronic obstructive pulmonary disease. A nonproportional Venn diagram shows subsets of patients with chronic bronchitis, emphysema, and asthma in three overlapping circles. Subset of patients lying within the rectangle have airways obstruction. Patients with asthma, subset 9, are defined as having completely reversible airways obstruction and lie entirely within the rectangle; their diagnosis is unequivocal. Patients in subsets 6 and 7 have reversible airways obstruction with chronic productive cough or emphysema, respectively. Patients in subset 8 have features of all three disorders. It may be difficult to be certain whether patients in subsets 6 and 8 indeed have asthma or whether they have developed bronchial hyperactivity as a complication of chronic bronchitis or emphysema; the history helps. Patients in subset 3 have chronic productive cough with airways obstruction but no emphysema; it is not known how large this subset is, since epidemiologic studies are not available using computed tomographic (CT) scan, the most sensitive in vivo imaging technique for diagnosing or excluding emphysema. It is much easier to identify patients with emphysema in the chest radiograph who do not have chronic bronchitis (subset 4). Most patients who require medical care for their disease fall into subsets 5 and 8. Patients in subsets 1 and 2 do not have airways obstruction as determined by the FEV$_1$ but have clinical or radiographic features of chronic bronchitis or emphysema, respectively. Because chronic obstructive pulmonary disease (COPD), when defined as a process, does not have airways obstruction as a defining characteristic, and because pure asthma is not included in the term COPD, patient subsets 1 through 8 are included within the area outlined by the shaded band that denotes COPD. (From Snider, GL: Chronic bronchitis and emphysema. In Murray, JF, and Nadel, JA: Textbook of Respiratory Medicine. WB Saunders, Philadelphia, p 1071, 1988, with permission.)

lung function[2-4] and a higher incidence of respiratory infections, chronic bronchitis, and emphysema. The differences between smokers and nonsmokers in terms of lung function increase as the quantity of cigarette consumption increases.[1] Pipe and cigar smokers have higher morbidity and mortality rates for COPD compared to nonsmokers, but lower rates compared to cigarette smokers.[1]

Because chronic bronchitis is less common among nonsmokers, it appears that factors other than smoking are much less important causes of chronic bronchitis.[1] Other factors may, however, be important in the overall decline of the chronic bronchitis patient's clinical condition. Factors such as infection (viral or bacterial), air pollution, and occupational exposure to irritants may play a key role in exacerbating chronic bronchitis.

Pathology and Pathophysiology

Chronic cigarette smoking causes the airways to undergo a variety of pathological changes. The bronchial mucous glands enlarge (hypertrophy) and the goblet cells increase in number,[1,5] resulting in an abnormal increase in **mucus** production. Increased mucus is hardly noticeable early in the disease, but as exposure to cigarette smoke continues, the airways produce increasing amounts of mucus. The bronchial walls often become inflamed and lose cilia either as a result of exposure to smoke or as a complication of airway infection. The combination of excessive mucus production and reduced ciliary function leads to mucus plugging of the smaller airways. Mucus plugging promotes infection.

Patients with chronic bronchitis may have only a minimal increase in airway resistance. Bronchial wall inflammation and excessive mucus decrease airflow through the larger bronchi as the bronchitis becomes more complicated. Mucus plugging and airway obstruction cause ventilation-perfusion ($\dot{V}/\dot{Q}$) mismatching, which leads to significant changes in gas exchange and hypoxemia. Exacerbations of chronic bronchitis are associated with a significant increase in airway eosinophilia and, to a lesser degree, neutrophilia.[6]

In response to hypoxemia, the pulmonary vasculature constricts (hypoxic vasoconstriction). Acidosis adds to the contraction of smooth muscles in the pulmonary blood vessels.[7] This added resistance to blood flow through the pulmonary circulatory system places an abnormally high work load on the right side of the heart. The added work load causes the right ventricle to hypertrophy and then dilate. If the problem continues for many months or years, the right ventricle will not be able to continue effectively pumping blood through the pulmonary circulation. This results in right heart failure due to chronic lung disease and is known as **cor pulmonale.**[8]

Clinical Features

Medical History

Patients with chronic bronchitis almost always admit having a chronic cough and sputum production. In many patients, the onset of these symptoms is very gradual, and as a result, the patient may not consider these symptoms serious or be able to identify the date of onset. The patient typically seeks medical attention when either a superimposed acute problem such as infection is present, or when the chronic problem becomes severe enough to cause concern. Dyspnea is often present during acute exacerbations, but it may not be a primary symptom when the patient is stable.

Mucus is usually white or mucoid in patients with stable chronic bronchitis. Infection changes the **mucoid sputum** to yellow-green and makes it thick and purulent. The change in color of mucus may also occur as a result of allergic reactions or stagnation of secretions within the airways. Microscopic examination of the sputum sample will help differentiate between infection and allergy when the mucus changes character.

Hemoptysis (coughing up blood from the lung) may occur in patients with chronic bronchitis.[1] Airway inflammation, coughing, and infection can contribute to the rupture of superficial blood vessels in the bronchi, which results in blood-streaked sputum. The patient with hemoptysis should be evaluated for lung cancer if there is also a significant history of smoking.

The interviewer should report the smoking history, which includes the age at which the patient started smoking, how many packs of cigarettes are typically smoked each day, whether there have been any attempts to stop smoking, and the duration of periods in which the patient refrained from smoking. It is also important to report the use of other forms of tobacco inhalation, such as pipes and cigars.

The family history is often positive for COPD, as the tendency to acquire this disease appears to be genetically transferable.[9] An occupational history should be obtained to identify any significant exposure to dusts or fumes in the work place that might contribute to the development of chronic bronchitis.

Physical Examination

No significant findings are discovered during the physical examination of patients with mild stable chronic bronchitis. More severe disease or acute exacerbations cause numerous abnormalities. Fever may indicate that an infection is present. Chest examination may reveal use of accessory muscles and a prolonged expiratory phase. Use of accessory muscles indicates diaphragmatic fatigue. Auscultation often reveals coarse crackles, expiratory wheezes, and rhonchi. The coarse crackles indicate excessive airway secretions, and the expiratory wheezes or rhonchi suggest partial airway obstruction. **Pulmonary hypertension** causes the pulmonary valve to close forcefully, which results in a **loud pulmonary valve sound** (P_2). Pulmonary hypertension severe enough and long-standing enough to cause right heart failure (cor pulmonale) will result in **jugular venous distention (JVD).** Elevated right heart pressures severe enough to cause right heart failure will also cause **pedal edema** and hepatomegaly (enlarged liver). Right ventricular hypertrophy caused by chronically elevated right heart pressures will cause the heart to bump against the chest wall at the left sternal border. The bumping can be felt on palpation of the chest wall and is called a **right ventricular heave.**

Cyanosis of the tongue and mucus membranes is often present in patients with complicated cases of chronic bronchitis and hypoxemia. Acute, severe hypoxemia and hypercapnia will change the patient's level of consciousness. Hypoxemia acts somewhat like alcohol in that it first may make the patient wild, but then eventually sedates the patient when it becomes severe. Hypercapnia acts much more like an anesthetic gas, sedating the patient more severely as the level rises. Chronic, compensated hypercapnia causes very few cognitive abnormalities.

Laboratory Evaluation

The complete blood count (CBC) generally reveals an elevated red blood cell (RBC) count if chronic hypoxemia is present. The white blood cell (WBC) count may increase if an infectious process such as pneumonia is present. Otherwise, the CBC is not significantly abnormal in most patients with chronic bronchitis.

The arterial blood gases (ABGs) are very useful for assessing oxygenation and acid-base status. ABGs are normal with mild chronic bronchitis. Hypoxemia is often severe, and respiratory acidosis is commonly seen with acute exacerbations complicating more advanced disease. Compensatory elevation of serum HCO_3^- occurs and the pH returns to near-normal after several days of increased Pa_{CO_2}.

The chest radiograph does not demonstrate obvious abnormalities in stable or mild cases of chronic bronchitis. In more severe cases, as during an exacerbation, the chest radiograph may demonstrate hyperinflation and increased lung markings. The increased lung markings refer to the radiologist's ability to identify airway walls within the chest that have enlarged as a result of bronchial wall thickening. The chest radiograph may also demonstrate an enlarged right heart when cor pulmonale is present. In any patient with an acute exacerbation of chronic bronchitis, the chest radiograph must be inspected for evidence of complications such as pneumonia.

Pulmonary function studies are useful for quantifying the severity of the disease and identifying the response to therapy. In mild chronic bronchitis, the routine pulmonary function study results are typically normal. With more significant disease, measurements of expiratory flow and vital capacity decrease and residual volume increases. If bronchospasm is also present, the expiratory flow rates may improve with bronchodilator therapy. The total lung capacity and diffusion capacity are usually normal in patients with chronic bronchitis. An electrocardiogram (ECG) may demonstrate right-axis deviation if right ventricular hypertrophy is present. The right-axis deviation is seen as a negative (downward) deflection of the QRS complex in lead I.

Treatment

Treatment of chronic bronchitis has two general goals: (1) to treat any superimposed acute medical problem such as congestive heart failure, infection, or bronchospasm; and (2) to attempt to slow the progress of the chronic bronchitis. Treating a superimposed medical problem initially requires identification of the problem. Once identified, the physician can begin appropriate treatment (e.g., furosemide [Lasix] for congestive heart failure, antibiotics for infection, bronchodilation for bronchospasm). These alone may significantly improve the clinical condition of the patient.

The progress of chronic bronchitis is best controlled by interventions designed to facilitate smoking cessation. Smoking cessation does not return lung function to normal, but it does decrease the rate of lung function deterioration to normal so that the patient has a better chance of survival to old age. The risk of smoking-related diseases such as lung cancer is reduced with smoking cessation and continues to drop as abstinence is maintained.[10] Smoking cessation is facilitated if the health care professionals provide counseling and support in addition to warning the patient about the health hazards associated with smoking.[11] Use of nicotine polacrilex (nicotine gum) and transdermal nicotine patches can be helpful in decreasing symptoms of smoking withdrawal, but they must be combined with counseling to obtain maximum results.[11]

Antibiotics, **sympathomimetics,** xanthines (theophylline), and corticosteroids may prove useful when infection and bronchospasm are present. Albuterol combined with ipratropium appears to be more effective than either medication alone.[12] Theophylline appears to be most useful not as a single therapy for treating COPD, but in combination with other bronchodilators.[13] Recent recommendations suggest using lower doses of theophylline aiming for serum levels of 5 to 15 μg/mL, thereby reducing the possibility of toxic side effects while maintaining the beneficial effects.[13] Postural drainage may be useful when sputum retention is a problem. Oxygen is useful when hypoxemia is present, but it does not help if the resting Pao_2 is greater than 60 mm Hg unless the patient can be shown to desaturate significantly during sleep. Long-term supplemental oxygen therapy is needed when the patient's Pao_2 is less than 55 mm Hg while breathing room air during stable conditions. A Pao_2 of 55 to 60 mm Hg coupled with evidence of cor pulmonale or polycythemia also suggests that home oxygen therapy may be of benefit. Long-term home oxygen therapy will most likely increase survival length in those COPD patients who have not developed significant pulmonary hypertension (mean arterial pressure less than 25 to 30 mm Hg).[14]

CASE STUDY

History

JL is a 54-year-old white man currently employed as a machinist. He was seen in the pulmonary outpatient clinic for the first time complaining of shortness of breath with exertion and a productive cough. JL states that his coughing had recently increased and was producing thick, yellow sputum. He states that his cough had been present for several years but was "usually not a problem." His cough has usually been productive of clear to white sputum in the morning. He had recently noticed more shortness of breath than usual and was now dyspneic at rest. JL did admit to feeling warm at times during the past few days but had not taken his temperature with a thermometer. He denied chest pain, hemoptysis, sinusitis, weight loss, allergies, night sweats, or chills.

JL admitted to smoking 2½ packs of cigarettes per day for the past 30 years. He had attempted to stop on several occasions, but was successful for no longer than 3 or 4 months. His machinist work had exposed him to many toxic fumes. His family history was positive for lung disease, as his father died of emphysema at the age of 64 years, which was 12 years earlier. His mother is alive and well at age 75. His sister is healthy at age 47, and his 51-year-old brother has diabetes.

QUESTIONS

1. What medical problems are suggested by the medical history, and what are the key symptoms to explore?
2. What is the significance of the patient's sputum color?
3. What is JL's smoking history in pack-years?
4. What is the significance of the family and occupational history?
5. What should the physical examination accomplish at this point in the assessment of the patient?

ANSWERS

1. The patient's medical history suggests chronic bronchitis exacerbated by a respiratory infection such as acute bronchitis, flu, bronchospasm, or pneumonia. The symptoms do not suggest congestive heart failure. JL's cough and shortness of breath need evaluation. The interviewer should determine the severity of the dyspnea by asking about the degree to which the dyspnea limits JL's daily routine. The changes in JL's dyspnea over the past years and factors that trigger the dyspnea are important in evaluating prognosis and avoiding exacerbation of the disease.
2. Uncomplicated chronic bronchitis most often causes clear or opaque sputum. Infection will most often cause the sputum to turn colored, but allergic reactions can also result in thick, yellow-green sputum.
3. JL's smoking history in pack-years is 75 pack-years (2.5 packs per day × 30 years = 75 pack-years).
4. JL's family history is significant, given that his father died of emphysema. It appears that the tendency for COPD is genetically transferable from parent to child, although the disease is not considered a hereditary disease.[9] The occupational exposure to irritant gases as a machinist may have also increased his risk for lung disease.

5. The physical examination should help determine the symptoms of JL's pulmonary dysfunction (e.g., cyanosis, cor pulmonale, crackles, wheeze, pedal edema); the severity of the pulmonary dysfunction; and the cause of the symptoms. The clinician can accomplish this by assessing parameters such as vital signs, sensorium, breath sounds, respiratory pattern, heart sounds, and ankle edema.

Physical Examination

General: Patient alert and oriented, but in moderate respiratory distress; uses choppy sentences because of dyspnea and frequent coughing, which produces thick, yellow sputum

Vital Signs: Temperature 38.1°C (100.6°F), respiratory rate 26/minute, blood pressure 144/90 mm Hg; pulse 120/minute

HEENT: Tongue and mucus membranes slightly cyanotic; pupils equal, round, and reactive to light and accommodation (PERRLA); sinuses nontender to palpation

Neck: Trachea midline and mobile; transmitted wheezes present, but no stridor present; carotids + + bilaterally with no bruits; JVD noted with head of bed elevated to a 45° angle; accessory muscles in neck tense with each inspiratory effort

Chest: Anteroposterior diameter large, and chest wall excursion small; generalized hyper-resonance but decreased resonance over right lower lobe noted on chest percussion; bilateral expiratory polyphonic wheezes, louder on right side, noted on auscultation of lungs; coarse crackles and bronchial breath sounds present over right lower lobe

Heart: Regular rhythm with rate of 120/minute; no murmurs or rubs noted; S_3 gallop and loud P_2 noted on auscultation of lungs; systolic heave noted at left sternal border; point of maximal impulse located in fifth intercostal space at midclavicular line on the left

Abdomen: Soft and nontender; hepatomegaly present, and hepatojugular reflex positive; no evidence of paradoxical respiratory movement

Extremities: No evidence of cyanosis or clubbing; pedal edema present and 2+ bilaterally in the lower extremities up to knee level; extremities dry and warm to touch

---

QUESTIONS

6. How do you interpret the vital signs?
7. What is indicated by cyanosis of the tongue and mucous membranes?
8. What are the possible causes of the expiratory polyphonic wheezes heard bilaterally and the bronchial breath sounds heard over the right lower lobe?
9. What is suggested by the loud P_2?
10. What pathophysiology could be causing the JVD, hepatomegaly, hepatojugular reflex, and pedal edema?
11. How is the hepatojugular reflex identified?
12. How is the severity of the pedal edema characterized?
13. What is the significance of the systolic heave located at the left sternal border?

14. What is indicated by the fact that JL's accessory respiratory muscles of the neck are tensing with each inspiratory effort?

ANSWERS

6. The patient's body temperature is elevated. Infections, either viral or bacterial, can cause fever. Fever increases the patient's oxygen consumption and places an increased demand on the cardiac and respiratory systems. The respiratory and heart rates are slightly elevated, which may be related to the fever or the hypoxemia, or both. Tachycardia and tachypnea help meet the increased need for oxygen consumption and CO_2 excretion associated with fever and help compensate for hypoxemia when present.

7. Cyanosis of the tongue and mucous membranes of the mouth indicates central cyanosis. Central cyanosis is caused by hypoxemia which turns the arterial blood dark. Polycythemia makes cyanosis more visible and anemia makes it difficult to recognize.

8. The expiratory polyphonic wheezes may be produced by one or more of the following: bronchospasm, mucosal edema, and excessive airway secretions. Intrathoracic airways tend to narrow slightly on exhalation owing to the additive effects of positive intrathoracic pressure and the decreased retractile forces of elastic fibers within the airway walls. When the airways are obstructed because of bronchospasm, edema, or secretions, exhalation can result in severe narrowing, resulting in vibration of the airway walls and therefore expiratory wheezes. Polyphonic wheezes suggest partial obstruction of many small airways, rather than one large upper airway.

   The bronchial breath sounds suggest consolidation in the right lower lobe. Normal lung tissue acts as a filter to sound, allowing only low-pitched sounds to pass. Consolidated lung allows the turbulent flow sounds of the larger airways to pass through the lung without filtering the high-pitched sounds. In such cases, the normal vesicular breath sound is replaced with a louder, higher pitched, bronchial-type breath sound over the area of the consolidated lung.

9. The loud P_2 suggests pulmonary hypertension. Pulmonary circulation pressures increase as the capillary smooth muscle constricts in response to hypoxemia. Eventually collagen tissue replaces the pulmonary arteriolar smooth muscle, causing irreversible pulmonary hypertension. The increase in pulmonary artery pressure causes the pulmonic valve to close more loudly than it would under normal conditions. A loud P_2 is best heard in the pulmonic area, which is located at the second left intercostal space near the sternal border (Fig. 5–2).

10. JVD, hepatomegaly, pedal edema, and the hepatojugular reflex are typically caused by right heart failure. Right heart failure may be the result of left heart failure, acute severe pulmonary embolism, or chronic hypoxemia. Right heart failure allows filling pressures of the right heart to increase and all venous pressures to rise. High venous pressures result in distended neck veins; an engorged, swollen liver; and an accumulation of fluid in the lower extremities.

11. Right heart failure increases venous pressure and causes liver engorgement. If pressure in the neck veins appears to increase while the physician is pressing gently but firmly on the liver (right upper quadrant of the patient's

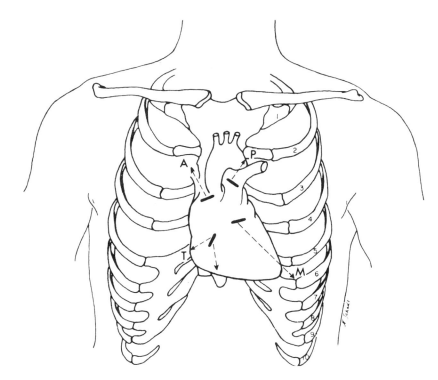

FIGURE 5–2   Diagram of the chest wall demonstrating the optimal locations for auscultating the various components of the heart sounds. The pulmonic valve is best heard over the second left intercostal space near the sternum and is known as the pulmonic area. The aortic valve is best heard in the second intercostal space on the right near the sternal border. This area is known as the aortic area. The mitral and tricuspid valves are loudest over the apex of the heart. (From Prior, JA, and Silberstein, JS: Physical examination: The History and Examination of the Patient, ed 6. CV Mosby, St Louis, 1982, p 267, with permission.)

abdomen), the **hepatojugular reflex** is present. The presence of this reflex is consistent with right heart failure.

12. The severity of the edema is graded on a scale of 1+ through 4+ on the basis of pitting produced by sustained, light pressure applied by the examiner over the tissue being examined.[15] Minimal pitting edema is indicated as 1+, whereas 4+ suggests severe pitting edema that "weeps" when the examiner presses on the edematous tissue. In this case, 2+ pitting edema indicates a moderate degree of ankle edema. The level to which the edema extends up the lower extremities also indicates the severity of the right heart failure. In this case, the edema is at the level of the knees, which implies moderate disease. More severe heart failure causes the edema to extend higher.

13. A heave at the left sternal border is usually produced by contraction of an enlarged right ventricle. Right ventricular hypertrophy often occurs when the right heart pumps against high pressures for many months (much like the biceps of a compulsive weight lifter). The heave at the sternal border along with the JVD, hepatomegaly, loud P_2, and pedal edema are evidence of cor pulmonale.[16] Right ventricular heave and a loud P_2 may be difficult to identify when the anteroposterior chest diameter is large. These findings of right heart failure suggest that the patient has had hypoxemia for many months or years.

14. Use of the accessory muscles of respiration indicates that the patient has respiratory distress and the diaphragm is no longer able to provide adequate respiratory support. This is a common finding in patients with acute exacerbation of lung disease and provides an objective parameter for monitoring the patient's condition and response to therapy.

Laboratory Evaluation

Chest Radiograph: (Fig. 5–3)

ABGs: pH 7.41, PaO_2 45 mm Hg on room air, $PaCO_2$ 44 mm Hg, HCO_3^- 28 mEq, $P(A-a)O_2$ 53 mm Hg, O_2 content 16.4 mL

Complete Blood Count:

	Observed	Normal
WBCs	16 thousand/mm³	4–11 thousand/mm³
RBCs	5.7 million/mm³	4.1–5.5 million/mm³
Hemoglobin (g)	17.5	14–16.5
Hematocrit (%)	56	37–50
Segmented neutrophils (%)	77	38–79
Bands (%)	10	0–7
Lymphocytes (%)	10	12–51
Eosinophils (%)	1	0–8
Monocytes (%)	1	0–10

Chemistry: All within normal limits except for CO_2 (slightly elevated at 34 mEq/liter)

QUESTIONS

15. How important is the chest radiograph in determining the cause of the patient's symptoms? What does it show to be the underlying condition of this patient's respiratory system?
16. How would you interpret the ABGs?
17. Should complete pulmonary function testing be done at this point?
18. How would you interpret the CBC? What could be causing the elevated WBC count? What is the most likely cause of the elevated RBC count?
19. What is the tentative diagnosis, and should the patient be admitted to the hospital?
20. What other diagnostic procedures should be ordered at this point?
21. What therapy should the physician order for the patient?

ANSWERS

15. The chest radiograph is very important, as it demonstrates an infiltrate typical of pneumonia in the right lower lobe. Respiratory infections are a common cause of exacerbation in patients with COPD.[17]

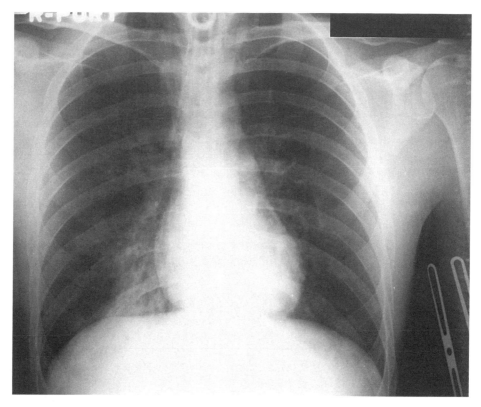

FIGURE 5-3   Chest radiograph taken a few hours after admission.

16. The ABG measurements reveal moderate hypoxemia on room air. This is a common finding in COPD patients, especially when an infection is present. The acid-base status shows both respiratory acidosis and metabolic alkalosis. Because the body never completely compensates for an acid-base disturbance and the pH is 7.41, there must be two simultaneous primary disturbances. It is possible that this patient's "normal" Pa_{CO_2} is greater than 45 mm Hg and is compensated for by an elevation of blood HCO_3^-. When an acute problem such as pneumonia occurs, significant hypoxemia can drive the patient's respiratory system to increase ventilation. This may result in relative hyperventilation, with the Pa_{CO_2} decreasing back to a more normal range, which causes acute respiratory alkalosis (even though the Pa_{CO_2} is normal) superimposed over chronic respiratory acidosis. If the patient had vomiting associated with his other symptoms, acute metabolic alkalosis might also have developed.

17. This is not a good time to have the patient perform additional pulmonary function testing, as he is acutely ill. After his condition stabilizes, complete pulmonary function testing will provide a better indication of his underlying pulmonary disease.

18. The CBC reveals elevated white and RBC counts. The leukocytosis is probably in response to the infiltrate seen on the chest radiograph. The elevation of the bands is known as a *left shift,* which indicates that immature WBCs are being released by the bone marrow in response to the acute

infection. The elevated RBC count indicates that polycythemia is present. This abnormality may be secondary to a chronically low Pao_2. Polycythemia helps to compensate for the hypoxemia by increasing the blood's oxygen-carrying capacity. Unfortunately, it also increases cardiac work load by increasing blood viscosity. Many pulmonary physicians will phlebotomize patients to a hematocrit of less than 55 percent in order to decrease right heart work load and to prevent RBC slugging and arteriolar obstruction.

19. The tentative diagnosis is acute exacerbation of chronic bronchitis and right heart failure caused by pneumonia. The patient should be admitted for close monitoring, intravenous (IV) bronchodilators, steroids, antibiotics, and possible phlebotomy.

20. Sputum analysis with a Gram stain and culture may be helpful in determining the cause of the pneumonia. An ECG may be helpful in ruling out cardiac ischemia.

21. Appropriate therapy for the patient at this point would include oxygen, antibiotics, bronchodilators, and steroids.

CASE STUDY—continued

The patient was admitted to the pulmonary care unit. The physician wrote orders for the following:

- Oxygen by nasal cannula 2 liters/minute titrated to achieve an arterial oxygen saturation (Sao_2) of greater than 90 percent.
- Medication nebulizer with albuterol (Ventolin/Proventil) 0.5 mL and ipratropium 2.5 mL every 4 hours
- Methylprednisolone (Solu-Medrol) 125 mg IV every 6 hours × 3, and then 60 mg IV
- Aminophylline at a rate of 25 to 30 mg/hour
- Cefuroxime 750 mg IV every 8 hours, and clarithromycin (Biaxin) 500 mg by mouth every 12 hours
- ECG
- Daily theophylline blood levels
- Sputum Gram stain, culture, and sensitivity

QUESTIONS

22. What is the goal of oxygen therapy in this case? What level of arterial oxygenation is appropriate? How should the oxygen therapy be evaluated? Once this patient is stable and ready to go home, should he be sent home on a regimen of oxygen therapy?

23. What abnormalities on the ECG would demonstrate right-axis deviation? What does this abnormality indicate?

24. What type of bronchodilators are albuterol and ipratropium, and what are the possible side effects of these medications? Why give both bronchodilators together?

25. What parameters should the respiratory care practitioner (RCP) monitor before, during, and after administration of the medication nebulizer treatments?

26. How should the overall effectiveness of the bronchodilators be evaluated?

27. What should the RCP do to improve the chances of obtaining an appropriate sputum sample for analysis?

28. What is the most important advice this patient's physician could give him with regard to his long-term respiratory health?

ANSWERS

22. The goal of oxygen therapy is to correct the hypoxemia. A PaO_2 of 55 to 65 mm Hg is an appropriate level of oxygenation in this case. The hemoglobin is more than 90 percent saturated under most conditions at a partial pressure of about 60 mm Hg. Elevating the PaO_2 above 65 mm Hg does not add significant oxygen content to the arterial blood, but does slightly increase the risk of oxygen-induced hypoventilation.

The RCP should evaluate the oxygen therapy by using a combination of parameters. Pulse oximetry is useful when changes in ventilation and therefore PCO_2 are not likely. The patient's mild hypoventilation makes it important to titrate the fraction of inspired oxygen (FIO_2) to result in a SaO_2 of 90 percent and to check ABGs to evaluate ventilatory and acid-base status.

The clinical findings of polycythemia and cor pulmonale strongly suggest that this patient would benefit from home oxygen therapy. If the patient's resting room air PaO_2 is less than 55 mm Hg at the time of discharge, home oxygen should be arranged. If the PaO_2 is 55 to 60 mm Hg, chronic home oxygen supplementation will be important, as the patient has both polycythemia and evidence of right heart failure. If the patient's resting PaO_2 is greater than 60 mm Hg, nocturnal desaturation may be demonstrated by nocturnal pulse oximetry monitoring and would indicate the need for oxygen during sleep.

23. The negative deflection of the P and QRS waves in lead I is consistent with right-axis deviation. This finding is typical for patients with cor pulmonale.[18] Normally the mean axis of electrical activity for the heart is between 0 and $+90°$. With pulmonary hypertension, enlargement of the right side of the heart causes the mean axis to shift to the right, somewhere between $+90°$ and $+180°$ (Fig. 5–4).

24. Albuterol is a sympathomimetic bronchodilator that has fewer side effects than isoproterenol.[19] It is available in oral, IV, or aerosol forms. When administered by aerosol it produces significant bronchodilatation within 15 minutes and continues to cause bronchodilatation for 3 to 4 hours.[20] Although tremors, nervousness, and cardiovascular side effects such as tachycardia and palpitations are possible with all β-agonists, they are less common in patients using this medication. Ipratropium is an anticholinergic bronchodilator that is more effective in causing bronchodilation when combined with albuterol than either agent used alone.[12]

25. RCPs should monitor the patient's vital signs, breath sounds, sensorium, and breathing pattern before, during, and after the treatment. Changes in these parameters will help assess the effectiveness of therapy and the onset of complications.

26. The patient's dyspnea should improve if the bronchodilators are proving beneficial. Changes in breath sounds that indicate bronchodilatation include

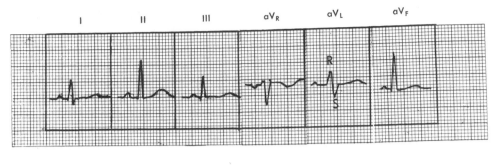

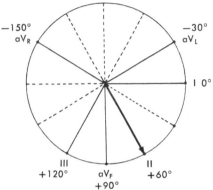

FIGURE 5-4   Hexaxial reference system used for assessment of the mean axis of electrical activity of the heart. Normal axis is between 0 and +90 degrees. Left-axis deviation exists when the mean axis is between 0 and −90 degrees. Right-axis deviation is present when the axis is between +90 and +180 degrees. To identify the axis, examine the limb leads to identify the lead with the largest (either positive or negative) deflection from baseline. Next use the hexaxial reference system to identify the position in the circle of the lead with the largest QRS complex. If the QRS complex is upright (positive) in the lead with the most voltage, the mean axis must be very close to the position of this lead on the circle. If the QRS complex is downward (negative), the mean axis must be located in the opposite direction from the location of this lead on the hexaxial circle. In this example the axis is located at +60 since lead II displays the most voltage and is upright. (From Goldberger, AL, and Goldberger, E: Clinical Electrocardiography, ed 3. CV Mosby, St. Louis, 1986, p 62, with permission.)

a decrease in the pitch, length, and intensity of the wheezing.[21] Changes in the patient's breathing pattern with less use of accessory muscles and a shorter expiratory time also indicate improvement.

27. The RCP obtaining the sputum sample should explain the procedure to the patient, emphasizing that a true sample of phlegm from the lungs is needed. Asking the patient to rinse his mouth and brush his teeth just before obtaining the sample is a useful way of reducing sputum contamination by oral bacteria. The sample should be collected in a sterile sputum cup and then transported to the laboratory with the lid tightly in place. The patient's name and identification number must be secured to the container.

28. The best advice health care personnel can give to this patient is to *stop smoking!* This advice is easy to give, but not as easy for the patient to follow. Many patients will stop smoking upon the firm recommendation of the physician. The physician may also recommend nicotine gum or nicotine patches. These are more effective in conjunction with a formal smoking cessation program. The American Lung Association and American Cancer Society have excellent smoking cessation programs.

CASE STUDY—continued

Over the next several days JL steadily improved. His initial ABG revealed a PaO_2 of 66 mm Hg on 2 liters/minute of oxygen by nasal cannula. His dyspnea improved to the point where he could walk around the unit without significant difficulty by the third hospital day. On the fifth day, he was discharged on a regimen of oral antibiotics and oxygen. The attending physician requested a follow-up appointment with JL at the pulmonary outpatient clinic in 1 week.

REFERENCES

1. Snider, GL: Chronic bronchitis and emphysema. In Murray, JF, and Nadel, JA: Textbook of Respiratory Medicine. WB Saunders, Philadelphia, 1988.
2. Camilli, AE, et al: Longitudinal changes in forced expiratory volume in one second in adults. Am Rev Respir Dis 135:794–799, 1987.
3. Beaty, TH, et al: Risk factors associated with longitudinal change in pulmonary function. Am Rev Respir Dis 129:660–667, 1984.
4. Samet, JM: The relationship of smoking to COPD. In Cherniak, NS (ed): Chronic Obstructive Pulmonary Disease. WB Saunders, Philadelphia, 1991, pp 249–258.
5. Thurlbeck, WM: Pathology of chronic airflow obstruction. In Cherniak, NS (ed): Chronic Obstructive Pulmonary Disease. WB Saunders, Philadelphia, 1991, pp 3–20.
6. Saetta, M, et al: Airway eosinophilia in chronic bronchitis during exacerbations. Am J Respir Crit Care Med 150:1646–1652, 1994.
7. Wiedemann, HP, and Matthay, RA: Treatment overview: Chronic hypercapnia and cor pulmonale. In Cherniak, NS (ed): Chronic Obstructive Pulmonary Disease. WB Saunders, Philadelphia, 1991, pp 429–442.
8. Wiedemann, HP, and Matthay, RA: Cor pulmonale in chronic obstructive pulmonary disease: Circulatory pathophysiology and new concepts of therapy. In Simmons, DH (ed): Current Pulmonology, Vol 8. Year Book, Chicago, 1987, pp 127–162.
9. Redline, S: The epidemiology of COPD. In Cherniak, NS (cd): Chronic Obstructive Pulmonary Disease. WB Saunders, Philadelphia, 1991, pp 225–234.
10. Samet, JM: Health benefits of smoking cessation. Clin Chest Med 12:669, 1991
11. Schwartz, JL: Methods for smoking cessation. Clin Chest Med 12:737, 1991
12. Petty, TL: The combination of ipratropium and albuterol is more effective than either agent alone. Chest (suppl)107:183S, 1995.
13. Ramsdell, J: Use of theophylline in the treatment of COPD. Chest (suppl)107:206S, 1995.
14. Oswald-Mammosser, M, et al: Prognostic factors in COPD patients receiving long-term oxygen therapy. Chest 107:1193–1198, 1995
15. Judge, RD, et al: Clinical Diagnosis, ed 4. Little, Brown & Co, Boston, 1982, p 223.
16. Georgopoulos, D, and Anthonisen, NR: Symptoms and signs of COPD. In Cherniak, NS (ed): Chronic Obstructive Pulmonary Disease. WB Saunders, Philadelphia, 1991, pp 357–362.
17. Reynolds, HY: Antibiotic treatment of bronchitis and chronic lung disease. In Cherniak, NS (ed): Chronic Obstructive Pulmonary Disease. WB Saunders, Philadelphia, 1991, pp 456–460.
18. Donahoe, M, and Rogers, RM: Laboratory evaluation of the patients with COPD. In Cherniak, NS (ed): Chronic Obstructive Pulmonary Disease. WB Saunders, Philadelphia, 1991, pp 373–385.
19. Peters, JA, and Peters, BA: Pharmacology for respiratory care. In Scanlon, CL, et al (eds): Egan's Fundamentals of Respiratory Care, ed 5. CV Mosby, St. Louis, 1990, pp 445–482.
20. Weiner, N: Norepinephrine, epinephrine, and the sympathomimetic amines. In Gilman, AG (eds): Goodman and Gilman's The Pharmacological Basis of Therapeutics, ed 7. New York, Macmillan, 1985
21. Baughman RP, Loudon RG: Quantification of wheezing in acute asthma. Chest 86:718–722, 1984.

CHAPTER **6**

Emphysema

Kenneth D. McCarty, MS, RRT

Key Terms

abdominal paradox	centrilobular	panlobular
α_1-protease inhibitor (αPI)	emphysema	pneumoplasty
barrel chest	Hoover's sign	

Definition

Pulmonary **emphysema,** from the Greek *emphysan* (to inflate), is an obstructive pulmonary disease characterized by dilation and destruction of lung units from the terminal bronchioles to the alveoli. Onset of the symptoms typically occurs after the age of 50 and affects men more often than women even when smoking is taken into account. Technically, confirmation of the pathology can be made only by a lung biopsy or postmortem examination; however, certain clinical and diagnostic findings are highly suggestive of the disease.

Emphysema can be classified according to its anatomic location of the pathology. **Panlobular** (panacinar) emphysema involves enlargement of all airspaces distal to the terminal bronchioles, including the respiratory bronchioles, alveolar ducts, and alveoli, and is most commonly caused by a deficiency in α_1**-protease inhibitor** (αPI). Conversely, **centrilobular** emphysema primarily involves the central acinar respiratory bronchioles, thus sparing distal lung units.[1]

Etiology

The two main etiologic factors identified in the progression of pulmonary emphysema are cigarette smoking and a genetic predisposition for the development of the disease. The most common factor associated with the development of emphysema is a history of cigarette smoking.[1,2] The exact role that cigarettes play in the development of the disease, as well as their mechanism of action, is unknown; however, the inhalation of cigarette smoke is known to increase protease activity, which destroys the terminal bronchioles and alveolar walls. Smoking also decreases mucociliary transport, leading to retention of secretions and increased susceptibility to pulmonary infections. Although smoking appears to be the chief cause of emphysema in the majority of cases, pulmonary emphysema does develop in a small number of persons with minimal or no smoking exposure as a result of an αPI deficiency.[1]

Normally the liver produces 200 to 400 μg/dL of αPI, which was previously called α_1-antitrypsin. αPI plays a role in inflammation and is mainly responsible for the inactivation of **neutrophil elastase,** an enzyme released from polymorphonuclear leukocytes (PMNs) that breaks down elastin during an inflammatory response. Therefore, a deficiency in αPI results in elastase-induced destruction of lung tissue, producing panlobular pulmonary emphysema. This occurs as a result of a genetically inherited homozygous trait that is present in approximately 1 percent of emphysema patients, who are initially symptomatic in the third to fourth decade of life. There is also evidence that cigarette smoking exacerbates the problem encountered in αPI deficiency.[1] Homozygous αPI deficiency is also characterized by liver disease manifested as hepatomegaly, cholestasis, and elevated liver enzymes in infancy.

Chronic respiratory infections during childhood may result in the development of obstructive pulmonary disease later in life, and inhaled pollutants, such as sulfur dioxide and ozone, may cause higher morbidity in patients with lung disease.[3] Although the exact role inhaled pollutants play in the etiology of pulmonary emphysema is unclear, exacerbations of the disease may result when pollutant levels are high.[1] Hence, to prevent exacerbations of their condition, patients with emphysema should avoid exposure to infections and inhaled irritants.

Pathophysiology

Because of the tissue destruction and loss of elastic recoil that occurs in pulmonary emphysema, limitations in exhaled flow and abnormalities in gas exchange exist. The main cause of an impairment in expiratory flow is the loss of elastic recoil by the lung tissue. This results in decreased driving pressure for exhaled gas, increased lung compliance, and increased collapsibility of the airway walls. These elements lead to air trapping during forced exhalation and an increase in functional residual capacity (FRC), residual volume (RV), and total lung capacity (TLC).[1,4]

Destruction of the alveolar capillary bed results in a reduced surface area, and airway dilation causes an increased distance for gaseous diffusion, both of which impair the efficiency of external respiration. These abnormalities cause ventilation-perfusion ($\dot{V}/\dot{Q}$) mismatching with large areas of dead-space ventilation and contribute to increased work of breathing.

Clinical Features

The clinical findings of emphysema usually occur in conjunction with those of chronic bronchitis.[1] For the purpose of this discussion, however, the signs and symptoms associated with emphysema will be emphasized. As stated previously, an official diagnosis can be made only after pathological examination of the patient's lung tissue; however, the medical history, physical examination, and diagnostic findings will often provide adequate information to confirm a clinical diagnosis of pulmonary emphysema. The patient with emphysema often complains of increasing shortness of breath occurring during exertion. Dyspnea at rest occurs relatively late in the disease process. Exacerbations of the disease typically occur with viral or bacterial respiratory tract infections, as a result of exposure to dust or pollutants, or in association with congestive heart failure (see Chapter 10). A history of cigarette smoking should alert the clinician as to the probability of developing not only emphysema, but also other smoking-related respiratory diseases, such as chronic bronchitis (see Chapter 5). A family history of αPI deficiency should also alert the clinician that signs and symptoms of emphysema may occur early in life.[1,3,5,6]

The physical examination may provide key information for establishing a clinical diagnosis of pulmonary emphysema. Inspection of the patient with pulmonary emphysema will frequently demonstrate tachypnea with a prolonged exhalation, use of accessory muscles of breathing, increased anteroposterior diameter of the chest (**barrel chest**), inward movement of the lower ribs, and narrowing of the subcostal angle (**Hoover's sign**) during inspiration, and perhaps pursed-lip breathing on exhalation. Paradoxical movement of the abdomen with breathing (**abdominal paradox**) suggests diaphragm fatigue. Patients with emphysema also often assume a body position in which they lean forward with their hands braced on their knees or their elbows braced on a table. This provides more optimal mechanical advantage for their respiratory musculature. Palpation usually reveals decreased tactile and vocal fremitus, whereas percussion reveals flattened, immobile hemidiaphragms and increased resonance over the lung fields. Auscultation findings include decreased breath sounds as well as decreased transmission of heart and voice sounds.[1,6]

Laboratory Evaluation

Evaluation of the chest radiograph shows hyperlucent, hyperexpanded lung fields with low, flattened diaphragms, and a small vertically oriented heart (Fig. 6–1). The lateral chest radiograph also frequently demonstrates an increased retrosternal airspace.[1,5,6,7] A pattern of arterial deficiency in which vascular shadows quickly taper and disappear is an important but somewhat subjective determination. The appearance of bullae is suggestive of local emphysematous changes.[1]

Pulmonary function studies, though not routinely done during an acute exacerbation, reveal increased RV, FRC, and TLC as a result of air trapping. Forced vital capacity (FVC), forced expiratory volume in 1 second (FEV_1), and FEV_1/FVC decrease because of airflow obstruction.[4] Decreases in diffusing capacity of carbon monoxide in the lung (D_{LCO}) reflect the loss of surface area due to alveolar and pulmonary vascular bed destruction.[4,8] A significant decrease in D_{LCO} is strong evidence for the presence of emphysema. The peak-expiratory flow rate correlates well with FEV_1, and although dependent on patient effort, can be used to assess changes in airflow obstruction and efficacy of therapy via disposable flowmeters.[1]

Arterial blood gases (ABGs) of the emphysematous patient typically do not reflect the severity of the pathological process. Common findings include respiratory alkalosis with moderate hypoxemia in mild to moderate emphysema. The development of respiratory acidosis with more severe hypoxemia generally occurs during acute exacerbations and the terminal stages of the disease.

Although an electrocardiographic (ECG) examination does not determine the di-

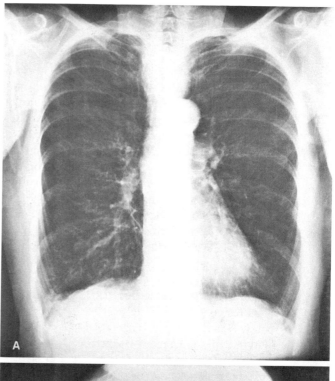

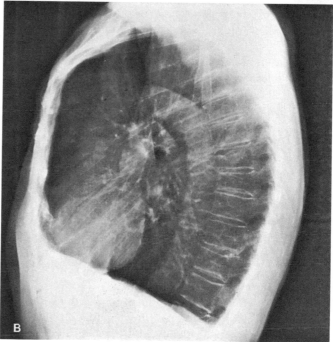

FIGURE 6-1 Chest radiograph typical for emphysema. *(A)* Posteroanterior (PA) view demonstrates hyperinflation of the lungs and a small, narrow heart. *(B)* Lateral view demonstrates a large retrosternal airspace and low, flat diaphragms.

agnosis of emphysema, it does provide valuable information about the patient. The more vertical position of the heart associated with marked hyperinflation of the lungs and flattening of the diaphragm causes a rightward shift of the P and QRS axes in the frontal plane. Lung hyperinflation also reduces the amplitude (voltage) of the limb leads.[6]

Treatment

Treatment of pulmonary emphysema includes both acute and supportive care. Therapy during an acute exacerbation should decrease the work of breathing and provide optimal oxygenation and ventilation. Long-term care is designed to decrease morbidity and increase patient autonomy and quality of life.

Pulmonary rehabilitation programs provide emphysematous patients with an opportunity to learn about their disease as well as a framework for long-term care. Careful long-term pulmonary management reduces symptoms and decreases in-hospital days. It also increases exercise tolerance and ease of performing activities of daily living, reduces anxiety and depression, and improves the quality of life.[9] Clinicians should counsel patients on how to stop smoking and how to avoid respiratory infections and irritants. The physician should encourage the patient to obtain an annual influenza shot, since an attack of the flu will often precipitate an exacerbation requiring hospitalization.[10] Proper nutritional status must also be emphasized, as it directly affects the patient's respiratory status and ability to perform activities of daily living.

Supplemental oxygen therapy is useful when the resting room air Pao_2 is less than 55 mm Hg or the Sao_2 is less than 90 percent. Adequate oxygenation can usually be accomplished with nasal cannula at a flow rate of less than 3 liters/minute in patients with emphysema. If an acute exacerbation is precipitated by pneumonia or congestive heart failure, hypoxemia may be severe and may require more significant elevation of Fio_2.

Treatment of the acute exacerbation involves stabilization of the patient's respiratory status and treatment of the exacerbating source. Sympathomimetic and methylxanthine bronchodilators are important agents for treatment of bronchospasm when associated with exacerbation of emphysema.[1,10] Methylxanthines also increase diaphragmatic contractility, decrease allergic mediator release, and increase medullary chemoreceptor sensitivity to carbon dioxide.[10,11] Steroids decrease inflammatory response in the airway and appear to be most effective in patients with a reversible airway obstruction component. In addition, anticholinergic bronchodilators are especially useful in the treatment of bronchospasm because they produce an increase in parasympathetic tone.[12] Antibiotics are indicated when a respiratory tract infection is present, typically seen as a change in sputum quantity, color, or consistency. Diuretics are useful when congestive heart failure is complicating the patient's clinical condition.

If secretion clearance becomes a problem during acute exacerbation, caregivers should employ techniques for improving pulmonary hygiene, such as chest physiotherapy and bland mist aerosol administration. Acute respiratory failure may require the initiation of continuous mechanical ventilation (CMV) to maintain adequate management of the patient's ventilatory status. CMV is most reasonable when the acute respiratory failure is the result of a reversible problem superimposed on the patient's chronic obstructive pulmonary disease (COPD).

In patients suffering from αPI deficiency, aerosol or intravenous (IV) αPI can be provided to limit enzyme degradation of the pulmonary parenchyma.[1,13] The American Thoracic Society guidelines for the administration of αPI state that supplemental αPI should be used only if serum levels are less than 11 μmol. Further, αPI supplementation should be used only in patients with emphysema caused by αPI deficiency. It should not be given to patients with αPI-deficient liver disease without emphysema.[14] Although αPI therapy is new and exciting, it is expensive and the benefits of long-term therapy have not yet been demonstrated.[11] Gene therapy is another treatment modality that looks promising for patients with αPI deficiency.[15]

Patients with severe emphysema usually have extreme dyspnea that often responds poorly to bronchodilator therapy. The administration of low-dose oral opiate preparations, such as hydrocodone, morphine, and dihydrocodeine, may help to alleviate the sensation of dyspnea in some patients.[1] It is necessary to monitor the patient carefully because these medications can induce hypoventilation.

Patients with severe emphysema may benefit from thoracic surgery that removes overdistended, poorly ventilated, functionless lung tissue.[16] Removal of severely hyperinflated lung tissue allows the surrounding, more healthy alveoli to provide gas exchange more efficiently. A recent study reported significant improvement in PaO_2, $PaCO_2$, FEV_1, and dyspnea in patients with emphysema who had received this lung-volume reduction surgery (**pneumoplasty**).[17] Criteria for determining which patients with emphysema may benefit from the surgery and long-term efficacy are not well established, suggesting a need for more studies.[18] Although mortality rates are low for lung-volume reduction surgery, persistent air leaks can be a problem in the postoperative period. A national, multicenter study is under way to determine criteria and long-term benefits.

CASE STUDY

History

Mrs. D.G., a 62-year-old white woman, is being seen in the emergency room for complaints of increasing shortness of breath. She states that she had the flu approximately 1½ weeks earlier and that her breathing has been more difficult since that time. Her ankles have been swollen for the first time, and sleeping during this time has required "two pillows to support her." She stated that occasionally she awakens in the middle of the night very short of breath. These episodes of nocturnal dyspnea are relieved by sitting up for several minutes. She has been producing ¼ cup of yellow sputum since the onset of the flu. Her exercise tolerance was 1 block but is now 20 feet. Mrs. D.G. stated that 7 years ago her family physician told her she had pulmonary emphysema. Mrs. D.G. started smoking at age 12 and smoked approximately 2 packs of cigarettes a day until she quit 2 years ago. Mrs. D.G. took the following home medications: small-volume nebulizer (SVN) with metaproterenol four times a day, theophylline (Theo-Dur tablets) 200 mg two times a day, and oxygen via nasal cannula at 1 liter/minute.

QUESTIONS

1. What symptoms should be explored in greater detail?

2. How many pack-years has this patient smoked, and how is this significant in terms of producing pulmonary symptoms?

3. What is the most likely cause of the patient's pulmonary emphysema?

4. What is the most likely cause of the patient's exacerbation?

5. What is the pathophysiological significance of the patient's orthopnea and paroxysmal nocturnal dyspnea (PND)?

ANSWERS

1. The key symptoms include increasing shortness of breath, exercise intolerance, orthopnea, PND, and sputum production. Because pulmonary emphysema is a progressive and chronic disease, gradual worsening of the pathology is expected. However, a sudden decline in respiratory status indicates an acute problem that is exacerbating the COPD. This patient

should be questioned about her salt intake, including foods such as olives, pickles, and potato chips; exposure to known respiratory irritants; evidence of infection; and compliance with her treatment program. She should be questioned about subjective evidence of changes in her cardiac status to determine the presence of chest pain, palpitations, or fainting spells.

2. A 96–pack-year smoking history is present (48 years $\times$ 2 packs per day). Generally a smoking history greater than 20 pack-years is required before symptoms of dyspnea and COPD begin to occur.

3. The most likely cause of the patient's pulmonary emphysema is cigarette smoking. Although men have historically outnumbered women in the development of smoking-related diseases, the increase in the number of female smokers since World War II has led to a related rise in the number of smoking-related diseases in women.

4. The patient's exacerbation is probably a result of her recent bout with influenza. Frequently, any acute illness will further compromise an already borderline respiratory status in COPD patients. They should be encouraged to get annual flu shots to minimize the chance of infection-induced exacerbations. This patient's dyspnea appears to be exacerbated by congestive heart failure (requiring several pillows for respiratory comfort at night).

5. Orthopnea and PND are generally caused by congestive heart failure.[7] These symptoms occur as pulmonary vascular congestion increases in the reclining position. The congestive heart failure may be caused by ischemic heart disease or cardiomyopathy.

Physical Examination

General: The patient is an alert, cachectic, white woman in moderate respiratory distress, sitting on the edge of her bed leaning forward with her elbows braced on the bedside table. She appears to have difficulty talking secondary to dyspnea and pursed-lip breathing.

Vital Signs: Temperature is 37.0°C (98.6°F) orally; respiratory rate is 28/minute; pulse is 108/minute; and blood pressure is 142/80 mm Hg.

HEENT: Unremarkable.

Neck: Trachea is midline without stridor or masses. Carotid pulses are $++$ without bruits; no lymphadenopathy or thyromegaly present; patient is using her sternocleidomastoid muscles during inspiration; no jugular venous distention is present.

Chest: Increased anteroposterior diameter, large supraclavicular fossae, and mild abdominal paradox during respiratory efforts are present; significant protrusion of the ribs with moderate retractions is present during inspiration, with narrowing of the subcostal angle; there is chest expansion of 3 cm at the eighth thoracic vertebra and a diffuse reduction in tactile fremitus on palpation; point of maximal impulse (PMI) is not identified with palpation; increased resonance bilaterally on percussion.

Heart: Heart sounds are very distant with a regular rate and rhythm of 108/minute without murmurs.

Lungs: There is bilateral reduction in breath sounds anteriorly and posteriorly with a prolonged expiratory phase on auscultation; occasional scattered expiratory wheezes are also present.

Abdomen: Soft, nondistended, and nontender with bowel sounds present; no masses or organomegaly present. The abdomen sinks inward with each inspiratory effort (abdominal paradox).

Extremities: No cyanosis, clubbing, or peripheral edema is present.

QUESTIONS

6. Why is the patient pursed-lip breathing, and what physiological effect does it produce?

7. Why is the patient leaning forward on her elbows to breathe?

8. What is the significance of abdominal paradox during respiratory efforts?

9. What pathophysiology accounts for the patient's increased resonance, decreased tactile fremitus and decreased heart sounds?

10. Why is the patient's PMI not felt? What is indicated when the PMI is in the epigastric area?

11. What is the significance of the chest expansion measurement?

12. What is the cause of the patient's decreased breath sounds?

13. What findings indicate the need for hospitalization?

ANSWERS

6. Pursed-lip breathing provides a positive intra-airway pressure that is thought to decrease airway closure and air trapping and to aid gas exchange.[7] Patients often discover this maneuver on their own or learn it through formal instruction by health-care providers, although the exact benefit of this technique has not been established.

7. By leaning forward on her elbows, the patient provides the accessory respiratory muscles with an optimal mechanical advantage by stabilizing the shoulder girdle to which they are attached. This makes the accessory muscles more efficient and may improve ventilation for patients with poor diaphragmatic function.

8. Paradoxical abdominal movement during breathing is indicative of diaphragmatic muscle fatigue.[7] When the diaphragm is fatigued, accessory muscles of respiration create a negative intrathoracic pressure, which pulls the fatigued diaphragm slightly upward and into the chest cage, causing the abdominal wall to sink inward rather than rise during inspiration.

9. The patient's increased resonance, decreased tactile fremitus, and decreased heart sounds are a result of the increased intrathoracic volume. The tissue destruction and hyperinflation caused by emphysema lead to poor sound transmission through the chest.[7]

10. Normally the PMI is located along the left midclavicular line at the level of the forth or fifth intercostal space. In emphysematous patients the loss of lung recoil allows the natural tension of the diaphragm to go unopposed and results in flattening of the diaphragms. As a result, the mediastinal structures are elongated and the PMI assumes a more centrally located position lower in the chest or in the epigastric area. The lung hyperinflation in emphysema may reduce the examiner's ability to feel the PMI.

11. Chest expansion as measured by palpation is normally 6 to 10 cm. In the case of emphysema, loss of elastic recoil causes chronic hyperinflation, which increases anteroposterior diameter to near maximum, resulting in the reduced ability of the chest cage to move with breathing.[7]

12. Decreased breath sounds in patients with pulmonary emphysema result from both decreased sound production and decreased sound transmission. Loss of elastic recoil results in reduced expiratory flow rates, which minimizes turbulent flow sounds during exhalation. The inspiratory sounds are effectively filtered by the relatively large distal airspaces in emphysema, resulting in poor sound transmission to the chest wall.[19]

13. The need for hospitalization of this patient is indicated by the signs of respiratory distress: (1) respiratory rate greater than 24/minute, (2) paradoxical breathing pattern, and (3) use of accessory muscles. In addition, the peripheral edema (ankle swelling) indicates compromise of right heart function.

Laboratory Evaluation

Chest Radiograph: (Figs. 6–2 and 6–3)

ABGs on 1 liter/minute:

pH 7.32

$Paco_2$ 62 mm Hg

Pao_2 50 mm Hg

HCO_3^- 30 mEq/liter

Base excess (BE) +5

Hb 13.1 g/100 mL

Sao_2 85.5 percent

Oxygen-carrying capacity (Cao_2) 15.2 vol%

Pulmonary Function Tests*:

FVC	1.90 liters	(58 percent of predicted)
FEV_1	1.02 liters	(39 percent of predicted)
$FEF_{25-75\%}$	0.74 liters	(31 percent of predicted)
TLC	5.87 liters	(117 percent of predicted)
RV	3.97 liters	(226 percent of predicted)
FRC	4.33 liters	(120 percent of predicted)
D_{LCO}	6.4 mL/minute per mm Hg	(26 percent of predicted)

*From a previous admission when patient was stable.

Complete Blood Count (CBC): Results pending

Chemistry: Results pending

Theophylline level: Results pending

ECG Findings: Sinus tachycardia with decreased voltage in the limb leads; tall, narrow P waves; Occasional premature ventricular contractions

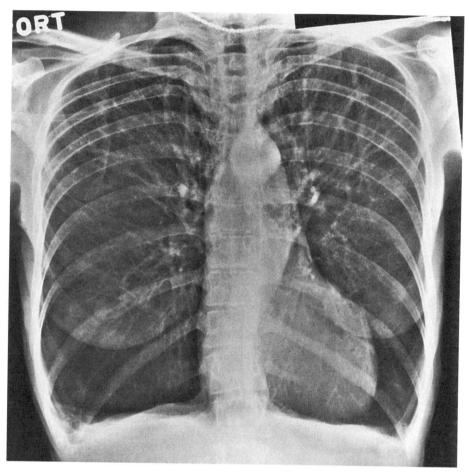

FIGURE 6-2   PA chest radiograph showing hyperinflation, flat diaphragms, decreased vascular markings, and narrow heart that are commonly seen in pulmonary emphysema.

QUESTIONS

15. What chest radiograph findings suggest hyperexpansion in this patient?

16. What is the significance of the decreased vascular markings on the chest radiograph?

17. What is the patient's acid-base and oxygenation status?

18. What is the cause of the decreased voltage and tall P waves in the limb leads, as noted on the ECG findings?

19. How do you interpret the pulmonary function test (PFT) results?

20. What pathology accounts for the decreased $D_{L}CO$?

21. What is your initial assessment of the patient's condition?

22. What treatment do you suggest?

23. Should the patient be monitored for any special adverse reactions to therapy?

24. Should high oxygen concentrations be administered to this patient if necessary?

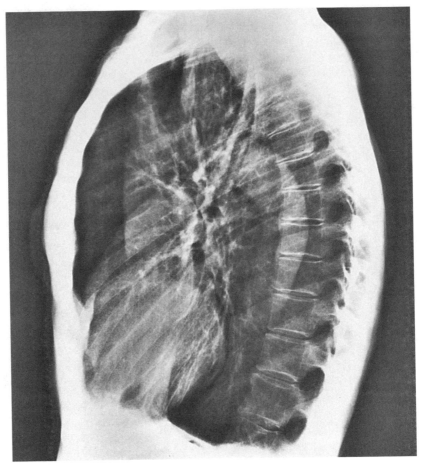

FIGURE 6-3   Lateral chest radiograph showing increased retrosternal airspace and flat hemidiaphragms.

ANSWERS

15. Hyperexpansion can be assessed by counting the number of ribs seen on the posteroanterior chest radiograph. Greater than 10 fully visualized posterior ribs, or 7 anterior ribs, indicates hyperexpansion. In addition, flattened diaphragms, increased intercostal spaces, and increased radiolucency indicate hyperexpansion. The lateral chest radiograph demonstrates flattened diaphragms and a large retrosternal airspace.

16. Decreased vascular markings on the chest radiograph occur as a result of the pulmonary parenchymal destruction involving not only terminal airspaces, but also pulmonary capillary vasculature. Excessive vascular tapering suggests a more severe case of emphysema.

17. The elevated $Paco_2$ and HCO_3^- indicate partially compensated respiratory acidosis. The patient has moderate hypoxemia on 1 liter/minute, and other indices of oxygenation are abnormally low. Since Cao_2 takes into account saturation, hemoglobin level, and Pao_2, it can be used to assess oxygen-carrying capacity. The Cao_2 of 15.2 vol% (normally 16 to 20 vol%) is slightly reduced, primarily owing to the low Sao_2.

18. Lung hyperinflation and flattening of the diaphragms result in a more vertical position of the heart and a clockwise rotation along its longitudinal axis. This may cause a rightward shift of the QRS axis as measured by the limb leads.

The mean QRS axis is also directed posteriorly and perpendicular to the frontal plane in emphysema. Electrical activity that is perpendicular to the frontal plane is not detected by the limb leads, which measure activity only in the frontal plane. As a result of the posterior shift of the mean QRS axis, the limb leads will reveal decreased amplitude. Hyperinflation also reduces the electrical conductivity of the lung, which adds to the decreased voltage seen in the limb leads of the ECG. Tall, narrow P waves (P pulmonale) indicate right atrial enlargement and are characteristic of severe pulmonary disease.

19. The PFT results are consistent with pulmonary emphysema. The loss of airway elasticity results in collapsible airways and air-trapping. The air trapping results in large lung volumes and capacities. The combination of a large intrathoracic volume, slow expiratory flow rates, and reduced diffusion capacity are typical of pulmonary emphysema.

20. The decreased DLCO is caused by the loss of pulmonary vascular bed resulting from tissue destruction and dilation of the terminal lung units. This results in a loss of alveolar surface area for diffusion.

21. The initial assessment of this patient is acute exacerbation of pulmonary emphysema secondary to influenza and heart failure.

22. Immediate treatment should consist of oxygen therapy at 1 to 2 liters/minute via nasal cannula in an attempt to increase the patient's PaO_2 to approximately 60 to 65 mm Hg. Aerosolized adrenergic bronchodilators may prove beneficial to relieve any airway obstruction caused by reactive airways, thus reducing the patient's work of breathing. These can be administered with a metered dose inhaler (MDI) or SVN if the patient can take a deep breath spontaneously (greater than 15 mL/kg). Intermittent positive-pressure breathing is rarely needed but may be beneficial if the patient is unable to take a deep spontaneous breath. IV aminophylline and corticosteroids may also prove useful if a reversible airway obstruction component is present. In this patient the scattered wheezing suggests that bronchodilators may be beneficial. Sputum collection for Gram stain and culture and sensitivity is warranted in light of the yellow sputum and low-grade fever. Other measures that might prove beneficial should the patient have trouble clearing secretions include bland aerosol therapy and chest physical therapy.

23. Yes, the caregivers should monitor the patient for certain side effects. The possible side effects of sympathomimetic bronchodilators include tachycardia, arrythmias, tremor, nervousness, and anxiety.[20] Aminophylline may cause nausea, tachycardia, tremor, and possible seizures. Since the patient is a chronic CO_2 retainer, the respiratory therapist should administer oxygen therapy carefully to avoid depressing the patient's hypoxic respiratory drive, thus inducing hypoventilation. The use of fixed-performance oxygen delivery devices that can administer precise oxygen percentages often can be used to carefully titrate oxygen delivery and minimize the chance of oxygen-induced hypoventilation.

24. High concentrations of oxygen may be lifesaving in certain situations. Oxygen should be administered judiciously to patients who are chronic CO_2 retainers; it should never be withheld for fear of dulling that drive at the expense of tissue oxygenation. Should the patient's drive to breathe diminish and result in an elevated $PaCO_2$ to the point where the pH is less than 7.25 or the patient's sensorium is abnormal, mechanical ventilation should be used to support ventilation until the patient's respiratory status improves.

CASE STUDY—continued

Patient was admitted to the respiratory intensive care unit and started on the following medications: oxygen therapy at 2 liters/minute via nasal cannula; aminophylline drip; methylprednisolone (Solu-Medrol) 120 mg IV every 6 hours; SVN with 0.5 mL 0.5 percent albuterol; and 2.5 mL 0.9 percent saline every 4 hours. Sputum for Gram stain and culture and sensitivity, theophylline level, and ABGs on 2 liters/minute were ordered.

Results of the sputum Gram stain showed 2+ pus cells, no epithelial cells, and a few very small gram-negative rods; the culture eventually grew predominantly *Haemophilus influenzae* sensitive to ampicillin. Theophylline level was 8.1 μg/mL. ABG results on 2 liters/minute were as follows: pH 7.33, $Paco_2$ 65 mm Hg, Pao_2 66 mm Hg, HCO_3^- 31 mEq/liter, BE +4, Hb 13.0 g/100 mL, Sao_2 91.2 %, Cao_2 16.2 vol%.

QUESTIONS

25. What is the significance of the sputum Gram stain and culture?

26. What antimicrobial agent is indicated?

27. What is the significance of the theophylline level?

28. How do you interpret the patient's acid-base and oxygenation status on 2 liters/minute of O_2?

29. Are any other changes in the patient's therapy indicated?

30. By what mechanism other than bronchodilation might theophylline be beneficial in the treatment of emphysema?

31. If a patient's dyspnea were severe despite bronchodilator therapy, what other therapy might be beneficial?

ANSWERS

25. The presence of pus cells in the sputum indicates inflammation or infection. The designations 1+, 2+, 3+, and 4+ are used to indicate the number of PMNs per oil immersion field (OIF), which the medical technologist determines in the following manner: 1+ = 1 to 5 PMNs per OIF; 2+ = 6 to 15 PMNs per OIF; 3+ = 16 to 50 PMNs per OIF; and 4+ = greater than 50 PMNs per OIF. In addition, the absence of epithelial cells indicates a specimen that was not significantly contaminated by oral secretions. Gram stain and culture are used to identify specific microbe characteristics and to allow selective antimicrobial treatment. *H. influenzae* is a common cause of infection among patients with obstructive lung disease. The sensitivity to ampicillin means that the infection should be easy to treat.

26. Ampicillin is a broad-spectrum antibiotic commonly used for the treatment of sensitive strains of *H. influenzae.* It is inexpensive and has few side effects. Chloramphenicol can also be used in the treatment of *H. influenzae.*

27. The therapeutic theophylline level is 10 to 20 μg/mL of plasma and a value of 8.1 μg/mL indicates that increasing the aminophylline drip might be helpful in relieving dyspnea. The serum level should be evaluated

periodically after changes in aminophylline administration to avoid toxicity and ensure therapeutic serum levels. Since toxic side effects of theophylline, such as tremors, insomnia, nausea, seizures, and atrial and ventricular arrhythmias, can be manifested within the therapeutic range, levels should be maintained on the low end of normal.[21]

28. The patient's ABGs show a partially compensated respiratory acidosis. The administration of oxygen has improved the patient's plasma oxygenation and CaO_2 to an acceptable level, considering the patient's age and disease state. Further increases in PaO_2 can depress the patient's respiratory drive without improving the patient's CaO_2 significantly.

29. The frequency of the patient's SVN treatments could be increased to every 2 to 3 hours to increase the bronchodilator effect if her pulse rate is not greater than 120/minute. Another method of increasing the bronchodilator response would be the administration of an anticholinergic agent, such as ipratropium bromide, in conjunction with the sympathomimetic therapy.[22]

30. In addition to bronchodilation, theophylline causes diaphragmatic stimulation,[23,24] and an increase in central respiratory drive,[25] both of which increase ventilation.

31. Low-dose opiate drugs might decrease the subjective sensation of dyspnea. These agents can also increase exercise tolerance in some patients.[1]

CASE STUDY—continued

The patient was started on ampicillin, and her aminophylline was increased. The frequency of the SVN treatments was changed to every 3 hours and prn, with an ipratropium bromide (Atrovent) MDI ordered to follow. During the day the patient's respiratory status improved, and she felt more comfortable. SVN and MDI were changed to every 4 hours while awake and prn at night. Subsequent follow-up revealed a therapeutic serum theophylline level of 13.5 µg/mL. Over the next 2 days (days 2 and 3), the patient's oxygen was reduced to 1 liter/min, and her aminophylline was changed to Theo-Dur. At this time her breath sounds were clear, though decreased bilaterally, and her cough produced only opaque-white secretions. The patient was discharged to home on day 5 with the following medications: Theo-Dur 200 mg twice a day; oxygen via nasal cannula at 1 liter/min; albuterol sulfate (Ventolin) via MDI 2 puffs every 4 hours and prn for dyspnea, with an Atrovent MDI to follow; and antibiotics. The patient was also encouraged to enter a pulmonary rehabilitation program to help manage her COPD optimally.

QUESTIONS

32. How could the patient's disease progress and response to bronchodilator therapy be cost-effectively assessed at home?

ANSWERS

32. The use of a disposable peak-expiratory flowmeter can be used to assess therapy response as well as changes in function that may signify exacerbation of the disease process.

REFERENCES

1. Snider, GL, et al: Chronic bronchitis and emphysema. In Murray, JF, and Nadel, JA (eds): Textbook of Respiratory Medicine, ed 2. WB Saunders, Philadelphia, 1994, p 1331.
2. US Surgeon General: The Health Consequences of Smoking: Chronic Obstructive Lung Disease. DHHS Publ No 84–50205. US Dept of Health and Human Services, Washington, DC, 1984, p 363.
3. Sherrill, DL, et al: Epidemiology of chronic obstructive pulmonary disease. In Weinberger, SE (ed): Clinics in Chest Medicine. WB Saunders, Philadelphia, 1990, p 375.
4. West J: Respiratory Physiology: The Essentials. Williams and Wilkins, Baltimore, 1995.
5. Clausen, JL: The diagnosis of emphysema. In Clinics in Chest Medicine. WB Saunders, Philadelphia, 1990, p 405.
6. Wilkins, RL, et al: Clinical Assessment in Respiratory Care, ed 3. Mosby-Yearbook, St. Louis, 1995.
7. Burki, NK: Roentgenologic diagnosis of emphysema. Chest 95:1178, 1989.
8. Morrison, NJ, et al: Comparison of single breath carbon monoxide diffusing capacity and pressure volume curves in detecting emphysema. Am Rev Respir Dis 139:1179, 1989.
9. Hodgkin, JE: Pulmonary rehabilitation. In Clinics in Chest Medicine. WB Saunders, Philadelphia, 1990, p 555.
10. Ziment, I: Pharmacologic therapy of obstructive airway disease. In Clinics in Chest Medicine. WB Saunders, Philadelphia, 1990, p 461.
11. Cottrell, GP, and Surkin, HB: Xanthine bronchodilators. In Pharmacology for Respiratory Care Practitioners. FA Davis, Philadelphia, 1995, p 175.
12. Tashkin, DP, et al: Comparison of the anticholinergic bronchodilator ipratropium bromide with metaproterenol in chronic obstructive pulmonary disease: A 90 day multicenter study. Am J Med 81:81, 1986.
13. Hubbard, RC, et al: Anti-neutrophil-elastase defenses of the lower respiratory tract in alpha-1-anti-trypsin deficiency directly augmented with an aerosol of alpha-1-antitrypsin. Ann Intern Med 111:206, 1989.
14. Buist, AS, et al: Guidelines for the approach to the individual with severe hereditary alpha-1-antitrypsin deficiency: An official statement of the American Thoracic Society. Am Rev Respir Dis 140:1494–1497, 1989.
15. Knoell, DL, and Wewers, MD: Clinical implications of gene therapy for alpha1-antitrypsin deficiency. Chest 107:535–545, 1995.
16. Snider, GL: Reduction pneumoplasty for bullous emphysema: implications for surgical treatment of nonbullous emphysema. Chest 109:540–548, 1996.
17. Cooper, JD, et al: Bilateral pneumonectomy (volume reduction) for chronic obstructive pulmonary disease. J Thorac Cardiovasc Surg 109:106, 1995.
18. Cutaia, M: Lung reduction surgery: Where are we heading? (editorial) Chest 109:866–868, 1996.
19. Ploysongsand, Y, et al: Lung sounds in patients with emphysema. Am Rev Respir Dis 124:45–49, 1981.
20. Rau, JL: Respiratory Care Pharmacology, ed 4. Mosby, St Louis, 1994, p 151.
21. Stoller, JK, and Aboussouan, LS: Chronic obstructive lung diseases: Emphysema, chronic bronchitis, bronchiectasis, cystic fibrosis. In George, RB, et al (eds): Chest Medicine: Essentials of Pulmonary and Critical Care Medicine. Williams & Wilkins, Baltimore, 1995.
22. Gross NJ, et al: Dose response to ipratropium as a nebulized solution in patients with chronic obstructive pulmonary disease. Am Rev Respir Dis 139:1185, 1989.
23. Supinski, GS, et al: The effects of caffeine and theophylline on diaphragm contractility. Am Rev Respir Dis 130:429, 1984.
24. Aubier M, et al: Aminophylline improves diaphragmatic contractility. N Engl J Med 305:249, 1981.
25. Murciano D, et al: A randomized, controlled trial of theophylline in patients with severe chronic obstructive pulmonary disease. N Engl J Med 320:1521, 1989.

CHAPTER 7

Cystic Fibrosis

N. Lennard Specht, MD

Key Terms

autosomal recessive
bronchiectasis
cor pulmonale

cystic fibrosis
exocrinopathy
nasal polyps

sweat chloride
tram tracks

Introduction

Cystic fibrosis is the most common lethal genetic disease in the United States, affecting as many as 1 in 2000 white children.[1] The disease is typically diagnosed in childhood and causes many organs of the body to malfunction (Table 7–1). The principal problems associated with the disease are **bronchiectasis** (abnormal dilation of a bronchus), pancreatic exocrine insufficiency, and an elevated sweat electrolyte concentration. Pulmonary disease causes the greatest problems for patients with cystic fibrosis and is the leading cause of mortality.[2]

Cystic fibrosis was first formally portrayed in 1936, when Fanconi and colleagues[3] described two children with "cystic fibrosis of the pancreas and bronchiectasis." Cystic fibrosis was probably just as frequent and lethal centuries before Fanconi published his landmark article. In 18th- and 19th-century European literature, there are numerous references to children with abnormalities suggestive of cystic fibrosis. Most of these reports noted a correlation between a child's salty taste when kissed and the likelihood the child would die at a very young age.[4]

Etiology

Cystic fibrosis is an inherited disease that affects primarily whites of European descent. The inheritance pattern is **autosomal recessive** and therefore patients affected by the disease have two genes for cystic fibrosis (one gene given by each parent). Those who have only one gene for cystic fibrosis are called *carriers*. Carriers show no evidence of cystic fibrosis and live healthy lives. If two carriers have a child, however, chances are

TABLE 7-1   **Organ Systems Involved in Cystic Fibrosis**

Lungs
>   Bronchiectasis
>   Bronchitis
>   Pneumonia
>   Atelectasis
>   Mucus plugging
>   Respiratory failure

Pancreas
>   Pancreatic exocrine insufficiency
>   Recurrent pancreatitis
>   Diabetes mellitus

Sweat glands
>   Increased electrolyte concentration in the sweat

Upper airway
>   Recurrent sinusitis
>   Nasal polyps

Intestines
>   Meconium plug
>   Meconium ileus
>   Intussusception

Liver
>   Cirrhosis
>   Neonatal jaundice

Gallbladder
>   Cholelithiasis

Salivary glands
>   Altered electrolyte concentration of secretions

Reproductive system
>   Obstructed vas deferens
>   Decreased female fertility

one in four that the child will have cystic fibrosis. It is estimated that between 1 in 16 to 1 in 25 white Americans carry the cystic fibrosis gene. The frequency of the cystic fibrosis gene among Asians and blacks is much lower than among whites.

The gene responsible for the development of cystic fibrosis has been identified on chromosome 7.[5,6] The gene may be altered (mutated) in at least 400 different ways; several of these mutations cause cystic fibrosis. The most common abnormality of the gene is deletion of three base pairs in the DNA. This three-base-pair deletion leads to the loss of one amino acid from the protein encoded by the gene. This mutation is known as ΔF508. The ΔF508 gene accounts for 70 to 75 percent of the genetic abnormalities responsible for cystic fibrosis. The severity of a patient's cystic fibrosis is partly related to the genetic form of the disease that he or she inherits.[7]

The cystic fibrosis gene contains the code for a large protein that regulates the flow of ions (salt) through glands that secrete fluids (exocrine glands).[8,9] As a result, cystic fibrosis patients have a malregulation of the salt composition of their secretions, which is responsible for most, if not all, of the problems that these patients face.

Pathology and Pathophysiology

Cystic fibrosis is characterized as a generalized **exocrinopathy.** To some degree, virtually all exocrine glands of the body are affected by the disease. The classic triad of exocrine abnormalities consists of pancreatic insufficiency, chronic recurrent pulmonary infections, and an elevated sweat electrolyte concentration.

In very young patients with cystic fibrosis, the pancreas appears normal. As the disease progresses, however, the pancreas becomes smaller and fibrotic. Microscopic examination of the pancreas reveals obstruction of the pancreatic ducts and ductules. This is followed by dilation of the glandular lumen and, eventually, replacement of the exocrine glands with fibrous connective tissue.

Lung disease causes the greatest morbidity and mortality for patients with cystic fibrosis. The three most common pulmonary problems that these patients face are recurrent pulmonary infections, bronchiectasis, and bronchial hyperactivity. These problems may be mild in young children, but their frequency and severity increase as the disease progresses.

In the earliest stages of cystic fibrosis, the lungs often appear normal. As patients mature, however, the lungs show a progressive increase in the size and number of bronchial goblet cells (mucous glands) and inflammation in the peribronchial tissue. The airway mucosa changes from normal epithelium to stratified squamous epithelium in a process called *squamous metaplasia.* In patients who have had pulmonry symptoms for several years, these findings are more widespread and severe. Emphysematous changes are frequently seen, and hemorrhage can be found within the lung. Mucus plugging is seen in small airways, and bronchiectasis is a universal finding.

During the end stages of the disease, obstructive emphysema is frequent, but destruction rarely involves more than 10 percent of the lung.[11] Mucus plugging is pronounced, and abscesses are found distal to these plugs. Lymph nodes in the hilum of the lung are enlarged.[12]

Clinical Features

Medical History

Cystic fibrosis is usually first recognized during infancy or childhood; however, a small number of patients are diagnosed as young adults. Cystic fibrosis patients frequently first present with recurrent pulmonary infections.[13] Children with cystic fibrosis have more frequent and more prolonged respiratory infections than normal children. Most infants with cystic fibrosis have a chronic cough and wheezing. As the disease progresses, symptoms of bronchiectasis and bronchial hyperactivity become more prominent. Clubbing of the digits and dyspnea on exertion are also seen. Fevers are at most mild during exacerbations of bronchiectasis, but may be very high during episodes of pneumonia. In advanced stages of the disease, complications of lung involvement include hemoptysis (which is occasionally massive), pneumothorax, atelactasis, cor pulmonale, and respiratory failure.

Pancreatic involvement with cystic fibrosis causes pancreatic exocrine insufficiency. The lack of pancreatic enzymes leads to maldigestion and malabsorption. Pancreatic exocrine insufficiency is associated with diarrhea and stools that contain large amounts of fat. These symptoms are frequently associated with crampy abdominal pain, malnutrition, and failure to maintain a normal growth rate.[14] Other less common gastrointestinal symptoms include meconium plug, intussusception (slipping of one part of the intestine into another part), rectal prolapse, intestinal obstruction, prolonged neonatal jaundice, hepatic cirrhosis, cholelithiasis (bile stones in gallbladder), recurrent pancreatitis, and diabetes mellitus.

Abnormalities of sweat production result in excessive concentrations of salt in sweat. This increase in salt leads a salty taste to the skin and the development of salt crystals on the skin or within clothing, particularly shoes and boots. Loss of electrolytes during warm months of the year can lead to heat intolerance, heat prostration, electrolyte depletion, and dehydration.

Upper respiratory symptoms associated with cystic fibrosis include recurrent sinusitis and the development of **nasal polyps.** Almost all men and most women with cystic fibrosis are sterile. If a woman with cystic fibrosis becomes pregnant, she is not likely to carry the infant to term. The infant will either have cystic fibrosis or be a carrier of the cystic fibrosis gene.

Physical Examination

The physical examination of affected patients is nearly always abnormal within a few years after the diagnosis is established. Cystic fibrosis patients are typically thin children or young adults. If respiratory distress is present, accessory muscles of respiration will be used. A productive cough is an almost universal finding. Examination of the extremities may disclose clubbing of the digits. The upper airway may reveal nasal polyps or tenderness over the sinuses. The chest will appear barrel shaped. The lungs usually have diffuse, coarse crackles and wheezes.

In advanced disease, cyanosis around the mouth is associated with hypoxemia. Auscultation of the heart may disclose a loud pulmonic component of the second heart sound (S_2), which is suggestive of pulmonary hypertension. Jugular venous distention and pedal edema are associated with the development of right heart failure (**cor pulmonale**).

Laboratory Evaluation

Arterial blood gases (ABGs) are nearly normal early in the disease, with an increase only in the alveolar-arterial oxygen gradient $P(A-a)O_2$. Hypoxemia on room air increases as the disease progresses. Hypercapnia and severe hypoxemia occur only with very advanced lung disease.

Serum chemistries and blood counts show no abnormalities unique to cystic fibrosis. Elevation of serum bicarbonate (HCO_3^-) is seen, however, as a result of chronic respiratory failure, and elevations of the hematocrit may reflect chronic hypoxemia. Acute bronchopneumonia can lead to an elevation of the white blood cell (WBC) count, with an accompanying shift to more immature granulocytes. Serum protein and albumin concentrations may be low if malnutrition is present.

The chest radiograph characteristically shows hyperinflation, seen as a flattening of the hemidiaphragms and an increase in the retrosternal airspace (Fig. 7–1). Bronchial wall thickening is commonly seen as parallel lines radiating outward from the hilum (**tram tracks**) (Fig. 7–2). Small, rounded opacities can be seen in the periphery of the lung, which may represent small abscesses distal to impacted airways. These areas of infection usually clear, leaving a residual of small cysts. Other abnormalities seen on chest radiographs include atelectasis, fibrosis, hilar adenopathy, acute bronchopneumonia, and pneumothorax (Fig. 7–3).

Pulmonary function testing is very useful for evaluating the extent of lung disease and following the rate of disease progression. By following the rate of disease progression, the clinician can increase therapy if lung function deteriorates unexpectedly. Spirometry typically reveals airway obstruction by demonstrating a reduction in forced expiratory volume in 1 second (FEV_1). Loss of forced vital capacity (FVC) is seen in advanced disease. Both of these changes may improve after the administration of bronchodilators. Residual volume increases early in the course of the disease and can be best measured via body plethysmography.

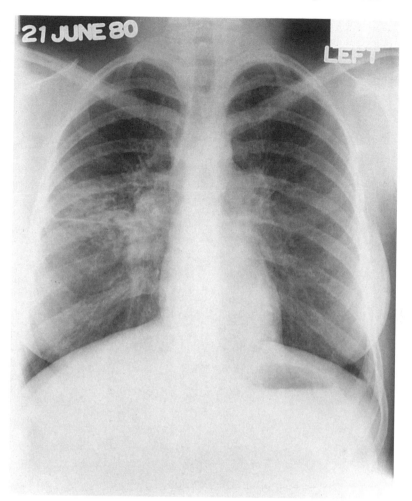

FIGURE 7-1   Chest radiograph of a patient with cystic fibrosis.

Sweat chloride measurement has been the standard technique for confirming the diagnosis of cystic fibrosis. Sweat secretion is stimulated, and sweat is collected under an airtight seal. After about 0.1 mL of sweat is collected, the electrolyte concentration is measured. In children, a **sweat chloride** concentration greater than 60 mEq/liter is consistent with the diagnosis of cystic fibrosis.[15] A concentration greater than 80 mEq/liter is usually required to confirm the diagnosis of cystic fibrosis in adults.[16] If the concentration is equivocal (50 to 80 mEq/liter), a repeat measurement will usually resolve the question. Although the sweat electrolyte concentration is useful for confirming the diagnosis of cystic fibrosis, it must be performed with meticulous attention to detail, or else the results may be misleading.[17]

Patients with cystic fibrosis typically have pathogenic organisms in their sputum. The three organisms most commonly found are *Staphylococcus aureus, Haemophilus influenzae,* and *Pseudomonas aeruginosa.* The strain of *P. aeruginosa* found in patients with cystic fibrosis typically produces mucin. This mucoid form of *P. aeruginosa* is virtually unique to cystic fibrosis. This strain is found almost exclusively in the airways of patients with advanced cystic fibrosis. Severe exacerbations may be caused by several different strains of mucin-producing *P. aeruginosa.*

Discovery of the cystic fibrosis gene has made it possible to perform diagnostic

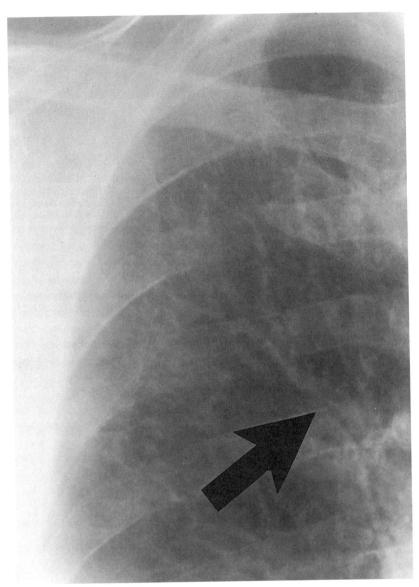

FIGURE 7-2 Close-up of bronchiectatic airway as seen on chest radiograph. Note that the thickened bronchial walls appear as parallel white lines, popularly called "tram tracks."

testing for some of the genetic abnormalities associated with cystic fibrosis. Testing for just the ΔF508 gene will identify about 70 percent of the abnormal genes or about 50 percent of affected patients. Testing for all currently known cystic fibrosis genes will identify the vast majority of the abnormal genes responsible for cystic fibrosis. Because routine genetic testing cannot identify 100 percent of the cystic fibrosis genes, it is best reserved for evaluation of patients with suspected cystic fibrosis who have equivocal results from sweat chloride testing, or subjects who require genetic counseling because they are at high risk for having children with cystic fibrosis.[18] If it is likely that a couple will have a child with cystic fibrosis, the fetus can be checked at the time of amniocentesis[19,20] or before implantation following in vitro fertilization.[21,22]

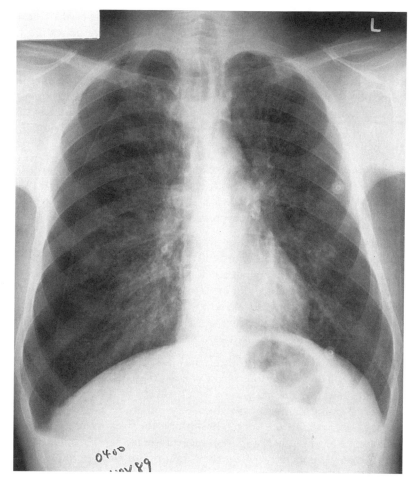

FIGURE 7-3   Chest radiograph of a patient with cystic fibrosis and a right pneumothorax. Note the pleural line visible in the right chest and the absence of lung markings beyond the line.

Treatment

Initiating early treatment in patients with cystic fibrosis leads to a decreased rate of lung volume loss, improved weight gain, and improved survival rate.[23] The diagnosis of cystic fibrosis can be established through neonatal screening before symptoms develop.

Reversal of the Defect

Cystic fibrosis lung disease is caused by the dysfunction of a protein that regulates electrolyte movement. Several strategies are being attempted to reverse the defective electrolyte transport in the lungs of these patients.

Virally Mediated Gene Transfer. The discovery of the gene that, when damaged, causes cystic fibrosis has led to the hope that the normal gene could be inserted into cells of cystic fibrosis patients. Insertion of the normal gene may reverse the electrolyte defect and stop progression of the respiratory disease. One of the most promising methods of inserting the gene into a cell accomplished by placing the gene in a virus that has had its DNA inactivated. When the virus is placed on a respiratory epithelium, it injects the gene into epithelial cells. If the genes are inserted into cells from a cystic fibrosis patient that have been grown in culture, the ability of the cells to control chloride movement becomes normal.[24] Introduction of these viruses into cystic fibrosis patients leads to a small number of cells expressing the gene. The physiological results of these trials has been inconsistent: In some patients, the electrolyte conductance of epithelial surface improves,[25] whereas others continue to show the electrolyte abnormalities of cystic fibrosis.[26] Virally mediated gene transfer causes few adverse effects.[27]

Transplantation. Heart-lung transplantation and bilateral lung transplants have been used successfully to treat patients with end-stage lung disease due to cystic fibrosis. Transplantation reverses the physiologic abnormalities that characterize cystic fibrosis lung disease[28] but requires immunosuppression, which can lead to opportunistic infections.[13]

Pharmacotherapy. Another approach to reversing the defect of cystic fibrosis is to give drugs that eliminate some or all of the abnormal electrolyte transport. Aerosolized amiloride[29-31] or triphosphate nucleotides[32] may overcome some of the ion transport abnormalities associated with cystic fibrosis. Early trials of these substances have been promising, but it is not known whether these agents alter the course of cystic fibrosis.

Respiratory Secretions

The most significant health threat to cystic fibrosis patients is recurrent respiratory infections. These infections are associated with increased production of mucinous secretions and the tendency to obstruct small- and medium-sized bronchi with mucus plugs. Postural drainage and chest physiotherapy assist patients in clearing mucus plugs. After administration of chest physiotherapy, there is an acute improvement in a number of pulmonary function measurements.[33,34] Autogenic drainage is a mechanism that patients use to clear their own pulmonary secretions[35]; it appears to be as effective in clearing secretions as chest physiotherapy and postural drainage.[36]

The breakdown of neutrophils is an important cause of sputum viscosity in patients with cystic fibrosis. The DNA of dying neutrophils is released into the sputum, increasing its viscosity. Breaking up the DNA with the recombinant human deoxyribonuclease (DNase) improves sputum viscosity and clearance. The improved ability to clear secretions may be responsible for the reduction in the number of exacerbations patients on inhaled DNase experience. DNase inhalation also improves FEV_1 pulmonary function and reduces the need for antibiotic therapy.[37-39] Additional therapies to assist in bronchial clearance include regular aerobic exercise, airway oscillators,[40] voluntary coughing,[41] and the use of a positive expiratory pressure (PEP) mask.[42]

Other treatments have been used to help cystic fibrosis patients clear secretions. Most of these therapies have not been shown to be clearly beneficial and have not been widely adopted. These procedures include the following:

1. Administration of mists and aerosols of saline or water to help hydrate secretions and make them easier to expectorate
2. Administration of mucolytic aerosols to liquefy mucus plugs
3. Bronchoscopy with bronchoalveolar lavage to clear mucus plugs from intermediate and small airways

Respiratory Infections

Repeated lung infections are almost universal in patients with cystic fibrosis. These infections lead to destruction of lung tissue and therefore to loss of pulmonary function. Antibiotics are a critical component of the treatment of these infections and therefore preservation of lung function. Although the exact timing for the initiation of antibiotics remains controversial, antibiotics are usually started when new symptoms develop that suggest respiratory infection. These symptoms may include change in cough, new onset of cough, change in character or consistency of sputum, sudden deterioration in pulmonary function, fever, chest radiograph changes, or lack of expected weight gain. The initial choice of antibiotics should be effective against organisms that commonly infect patients with cystic fibrosis. The antibiotic coverage is adjusted once the sputum culture discloses a predominant organism. Serious infections may require intravenous (IV) antibiotics. Prolonged courses of IV antibiotics usually begin in the hospital, but may be continued at home after the patient or family has learned to administer the antibiotics.

Oral antibiotics are frequently used for less severe respiratory infections. Fluorinated quinolones belong to a potent new class of oral antibiotics, many of which have acceptable activity against *P. aeruginosa*. These new oral antibiotics are highly effective at controlling exacerbations of cystic fibrosis, but antibiotic-resistant strains may become a significant problem.[43]

Inhaled antibiotics, most commonly gentamicin, are occasionally used to suppress airway infections. The dose of inhaled gentamicin typically varies from 60 to 80 mg two to four times daily.[44,45] Aerosolized tobramycin has recently been shown to be well tolerated by children and adults with cystic fibrosis.[46] It has been shown to reduce the frequency of exacerbations and to improve lung function in cystic fibrosis patient with stable disease.

Bronchial Hyperactivity

A large number of patients with cystic fibrosis have bronchial hyperactivity similar to asthma (see Chapter 4); thus, the symptoms of bronchial hyperactivity are usually treated with agents used to treat asthma. Treatment includes the administration of inhaled or oral β-agonists and theophylline. Anti-inflammatory agents (e.g., cromolyn sodium, inhaled or oral corticosteroids) have been helpful in some cases.

Pancreatic Insufficiency

Patients with cystic fibrosis are frequently malnourished because of pancreatic exocrine insufficiency, inadequate food intake,[47] and the high metabolic demands associated with infection.

Pancreatic enzyme replacement is standard therapy for relieving the symptoms of pancreatic exocrine insufficiency. The enzymes are usually given as capsules or pills before every meal and are adjusted to relieve steatorrhea (fatty stools). In addition, fat-soluble vitamins (A, D, E, and K) are routinely supplemented. Patients should be encouraged to eat a balanced diet and avoid excessive fat intake.[48]

Prognosis

The prognosis for patients with cystic fibrosis is steadily improving. At one time, most patients would not live beyond their 10th birthday. Now, with aggressive treatment of this multisystem disease, most cystic fibrosis patients live to age 30.[49]

CASE STUDY

History

MB is a 26-year-old woman who presented to the pulmonary clinic for the first time with complaints of dyspnea on exertion and a productive cough. She had had a productive cough for many years and periodically developed yellow or green sputum and occasional hemoptysis. These symptoms were attributed to bronchiectasis. When she was a child, her parents were told she had asthma. She also had many childhood respiratory infections requiring hospitalization. At age 11, she was told she had bronchiectasis. Since that time her therapy included inhaled metaproterenol and occasional antibiotic therapy. She had no regular pulmonary hygiene program.

Three weeks before admission, an increasingly severe cough producing greenish sputum developed. She also noticed increasing dyspnea on exertion, and wheezing. Her family physician gave her a prescription for ciprofloxacin 750 mg twice daily, but her symptoms progressed despite this therapy. Her current symptoms increased to such a degree that she requested sick leave from her job as a secretary.

This was the third such episode MB experienced in the last year. Her previous episodes were successfully treated with oral ciprofloxacin. She chronically heard wheezing and crackles with breathing, particularly when she went to bed at night. She also had difficulty maintaining weight and felt she was far below her ideal weight. She did not have fever, chills, pharyngitis, cordon (clear nasal discharge), or purulent nasal discharge. She had no problems with steatorrhea (fatty stools), nasal polyps, or sinus infections.

MB never smoked. She has two younger sisters who have cystic fibrosis and an older brother who is healthy. Her father had a chronic problem with bronchiectasis that began as a teenager. MB had been tested for cystic fibrosis using a sweat chloride concentration when she was first diagnosed with bronchiectasis at age 11. Her sweat chloride concentration was 57 mEq/liter.

QUESTIONS

1. What features of this patient's history support the diagnosis of cystic fibrosis?
2. Which parts of the MB's history suggest that she does not have cystic fibrosis?
3. Does her sweat chloride concentration help to clarify whether or not she has cystic fibrosis?
4. What findings would you expect on physical examination if this patient has cystic fibrosis?
5. What additional testing would be appropriate to support or refute the diagnosis of cystic fibrosis?

ANSWERS

1. A number of features in the history support the suspicion that this woman has cystic fibrosis. The development of bronchiectasis at a young age, particularly in an area of the world where antibiotics are readily available, suggests cystic fibrosis. Children with cystic fibrosis are occasionally misdiagnosed in infancy as having asthma. Her weight loss and inability to maintain a normal body weight are indicative of cystic fibrosis, as are her symptoms of asthma and recurrent pulmonary infections in childhood. Perhaps the most important

feature of the history, however, is that she has siblings with cystic fibrosis. If one child in a family has cystic fibrosis, each sibling has a one in four chance of also having the disease.

2. This patient lacks certain classic characteristics of cystic fibrosis. She does not have diarrhea or symptoms of malabsorption that suggest pancreatic exocrine insufficiency, and she lacks a history of sinus difficulties or nasal polyps.

3. No, a sweat chloride value of between 50 and 80 mEq/liter is considered equivocal.

4. You would expect to find a thin, underweight woman with an increased anteroposterior (AP) chest dimension. Her fingers would show clubbing, and if the lung disease were very advanced, she would have some cyanosis. Auscultation of breath sounds would reveal inspiratory crackles and expiratory wheezing. If cor pulmonale were present, one would see distended neck veins and edema in the lower extremities.

5. Because the sweat chloride test done in childhood was equivocal, a repeat sweat chloride test should be performed. If the repeated sweat chloride concentrations are equivocal, then gene probes may be useful to determine whether she is homozygous for the cystic fibrosis genes.

Physical Examination

General: A thin, young, white woman with a productive cough; uses accessory muscles of respiration, but appears to be breathing comfortably and can converse without apparent dyspnea

Vital Signs: Temperature 37.2°C; (99.0°F), pulse 71/minute, respiratory rate 19/minute; blood pressure 105/72 mm Hg

HEENT: Nasal polyp seen in left nares; no sinus tenderness noted; oral examination normal and mucous membranes moist; eye and ear examinations normal

Neck: Trachea in midline position; both carotid impulses normal in contour and intensity; no jugular venous distention

Chest: AP dimensions of chest increased; diffuse inspiratory and expiratory crackles with polyphonic expiratory wheezing heard over both lungs; hyper-resonance noted with chest percussion

Heart: Regular rate with loud P_2 component of S_2 noted on cardiac auscultation; no murmurs or gallops noted; point of maximum impulse (PMI) difficult to appreciate but located in the fifth interspace 2 to 3 cm lateral to sternal border

Abdomen: Bowel sounds active, with no guarding or tenderness; liver 8 cm in the midclavicular line; no masses palpated

Extremities: Digital clubbing, but no cyanosis or edema; pulses equal and symmetrical

---

QUESTIONS

6. This patient does not have a fever at the time of examination or a history of fever before this visit. Does the lack of fever indicate that the patient does not have a significant exacerbation of her lung disease?

7. What is the significance of MB's underweight appearance?

8. What is a nasal polyp, and what respiratory problems may it create?

9. What is indicated by an increase in the AP dimension of the chest?

10. What is the significance of the crackles heard over the lungs?

11. The S_2 has two components: an aortic sound (A_2) and a pulmonic sound (P_2). Describe the source of these heart sounds and the meaning of a loud P_2.

12. Why does this patient have a cardiac PMI that is decreased in intensity and displaced from the normal position?

13. This patient demonstrates clubbing of the digits. What does clubbing of the fingers look like, and what it may indicate?

14. What laboratory work should be ordered at this time?

ANSWERS

6. No. Patients with exacerbations of bronchiectasis typically complain of copious, grossly purulent secretions and dyspnea; however, is infrequent during bronchiectatic exacerbations. The best guide to determine the severity of a bronchiectatic exacerbation is the nature and severity of the symptoms. Fever is commonly found with pneumonia or viral respiratory infections; thus, if MB had presented with a fever, pneumonia or viral illness would have been the most likely cause.

7. The underweight appearance is suggestive of cystic fibrosis in patients with symptoms such as these. Malnutrition develops in these patients as a result of (1) malabsorption due to pancreatic exocrine insufficiency; (2) a lower than normal caloric intake; and (3) increased metabolic demands due to respiratory effort and recurrent infections.

8. A nasal polyp is an overgrowth of mucosa in the nose that leads to a fingerlike growth. These polyps tend to form in cyptic fibrosis patients, and they may become so numerous or large that they completely block the nasal passages.

9. When the lungs become hyperexpanded because of air trapping the chest enlarges, particularly in the AP dimension. This increase in chest diameter is associated with emphysema, chronic bronchitis, asthma, and cystic fibrosis.

10. Crackles are associated with increased pulmonary secretions. In advanced cases of cystic fibrosis, the lung examination will almost always disclose crackles. The presence of crackles in this case does not necessarily represent pulmonary edema or pneumonia.

11. The S_2 has two components. One is created when the aortic valve closes (A_2) and the other is produced when the pulmonic valve closes (P_2). Normally, A_2 is louder than P_2; the reverse is suggestive of pulmonary hypertension.

12. As the lungs hyperexpand because of obstructive lung disease, the heart is forced to assume a more vertical and central position in the chest. This change in position can be seen on physical examination by a movement of the PMI centrally and toward the epigastrium.

13. Clubbing is enlargement of the tips of the fingers and toes; it is associated with convexity of the nails and is often seen in patients with chronic lung disease. It is unclear why clubbing develops in these patients.

14. Several questions should be clarified before the optimum treatment program can be initiated:
   a. Does she have pneumonia or just an exacerbation of her bronchiectasis?
   b. Is her dyspnea due, in part, to hypoxemia?
   c. Is her nutrition adequate?

To evaluate for pneumonia, a chest radiograph plus a WBC count and differential should be ordered. Hypoxemia can be identified by ABG analysis. If chronic hypoxemia is present, there is usually an elevation of the hemoglobin concentration or the hematocrit. Malnutrition can be evaluated by measurements of serum proteins such as albumin or total protein.

Laboratory Evaluation

Chest Radiograph: See Figure 7–4

ABGs (on room air): pH 7.42, $Paco_2$ 34 mm Hg, Pao_2 67 mm Hg, HCO_3^- 21 mEq/liter, $P(A-a)o_2$ 39 mm Hg, O_2 content 17.5 mL/dL

Complete Blood Count:

	Observed	Normal
WBCs/mL	12,400	4,000–11,000
Red blood cells (M/mL)	4.7	4.1–5.5
Hemoglobin (g/dL)	14.2	14–16.5
Hematocrit (%)	43	37–50
Differential		
Segmented neutrophils (%)	72	38–79
Band neutrophils (%)	12	0–7
Lymphocytes (%)	13	12–51
Monocytes (%)	1	0–10
Eosinophils (%)	1	0–8
Basophils (%)	1	0–2

Chemistry:

	Observed	Normal
Na^+ (mEq/liter)	138	136–146
K^+ (mEq/liter)	4.6	3.5–5.1
Cl^- (mmol/dL)	106	98–106
HCO_3^- (mm/L)	20	22–29
Blood urea nitrogen (mg/dL)	13	7–18
Creatinine (mg/dL)	0.7	0.5–11
Calcium (mmol/liter)	2.1	2.1–255
Phosphate (mg/dL)	2.7	2.7–4.5
Uric acid (mg/dL)	3.4	4.5–8.2
Albumin (g/dL)	3.1	3.5–5.0
Protein (g/dL)	6.0	6.4–8.3

QUESTIONS

15. How would you correlate MB's chest radiograph with her condition (Fig. 7-4)?

16. How would you interpret the ABGs?

17. Why are the WBC count and the number of band neutrophils elevated?

18. What do a low albumin and total protein level indicate?

19. What additional diagnostic tests would be important to obtain?

20. If the physician decides to admit this patient to the hospital, what respiratory therapy orders would you suggest?

ANSWERS

15. Scoliosis is noted in the thoracic and lumbar spine. The lungs are hyperexpanded with diffuse reticular nodular opacities throughout both lungs. Numerous cystic airspaces are seen, as are occasional thickened bronchial walls. This radiograph is consistent with a patient with bronchiectasis or cystic fibrosis. Although the disease is more pronounced in the right lung, no focal areas of pneumonia are seen. This woman appears very thin, with no excessive soft tissue shadows.

16. MB has a chronic respiratory alkalosis and a widened $P(A-a)O_2$. Mild hypoxemia is present.

17. An acute infection of any type can elevate the WBC count and lead the bone marrow to release immature neutrophils (bands) into the blood to help fight the infection. In this case, the elevation is most likely due to either pneumonia or an exacerbation of bronchiectasis.

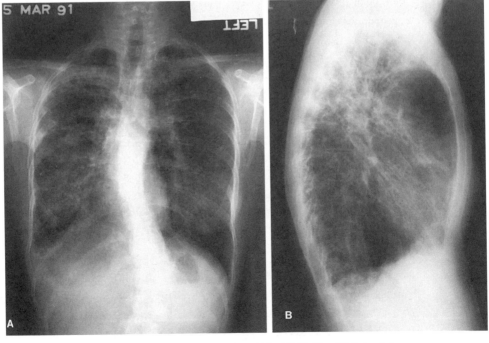

FIGURE 7-4　Chest radiograph from M.B. (*A*) PA film. (*B*) Lateral view.

18. Both of these serum proteins are likely to be depressed in the setting of malnutrition.

19. With any infection, selection of the appropriate antibiotic is easiest if the physician knows the offending organism. It is important to culture the sputum to determine, if possible, which organism is causing her infection. Identifying the infecting organism in this case is very important, because MB has already failed to respond to one course of antibiotics.

20. Respiratory therapy should aim to reverse bronchospasm and assist in the clearance of secretions. Inhaled β-agonists will help reverse bronchospasm. The optimum method of delivering β-agonists is not clearly defined. Either a metered-dose inhaler (MDI) or a nebulized solution would be appropriate. To help clear secretions, chest physiotherapy and postural drainage should also be started. Other therapies, such as mist tents, bland aerosol therapy, and N-acetyl-L-cysteine, have been used to help these patients clear pulmonary secretions, but they have not proved effective.

CASE STUDY—continued

Because MB failed to improve on oral antibiotics, her physician admitted her to the medicine service for more aggressive treatment. The admitting orders included the following:

> Supplemental vitamins, A, D, E, and K
>
> Aminophylline 1 g in 0.25 liter normal saline: an initial IV infusion of 5 mg/kg over 30 minutes, then constant infusion at a rate of 0.5 mg/kg per hour
>
> Piperacillin IV 1 g every 6 hours
>
> Amikacin 225 mg IV every 8 hours
>
> Medication nebulizer treatments with 0.3 mL metaproterenol (Alupent) in 3 mL normal saline every 6 hours
>
> Chest physiotherapy and postural drainage every 6 hours
>
> Theophylline level on the second hospital day
>
> Amikacin level before and after the third dose of amikacin
>
> A sputum Gram stain and culture
>
> Sweat chloride concentration
>
> Gene probe for the ΔF508 gene

QUESTIONS

21. The admitting physician believes that MB may have cystic fibrosis. Why did the physician prescribe the supplemental A, D, E, and K vitamins?

22. What is metaproterenol? What are the potential side effects?

23. Is the prescribed chest physiotherapy and postural drainage important for this patient, or should you recommend that it be discontinued? Why?

24. What is the most important thing that you as a respiratory care practitioner could teach this patient to help in her long-term health?

25. If this patient is found to have cystic fibrosis, what organisms would you expect to find on the sputum culture?

26. One of the microorganisms that patients with cystic fibrosis commonly have as a respiratory pathogen has a unique characteristic. What is unique about the *P. aeruginosa* found in cystic fibrosis patients?

27. If MG is found to have cystic fibrosis, what are the odds that she will have both copies of the ΔF508 gene?

ANSWERS

21. MB appears mildly malnourished on physical examination and on her admitting laboratory work-up. If she has cystic fibrosis she may have difficulty absorbing fat and the fat-soluble vitamins. To overcome the vitamin deficiency, these patients are generally given the supplemental fat-soluble vitamins A, D, E, and K.

22. Metaproterenol is an inhaled β-agonist. The purpose of giving it to this patient is to reverse bronchospasm, which is the cause of her wheezing and some of her dyspnea. The primary side effects of metaproterenol are tachycardia, tachyarrhythmias, and tremors.

23. Chest physiotherapy is very important for patients with bronchiectasis and cystic fibrosis. Mucus plugs in the distal airways may obstruct these airways and cause right-to-left shunting, leading to small, distal abscesses. Therefore, clearance of mucus plugs is very important for patients with cystic fibrosis. Chest physiotherapy and postural drainage will help move these mucus plugs from the distal airways to the large central airways, from which they can be expectorated.

24. MG has had no program of bronchial hygiene. She should be instructed in postural drainage and a family member taught to perform chest physiotherapy. Other therapies that may assist bronchial hygiene include regular exercise and the use of PEP by mask or mouthpiece.

25. The three organisms most commonly found in the tracheal secretions of patients with cystic fibrosis include: *H. influenzae, S. aureus,* and *P. aeruginosa.*

26. The *P. aeruginosa* organism that infects patients with cystic fibrosis differs from the vast majority of *P. aeruginosa* isolates in that it produces mucin.

27. The ΔF508 gene accounts for about 70 percent of the abnormal genes that cause cystic fibrosis. To have the disease, the affected individual must have two genes that cause cystic fibrosis. The chance that an individual with cystic fibrosis has both delta F508 genes is $0.7 \times 0.7 \times 100 = 49$ percent.

CASE STUDY—continued

MB is a typical example of an older patient with cystic fibrosis: She has many classic features of the disease, but also lacks a significant number of common abnormalities. Pancreatic exocrine insufficiency is one classic finding that she does not have. Patients with normal pancreatic exocrine function have a better prognosis than those with pancreatic dysfunction.[50]

QUESTIONS

28. What effect does inhaled DNase have on the sputum of patients with cystic fibrosis?

29. Does MB have cystic fibrosis?

ANSWERS

28. DNase breaks up the DNA in the sputum of patients with cystic fibrosis. This effect decreases the viscosity of the sputum and makes it easier to expectorate. The administration of inhaled DNase in patients with cystic fibrosis has been shown to improve FEV_1, prolong the time between respiratory exacerbations, and improve survival.

29. Yes, the elevation of sweat chloride to 103 mEq/liter confirms that MB, like her sisters, has cystic fibrosis. The gene probe found that MB was heterozygous for the ΔF508 gene; however, there are several mutations of the gene other than ΔF508 that can lead to cystic fibrosis. The ΔF508 gene accounts for only 70 percent of the genes causing cystic fibrosis. Therefore, it is not surprising that MB has only one of the ΔF508 genes yet still has cystic fibrosis.

CASE STUDY—continued

MB was hospitalized for 5 days. During this time she received antibiotics, bronchodilators, inhaled DNase, and chest physiotherapy. Her symptoms improved greatly showing marked reduction in coughing and dyspnea. She now produces far less sputum, and the color is a light yellow. She has been trained to administer her own IV antibiotics and to perform postural drainage; her husband has been trained to deliver chest percussion. The sputum culture grew a mucinous strain of *P. aeruginosa* that was resistant to ciprofloxacin. Her sweat chloride concentration was 103 mEq/liter. The gene probe revealed that MB had only one copy of the ΔF508 gene.

REFERENCES

1. Conneally, PM, et al: Cystic fibrosis: Population genetics. Tex Reprod Biol Med 31:639, 1973.
2. Levison, H, and Tabachnik, E: Pulmonary physiology. In Hodson, ME, et al (eds): Cystic Fibrosis. Baillière Tindall, London, 1983, pp 52–81.
3. Fanconi, G, et al: Das coeliakiesyndrom bei angeborener zysticher pankreasfibromatose und bronchiektasien. Wein Med Wochnschr 86:753, 1936.
4. Taussig, LM: Cystic Fibrosis. Thieme-Stratton, New York, 1984.
5. Riordan, JR, et al: Identification of the cystic fibrosis gene: Cloning and characterization of the complementary DNA. Science 245:1066, 1989.
6. Rommens, JM, et al: Identification of the cystic fibrosis gene: Chromosome walking and jumping. Science 245:1059, 1989.
7. Kerem, E, et al: The relation between genotype and phenotype in cystic fibrosis of the most common mutation (delta F508). N Engl J Med 323:1517,1990.
8. Rich, DP, et al: Expression of cystic fibrosis transmembrane conductance regulator corrects defective chloride channel regulation in cystic fibrosis airway epithelial cells. Nature 347:358, 1990.
9. Anderson, MP, et al: Generation of cAMP-activated chloride currents by expression of CFTR. Science 251:679, 1991.
10. Quinton, PM, and Bijman, J: Higher bioelectric potentials due to decreased chloride absorption in the sweat glands of patients with cystic fibrosis. N Engl J Med 308:1185, 1983.
11. Esterly, JR, and Oppenheimer, EH: Observations in cystic fibrosis of the pancreas. Part III: Pulmonary lesions. Johns Hopkins Med J 122:94, 1968.
12. Bedrossian, CWM, et al: The lung in cystic fibrosis: A quantitative study including preva-

lence of pathologic findings among different age groups. Hum Pathol 7:195, 1976.

13. Rosenstein, BJ, and Langbaum, TS: Diagnosis. In Taussig, LM (ed): Cystic Fibrosis. Thieme Stratton, New York, 1984.

14. Schwachman, H: Gastrointestinal manifestations of cystic fibrosis. Pediatr Clin North Am 22:787, 1975.

15. Gibson, LE, and Cook, RE: A test of concentration of electrolytes in sweat in cystic fibrosis of the pancreas utilizing pilocarpine iontophoresis. Pediatrics 23:545, 1959.

16. Report of the Committee for a Study for Evaluation of Testing for Cystic Fibrosis. National Academy of Sciences, Washington, DC, 1975.

17. Rosenstein, BJ, et al: Cystic fibrosis: Problems encountered with sweat testing. JAMA 240:1987, 1978.

18. Statement from the National Institutes of Health Workshop in Population Screening for the Cystic Fibrosis Gene. N Engl J Med 323:70, 1990.

19. Jedlicka-Kohler, I, et al: Utilization of prenatal diagnosis for cystic fibrosis over the past seven years. Pediatrics 94:13, 1994.

20. Wertz, DC, et al: Attitudes toward the prenatal diagnosis of cystic fibrosis: Factors in decision making among affected families. Hum Genet 50:1077, 1992.

21. Cui, KH, et al: Optimal polymerase chain reaction amplification for preimplantation diagnosis in cystic fibrosis (delta F508). BMJ 311:536, 1995.

22. Storm, CM, et al: Reliability of polymerase chain reaction (PCR) analysis of single cells for preimplantation genetic diagnosis. J Assist Reprod Gent 11:55, 1994.

23. Dankert-Roelse, JE, and te Meerman, GJ: Long term prognosis of patients with cystic fibrosis in relation to early detection by neaonatal screening. Thorax 50:712, 1995.

24. Drumm, ML, et al. Correction of cystic fibrosis defect in vitro by retrovirus mediated gene transfer. Cell 74:215, 1993.

25. Hay, JG, et al: Modification of nasal epithelial potential differences of individuals with cystic fibrosis consequent to local administration of normal CFTR cDNA adenovirus gene transfer vector. Hum Gene Ther 6:1487, 1995.

26. Knowles, MR, et al: A controlled study of adenoviral-vector-mediated gene transfer in the nasal epithelium of patients with cystic fibrosis. New Engl J Med 333:823, 1995.

27. Crystal, RG, et al: Administration of an adenovirus containing the human CFTR cDNA to the respiratory tract of individuals with cystic fibrosis. Nat Genet 8:42, 1992.

28. Alton, EW, et al: Effect of heart lung transplantation on airway potential difference in patients with and without cystic fibrosis. Eur Respir J 4:5, 1991.

29. Higenbottam, TW, et al: Mortality and morbidity following heart-lung transplantation for cystic fibrosis. Am Rev Respir Dis 141:605, 1990.

30. App, EM, et al: Acute and long term amiloride inhalation in cystic fibrosis lung disease: A rational approach to cystic fibrosis therapy. Am Rev Respir Dis 141:605, 1990.

31. Knowles, MR, et al: A pilot study of aerosolized amiloride for treatment of lung disease in cystic fibrosis. N Engl J Med 322:1189, 1990.

32. Knowles, MR, et al: Activation by extracellular nucleotides of chloride secretion in the airway epithelia of patients with cystic fibrosis. N Engl J Med 325:533, 1991.

33. Desmond, KJ, et al: Immediate and long term effects of chest physiotherapy in patients with cystic fibrosis. J Pediatr 103:538, 1983.

34. Maxwell, M, and Redmond, AO: Comparative trial of manual and mechanical percussion technique with gravity-assisted bronchial drainage in patients with cystic fibrosis. Arch Dis Child 54:542, 1979.

35. Partridge, C, et al: Characteristics of the forced expiration technique. Physiotherapy 75:193, 1989.

36. Giles, DR, et al: Short-term effects of postural drainage with clapping vs autogenic drainage on oxygen saturation and sputum recovery in patients with cystic fibrosis. Chest 108:952, 1995.

37. Hubbard, RC, et al: A preliminary study of aerosolized recombinant deoxyribonuclease I in the treatment of cystic fibrosis. N Engl J Med 326:812, 1992.

38. Aitken, ML, et al: Recombinant human DNase inhalation in normal subjects and patients with cystic fibrosis. JAMA 267:1947, 1992.

39. Fuchs, HJ, et al: Effect of aerosolized recombinant human DNase on exacerbations of respiratory symptoms and on pulmonary function in patients with cystic fibrosis: The Pulmozyme Study Group. N Engl J Med 331:637, 1994.

40. Konstan, MW, et al: Efficacy of the Flutterdevice for mucous clearance in patients with cystic fibrosis. J Pediatr 124:689, 1994.

41. Zimman, R: Cough versus chest physiotherapy: A comparison of the acute effects on pulmonary function in patients with cystic fibrosis. Am Rev Respir Dis 129:182, 1984.

42. Steen, HJ, et al: Evaluation of the PEP mask in cystic fibrosis. Acta Paediatr Scand 51, 1991.

43. Radberg, G, et al: Development of quinolone-imipenem cross resistance in *Pseudomonas aeruginosa* during exposure to ciprofloxacin. Antimicrob Agents Chemother 34:2142, 1990.

44. Hodson, ME, et al: Aerosol carbenicillin and gentamicin treatment of *Pseudomonas aeruginosa* infection in patients with cystic fibrosis. Lancet 2:1137, 1981.

45. Nolan, G, et al: Antibiotic prophylaxis in cystic fibrosis: Inhaled cephaloridine as an adjunct to oral cloxacillin. J Pediatr 101:626, 1982.

46. Fiel, SB: Aerosol delivery of antibiotics to the lower airways of patients with cystic fibrosis. Chest 107:615, 1995.

47. Hubbard, VS, and Mangrum, PJ: Energy intake and nutritional counseling in cystic fibrosis. J Am Diet Assoc 80:127, 1982.

48. Dodge, JA: Nutrition. In Hodson, ME, et al (eds): Cystic Fibrosis. Baillière Tindall, London, 1983, pp 132–141.

49. Patient Registry, Cystic Fibrosis Foundation, through 1995.

50. Gaskin, K, et al: Improved respiratory prognosis in patients with cystic fibrosis with normal fat absorption. J Pediatr 100:857, 1982.

CHAPTER **8**

Hemodynamic Monitoring and Shock

Robert L. Wilkins, PhD, RRT
James R. Dexter, MD, FCCP

Key Terms

afterload
cardiac index
cardiac output
circulatory failure
contractility

hypovolemic shock
inotropes
mixed venous oxygen
 tension
perfusion

preload
septic shock
shock
stroke volume

Introduction

The circulatory system is composed of the heart, blood vessels, and the blood. Each component plays a vital role in the process of circulation. The heart is the pump that provides the power to move blood throughout the blood vessels (**perfusion**). The blood vessels direct the blood from the heart to the tissues through arteries and back to the heart through veins. The arteries are endowed with smooth muscle, which provides variable resistance to flow to help maintain the blood pressure (BP) needed for perfusion. Blood is the medium in which oxygen and other nutrients are carried to the tissues.

Supplementary organs involved in circulation include the lungs, which provide oxygen; the bone marrow, which provides red blood cells; the liver, which processes nutrients from the digestive tract; and the nervous system, which regulates muscle tone in the arteries.

The circulatory system can be divided into two major parts: the *pulmonary system* and the *systemic system*. The pulmonary system is made up of the right side of the heart (right atrium and right ventricle), pulmonary arteries, and pulmonary veins. The pulmonary arteries direct blood from the right ventricle to the lungs for gas exchange. The pulmonary veins conduct the oxygenated blood from the lungs back to the left side of the heart. The systemic system is made up of the left side of the heart (left atrium and left ventricle), the arteries, and the veins. The systemic arteries carry oxygenated blood from the left heart to the different organ systems, where oxygen and nutrients are given up to the tissues and metabolic waste products are removed. The veins return the partially deoxygenated blood back to the right side of the heart.

Because the purpose of circulation is to provide the organs of the body with oxygen and other vital nutrients, **circulatory failure** is defined in terms of vital organ system dysfunction. When circulation is not sufficient to meet the metabolic needs of vital organs such as the brain, heart, and kidneys, the patient is said to be suffering from circulatory failure or **shock.** Although many parameters may indicate that circulation may not be optimal (e.g., hypotension, elevated lactic acid level), shock is present only when there is evidence of vital organ dysfunction (e.g., abnormal sensorium, decreased urine output).

What Is Cardiac Output?

The pumping function of the left ventricle is very important, since it moves the oxygenated blood to all areas of the body. The quantity of blood pumped out of the left ventricle each minute is known as the **cardiac output.** Normally the adult cardiac output is 4 to 8 liters/minute. Since normal cardiac output is dependent on the size and metabolic rate of the patient, clinicians must interpret it in relation to the patient's body mass and metabolic rate. A cardiac output of 3.5 liters/minute might be acceptable for a petite, afebrile, resting woman, whereas this same value could represent a circulatory crisis for a large, male patient with a fever.

Cardiac index (cardiac output/body surface area) is a useful parameter because it accounts for the variations in body size. The patient's body surface area in square meters can be determined from standard nomograms and is divided into the cardiac output to determine cardiac index. A normal index is 2.5 to 4.0 liters/minute per m^2.

What Determines Cardiac Output?

Cardiac output is the product of heart rate and **stroke volume** (the volume of blood ejected by the ventricle with each contraction). Heart rate is strongly influenced by the sympathetic and parasympathetic nervous systems. Activation of the sympathetic nervous systems leads to tachycardia and usually increases cardiac output except at extremes. Stimulation of the parasympathetic nervous system promotes bradycardia, and profound bradycardia may reduce cardiac output.

Stroke volume is a function of three important factors: filling volume of the ventricle (**preload**), arterial resistance to flow out of the ventricle during contraction (**afterload**), and cardiac **contractility** (Fig. 8–1). Bedside clinicians must evaluate all three factors in patients suffering from circulatory insufficiency.

Preload

The strength of myocardial muscle contraction is directly related (within limits) to the amount of stretch applied to the muscle prior to contraction. This precontraction stretch is known as preload and is primarily a function of venous pressure,

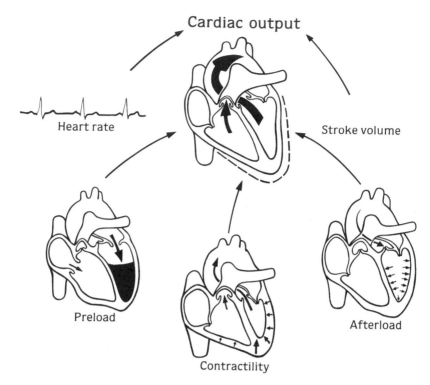

FIGURE 8-1   Factors determining cardiac output are stroke volume and heart rate. Stroke volume is determined by preload, afterload, and contractility. (From Wilkins, RL, Sheldon, RL, and Krider, SJ: Clinical Assessment in Respiratory Care, Mosby–Year Book, St. Louis, 1995, p 279, with permission.)

which determines the volume in the ventricle just prior to contraction. Up to a certain point the more the ventricle is stretched during ventricular filling (diastole), the greater the force of the subsequent contraction and the greater the stroke volume (Fig. 8–2). If the filling of the ventricle is minimal (as in hypovolemia) the subsequent contraction will result in a reduced stroke volume. Excessive overfilling of the ventricle will also lead to a reduced stroke volume as a result of overstretching of the myocardium (Fig. 8–2). The point at which optimal filling of the heart occurs varies from patient to patient, depending on the compliance of the ventricles.

At the bedside, clinicians look at the patient's neck veins and measure central venous pressure (CVP) to evaluate right heart filling pressure. Clinicians measure the pulmonary capillary wedge pressure (PCWP) to assess preload for the left ventricle. Physicians place a balloon-tipped catheter into the pulmonary artery (PA) to obtain this measurement (Fig. 8–3). Indications for the use of a PA catheter are described below in the Treatment section. Normal CVP is 2 to 6 mm Hg, and normal PCWP is 4 to 12 mm Hg.[1]

Afterload

The tension created by the cardiac muscle fibers during contraction to overcome impedance to flow out of the ventricle is known as afterload. Since ventricular wall tension is very difficult to measure, other parameters are used to reflect afterload.

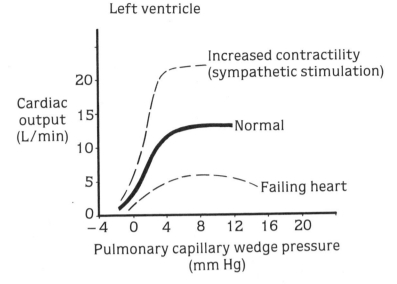

FIGURE 8-2 Ventricular function curves for left ventricle. Note how the stroke volume increases with an increase in filling pressure, up to a certain point. Overfilling of the ventricle results in a decrease in stroke volume, especially in the failing heart. (From Wilkins, RL, Sheldon, RL, and Krider, SJ: Clinical Assessment in Respiratory Care, Mosby–Year Book, St. Louis, 1995, p 280, with permission.)

Systemic vascular resistance (SVR) indicates afterload for the left ventricle; pulmonary vascular resistance (PVR) indicates afterload for the right ventricle (see Table 8–1 for normal values). Afterload for the left ventricle increases with systemic vasoconstriction and decreases with peripheral vasodilatation. Afterload increases for the right ventricle with pulmonary vasoconstriction and decreases with pulmonary vasodilatation. The interaction between cardiac output and afterload determines BP.

The calculation of resistance requires measurement of the driving pressure across the circuit. For SVR this driving pressure is the difference between mean arterial pressure (MAP) and CVP; for PVR the driving pressure is the difference between

TABLE 8-1 **Hemodynamic Parameters**

Parameter	*Normal Range*	*Indication*
CO	4–8 liters/minute	Total blood flow
CI	2.5–4.0 liters/minute per m^2	Blood flow for size of patient
CVP	0–6 mm Hg	Right ventricular preload
PCWP	6–12 mm Hg	Left ventricular preload
SVR	900–1400 dynes-sec/cm^5	Left ventricular afterload
PVR	200–450 dynes-sec/cm^5	Right ventricular afterload
MAP	80–100 mm Hg	Perfusion pressure
P$\bar{v}O_2$	35–45 mm Hg	Tissue oxygenation
PAP	20–30/6–15 mm Hg	Pulmonary artery pressure

CO = cardiac output; CI = cardiac index; CVP = central venous pressure; PCWP = pulmonary capillary wedge pressure; SVR = systemic vascular resistance; PVR = pulmonary vascular resistance; MAP = mean arterial pressure; P$\bar{v}O_2$ = mixed venous oxygen tension; PAP = pulmonary artery pressure

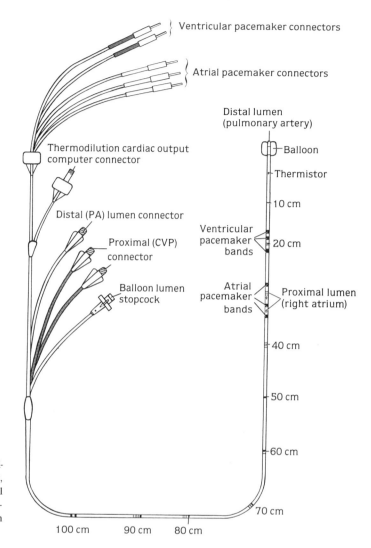

FIGURE 8-3 Illustration of a pulmonary artery catheter. (From Wilkins, RL, Sheldon, RL, and Krider, SJ: Clinical Assessment in Respiratory Care, Mosby-Year Book, St. Louis, 1995, p 310, with permission.)

mean pulmonary artery pressure (PAP) minus left atrial pressure (PCWP). Once the driving pressure is determined, the resistance can be calculated by dividing the cardiac output into the pressure difference:

$$SVR = \frac{MAP \ (mm \ Hg) - CVP \ (mm \ Hg)}{Cardiac \ output \ (liters/minute)} \times 80^*$$

$$PVR = \frac{PAP \ (mm \ Hg) - PCWP \ (mm \ Hg)}{Cardiac \ output \ (liters/minute)} \times 80^*$$

An appropriate level of afterload for the left ventricle is essential to maintain adequate perfusion pressures throughout the body. Decreases in afterload (peripheral

---

*Used to convert the units to dynes-sec/cm [5].

vasodilatation) will cause the BP to drop. The decrease in BP will stimulate the heart to increase cardiac output in an effort to maintain circulation. If the drop in afterload is excessive and the compensatory mechanisms are inadequate, BP may be inadequate for perfusion of vital organs (shock).

Contractility

The forcefulness of myocardial contraction is known as contractility. Even if the ventricle is adequately filled and resistance to outflow optimal, cardiac output will not be adequate if contractility is poor. Common vascular responses to decreased cardiac contractility include an increased afterload (elevated SVR) and increased preload (elevated CVP and PCWP). Factors that reduce cardiac contractility are called **negative inotropes** and include hypoxemia, acidosis, and medications such as β-blockers. Damage to the myocardium as with myocardial infarction will also reduce cardiac contractility. Factors that increase contractility are called **positive inotropes** and include certain β-adrenergics (e.g., Isuprel) and parasympatholytics (e.g., Atropine).

Etiology

Circulatory shock results from inadequate cardiac contractility, failure of vascular tone (inadequate afterload), or hypovolemia (inadequate preload). For example, myocardial infarction may cause inadequate cardiac contractility and shock (see Chapter 10). Sepsis (infection in the blood stream) may cause vasodilatation with decreased afterload and shock. Bleeding from trauma or surgery and dehydration may result in significant hypovolemia (a decrease in circulating blood volume). This can precipitate **hypovolemic shock** when the circulating blood volume is inadequate to meet the metabolic needs of the body. This typically requires a loss of more than 20 to 25 percent of the circulating blood volume.[2] Other causes of shock include those that obstruct the flow of blood (e.g., massive pulmonary embolism causing high afterload for the right heart and inadequate preload to the left heart), and those that cause inadequate contractility by restricting the function of the heart (e.g., constrictive pericarditis, pericardial tamponade).

The most complex forms of shock are those caused by maldistribution of blood flow. This category of circulatory failure includes **septic shock,** *toxic shock, anaphylactic shock,* and *neurogenic shock.* In each case perfusion of vital organs is diminished because of loss of peripheral resistance from vasodilatation and hypotension. Of these different types of shock due to failure of vascular tone, septic shock is the most common.[3] Septic shock produces a syndrome that affects the heart, vascular system, and most organs of the body. Although gram-negative bacteria are the most common cause of septic shock, a vast number of microorganisms can cause it by releasing toxins into the blood.[2]

The role of metabolism in the evaluation of patients with circulatory failure is important to consider. Anything that increases the metabolic rate of a patient will potentially increase the incidence and severity of shock. For example, fever increases oxygen consumption and may result in shock in the patient with marginal cardiac function.

Pathophysiology

The majority of organ systems in the body are affected by circulatory failure. Reduced perfusion to the brain initially results in diminished cognitive function and alertness, and eventually results in coma. Urine output will decrease in response to inadequate renal circulation. The skin typically becomes cool and clammy to the touch as peripheral vasoconstriction is induced in an effort to preserve blood flow to the vital organs. Shock associated with loss of vascular tone is most often caused by sepsis. Toxins produced by bacteria cause the blood vessels to relax, which decreases BP and may directly injure the capillaries of the lung, causing adult respiratory distress syndrome (ARDS). Another effect of bacterial toxins may be to disorganize the blood clotting system, resulting in *disseminated intravascular coagulation* (DIC).[4] DIC is a complex medical problem that results in hemorrhage due to unimpeded clotting and the consumption of platelets and clotting factors to the point where clotting is no longer possible.

The lungs are also affected when circulatory failure is present. The type of shock present determines the effect of the circulatory problem on the lungs. When the left ventricle is unable to pump effectively (decreased contractility), BP increases in the pulmonary circulation, causing fluid to leak into the lung tissue (pulmonary edema) and is known as *congestive heart failure* (see Chapter 10). When the shock is due to hypovolemia, there is little pulmonary consequence except under the most severe circumstances, where underperfusion of the lungs leads to ARDS (see Chapter 13).

Clinical Features

Shock typically produces a similar clinical picture in most patients, regardless of the cause. Patients in shock usually have hypotension, tachypnea, and tachycardia. The peripheral pulses are typically weak or "thready" as a result of the reduced stroke volume associated with shock. Signs of organ dysfunction are present and include oliguria (diminished urine output), altered sensorium, and hypoxemia.[5] The skin often becomes cool and clammy as epinephrine is released, causing peripheral vasoconstriction in an attempt to compensate for the hypotension.

As shock becomes more severe and tissue perfusion decreases, the tissues switch to anaerobic metabolism and lactate builds up, which causes metabolic acidosis.[2] This is often (but not always) accompanied by a decrease in **mixed venous oxygen tension** ($P\bar{v}o_2$). The decrease in $P\bar{v}o_2$ occurs as tissues extract more than the usual amounts of oxygen from the slowly passing blood to compensate for the reduced cardiac output. Sepsis may paradoxically raise $P\bar{v}o_2$ by causing precapillary arterial-venous (AV) shunting and by disrupting the tissues' ability to use oxygen.

Evaluation of serum electrolytes is useful in patients in shock because significant defects (e.g., low potassium) may contribute to the cardiovascular compromise and can be easily corrected. This evaluation is also useful in calculating the anion gap, which is used to detect the onset of lactic acidosis due to lactic acid production from anaerobic metabolism. To calculate the anion gap, the Cl^- and HCO_3^- values are added, and the total is subtracted from the Na^+ value. Normal values are 8 to 16 mEq/liter. An anion gap above 16 mEq/liter in the patient with shock indicates that the shock is severe enough to cause lactic acidosis.

Patients with failure of vascular tone (e.g., septic shock, toxic shock) typically

TABLE 8-2   **Assessment of the Type of Shock**

Parameter	*Hypovolemic*	*Septic*	*Pump Failure*
CO/CI	Decreased	Increased*	Decreased
CVP	Decreased	Normal to low	Increased
PCWP	Decreased	Normal to low	Increased
SVR	Increased	Decreased	Increased
MAP	Normal/low	Decreased	Decreased
$P\bar{v}O_2$	Decreased	Normal	Decreased

*Cardiac output/index is often increased in the early phase of septic shock but may decrease later.
CO = cardiac output; CI = cardiac index; CVP = central venous pressure; PCWP = pulmonary capillary wedge pressure; SVR = systemic vascular resistance; MAP = mean arterial pressure; $P\bar{v}O_2$ = mixed venous oxygen tension

demonstrate fever or hypothermia and leukocytosis.[6] Because the patient with septic shock often has peripheral vasodilation, the extremities may remain warm and pink despite poor circulation to the vital organs. Hemodynamic monitoring of the patient with septic shock reveals an increased cardiac output, reduced SVR, and a low to normal PCWP in the hyperdynamic phase of this syndrome (Table 8-2). $P\bar{v}O_2$ may be normal despite inadequate tissue oxygenation. As mentioned above, the reason for the normal $P\bar{v}O_2$ in septic shock is probably due to decreased peripheral utilization of oxygen and peripheral AV shunts.[1] Later the myocardium often becomes depressed and cardiac output decreases.

Patients in hypovolemic shock typically have poor perfusion to the extremities, which results in a slow capillary refill, peripheral cyanosis, and cool digits. Hemodynamic monitoring reveals reduced filling pressures of the heart (low CVP and PCWP), low cardiac output, and high SVR. Urine output decreases in hypovolemic shock, as the kidneys try to conserve body fluids.

The electrocardiogram (ECG) most commonly shows tachycardia, although abnormal rhythms may be seen when coronary perfusion is inadequate. When coronary artery perfusion is inadequate the ECG will demonstrate ST-segment elevation or depression or T-wave inversion, or both (Fig. 8-4).[2] When considering the use of a vasopressor to correct hypotension, abnormal ST segments or T waves on the ECG suggest that the patient's heart may not tolerate the strain on it associated with an increased afterload from the vasopressor.

Chapter 10 reviews the clinical findings typical of cardiogenic shock resulting from left heart failure.

Treatment

A few general guidelines apply to treating all patients in shock. Oxygen therapy is needed to treat hypoxemia and maximize efficiency of circulation. Oxygen may be required in high concentrations (greater than 40 percent), especially if pulmonary edema is present. Endotracheal intubation is required when the patient's sensorium is depressed to the point where aspiration of gastric contents might occur when respiratory muscle fatigue requires mechanical ventilation or when hypoxemia requires positive end-expiratory pressure (PEEP).[2]

Mechanical ventilation is often helpful in treating the patient in shock, as it reduces oxygen consumption of the respiratory muscles and circulatory demands as

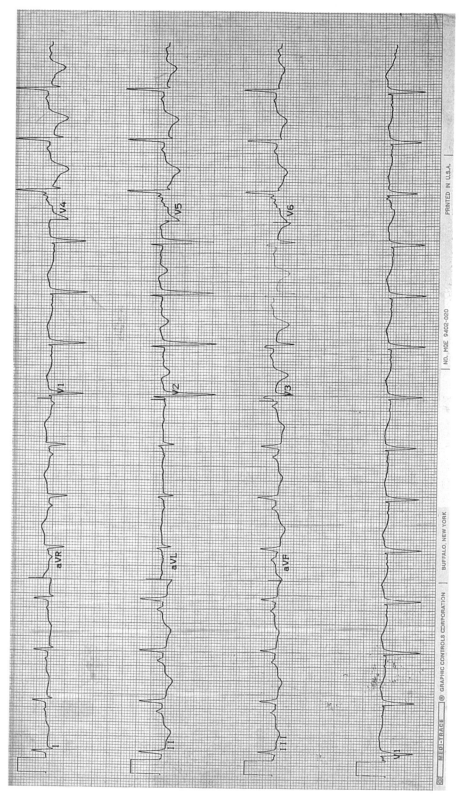

FIGURE 8–4   Electrocardiogram (ECG) illustrating ST-segment and T-wave abnormalities typical for myocardial ischemia. Note the ST-segment depression and T-wave inversion in leads V_3, V_4, V_5, and V_6. Also note the T-wave inversion in leads II, III, and aVF. (Courtesy of Ken Jutzy, MD.)

well as treats the respiratory failure. The use of PEEP may be needed when the Pa_{O_2} is less than 60 mm Hg on an F_{IO_2} greater than 0.50. Close monitoring of the patient in an intensive care unit (ICU) is important, and a PA catheter allows accurate assessment of the cause of the circulatory problems and the patient's response to therapy. A list of the hemodynamic parameters useful in monitoring patients in shock is provided in Table 8–1.

For patients in hypovolemic shock, rapid replacement of circulating blood volume is crucial. As a general rule, fluid resuscitation is needed whenever the systolic BP is below 90 mm Hg and there are signs of vital organ dysfunction (e.g., abnormal sensorium).[2] When the patient has lost large amounts of blood, it is ideal to use blood as the replacement. When there is no time to type and cross-match blood, rapid infusion of a volume expander (e.g., Ringer's lactate, normal saline, hetastarch) supports circulation until definitive treatment is available.

Antibiotics and volume expansion are essential for patients in septic shock. The source of the infection should be sought and may include surgical sites, wounds, indwelling catheters, and tubes, in addition to common infections such as pneumonia, urinary tract infection, and sinusitis. Volume expansion improves BP by filling the void created by the peripheral vasodilatation associated with sepsis. Vasopressors such as dopamine or norepinephrine improve hypotension by partially reversing the vasodilatation caused by sepsis and by stimulating cardiac contractility and therefore improving cardiac output. (See Chapter 10 for a discussion on the treatment of heart failure.)

CASE STUDY

History

Mr. E is 46-year-old white man brought to the emergency room by ambulance following a gunshot wound to the abdomen. The patient was found by the emergency medical technicians outside a local bar lying on his side in a pool of blood. At the scene of the shooting, the patient was found semiconscious with a pulse rate of 128/minute, a breathing rate of 32/minute, and a BP of 95/60 mm Hg. The single gunshot wound was stabilized by the ambulance crew and an intravenous (IV) infusion with normal saline was initiated prior to transfer to the hospital. At the emergency room Mr. E's vitals were as follows: pulse thready at 130/minute, respiratory rate 34/minute, and BP 80/50 mm Hg. Mr. E was semiconscious and disoriented. His skin was cool and clammy to the touch with peripheral cyanosis noted. Breath sounds and heart sounds were normal. His abdomen was distended and bowel sounds were absent. Neurologic status was grossly intact. Past medical and family history was not available.

QUESTIONS

1. What is indicated by the cool, cyanotic extremities? What is suggested by the thready pulse?
2. What is indicated by the abnormal sensorium?
3. Is oxygen therapy indicated, and if so, at what F_{IO_2}?
4. What is your assessment of the patient's condition? Is shock present? If shock is present, what is the most likely type of shock?

5. Should the patient be intubated and mechanically ventilated?

6. What is the patient's most urgent need for care at this point?

ANSWERS

1. Cool, cyanotic extremities indicate poor perfusion. Peripheral vasoconstriction is a compensatory mechanism in which the body attempts to preserve blood flow to the central, vital organs whenever BP decreases below a critical level. This results in the patient's feet and hands feeling cool to the touch. Peripheral cyanosis occurs when the tissues extract excessive amounts of oxygen from the slowly passing blood, leaving it very desaturated. The thready pulse indicates that this patient's stroke volume is abnormally low.

2. The abnormal sensorium may indicate that the brain is not receiving optimal oxygenation. In this case this is probably the result of inadequate perfusion to the brain, which occurs when the MAP drops below 90 mm Hg.[2]

3. Oxygen therapy is useful whenever the patient demonstrates signs of circulatory or respiratory failure. An FIO_2 of ≥ 0.40 would be most appropriate.

4. There is evidence of vital organ dysfunction (an abnormal sensorium), most likely as a result of poor circulation. The patient is most likely suffering from hypovolemic shock due to blood loss from the gunshot wound (Table 8-2).

5. Mechanical ventilation is not indicated at this point, since there is no evidence of respiratory failure and the patient may respond rapidly to treatment. Intubation may be useful if the patient's mental status deteriorates to the point that he may aspirate if vomiting occurs.

6. The patient's most urgent need is surgical repair of internal bleeding and replacement of the blood lost by hemorrhage. A blood sample should be obtained immediately for cross-matching so that the appropriate blood type can be given. A volume-expanding fluid must be given in large amounts until the cross-matching has been done. Additionally, the patient will need to be taken to the operating room to repair internal injuries related to the gunshot wound.

CASE STUDY—continued

The patient was given oxygen via simple face mask, and a follow-up arterial blood gas (ABG) revealed: pH 7.41, PCO_2 34 mm Hg, PO_2 98 mm Hg. A CVP catheter was placed and demonstrated a reading of 2 cm H_2O. The patient was taken to the operating room, where the inferior vena cava and portions of the small bowel were repaired. A total of 4 units of whole blood and 3 liters of normal saline were given to the patient.

Upon return to the ICU the patient assessment revealed the following: BP 125/75 mm Hg; pulse 96/minute; respiratory rate 14/minute via mechanical ventilation with a tidal volume of 1000 mL; and an FIO_2 of 0.45. ABGs showed a pH of 7.47, a PCO_2 of 33 mm Hg, and a PaO_2 of 110 mm Hg. CVP was 6 cm H_2O, and his body temperature via rectal probe was 36.5°C (97.7°F). A urinary catheter was in place, and urine output was 50 mL for the 2 hours of surgery. The patient was nonresponsive because of the effects of general anesthesia. His peripheral pulses were normal, and his hands and feet were warmer than they had been before surgery.

QUESTIONS

7. What is your assessment of Mr. E's circulatory status following the surgery?

8. Interpret the ABG findings following surgery. What changes in the ventilator settings do you recommend?

9. When should weaning from the mechanical ventilation begin?

10. What are complications of circulatory shock that might occur in this patient?

ANSWERS

7. Mr. E's circulatory status following surgery appears to be improved. This is based on the fact that his peripheral pulses, BP, CVP, and urine output are adequate and his extremities warmer.

8. The ABGs reveal a respiratory alkalosis with a supernormal oxygenation on a FIO_2 of 0.45. This suggests that the FIO_2 and the minute volume could be decreased. A decrease in the minute volume can be accomplished by decreasing the tidal volume or by decreasing the ventilator rate. Keeping the tidal volume in the range of 10 to 15 mL/kg is helpful in reducing the incidence of atelectasis. For this reason, reducing the ventilator rate would probably be optimal in this case.

9. Weaning from mechanical ventilation can begin as soon as the patient recovers from the effects of the general anesthesia. Evidence of recovery includes increased mental acuity, ability to follow commands, and a return of reflexes (e.g., gag reflex). Since there is no evidence of prior respiratory disease, the patient will probably not need the ventilator after he wakes up from the anesthesia.

10. The patient is at risk for ARDS (see Chapter 13), DIC, renal failure, sepsis, and postoperative atelectasis (see Chapter 15 for a discussion of postoperative atelectasis).

CASE STUDY—continued

Mr. E was weaned from mechanical ventilation during the next 3 hours without difficulties. ABGs on a FIO_2 of 0.35 via entrainment mask demonstrated a pH of 7.43, PCO_2 of 36 mm Hg, and a PO_2 of 88 mm Hg. Because of the injury to his intestinal tract, Mr. E was given IV feeding to meet his nutritional needs. Mr. E's only complaint at this time was abdominal pain related to the gunshot and subsequent surgery. The pain was controlled by IV morphine.

Over the next 3 days Mr. E continued to improve. His hemodynamic status was stable with normal sensorium, BP, urine output, and vital signs. At the end of the third hospital day, Mr. E began to complain of intermittent fever, chills, and general malaise. He subsequently became restless and somewhat confused. Physical examination at this time revealed the following findings.

Physical Examination

General: Patient awake but slow to respond and confused; appears to be in mild respiratory distress.

Vital Signs: Body temperature 38.5°C (101.3°F), respiratory rate 32/minute, pulse rate 124/minute, and BP 85/50 mm Hg.

HEENT: Normal findings.

Neck: Trachea midline, mobile, with no stridor; carotid pulses ++ with no bruits; no lymphadenopathy, thyromegaly, or jugular venous distention noted; accessory muscles of breathing not being used.

Chest: Normal anteroposterior diameter and bilateral expansion noted with breathing; resonance to percussion normal bilaterally.

Lungs: Rapid, shallow breathing noted; breath sounds normal in the mid and upper lung regions but diminished in the bases posteriorly with end-inspiratory crackles.

Heart: Regular rhythm with a rate of 124/minute; no murmurs or heaves noted; point of maximum impulse not palpable.

Abdomen: Slightly distended, tender, and no bowel sounds noted; no masses or organomegaly noted.

Extremities: No clubbing, cyanosis, or edema; pulses weak but present bilaterally; extremities warm to the touch

Because of the concern for Mr. E's hemodynamic status, a PA catheter was inserted. Hemodynamic and clinical measurements at this time revealed the following:

Cardiac Output: 6.0 liters/minute

Urine Output: 15 mL/hour

Plasma Lactate: 3.5 mg/dL

Pao_2: 70 mm Hg on Fio_2 of 0.35

$Paco_2$: 26 mm Hg

Plasma Bicarbonate: 16 mEq/liter

Arterial pH: 7.32

SVR: 675 dynes-sec/cm^5

PCWP: 7 mm Hg

CVP: 4 mm Hg

QUESTIONS

11. Is there evidence of circulatory failure? If so, what is it?
12. What do the ABG findings suggest? Are they consistent with the circulatory picture? If so, how? Does the acid-base status influence cardiac performance?
13. How do you interpret the SVR? What could cause this finding?
14. How do you interpret the PCWP?
15. How would you classify this type of circulatory problem?
16. What therapy is indicated at this time?
17. What laboratory tests would you suggest be obtained at this time?
18. If Mr. E's body surface area is 1.7 m^2, what is his cardiac index? If cardiac output is 6.0 liters/minute and heart rate 124/minute, what is the stroke volume?

ANSWERS

11. Circulatory failure is present despite the normal cardiac output. Evidence to support this is found in the abnormal sensorium, reduced urine output, and elevated plasma lactate.

12. The ABGs suggest metabolic acidosis partially compensated for by hyperventilation. The patient also suffers from mild hypoxemia on 35 percent oxygen. The metabolic acidosis and hypoxemia are consistent with circulatory failure. Lactic acidosis due to anaerobic metabolism is common in circulatory failure and suggests a more severe case. Metabolic acidosis has a negative inotropic effect on the heart. Hypoxemia is common in patients in shock and in those who are bedridden following surgery. In this case, the hypoxia is probably the result of atelectasis and shunting.

13. The SVR is markedly reduced. The peripheral vasodilatation is probably due to the release of chemical mediators (endotoxins) into the circulation from the infecting microorganism.

14. The PCWP is at the lower end of normal limits. Most patients will have a better stroke volume if the PCWP is in the range of 12 to 16 mm Hg.

15. This type of clinical picture suggests circulatory failure due to sepsis or septic shock. This assessment is based on the fever, low SVR, and high cardiac output (Table 8–2).

16. Therapy should be aimed at improving the perfusion of vital organs. Even though the cardiac output is in normal range, blood flow to many organs is insufficient as a result of the vasodilatation and precapillary AV shunting. Giving IV fluids could help to increase the MAP and perfusion pressure by improving preload. Antibiotics are needed to treat the sepsis. Increasing the FIO_2 is needed to correct the hypoxemia. A vasopressor such as dopamine may be useful to increase the perfusion pressure if the patient does not respond adequately to fluid therapy. This patient will need close monitoring, since he is at high risk for respiratory failure and would then need intubation and positive pressure breathing (see Chapter 13).

17. Laboratory tests that could be useful to assess this patient include an ECG, chest x-ray, complete blood count (CBC), blood cultures, and electrolytes. ABGs should be repeated if there is evidence of respiratory problems.

18. Mr. E's cardiac index (CI) is 3.5 liters/minute per m². This is calculated by dividing the body surface area (BSA) into the cardiac output (CO), as follows:

$$CI = \frac{CO}{BSA} = \frac{6.0 \text{ liters/minute}}{1.7 \text{ m}^2} = 3.5 \text{ liters/minute per m}^2$$

The stroke volume (SV) is calculated by dividing the heart rate into the cardiac output:

$$SV = \frac{6000 \text{ mL/minute}}{124/\text{minute}} = 48 \text{ mL}$$

Laboratory Evaluation

ECG: Sinus tachycardia with no evidence of ST-segment depression or elevation.

Chest X-ray: Diminished lung volumes with normal heart size. No evidence of infiltrates or pulmonary edema.

Electrolytes:

Na^+ 140 mEq/L

K^+ 3.6 mEq/L

HCO_3^- 17 mEq/L

Cl^- 102 mEq mEq/L

CBC:

WBC 18,500/mm^3

60 percent segmented neutrophils

8 percent bands

CASE STUDY—continued

Following the administration of fluids, the patient's PCWP increased to 12 cm H_2O and cardiac output increased to 6.5 liters/minute. SVR was measured at 660 dynes/sec per cm^5. Intravenous gentamicin and piperacillin were started. $P\bar{v}O_2$ was measured at 42 mm Hg. The patient remained semiconscious with a BP of 90/52 mm Hg, respiratory rate of 34/minute, and a pulse rate of 130/minute. His rectal temperature was measured at 38.5°C (101.3°F).

QUESTIONS

19. Calculate the anion gap for this patient and state what the results indicate.
20. What are the potential sources of the infection?
21. Should the patient be intubated and mechanically ventilated?
22. How is the effectiveness of the fluid therapy evaluated?
23. What is indicated by the $P\bar{v}O_2$ of 42 mm Hg?
24. What is the significance of the patient having a elevated body temperature? How does this influence his clinical condition?
25. What therapy is needed at this point?

ANSWERS

19. The anion gap is calculated by subtracting the HCO_3^- and Cl^- from the Na^+ (140 − 102 − 17 = 21). An anion gap of 21 is elevated above normal and indicates the presence of metabolic acidosis due to (in this case) lactic acidosis.
20. Potential sources of the infection include the abdominal wound and the IV feeding line.
21. Since this patient is not expected to recover quickly and oxygenation is marginal on supplemental oxygen, this patient could benefit from intubation and mechanical ventilation.
22. The fluid therapy is evaluated with a combination of hemodynamic parameters such as PCWP, BP, and cardiac output and by looking for evidence of improved organ perfusion (e.g., increased urine output).

Evidence of better vital organ perfusion includes improved urine output and sensorium. In this case it appears that the fluid therapy did not improve BP and vital organ perfusion despite an increase in cardiac output. This is typical for septic shock, in which maldistribution of circulation is prevalent.

23. A $P\bar{v}O_2$ of 42 mm Hg is considered in the normal range and often indicates that tissue oxygenation is optimal. In this case, however, the normal $P\bar{v}O_2$ may be misleading because septic shock causes precapillary shunting and often results in an inappropriately increased $P\bar{v}O_2$ Since there is evidence that tissue oxygenation is less than optimal in this case, the $P\bar{v}O_2$ must be inappropriately elevated.

24. The elevated body temperature is significant because this results in an increased metabolic rate and adds to the problems created by circulatory failure.

25. Since volume expansion alone did not significantly improve BP, the use of a vasopressor is needed. Dopamine would be a good vasopressor at this time because it would also increase cardiac contractility and blood flow to the kidneys.

CASE STUDY—continued

Over the next several days the patient responded well to therapy despite the onset of respiratory failure due to ARDS (see Chapter 13). His hemodynamic status improved with the use of vasopressors and fluid therapy. He was eventually weaned from vasopressors and mechanical ventilation and transferred to the general care unit on the 12th hospital day.

REFERENCES

1. Daily, EK, and Schroeder, JP: Techniques in Bedside Hemodynamic Monitoring, ed 4., CV Mosby, St. Louis, 1989, pp 88–150.
2. Schuster, DP, and Lefrak, SS: Shock. In Civetta, JM, et al (eds): Critical Care. JB Lippincott, Philadelphia, 1988, pp 891–908.
3. Parillo, JE: Septic shock in humans: Clinical evaluation, pathogenesis, and therapeutic approach. In Shoemaker, WC (ed): Textbook of Critical Care, ed 2. WB Saunders, Philadelphia, 1989, pp 1006–1023.
4. Marini, JJ, and Wheeler, AP: Critical Care Medicine: The Essentials. Williams & Wilkins, Baltimore, 1989, p 31.
5. Shoemaker, WC: Shock states: Pathophysiology, monitoring, outcome prediction and therapy. In Shoemaker, WC (ed): Textbook of Critical Care, ed 2. WB Saunders, Philadelphia, 1989, pp 977–992.
6. Marino, PL: The ICU Book. Philadelphia, Lea & Febiger, 1991, p 174.

CHAPTER **9**

Pulmonary Thromboembolic Disease

Kenneth D. McCarty, MS, RRT

Key Terms

angiography
anticoagulation
heparin

infarction
pulmonary
  thromboembolism

thrombi
thrombosis

Introduction

Pulmonary thromboembolism is a relatively common disorder affecting approximately 500,000 persons a year in the United States.[1] Pulmonary thromboembolism refers to the vascular obstruction (embolization) of the pulmonary vessels by blood clots (**thrombi**) that have traveled through the venous system to the lungs. Other materials such as fat deposits, air, tumor fragments, and amniotic fluid can produce an embolus.[1,2] This chapter discusses the most common form of embolism, thromboembolism.

Etiology and Pathology

Three main factors are associated with the formation of deep venous thrombi: hypercoagulability, damage to the endothelial wall of the blood vessel, and venostasis.[1,2] *Hypercoagulability* is a factor in emboli caused by genetic deficiencies in antithrombin III, protein S, and protein C, and lupus anticoagulant; in rare cases, it occurs in patients with homocystinuria and fibrinolytic abnormalities.[1,3-6] Fractures and surgical procedures, along with trauma, are common causes of *venous blood vessel damage.* Stasis of venous blood flow (*venostasis*) is common in many circumstances that promote physical immobilization, such as surgery, fractures, and prolonged illness.

Risk factors for deep venous **thrombosis** (DVT) include age (greater than 70 years old), obesity, congestive heart failure, malignancy, burns, use of estrogen-containing drugs, and postoperative and postpartum states. These factors are additive in effect.[1]

Although thromboemboli may form at almost any site, approximately 95 percent originate in the deep veins of the lower extremities, the remainder forming in pelvic veins. Emboli rarely arise from the upper extremities or as a result of indwelling cardiac catheters.[7] The embolic risk increases if thrombosis occurs in veins above the knee.[8,9] Thrombi generally occur at the site of turbulent blood flow at the venous valves or at sites of endothelial (intimal) damage. With stasis, coagulation activity is localized, and hence produces a red-fibrin thrombosis. This thrombus may then be dislodged and carried to the lungs. Risk of embolism appears highest within 72 hours after the development of DVT.[1]

The pathologic changes in the lung are related to both the magnitude of the occlusion and the subsequent degree of compromised pulmonary blood supply. Small thromboemboli may cause little or no injury to the distal lung tissue, whereas large thromboemboli may disrupt blood flow enough to injure lung parenchyma (*infarction*).

Pathophysiology

Pulmonary vascular obstruction due to thromboembolism may affect both respiratory and hemodynamic systems.[1] Vascular occlusion by a large thrombus decreases perfusion of the affected pulmonary vascular bed and initially leads to parenchymal areas with more ventilation than perfusion (alveolar dead space). Local bronchoconstriction also typically accompanies pulmonary embolism.[1] The release of cellular mediators such as serotonin, histamine, and prostaglandins from platelets, local areas of alveolar hypocapnia, and hypoxemia are thought to be involved in causing the bronchoconstriction, although the exact etiology is unknown.[1,10,11]

Bronchospasm may also cause hypoxemia during a pulmonary embolism by producing ventilation-perfusion ($\dot{V}/\dot{Q}$) mismatching. Although the entire cause of emboli-induced hypoxemia is unclear, many factors are probably involved, including venous shunting and reduced cardiac output resulting in an increased arterial-venous oxygen difference and worsened venous admixture.[1] Obstruction of blood flow to the lung tissue results in a decrease in surfactant production about 24 hours after the embolization.[12] This leads to decreased pulmonary compliance, atelectasis, and further $\dot{V}/\dot{Q}$ mismatching and hypoxemia.

Vascular occlusion and vasoconstriction cause an increase in pulmonary vascular resistance (PVR).[1] Cardiac output is maintained only by increased right ventricular work and hence pulmonary artery pressures (PAPs). If the output of the right ventricle falls, filling of the left heart diminishes, resulting in systemic hypotension and eventual cardiovascular collapse. Approximately 50 percent or more occlusion of the pulmonary vasculature, however, must occur in previously healthy individuals before sustained pulmonary hypertension develops and cardiac output falls.[13]

The severity of the hemodynamic compromise depends not only on the magnitude of the embolism but also on the patient's preexisting cardiovascular and pulmonary status.[14] Pulmonary or cardiovascular diseases that limit the pulmonary vascular reserve, such as congestive heart failure, chronic obstructive pulmonary disease (COPD), and aortic or mitral valve disease, frequently result in greater than expected pulmonary hypertension compared to otherwise healthy patients.

Although pulmonary infarction is a potential consequence of thromboembolism, death of lung tissue owing to ischemia is uncommon because there is usually some perfusion past the embolus, collateral blood flow via bronchial arteries, and oxygenation from the airways.[1] Pulmonary infarction is more likely in patients with left ventricular failure or COPD,[15] probably because of reduced cardiac output or reduced collateral blood flow, respectively.[13,16]

Natural resolution of the thromboembolus begins shortly after the clot lodges in the lung.[1,10] *Fibrinolysis* is the process of clot destruction in which blood-borne and vascular endothelial factors, such as tissue plasminogen activator, act to dissolve the clot. Clot resolution involves organization of the thrombus, attachment to the vascular wall, and return of blood flow. Resolution usually results in complete or partial return of flow within 7 to 10 days. Perfusion can be restored with as little as 20 percent of the vessel diameter being patent.[1]

Clinical Features

The clinical symptoms of pulmonary thromboembolism are nonspecific, and emboli may occur without causing symptoms.[1,13,16] Therefore it is important to have a high index of suspicion, especially if risk factors are present.[1,17]

The most common symptom associated with pulmonary embolism is transient acute dyspnea (Table 9-1).[18] Although rare, pleuritic chest pain and hemoptysis indicate pulmonary infarction and pleural involvement. Syncope, although uncommon, suggests large clots and severe hemodynamic compromise.[10] A sense of impending doom is a potential symptom and may be associated with large emboli and hypotension.[1]

Physical examination of the patient with thromboembolism most commonly reveals tachypnea, tachycardia, and mild fever (Table 9-2).[18] Inspection of the patient is most often normal, but if clots are large, there may be findings suggesting right ven-

TABLE 9-1 **Common Symptoms in Pulmonary Thromboembolism**

Symptom	*% Occurrence*
Dyspnea	73
Pleuritic pain	66
Cough	37
Leg swelling	28
Leg pain	26
Hemoptysis	13
Palpitations	10
Wheezing	9
Angina-like pain	4

SOURCE: Adapted from and used by permission of Stein, PD, et al: Clinical, laboratory, roentgenographic, and electrocardiographic findings in patients with acute pulmonary embolism and no pre-existing cardiac or pulmonary disease. Chest 100(3):598, 1991.

TABLE 9-2   **Common Signs of Pulmonary Thromboembolism**

Sign	% Occurrence
Tachypnea ($\geq$20/minute)	70
Crackles	51
Tachycardia ($\geq$100/minute)	30
Increased P_2	23
Diaphoresis	11
Fever	7
Pleural friction rub	3
Cyanosis	1

SOURCE: Adapted from and used by permission of Stein, PD, et al: Clinical, laboratory, roentgenographic, and electrocardiographic findings in patients with acute pulmonary embolism and no pre-existing cardiac or pulmonary disease. Chest 100(3):598, 1991.

tricular strain (e.g., jugular venous distention). The lower extremities are often normal but may reveal swelling and tenderness associated with DVT. The patient's breath sounds may be normal or may reveal localized wheezing or crackles.[18] A pleural friction rub may also be heard, particularly if infarction involving the pleura is present. Percussion of the chest wall is usually normal. Auscultation of the heart may identify loud pulmonic valve closure (P_2) as part of the second heart sound (S_2), S_2 splitting, and a possible S_3 or S_4.[18]

Hemodynamic and Laboratory Data

The insertion of a balloon-tipped, flow-directed catheter classically reveals an increased PAP, and central venous pressure (CVP), and a normal or low pulmonary capillary wedge pressure (PCWP). A low PCWP occurs when significant occlusion of the pulmonary vasculature leads to inadequate filling of the left side of the heart.

The chest radiograph is often normal, or it may show only nonspecific abnormalities such as signs of volume loss or pleural effusion, which are most often located in the mid to lower lung fields (Fig. 9-1). Pulmonary vascular distention may be caused by pulmonary hypertension. A subtle, localized vascular narrowing in the area of decreased perfusion distal to the emboli may be evident ("Westermark's sign").[10,18]

Arterial blood gases (ABGs) commonly show an uncompensated respiratory alkalosis with mild to moderate hypoxemia on room air and an increased alveolar-arterial oxygen gradient.[1,10] The electrocardiogram is useful in determining the differential diagnosis, particularly in ruling out a myocardial infarction.[1] In pulmonary embolism it is frequently normal or reveals sinus tachycardia.[1,18] Changes indicating acute right heart strain, such as right axis deviation and P pulmonale, occur relatively infrequently, whereas the presence of premature ventricular contractions is a more common finding.[10,18]

$\dot{V}/\dot{Q}$ scans demonstrate the difference between the alveolar distribution of inhaled radioactive xenon-133 and pulmonary capillary distribution of albumin radioactively labeled with iodine or technetium. Healthy patients have an even distribution of ventilation and perfusion. Typical findings of a pulmonary embolus include normal ventilation, but segmental or lobar defects in perfusion. Matching defects in ventilation and perfusion, such as those that occur with pneumonia, are nondiagnostic of pulmonary embolism. A normal perfusion scan effectively rules out thromboembolism.[1,19] Normal ventilation in the presence of at least two segmental defects or one lobar defect in perfusion indicates a high probability that pulmonary embolism is present.[1]

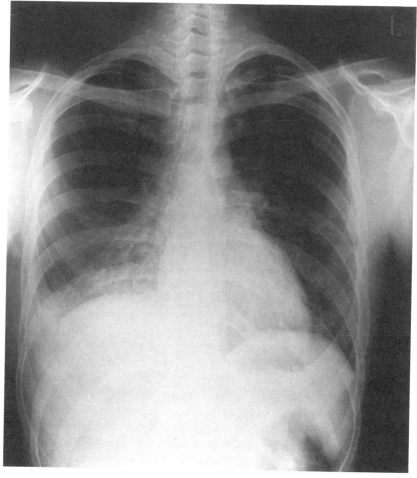

FIGURE 9-1   Chest radiograph of a patient with pulmonary embolism showing right hemidiaphragm elevation and right lower lobe radiopacity as a result of atelectasis.

Pulmonary angiography is the diagnostic gold standard and also demonstrates the extent of vascular involvement. A radiopaque contrast is introduced via catheter into the pulmonary artery (PA), and radiographs are taken as it circulates. Two signs are diagnostic of pulmonary emboli: (1) abrupt cut-off of a vessel and (2) intraluminal filling defects.[20] Angiography requires catheterization of large veins and catheter manipulation through the right heart. Because of complications such as dysrhythmias and hemorrhage associated with these maneuvers, pulmonary angiography should be used as a last resort. Newer diagnostic procedures being investigated include digital angiography, chest computed tomography, and fiberoptic angioscopy.[1]

Treatment and Prevention

Pulmonary thromboembolism therapy is aimed at treating the vascular occlusion and its pulmonary and hemodynamic consequences, and preventing the reoccurrence of emboli.

Anticoagulant therapy using subcutaneous or intravenous (IV) **heparin** is the most common initial form of treatment.[1] Heparin inactivates thrombin and clotting factor X and inhibits platelet aggregation, thereby inhibiting the formation of new thrombi.[21] Oral anticoagulants, such as the coumarin derivatives sodium warfarin (Coumadin) and dicumarol, inactivate the vitamin K-dependent clotting factors II, VII, IX, and X and are used for long-term therapy.[22] **Anticoagulation** caused by heparin therapy is monitored by the partial thromboplastin time (PTT); anticoagulation caused by the oral anticoagulants is monitored by the prothrombin time (PT).[10] Heparin is used initially and usually continued for 5 to 10 days until the PTT is stabilized in the therapeutic range. The duration of coumarin therapy varies, depending on the likelihood of clot recurrence. Patients with clots caused by easily identifiable insults and not associated with risk factors for recurrence are usually treated for 3 to 6 months, whereas recurrent clots may require years of therapy.

Although anticoagulants prevent new clot formation and the growth of already existing thrombi, they do relatively little to dissolve existing clots.[1] Thrombolytic agents such as streptokinase, urokinase, and tissue plasminogen activator dissolve fresh clots and help restore vascular patency. Since these agents affect any recently formed clots and therefore increase the risk of bleeding,[23] relative contraindications to their use include recent surgical procedures, ulcers, stroke, and childbirth. Thrombolytic agents are most often used in patients with thrombi causing significant hemodynamic compromise.[10] Thrombus treatment is most effective during the first 5 days after the embolus and is usually followed by heparin and then sodium warfarin therapy.

Surgical removal of massive pulmonary emboli is probably not more effective than thrombolytic therapy. It is used only as a last resort because the mortality rate following this procedure is approximately 60 percent.[10]

Since the advent of modern anticoagulant therapy, inferior vena caval interruption by surgical ligation, clips, or vena caval umbrella is less frequently performed. These procedures limit the entry of clots into the pulmonary vasculature by blocking their path of entry from the lower extremities.[1] Vena caval interruption is most useful if emboli recur after anticoagulation, or when anticoagulant therapy is contraindicated.[10]

In addition to specific therapy, patients with pulmonary thromboembolism may need additional supportive treatment. Respiratory care practitioners administer oxygen when hypoxemia is present. The elimination of carbon dioxide is rarely a problem; however, the patient may benefit from intubation and mechanical ventilation if a massive embolus causes respiratory failure. If hypotension develops, volume expansion and dopamine can be used to maintain adequate perfusing pressure.[10]

Because pulmonary thromboembolism is a relatively common and potentially severe problem, prophylaxis is important in high-risk patients. There is no proven prophylactic benefit to wearing standard elastic stockings and ambulating early after surgical procedures.[1] Three factors that have proved useful in preventing thromboembolism include low-dose heparin, sodium warfarin, and venous compression devices.[1] Two to three doses of heparin each day administered subcutaneously is effective in many patients at risk because of surgical immobilization and myocardial infarction. Likewise, sodium warfarin is commonly used after the initial heparin therapy to prevent recurring thrombosis. External venous compression devices, in which an air-filled cuff is alternately inflated and deflated, are effective in reducing thrombi formation in the lower legs. This modality is especially useful in patients who are at increased risk of bleeding as a result of anticoagulant therapy.

CASE STUDY

History

Mr. H is a 52-year-old Asian man who presents to the emergency room. His left leg is in a cast, and he states that 1 week ago he was in an automobile accident and broke his upper leg. Since that time he has had difficulty "getting around" and has mostly been lying on the couch watching television. On the evening of admission he noticed a sudden onset of dyspnea and chest pain. He denies having orthopnea, cough, hemoptysis, or wheezing. He routinely took iron supplements and occasionally aspirin, but no other medications. He smoked two packs of cigarettes a day for 19 years but quit 3 years ago.

QUESTIONS

1. What are the key pulmonary symptom(s) that the attending physician should explore in greater detail, and what problems do these symptoms suggest?

2. What further questions should the physician ask of the patient to aid in the differential diagnosis?

3. Why is the diagnosis of pulmonary embolism most likely?

ANSWERS

1. The key pulmonary symptoms in this case are dyspnea and chest pain. The sudden onset of the dyspnea and chest pain indicate an acute problem, rather than a chronic condition. Dyspnea and chest pain occur with pulmonary thromboemboli, pneumonia, myocardial infarction, and pneumothorax (Table 9–3).[13] Differentiation among these medical problems is extremely important because they are all potentially fatal diseases with similar symptoms, yet they require different treatment.

2. Pertinent questions should attempt to differentiate between the problems that cause chest pain and those that cause dyspnea. The interviewer should identify the risk factors and other symptoms present in this patient for each of the diseases listed in the differential diagnosis. Risk factors for DVT include those that promote stasis, injury to blood vessels, or increased coagulability of the blood. Other symptoms associated with DVT include fever, leg tenderness, and hemoptysis. Risk factors for heart disease include hypertension, smoking, high cholesterol, a high-stress life style, and lack of exercise. Other symptoms associated with heart disease include nausea,

TABLE 9–3   **Differential Diagnosis of Pulmonary Thromboembolism**

Pneumonia (bacterial or viral)
Pneumothorax
Aortic dissection
Tuberculosis
Acute pleuritis from:
    Collagen vascular disease
    Viral pleurisy
Myocardial infarction

diaphoresis, radiation of the chest pain to the shoulder or jaw, and exercise-related pain. Risk factors for pneumonia include immune deficiency disorders, poor nutrition, chronic lung disease, head injuries, and chronic health problems. Other symptoms associated with pneumonia include cough, fever, and sputum production. Pneumothorax may present with only pleuritic chest pain and dyspnea.

3. Two factors in the patient's history that favor the diagnosis of pulmonary embolism are trauma and immobilization. Trauma damages blood vessels and releases endothelial factors that promote clotting, whereas immobilization predisposes the patient to blood stasis.

Physical Examination

General: A well-nourished Asian male who is alert and oriented, anxious, and in mild respiratory distress

Vital Signs: Temperature 37.6°C (99.7°F) orally, respiratory rate 26/minute, pulse 110/minute, blood pressure 134/88 mm Hg

HEENT: Unremarkable

Neck: Supple with full active range of motion; trachea midline, mobile, and without stridor or wheezes; carotid pulses 3+, symmetric, and without bruits; no thryomegaly, jugular venous distention, or lymphadenopathy

Chest: Normal configuration and expansion with breathing

Lungs: Right middle lobe and right lower lobe late-inspiratory crackles revealed on auscultation

Heart: Regular rhythm, with a rate of 110/minute; a slightly increased S_2 (P_2) heard at the second intercostal space at the left sternal border; systolic heave located at the fourth intercostal space near the left border of the sternum

Abdomen: Nondistended, soft, nontender with no masses or organomegaly

Extremities: No cyanosis, digital clubbing, or peripheral edema; left leg in a cast

---

QUESTIONS

4. What is the significance of the patient's anxiety?

5. What is the significance of the patient's temperature?

6. What is the significance of the systolic heave noted at the left sternal border?

7. What is the cause of the patient's crackles?

8. What pathophysiology accounts for the louder P_2 component of the second heart sound?

9. What findings, if any, indicate the presence of hypoxemia?

ANSWERS

4. Anxiety and apprehension may be produced by any medical condition. They are relatively common symptoms of pulmonary emboli and are usually displayed by restlessness and irritability.[1,24] The etiology of these symptoms is unknown.

5. Although the presence of a fever is common with infections such as pneumonia, a low-grade fever is also a common finding in pulmonary embolism[1] and may help rule out other differential diagnoses, such as pneumothorax.

6. A heave is an abnormal pulsation occurring on the precordium, and when palpated at the left sternal border, is often caused by right ventricular hypertrophy. A right ventricular heave is indicative of pulmonary hypertension.[25] Many pulmonary vessels must be occluded before pulmonary hypertension develops. Therefore, a right ventricular heave indicates relatively severe disease.

7. Crackles are a common finding in patients with pulmonary emboli. Atelectasis is a common result of pulmonary embolism and is most likely responsible for the inspiratory crackles. Atelectasis may also be the cause of the fever if infection is present.

8. The P_2 portion of the second heart sound (S_2) represents pulmonic valve closure. An increased intensity of the P_2 portion of that sound is indicative of more forceful valve closure caused by pulmonary vascular hypertension. Obstruction of the pulmonary vessels by thromboemboli causes an increase in PAP, which results in the valve's snapping shut with more force.[25]

9. Although the patient is not cyanotic, more subtle signs of acute hypoxemia are present. Tachycardia and tachypnea are nonspecific cardiovascular and pulmonary responses to hypoxemia. The patient's anxiety might also indicate that he is hypoxemic.[25]

Laboratory Evaluation

Chest Radiograph: (Figs. 9–2 and 9–3)

ABGs (on Room Air):

pH 7.51

$Paco_2$ 30 mm Hg

Po_2 60 mm Hg

HCO_3^- 24 mEq/liter

base excess (BE) −1

Hb 13.1 g/100 mL

Sao_2 87.8 percent

Cao_2 15.6 vol%

$(A - a)o_2$ 52 mm Hg

Complete Blood Count: Results pending

Chemistry: Results pending

Electrocardiogram (ECG): Sinus tachycardia

QUESTIONS

10. What chest radiograph findings are consistent with pulmonary embolism? How do you interpret the chest radiographs (Figs. 9–2 and 9–3)?

11. What is the patient's acid-base and oxygenation status?

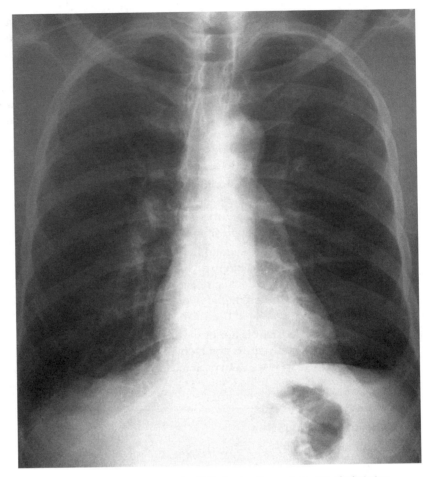

FIGURE 9-2 Anteroposterior (AP) chest radiograph on day of admission.

12. What treatment would you suggest at this time?

13. What other diagnostic information would be useful?

ANSWERS

10. Although the findings on the chest radiographs are frequently nonspecific for thromboembolism, hemidiaphragm elevation is common and is probably indicative of atelectasis.[1] The atelectasis is thought to occur as a result of bronchospasm, surfactant depletion, and underperfusion of alveolar spaces. Normally, most of the pulmonary perfusion is to the middle and lower lung fields. Most clots follow the perfusion to these areas, and as a result, atelectasis is most often found in the middle to lower lung fields.[1]

    Figures 9-2 and 9-3 demonstrate no significant abnormality, which is common for patients with pulmonary embolism.

11. The patient's acid-base status shows acute respiratory alkalosis. Moderate hypoxemia on room air is also present, which is common in patients with emboli. In addition, the arterial oxygen saturation (Sao_2) is low and the arterial oxygen content (Cao_2) slightly reduced. Because the calculation of Cao_2 includes Sao_2, Pao_2, and hemoglobin, it reflects oxygen-carrying

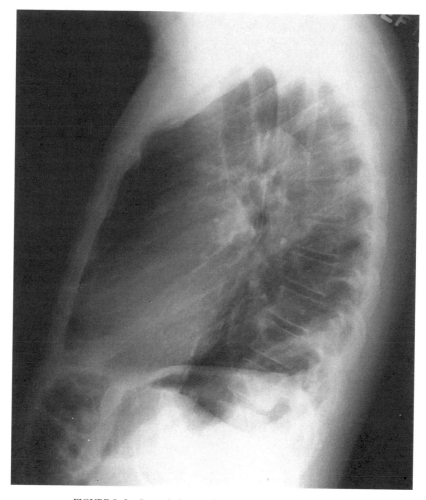

FIGURE 9-3   Lateral chest radiograph on day of admission.

capacity, which in this case is mildly reduced mostly owing to the low Sao_2. The alveolar-arterial oxygen gradient is increased as a result of the ventilated but underperfused regions of the lung affected by the embolus (dead space ventilation), resulting in $\dot{V}/\dot{Q}$ mismatch.

12. Treatment at this time should consist of oxygen therapy administered via nasal cannula to increase the patient's Pao_2 above 80 mm Hg. The physician should order IV anticoagulant therapy to prevent further thrombi. The use of thrombolytic agents is not indicated because of the relatively limited lung involvement and the absence of systemic hypotension. Should further embolization occur and cause hemodynamic compromise, the use of thrombolytic agents might be warranted.

13. The patient's history, physical, and diagnostic findings provide a presumptive diagnosis of pulmonary embolism. A $\dot{V}/\dot{Q}$ scan might be useful to confirm the diagnosis. Pulmonary angiography would better document the exact location and extent of the embolism, but is not necessary under these circumstances.

A day later, after having a V̇/Q̇ scan (Fig. 9–4) and while ambulating around the unit, the patient stated that he was feeling "worse" and having trouble breathing. He was acting very agitated and was slightly confused. There was no change in the physical examination findings, except that he was pale, his skin was cool and clammy, and his blood pressure was 88/45 mm Hg.

QUESTIONS

14. What is the significance of the results of the V̇/Q̇ scan?
15. Of what significance is the change in the patient's mental status?
16. What pathophysiology accounts for the patient's hypotension?
17. What therapy is indicated at this time?
18. Should the patient be admitted to the ICU?

ANSWERS

14. V̇/Q̇ scans depict the relative matching of ventilation to perfusion in the lung. In this case, segmental decrease in perfusion compared to ventilation in otherwise healthy lungs suggests vascular occlusion by pulmonary emboli. Unfortunately, other problems such as vasculitis, vasospasm, vessel

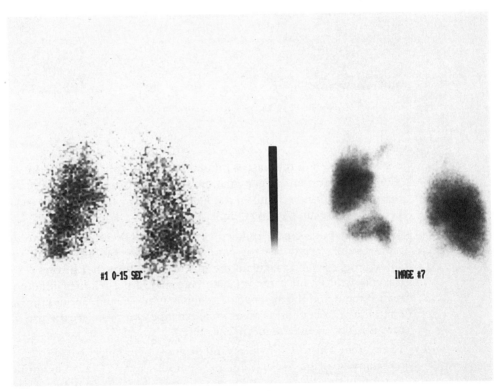

FIGURE 9–4 Ventilation-perfusion (V̇/Q̇) scan (ventilation scan on left, perfusion scan on right) one day after admission, showing scattered reduced perfusion compared to ventilation on the right and left sides.

destruction, and neoplastic vascular compression can reduce perfusion and result in similar findings during $\dot{V}/\dot{Q}$ scanning.[10]

15. Agitation, confusion, anxiety, and restlessness are all nonspecific symptoms associated with severe diseases, including pulmonary embolism. The sudden change in mental status most likely indicates a deterioration in perfusion and oxygenation of the brain and in this case most likely represents the formation of another pulmonary embolus.

16. Systemic hypotension in this case is a result of pulmonary vascular occlusion by thrombi. The vascular occlusion causes increased PVR, reduced right ventricular output, and corresponding decrease in left ventricular filling, cardiac output, and systemic blood pressure.

17. Oxygen therapy and anticoagulant therapy are still indicated. An increased fraction of inspired oxygen (FIO_2) is useful in this case because hemodynamics are marginal. In addition, thrombolytics may be necessary to induce rapid clot breakdown and aid the maintenance of cardiovascular hemodynamics.

18. The patient should be admitted to the intensive care unit (ICU) for close monitoring and definitive therapy. Massive pulmonary emboli are life threatening and require aggressive treatment.

Laboratory Evaluation

The attending physician inserted a PA catheter and ordered another chest radiograph and ABG analysis. The results were as follows:

PA Catheter Data:

CVP = 16 mm Hg

PAP = 45/32 mm Hg

PCWP = 4 mm Hg

Cardiac output 2.7 liters/minute

Cardiac index 1.6 liters/minute per m²

ABGs: (on 6 liters/minute O_2 by simple mask)

pH 7.37

$PaCO_2$ 30 mm Hg

PaO_2 54 mm Hg

BE −5

HCO_3^- 16 mEq/liter

Hb 13.5 g/100 mL

SaO_2 86 percent

CaO_2 15.8 vol%

QUESTIONS

19. What is the significance of the PA catheter measurements, and why is the cardiac output low?

20. What is the patient's prognosis?

21. What could explain the metabolic acidosis shown by the ABGs?

ANSWERS

19. The CVP and PAP are both elevated as a result of the pulmonary vascular obstruction that causes pulmonary hypertension. This causes an acute increase in right ventricular work and predisposes the patient to right ventricular failure. Cardiac output and cardiac index are reduced as a result of acute right ventricular failure, which reduces left ventricular filling (as evidenced by the low PCWP). These measurements indicate life-threatening disease with right heart failure.

20. The patient has a life-threatening problem that requires urgent treatment. Fatalities usually occur within the first hour after the embolus occurs. If the patient survives longer than 1 hour and appropriate treatment is initiated, there is relatively good chance of survival.[24]

21. The metabolic acidosis is most likely due to lactic acidosis. This is common in patients who have reduced cardiac output and tissue hypoxia, which leads to anaerobic metabolism and the production of lactic acid.

CASE STUDY—continued

The patient was admitted to the ICU and started on thrombolytic therapy, low-dose heparin therapy, and high-flow oxygen therapy. Within 24 hours of initiating thrombolytic therapy, the patient's hemodynamic parameters normalized. Over the next several days the patient gradually improved, and on day 4 he was able to maintain adequate oxygenation via nasal cannula at 3 liters/minute. The remainder of his hospital stay was uneventful, and on day 7 he was discharged on a regimen of sodium warfarin therapy.

REFERENCES

1. Moser, KM: Pulmonary embolism. In Murray, JF, and Nadel, JA (eds): Textbook of Respiratory Medicine. WB Saunders, Philadelphia, 1994, p 1652.
2. Mergher, WJ, and Trump, BF: Hemodynamic disorders. In Rubin, E, and Farber, JI (eds): Pathology, ed 3. JB Lippincott, Philadelphia, 1994, p 264.
3. Griffin, JH, et al.: Deficiency of protein C in congenital thrombotic disease. J Clin Invest 68:1370, 1981.
4. Comp, PC, and Esmon, CT: Recurrent venous thrombosis in patients with a partial deficiency of protein S. N Engl J Med 311:1525, 1984.
5. Egeberg, O: Inherited antithrombin deficiency causing thrombophilia. Thromb Diath Haem 13:516, 1965.
6. Wohl, RC, et al.: Physiologic activation of the human fibrinolytic system: Isolation and characterization of human plasminogen variants. J Biol Chem 254:9063, 1979.
7. Monreal, M, et al: Upper extremity deep venous thrombosis and pulmonary embolism. Chest 99:280, 1991.
8. Havig, GO: Source of pulmonary emboli. Acta Chir Scand 478:42, 1977.
9. Moser, KM, and LeMoine, JR: Is embolic risk conditioned by location of deep venous thrombosis? Ann Intern Med 94:439, 1981.
10. West, JW: Pulmonary embolism. In Wu, K (ed): Pathophysiology and Management of Thromboembolic Disorders. PGS Publishing, Littleton, MA, 1984, p 351.
11. Severinghaus, JW, et al.: Unilateral hypoventilation produced by occlusion of one pulmonary artery. J Appl Physiol 16:53, 1961.
12. Chernik, V, et al.: Effect of chronic pulmonary artery ligation on pulmonary mechanics and surfactant. J Appl Physiol 21:1315, 1966.
13. Moser, KM: Pulmonary embolism. Am Rev Respir Dis 115:829, 1977.
14. McIntyre, KM, and Sasahara, AA: Determinants of right ventricular function and hemodynamics after pulmonary embolism. Chest 65:534, 1974.
15. Dalen, JE, et al.: Pulmonary embolism, pulmonary hemorrhage, and pulmonary infarction. N Engl J Med 296:1431, 1977.
16. LeMoine, JR, and Moser, KM: Leg scanning with radioisotope-labeled fibrinogen in patients undergoing hip surgery. JAMA 243:2035, 1980.
17. Dalen, JE: Clinical diagnosis of acute pulmonary embolism: When should a scan be ordered? Chest 100(5):1185, 1991.
18. Stein, PD, et al.: Clinical, laboratory, roentgenographic, and electrocardiographic findings in

patients with acute pulmonary embolism and no pre-existing cardiac or pulmonary disease. Chest 100(3):598, 1991.

19. Kipper, MS, et al: Long-term follow up of patients with suspected embolism and a normal lung scan. Chest 82:411, 1982.

20. Sharma, GV, and Sasahara, AA: Diagnosis and treatment of pulmonary embolism. Med Clin North Am 63:239, 1979.

21. Wessler, S, and Gitel, SN: Heparin: New concepts relevant to clinical use. Blood 53:525, 1979.

22. Moser, KM, and Fedullo, PF: Venous thromboembolism: three simple decisions. Chest

83:117, 256, 1983.

23. Goldhaber, SZ, et al: Pooled analysis of randomized trials of streptokinase and heparin in phlebographically documented acute deep venous thrombosis. Am J Med 76:393, 1984.

24. Hinshaw, HC, and Murray, JF: Pulmonary thromboembolism. In Hinshaw, HC, and Murray, JF (eds): Diseases of the Chest. Philadelphia, WB Saunders, 1979, p 653.

25. Wilkins, RL: Techniques of physical examination. In Wilkins, RL, et al (eds): Clinical Assessment in Respiratory Care, ed 3. CV Mosby, St Louis, 1995.

CHAPTER **10**

Heart Failure

George H. Hicks, MS, RRT

Key Terms

cardiac output ($\dot{Q}_T$)
cardiomegaly
congestive heart failure
 (CHF)
cor pulmonale

diuretics
edema
Frank-Starling response
inotropic drugs
nocturnal dyspnea

orthopnea
pedal edema
stroke volume (SV)
ventricular hypertrophy

Introduction

Heart failure is a condition that results in the heart's inability to pump adequate blood flow to meet the metabolic needs of the body. In the United States, about 400,000 cases of heart diseases are diagnosed annually, and more than 4 million people are thought to suffer from heart failure and its complications.[1,2] Approximately 50 percent of those with heart failure die within the first 2 years after diagnosis.[3] This mortality rate is associated with multiorgan failure secondary to poor blood flow and organ congestion.

Physiologically, the heart in failure is unable to maintain an adequate cardiac output despite appropriate venous return. As a consequence, hypoperfusion and vascular congestion occur. The clinical manifestations are dependent on which side of the heart (left or right) is in failure and to what extent the cardiovascular system has been able to compensate. Patients in heart failure can therefore have varying degrees of acute or chronic conditions, depending on the magnitude of failure and their bodies' ability to compensate for the failure.

The term **congestive heart failure (CHF)** is frequently used in making the diagnosis of heart failure due to a large set of symptoms resulting from many different causes and triggering factors. In general, CHF results in an accumulation of fluid in the lungs (pulmonary edema) and dependent extremities as a consequence of left heart failure. **Cor pulmonale** is the term used to describe right heart enlargement and failure as a result of primary pulmonary disease.

Etiology

The factors that increase a person's risk for heart disease and failure include hypertension, diabetes, smoking, obesity, a high-fat diet, and family history of heart disease.[4,5] The Framingham 20-year follow-up study has established that more than 60 percent of heart-failure cases are caused by hypertension and coronary artery disease.[5,6] Idiopathic dilated cardiomyopathy or primary myocardial disease causes 30 to 40 percent of cases[1]; valvular heart disease causes less than 20 percent.[6] Table 10-1 lists the various causes of heart failure.

Most of all acute episodes of heart failure are caused by one or more precipitating factors that lead to cardiac decompensation. These factors interfere with one or more of the compensatory mechanisms that are supporting appropriate cardiovascular function. Knowledge of these various precipitating factors may greatly improve the recognition and treatment of heart failure. The more common factors are listed in Table 10-2.

Acute cor pulmonale is most frequently associated with an abrupt elevation of pulmonary artery pressure.[7] This can be caused by massive pulmonary embolism; severe hypoxemic pulmonary vasoconstriction due to acute hypoventilation or adult respiratory distress syndrome (ARDS), or both; or mechanical constriction of the pulmonary vasculature secondary to bilateral pneumothoraces. Chronic cor pulmonale is actually responsible for 10 to 30 percent of admissions for presumed CHF and is primarily caused by chronic obstructive pulmonary diseases (COPDs) such as chronic bronchitis, emphysema, and cystic fibrosis.[7]

TABLE 10-1   **The Etiologic Factors of Heart Failure**

Coronary artery disease
Hypertension
Primary or idiopathic dilated cardiomyopathy
Valvular abnormalities: regurgitation and stenosis
Congenital cardiac defects
Chronic pulmonary disease
Drugs: amphetamines, heroin, cocaine, anti-TB combinations, high-dose cancer chemotherapy combinations
Infectious myocardial inflammation
    Viral (e.g., influenza, mumps, and rabies)
    Bacterial (e.g., streptococcal—rheumatic heart disease)
    Mycotic (e.g., histoplasmosis)
Other causes
    Chronic alcohol ingestion
    Acute leukemia
    Metal poisonings (e.g., cobalt, iron, and lead)
    Metabolic defects (e.g., myxedema)
    Neurologic disorders (e.g., Duchenne's muscular dystrophy)
    Trauma (e.g., cardiac tamponade)

SOURCE: Modified from Chesebro, JH, and Burnett, JC: Cardiac failure: Characteristics and clinical manifestations. In Brandenburg, RO, Fuster, V, Giuliani, ER and McGoon, DC (eds): Cardiology: Fundamentals and Practice. Year Book, Chicago, 1987, p. 646, with permission.

TABLE 10-2   **Acute Precipitating Factors of Heart Failure**

Patient-induced factors
    Failure to take medications
    Excessive sodium consumption
    High alcohol ingestion
    Physical inactivity or overactivity
    Emotional stress
Infection: viral and/or bacterial
Arrhythmias
    Premature ventricular contractions (PVCs)
    AV block
    Bradycardia
    Tachycardia
Excessive fluid administration
Pulmonary embolism
High cardiac output demand
    Fever
    Anemia
    Pregnancy
    Hypermetabolism
Acute myocardial infarction or ischemia
Renal failure
Respiratory failure
Liver disease
Drug-induced failure
Environmental stress: hyperthermia or hypothermia

SOURCE: Adapted from Chesebro, JH, and Burnett, JC: Cardiac failure: Characteristics and clinical manifestations. In Brandenburg, RO, Fuster, V, Giuliani, ER, and McGoon, DC (eds): Cardiology: Fundamentals and Practice. Year Book, Chicago, 1987, p. 652.

Pathophysiology

The product of cardiac pump performance is the **cardiac output ($\dot{Q}$T),** which is commonly measured as the flow of blood from one ventricle in liters per minute. Cardiac
output is primarily influenced by heart rate (HR) and stroke volume (SV). The following equation describes this relationship:

$$\dot{Q}T = HR \times SV$$

Heart rate is regulated by the pacing system of the heart and influenced by the
neurotransmitters (norepinephrine and acetylcholine) released by the autonomic nervous system. **Stroke volume** is influenced by venous return (preload pressure),
downstream resistance (afterload pressure), myocardial contractility, and ventricular
compliance. A more complete discussion of these factors and their interrelationships
can be found in Chapter 8.

In the normal heart, there is an exceptional degree of autoregulation of cardiac
output to prevent an imbalance in output between the right heart and the left heart.
A difference of as little as 1 mL/minute can lead to venous congestion upstream from
the failing ventricle.[8] The smaller pulmonary circuit that is upstream from the left
heart produces more symptoms with milder degrees of failure compared to similar
degrees of right heart failure. The more muscular wall of the left heart, however, is
capable of doing much greater work compared to the less muscular right heart. The
more limited functional capacity of the right heart predisposes it to failure when chal-

lenged with increasing preloads or afterloads, or both. As a consequence, right heart failure commonly follows primary left heart failure.[7] Interestingly, secondary right heart failure actually reduces the pulmonary congestion and the preload of the failing left ventricle, which provides a type of compensation. Rarely does primary right heart failure lead to left side failure.[7]

A variety of functional changes in heart failure involve myocardial performance, circulatory changes, fluid and electrolyte imbalance, and pulmonary dysfunction.

Myocardial Performance

The myocardial fibers in heart failure are less numerous and have decreased length-tension and force-velocity capabilities when stimulated to contract.[8,9] This demonstrates the heart's reduced inotropic capacity and reduced ability to generate a normal ejection fraction (the percentage of end-diastolic ventricular volume pumped out in one stroke volume). The ejection fraction can fall from a normal value of approximately 70 percent to 20 percent in severe failure. These deficits produce reductions in contractility and the myocardium's ability to do work with varying degrees of loading.

Three types of cardiac compensatory mechanisms improve myocardial performance during greater demands and in failure[8-12]:

1. **Autoregulation of the Heart:** As the myocardial fibers are stretched by increasing the end-diastolic ventricular pressure and volume, the fibers contract with greater force (**Frank-Starling Response**).[8,12] Figure 10-1 illustrates

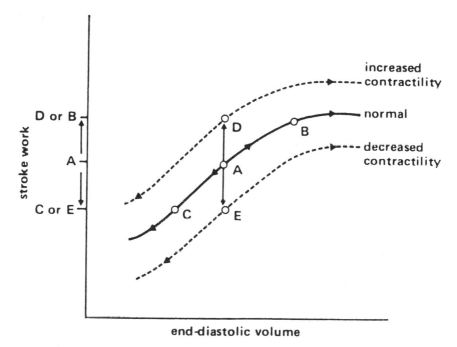

FIGURE 10-1 Frank-Starling ventricular function curves relating output (stroke work) and end-diastolic volume in three myocardial states of contractility. Output is varied along a single curve (e.g., A to B or A to C) as end-diastolic volume is altered by venous return. Output may also be changed by shifting from one curve to another (e.g., A to D or A to E) as the contractile or inotropic state of the ventricle is altered. Increased contractility can be brought about by hormonal or drug action while decreased contractility is typical of heart failure. (From Katz, AM: Physiology of the Heart. Raven Press, 1977, p 225, with permission.)

this relationship in both the normal and failing heart. In the normal heart, the attendant increase in venous return and ventricular filling associated with exercise or other forms of stress is easily compensated for through this mechanism. Failure of a ventricle results in a progressive increase in end-diastolic volume and ventricular dilation. The Frank-Starling response improves myocardial performance in heart failure, but this improvement leads to vascular engorgement that backs up into the pulmonary or systemic venous systems in left or right heart failure, respectively. To complicate cardiac performance further, an overly elevated end-diastolic volume reduces the compliance of the ventricle, which reduces contractility and nullifies or greatly reduces the Frank-Starling response and further contributes to CHF.

2. **Sympathetic Nervous Response:** During times of stress or hypotension, the sympathetic nervous system releases norepinephrine, which stimulates the β-receptors of the cardiac pacing system and myocardium. This results in greater heart rate and greater contraction strength, respectively, which in turn improve cardiac output. During heart failure, there is increased sympathetic activity and greater concentrations of norepinephrine in plasma during conditions of rest and exercise.[9,11] This response improves cardiac performance initially, but diminishes over time. Later, sympathetic stimulation can provoke ischemic symptoms as the myocardium's metabolic rate is stimulated beyond the coronary circulation's capacity to supply adequate blood flow to the myocardium. In long-term failure, persistent tachycardia lacking a parasympathetic bradycardic response develops, resulting in a reduction in the heart's ability to alter its rate from rest to exercise.[9]

3. **Ventricular Hypertrophy:** Ventricular hypertrophy is an increase in myocardial muscle thickness and mass produced by chronic exposure to elevated vascular pressure, greater blood volume, and elevated sympathetic nervous system release of neurotransmitters (e.g., norepinephrine, dopamine).[8,9] While the hypertrophy is beneficial for improving the strength of contraction in the early stages of heart failure, this benefit is eventually offset by a decreasing ventricular compliance. This condition is often further exacerbated by ischemic changes, which are brought about by inadequate oxygen delivery to an enlarged myocardium during conditions of increased myocardial work. Hypertrophy is not necessarily permanent if produced over a short period of time and then corrected. This reversal is common after surgical prosthetic replacement of a stenotic aortic valve.

Peripheral and Pulmonary Circulation

Significant systemic redistribution of blood flow occurs in CHF as an important compensatory mechanism. This adjustment results in a diversion of the already reduced cardiac output away from renal and cutaneous tissues to the more important coronary and cerebral circulations.[8,13] These adjustments occur during rest, but they are also further intensified during exercise and other forms of increased metabolism through the influence of the sympathetic nervous system.

During heart failure, the systemic vascular resistance is generally increased through the vasoactive effects of an elevated plasma norepinephrine concentration and vessel wall engorgement due to sodium and water absorption.[8,9] This results in a generalized inability of the heart to undergo vasodilation, which in turn limits its ability to increase oxygen transport and dissipate heat during exercise or other forms of stress. Thus, these patients are often very sensitive to heat and have reduced exercise tolerance.

Right heart failure results in systemic venous and capillary congestion and hypertension. This leads to liver engorgement, portal hypertension, reduced lymph duct drainage back to the venous system, and often fluid retention in various third spaces (e.g., dependent joint capsules, peritoneal cavity, pleural space).

Failure of the left heart produces pulmonary engorgement and hypertension. Initially, pulmonary artery diastolic pressure increases to around 12 to 18 mm Hg. This leads to increased blood flow to the upper lung or nondependent zones. Further failure results in greater pressures that can lead to pulmonary congestion and edema.

Fluid and Electrolyte Balance

In heart failure, reduced cardiac output and generalized vasoconstriction result in renal hypoperfusion.[8,9,14] This results in reduced glomerular filtration and subsequent sodium and water retention. Systemic venous congestion during right heart failure can lead to renal venous hypertension, which, in turn, can cause reductions in glomerular filtration and increase tubular reabsorption of sodium.[14] Thus, arterial hypoperfusion or venous hypertension, or both, can lead to renal responses that compound the congestive component of failure.

In addition to the renal vascular changes brought about by increased plasma concentrations of norepinephrine during heart failure, a variety of other hormonal adjustments induce further changes in renal function.[15] Reduced renal perfusion triggers the kidneys' production of renin, which, in turn, stimulates the production of angiotensin I. Angiotensin I is converted to angiotensin II during transit through the pulmonary circulation. Angiotensin II stimulates renal tubular sodium reabsorption; causes vasoconstriction, which intensifies renal hypoperfusion; and stimulates adrenal gland secretion of aldosterone. Aldosterone induces further renal retention of sodium. Atrial natriuretic peptide (ANP), a small protein hormone produced by specialized stretch receptor cells in the atria, is secreted in greater quantities during heart failure.[16] Increasing levels of ANP stimulate the kidneys to excrete sodium. This effectively antagonizes the effects of aldosterone and helps limit the sodium and water retention common in heart failure.

As a result of these renal changes, patients in heart failure generally have increased blood volume, interstitial fluid volume, and total body sodium. This altered fluid and electrolyte balance, coupled with poor cardiac performance, can easily lead to the development of systemic and pulmonary edema.

Edema Formation

The movement of fluid back and forth between the vascular and interstitial spaces is a normal phenomenon. The movement of water is governed by the permeability of the capillary wall, capillary blood pressure, interstitial fluid pressure, and oncotic pressure (primarily the osmotic force generated by proteins) of blood and interstitial fluid. These forces are brought together in Starling's law of the capillary:

$$\text{Fluid movement across the capillary wall} = K[(P_c - P_i) - (\pi_p - \pi_i)]$$

where K is the permeability constant for the capillary, P_c is the blood pressure within the capillary, π_p is the oncotic pressure exerted by interstitial fluid, P_i is the pressure of interstitial fluid, and π_i is the oncotic pressure exerted by blood. Normally these forces result in the net movement of about 150 mL of fluid into the interstitial space per hour. This fluid is absorbed by the lymphatics and returned to the systemic venous circulation and results in a stable interstitial fluid volume. When this natural drainage mechanism fails, excessive fluid collects in the interstitial space.

Edema is the term used to describe the clinical appearance of accumulated fluid in the interstitial spaces of the body. A variety of conditions can lead to the formation of edema:

1. Increased capillary permeability (e.g., effects of sepsis)
2. Increased capillary blood pressure
3. Reduced blood protein concentration (e.g., hypoalbuminemia), which results in reduced oncotic retention of intravascular water
4. Lymphatic obstruction[8]

Fluid retention and increased capillary blood pressure occurs in CHF.[8] Right heart failure causes systemic venous and capillary hypertension, which leads to systemic organ and dependent limb edema.[9,13] During left heart failure, pulmonary circuit blood pressure increases as blood collects upstream from the failing left ventricle. Pulmonary capillary pressures begin to increase, and interstitial fluid accumulates along the vessel walls, around the small airways, and in the pleural space.[8,9] This initially occurs in the dependent regions of the lung, where capillary pressures are the highest. As the severity of left heart failure increases, pulmonary edema occurs throughout the lung in those regions where pulmonary capillary pressures exceed 25 mm Hg.

Pulmonary Dysfunction

Pulmonary function is often disturbed during left ventricular failure (Table 10-3).[17,18] Advanced CHF produces marked impairment in pulmonary function; early left heart failure, with its attendant mild pulmonary hypertension (e.g., pulmonary artery wedge pressure

TABLE 10-3 **Pulmonary Dysfunction During Left Heart Failure**

Severity	Pathophysiology	Pulmonary Abnormalities
Mild	Pulmonary vascular congestion	↑ D_{LCO} ↑ Pa_{O_2} Pa_{CO_2} and pH are normal
Moderate	Pulmonary interstitial edema	↓ FVC or unchanged ↓ FEV_1 or unchanged ↑ Closing volume ↑ V_D/V_T ↓ $\dot{V}/\dot{Q}$ matching ↓ D_{LCO} ↓ Pa_{O_2} ↓ Pa_{CO_2} and ↑ pH
Severe	Alveolar flooding	↓↓ FVC ↓↓ FEV_1 ↓↓ Compliance ↑↑ Closing volume ↑↑ V_D/V_T ↑↑ $\dot{V}/\dot{Q}$ matching ↓↓ D_{LCO} ↓↓ Pa_{O_2} ↑ Pa_{CO_2} and ↓ pH

D_{LCO} = carbon monoxide diffusing capacity of the lung; FVC = forced vital capacity; FEV_1 = forced expiratory volume in 1 second; V_D/V_T = ratio of volume of dead space to tidal volume; $\dot{V}/\dot{Q}$ = ventilation-perfusion ratio.
SOURCE: Pastore, JO: Cardiac disease in respiratory patients in the intensive care unit. In MacDonnell, KF, Fahey, FJ, and Segal, MS (eds): Respiratory Intensive Care, Little, Brown & Co, Boston, 1987, p 377.

[PAWP] of 15 to 20 mm Hg), actually improves gas exchange through an increased pulmonary blood volume and improved ventilation-perfusion ($\dot{V}/\dot{Q}$) matching. As failure advances and increasing pulmonary congestion occurs, lung water increases. This causes decreases in lung volume and diffusion capacity and increases in airway resistance and $\dot{V}/\dot{Q}$ mismatching. Severe failure and frank alveolar flooding are often accompanied by a dramatic deterioration in forced vital capacity (FVC), forced expiratory volume in 1 second (FEV_1), lung compliance, and gas exchange, as well as a mixed respiratory and metabolic acidosis.[17,18] These changes can cause further heart failure, which, in turn, causes further pulmonary dysfunction, and thus a vicious circle of failure begins.

Clinical Features and Laboratory Findings

There are two major clinical manifestations of heart failure: (1) fluid retention and peripheral edema (associated with right heart failure); and (2) pulmonary vascular congestion (caused by left heart failure). This division is clinically useful but potentially misleading, since biventricular failure often occurs as one ventricle fails primarily and precipitates failure of the other. Cor pulmonale is difficult to recognize because the clinical picture is almost always dominated by chronic pulmonary disease. The clinical manifestations vary not only with the major form of heart failure present, but also with the patient's ability to compensate or as they respond to therapy.

The morbidity and mortality associated with heart failure necessitates early recognition and treatment. If the patient has a history of one or more of the triggering factors (Table 10-2), it is very useful to determine whether the heart failure is the primary or a contributing cause of the patient's complaints or condition.

The patient in left heart failure often has dyspnea, adventitious breath sounds, cough, reduced exercise tolerance, delirium, anxiety, and occasionally psychosis during moderate to severe failure (Table 10-4).[9,19] The increased sympathetic activity

TABLE 10-4   **New York Heart Association Functional Classification of Heart Disease Correlated with Mortality**

Functional Class	Definition	Manifestation	1-Year Mortality (%)
I	Patients with cardiac disease but without physical limitation	Ordinary activity does not cause undue fatigue, palpitations, dyspnea, or angina	0-5
II	Patients with cardiac disease that results in slight limitation; comfortable at rest	Ordinary physical activity results in fatigue, palpitations, dyspnea or angina	10-20
III	Patients with cardiac disease resulting in marked limitation of physical activity; comfortable at rest	Less than ordinary physical activity results in fatigue, palpitations, dyspnea, and angina	35-45
IV	Patients with cardiac disease resulting in an inability to carry out any physical activity without discomfort	Symptoms of cardiac insufficiency or angina may be present, even at rest	85-95

and release of norepinephrine combined with poor cardiac output leads to poor peripheral circulation. This often produces cool skin, diaphoresis, cyanosis of the digits, and peripheral pallor. Distended jugular veins, abdominal distention, and peripheral edema of the ankles are common findings of right ventricular failure.[9,19]

Dyspnea at rest and with minimal exertion is frequently seen during significant failure. The dyspnea commonly becomes worse when the patient is lying flat (**orthopnea**) and at night (**nocturnal dyspnea**). For this reason, these patients often report that their sleep is disturbed and that they sleep better with numerous pillows. Tachypnea is a compensatory breathing pattern that these patients often adopt. In patients with severe failure leading to prolonged circulation time between the lungs and the chemoreceptors of the nervous system, Cheyne-Stokes breathing may occur.[9]

Tachycardia is a common finding and represents a compensatory mechanism for maintaining cardiac output in the face of a poor stroke volume. Alterations in beat-to-beat blood pressure (pulsus alternans) may be detected, indicating severe myocardial disease. Tachycardia (heart rate greater than 130/minute) and arrhythmias may contribute to the degree of heart failure and may be a sign of secondary electrolyte imbalance or drug toxicity.[9] For these reasons, continuous electrocardiographic (ECG) monitoring is a standard of care during the acute phase of treatment.

Compensatory sympathetic vasoconstriction may maintain a normal blood pressure, but in severe failure the systolic and mean arterial pressures will be reduced. The patient's peripheral skin temperature is frequently reduced, whereas their core temperatures may actually be elevated as a result of impaired heat dissipation.

Auscultation of the chest during left heart failure often reveals inspiratory crackles (which sound like the high-pitched snapping sound of a Velcro fastener being separated) and polyphonic expiratory (cardiac) wheezes.[9] Crackles occur as small airways of atelectatic regions "pop" open upon inspiration. Wheezes are caused by airflow through airways that are narrowed by fluid accumulation in the surrounding airway wall. These findings are often heard over the lung bases of the patient in moderate failure and further up into the mid-lung and apical regions of the chest as failure worsens. Cardiac gallops and murmurs are common findings and may be more evident with exercise.[9]

Peripheral edema, abdominal distention, and superficial abdominal vein distention are common findings of right and biventricular chronic heart failure. Liver congestion (hepatomegaly) and excessive peritoneal fluid retention (ascites) cause abdominal distention as a result of chronic venous hypertension and impaired lymphatic drainage.[9,20] In most adults, fluid retention of approximately 5 liters must occur before peripheral edema is detectable.[9] Edematous fluids collect in the most dependent regions of the body, such as the ankles in the upright patient (**pedal edema**). The edema formation may become so severe that the skin will pit upon pressing on it. In those patients who are unable to get out of bed, edema rarely forms in the face but more often in the posterior parts of the arms, thighs, and legs.

Specific radiographic changes are associated with the three degrees of left heart failure, as follows[17,18]:

Mild Failure: Pulmonary venous congestion with widening of pulmonary arteries; redistribution of pulmonary blood flow to the upper lung fields

Moderate Failure: Cardiomegaly (heart greater than half the diameter of the thorax); pulmonary artery engorgement; interstitial pulmonary edema (presence of Kerley's A lines—1 to 2 cm lines of interstitial edema out from the hilum; and Kerley's B lines—short, thin, and flattened U-shaped streaks of interstitial edema outlining the lymphatics of a subsegmental region of lung that extends from the pleural surface)

Severe Failure: Cardiomegaly; pulmonary artery engorgement; interstitial pulmonary edema; fluffy, patchy alveolar edema (often in a "butterfly" pattern that radiates out from the perihilar region); pleural effusion

In right heart failure, the chest radiographs are generally normal unless pulmonary disease is present.

A variety of cardiac rhythm disturbances are frequently found during heart failure.[9] Sinus tachycardia is the most common ECG abnormality. Excessive premature ventricular contractions and atrial fibrillation may contribute to failure or be a result of it. Bundle branch blocks and axis deviations are common in cardiac hypertrophy. QT-wave changes are frequently present and suggest myocardial hypoxia or infarction, or both. Those patients with chronic heart failure are at increased risk for sudden death with increasing QT dispersion and variation.[21] Changes in R wave, right axis, or right bundle branch block are more common during right heart failure.[9]

Arterial blood gas (ABG) analysis is useful for determining the degree of gas exchange derangement and the trend in the patient's pulmonary status.[17,18] Reduced PaO_2, increased alveolar-arterial oxygen gradient ($P[A - a]O_2$), or reduced ratio of PaO_2 to fraction of inspired oxygen (FIO_2) are the most practical and sensitive signs of respiratory impairment during left heart failure. These changes indicate the magnitude of $\dot{V}/\dot{Q}$ mismatching and diffusion defects that are occurring as a result of pulmonary engorgement and edema. Respiratory alkalosis is frequently found in the early period of failure and often continues until the patient is unable to continue to compensate. With the onset of severe left heart failure and frank pulmonary edema, ventilatory failure is likely, and a combination of severe hypoxemia, carbon dioxide retention, and respiratory acidosis often occurs. A mixed respiratory and metabolic acidosis is not uncommon in severe failure as the result of anaerobic metabolism, which is caused by poor circulation and ventilatory failure.

Routine laboratory studies are seldom useful in establishing heart failure as the cause of patients' complaints, but some tests are useful. With chronic cor pulmonale, the hematocrit (Hct), hemoglobin (Hb) concentration, and erythrocyte count are frequently elevated 10 to 25 percent above normal values as the result of compensation for chronic hypoxia.[7] Hyponatremia and hypokalemia are often seen in patients with CHF; they may be the result of excessive fluid retention or diuretic therapy.[9] In right heart failure with excessive liver engorgement, the bilirubin and liver enzymes (e.g., aspartate aminotransferase, AST) may be elevated.[19]

An elevated ANP level is strongly associated with left heart failure. A finding of levels greater than 54 pmol/liter is highly (greater than 90 percent) sensitive and specific in detecting individuals with asymptomatic heart failure.[16]

The echocardiogram, Doppler flow, and radionuclide studies are useful in establishing the anatomic changes in heart structure and motion typically found in failure. Often the findings include dilated end-diastolic ventricular dimensions, hypertrophic myocardial changes, valvular dysfunction, and reduced ventricular motion and ejection fraction.[9]

Pulmonary artery catheterization is useful for evaluating the degree of pulmonary hypertension and the cardiac output. It also helps guide therapy in patients who are in severe heart failure.[22] Table 10–5 lists the combinations of physical findings and hemodynamic data that predict the severity of heart failure and patient outcome after a myocardial infarction (MI).

Aerobic exercise capacity is frequently diminished in patients with chronic heart failure.[23] This impairment is associated with inadequate oxygen delivery to skeletal muscles and their subsequent shift to anaerobic metabolism and fatigue.[24,25] As heart failure increases, exercise capacity and maximum oxygen utilization decrease as max-

TABLE 10-5   **Hemodynamic and Physical Finding Subsets After Heart Failure from Acute Myocardial Infarction**

Subset	PAWP (mm Hg)	Cardiac Index (liters/minute/m²)	Mortality (%)
I. No pulmonary congestion and no peripheral hypoperfusion	≤18	>2.2	3
II. Pulmonary congestion and no peripheral hypoperfusion	>18	>2.2	9
III. Peripheral hypoperfusion and no pulmonary congestion	≤18	≤2.2	23
IV. Pulmonary congestion and peripheral hypoperfusion	>18	≤2.2	51

PAWP = pulmonary artery wedge pressure
SOURCE: Adapted from Forrester, JS, et al: Medical therapy of acute myocardial infarction by application of hemodynamic subsets. N Engl J Med 295:1404–1413, 1976.

imum cardiac output decreases. Approximately 30 percent of patients with severe left heart failure are capable of performing near-normal exercise for their age and sex.[25] This tolerance appears to be the result of the body's compensatory ability to increase heart rate to preserve cardiac output, tolerate pulmonary hypertension without excessive dyspnea, and decrease vascular resistance. Patients with the poorest performance are at highest risk for complications, the need for hospitalization, and death.[26]

The combination of physical assessment, chest radiography, ABG analysis, ECG, and hemodynamic monitoring forms the core of early detection and management.

Treatment

Therapy for heart failure is chosen on the basis of the cause of failure, its severity, and the secondary complications. Therefore, treatment focuses on eliminating the cause of failure, reducing cardiac work load, and supporting the function of other organs. Table 10-6 summarizes the approaches commonly used to manage heart failure.

Reduction of Cardiac Work Load

Cardiac function can be improved by reducing myocardial work load and enhancing contractility.[27] The most effective approach to reducing cardiac work is *afterload reduction.* This can be achieved via lifestyle changes and certain medications. Lifestyle changes that reduce cardiac work include engaging in appropriate physical activity, reducing emotional stress, losing weight (if patient is overweight), and eating a low-salt diet. Bed rest and sedation with appropriate drugs (e.g., morphine, midazolam [Versed]) may be necessary to reduce anxiety and agitation, which cause cardiac stimulation. Afterload reduction can be induced with direct-acting vasodilators (e.g., nitroglycerin, nitroprusside, isosorbide, hydralazine, minoxidil). Decreasing the vaso-

TABLE 10-6 **Goals of Managing Heart Failure**

Goals	Methods
Reduce cardiac work load	Appropriate physical activity
	Stress reduction
	Vasodilation
	Assisted circulation
Improve cardiac pump performance	Digitalis
	β-Adrenergic stimulation
	Oxygen therapy
Prevent arrhythmias	Antiarrhythmic agents
Control sodium and fluid retention	Low-sodium diet
	Diuretic therapy
Prevent thromboembolism	Heparin and warfarin therapy
Provide support for secondary organ dysfunction	

constrictive effects of norepinephrine with an α-adrenergic receptor blocking agent (e.g., prazosin, trimazosin) is also useful to achieve indirect vasodilation. Vasodilation and afterload reduction occurs with the suppression of angiotensin II production. Angiotensin II is a powerful vasoconstrictive hormone produced from angiotensin I by angiotensin-converting enzyme (ACE). Use of an ACE inhibitor (e.g., captopril) results in generalized vasodilation and reduced blood pressure. Another approach to vasodilation and afterload reduction is the use of calcium channel blockers (e.g., verapamil, nifedipine). Calcium channel blockers inhibit the action of vasoconstrictive mechanisms and are also useful in controlling tachyarrhythmias. Recent evidence, however, reveals that high doses of short-acting calcium channel blockers may actually increase the risk of MI.[28] Each patient's response to lifestyle changes and drug-induced afterload reduction is variable and requires careful reevaluation to avoid hypotension or other complications.

Despite drug therapy, the mortality rate for patients in end-stage heart failure and cardiogenic shock ranges from 80 to 90 percent or higher. This has driven the need for other ways of reducing cardiac work and improving the basic problem of poor blood flow. Circulatory assistance is a mechanical approach to improving blood flow and reducing cardiac work. Such devices include the intra-aortic balloon pump, ventricular assist devices, and a total artificial heart. These devices can correct the acute problem of poor blood flow and give the patient time to respond to drug therapy or survive long enough for a heart transplant.

Improvement of Cardiac Pump Performance

Inotropic drugs (e.g., digitalis, dopamine, dobutamine, amrinone) are used to improve ventricular function by increasing contractility. This action, in turn, improves cardiac output and reduces congestion.[27] Digitalis remains the most frequently prescribed inotropic agent for heart failure and is the drug of choice. Patients with chronic heart failure due to systolic dysfunction are the most responsive. *Digitalis intoxication* can occur in up to 30 percent of patients.[29] The classic signs and symptoms include nausea, vomiting, insomnia, altered color vision, and irregular cardiac rhythm (e.g., frequent premature ventricular contractions).

Myocardial contraction is a highly aerobic process that requires an ample and stable supply of oxygen. Frequently the patient with heart failure has a compromised coronary circulation. This defect may be the primary trigger for failure or will limit the ability of the heart to compensate, or both. Supplemental oxygen is frequently employed to improve oxygen delivery to the myocardium.

Prevention of Arrhythmia

Cardiac arrhythmias can cause or exacerbate heart failure. The use of antiarrhythmic drugs to control bradycardia (e.g., atropine) and tachycardia (e.g., procainamide, metoprolol, bretylium) is frequently necessary.

Control of Sodium and Fluid Retention

Sodium and water retention can be improved with bed rest, which induces a natural diuresis by the kidneys.[27] Upright positions decrease sodium and water excretion and should be restricted until fluid and electrolyte balance is more acceptable. Dietary restriction of sodium and water are the next steps toward reduction of fluid retention. **Diuretics** such as loop of Henle agents (e.g., furosemide [Lasix]), thiazides (e.g., metolazone), and potassium-sparing agents (e.g., spironolactone) are useful in controlling water retention.[27]

High-dose diuretic therapy is usually started at the beginning of severe CHF and then tapered as the patient responds. The endpoint of diuretic therapy is frequently the fluid volume status that gives maximal cardiac output without causing pulmonary congestion. This usually results in a targeted PAWP (preload pressure) of 15 to 18 mm Hg. It frequently takes as much as 24 hours after the optimal preload pressure is achieved for the inspiratory crackles and radiographic signs of pulmonary edema to disappear. Careful use of these agents is necessary to avoid overdiuresis, which could lead to electrolyte imbalance and rebound hypotension. Careful fluid replacement and potassium therapy is almost always necessary to avoid hypokalemia and fluid imbalance.

Prevention of Thromboembolism

Patients in heart failure are at high risk for clotting disorders and development of emboli.[27,30] The potential for devastating systemic or pulmonary embolization necessitates the use of prophylactic anticoagulants (e.g., heparin). Long-term anticoagulant therapy reduces the risk of embolization by reducing the viscosity of blood, which, in turn, reduces the myocardial work load.

In cases of severe CHF, patients require most, if not all, of the above measures to correct their condition. The actions of these agents can be seen in Figure 10–2, which shows a family of Frank-Starling cardiac output and left ventricular filling pressure (preload) curves. The diuretics reduce preload and venous congestion but do not directly improve cardiac output. Vasodilators reduce afterload and improve cardiac output. Inotropic agents improve contractility and reduce preload when used with vasodilators. This results in improved cardiac performance and reduced venous congestion.

Surgical treatment of heart failure is directed toward specific repair of the cause. This includes valvular repair or replacement and coronary artery bypass grafting for coronary artery disease. Patients with severe left ventricular dysfunction, however, generally have higher mortality rates after surgery.[31] For younger patients, cardiac transplantation offers the best hope for long-term treatment of severe chronic heart failure.

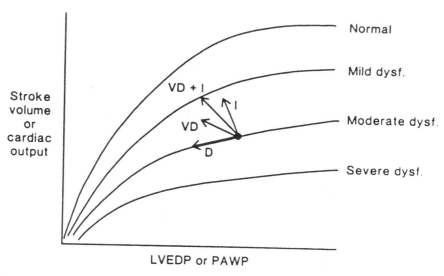

FIGURE 10-2   Frank-Starling left ventricular function curves relating preload pressure (left ventricular end-diastolic pressure [LVEDP] or pulmonary artery wedge pressure [PAWP] and stroke volume or cardiac output. Curves showing normal and various degrees of dysfunction (dysf) are shown. Diuretics (D) are shown to reduce preload and venous congestion without acutely improving cardiac output. Inotropic drugs (I) or vasodilators (VD) and especially the combination of these two (VD + I) act to shift heart function toward better cardiac output with reduced preload. (From Chesebro, JH: Cardiac failure: medical management. In Brandenburg, RO, Fuster, V, Giuliani, ER, and McGoon, DC (eds): Cardiology: Fundamentals and Practice. Year Book Medical, Chicago, 1987, with permission.)

Respiratory Care for Cardiogenic Pulmonary Edema

Initial treatment with oxygen therapy is necessary to improve arterial oxygenation, which will, in turn, improve cardiac function. Low-flow oxygen therapy with a nasal cannula is frequently the starting point if the patient is conscious and is responding to the medical management described earlier. A non-rebreathing mask with adequate flow should be administered if the patient presents with severe hypoxemia or frank pulmonary edema.

High-flow continuous positive airway pressure via mask (mask CPAP) has been used sporadically for heart failure–induced "cardiac asthma" since its initial description more than 50 years ago.[32] More recently, it has been shown that patients with cardiogenic pulmonary edema, serious tachypnea (respiratory rate greater than 25/minute), and $\dot{V}/\dot{Q}$ mismatching (Pao_2/Fio_2 less than 200) had a significant and rapid improvement in oxygenation and reductions in respiratory and heart rates with the use of mask CPAP.[33] Although hypoventilation and subsequent hypercapnia are potential contraindications to the use of mask CPAP, they have not detracted from its effective use in treating hypoxemia induced by heart failure.[34] The suggested mechanism behind the effectiveness of mask CPAP in this setting is improved lung compliance, reduced work of breathing, improved gas exchange, and reduced vascular congestion.[32] Mask CPAP should be used with a nasogastric tube in place. It should be avoided if the patient is at high risk for vomiting or has severe respiratory acidosis (pH less than 7.20).

Intubation and ventilatory support will become necessary if the patient exhibits a grave clinical picture of poor respiratory function (e.g., cyanosis and periodic breathing pattern) or evidence of severe respiratory failure (pH less than 7.20, $Paco_2$ greater than 50, Pao_2 less than 50) while receiving oxygen therapy. Initial ventilator settings should be assist/control mode, 100 percent F_{IO_2}, $V_T = 8$ to 10 mL/kg (ideal body weight), respiratory rate = 15/minute, and sensitivity of -2 cm H_2O. The addition of positive end-expiratory pressure (PEEP; 5 to 15 cm H_2O) is appropriate if the oxygenation and lung mechanics remain poor despite ventilatory support with an elevated F_{IO_2} (e.g., greater than 50 percent). Care must be given to the application of positive pressure ventilation with PEEP in these patients because of their precarious cardiac function. Use of a pulmonary artery catheter may be necessary to guide therapy and avoid decompensating the heart.[22,27]

Special attention to airway care is necessary after intubation in patients with frank pulmonary edema. Edema foam must be cleared rapidly to improve the effectiveness of the oxygen therapy and ventilatory support. In the past, aerosolized ethyl alcohol (20 to 40 percent) was used to reduce the pulmonary edema foam, but this has been abandoned because of its bronchial irritation and the more direct response to airway suctioning and application of high-dose diuretics.

Aerosolized bronchodilators (e.g., albuterol) should be used in patients who have a compounding component of asthma or bronchitis, or both. Incentive spirometry is also useful during the recovery phase to promote lung expansion and airway clearance.

CASE STUDY

History

Mr. N, a 64-year-old man, is a retired concession operator with a history of coronary artery disease, arrhythmia, COPD, and a recent episode of pneumonia and a small anterior wall MI, which required a 1-month hospitalization at a Veterans Administration (VA) hospital. He was discharged 4 days ago with an extensive assortment of medications to maintain his cardiac, renal, and pulmonary function. While at home he experienced a coughing spell that led to increasing shortness of breath and mild substernal pressure. He became increasingly anxious and requested that the paramedics be called and that he be taken to the hospital immediately because he could not "catch his breath" and that his "heart would not slow down." He was brought to the hospital and treated with oxygen via nasal cannula at 4 liters/minute.

QUESTIONS

1. What signs and symptoms should you evaluate immediately upon his arrival?
2. What diagnostic techniques could you use to help determine the nature of his shortness of breath?
3. What therapeutic techniques should be readily available upon his arrival?

ANSWERS

1. You should evaluate level of consciousness, signs of delirium, signs of a patent airway, spontaneous breathing and chest motion, quality of breath sounds and their symmetry, pulse rate, blood pressure, and temperature. You should also look for symptoms of respiratory distress, shock, and mental impairment.
2. You could evaluate the severity and origin of his shortness of breath by taking a rapid history, if possible, to determine the triggering factors that led

to the sudden exacerbation. After you perform a careful and rapid physical evaluation followed by appropriate laboratory studies, you should sort out the source of the dyspnea (pulmonary versus cardiac).

3. Oxygen therapy (via cannula, Venturi mask, and non-rebreathing mask), intubation equipment, manual resuscitation bag with proper mask, oxygen reservoir, venous and arterial line placement equipment, various fluids for vascular support, appropriate resuscitation drugs, and medications for pain and agitation should be readily available.

Physical Examination

General: An obese, elderly man with an approximate weight of 110 kg who is alert and in obvious respiratory distress while sitting up despite oxygen therapy via nasal cannula at 4 liters/minute; wife states, and patient confirms, history of heavy smoking for 26 years and cessation 12 years ago; history of MI 10 years ago, multiple hernia operations 10 years ago, chronic lung disease; recently hospitalized for pneumonia and heart disease; indicates compliance with medications and low-salt, low-fat diet

Vital Signs: Temperature 37.5°C (99.5°F); respiratory rate 31/minute, blood pressure 100/70 mm Hg; heart rate 160/minute, nail bed refill 5 seconds

HEENT: Pupils equal and reactive to light; some nasal flaring; normal oral structures

Neck: Trachea in midline; no signs of inspiratory stridor or laryngeal abnormality; carotid pulses + + bilaterally without bruit; no signs of lymphadenopathy or thyroidomegaly; noticeable jugular venous distention; some tensing of sternocleidomastoid and scalene muscles during inspiration

Chest: Normal chest configuration; no scars; some diminished motion noted; bilateral inspiratory crackles from bases midway up chest, with some scattered expiratory wheezes; some thoracoabdominal paradoxical motion noted

Heart: Heart tones diminished; point of maximal impulse not palpable; no murmurs, rub, or gallop

Abdomen: Obese and soft; no hepatomegaly; bowel sounds not heard clearly

Extremities: Moving all extremities; +2 pulses felt throughout; +2 pitting edema in both ankles; no clubbing; skin cool and diaphoretic with some digital cyanosis

---

QUESTIONS

4. What are the possible causes of his respiratory distress?
5. What signs and symptoms indicate CHF?
6. How will left heart failure influence respiratory function?
7. What diagnostic techniques should you use to further evaluate his cardiorespiratory distress?

ANSWERS

4. His respiratory distress may be caused by:
   a. Pulmonary edema due to heart failure
   b. Exacerbation of his COPD

    c. MI

    d. Pulmonary infection

5. His signs and symptoms of CHF include the following:

    a. Rapid onset of dyspnea

    b. Anxiety

    c. Disproportionate tachycardia and relatively low blood pressure

    d. Inspiratory crackles in the dependent lung regions

    e. Jugular venous distention

    f. Cool, diaphoretic skin and poor peripheral circulation

    g. Ankle edema

6. Left heart failure can induce the following:

    a. Pulmonary hypertension

    b. Increased lung water

    c. Increased airway resistance

    d. Alveolar edema

    e. Increased work of breathing

    f. Decreasing pulmonary compliance

    g. $\dot{V}/\dot{Q}$ mismatching

    h. Diffusion defect

    i. Hypoxemia

    j. Ventilatory failure

7. For further evaluation of his cardiorespiratory distress, ABGs, chest radiograph, and a 12-lead ECG with subsequent ECG monitoring are needed immediately. Continuous noninvasive monitoring of his oxyhemoglobin saturation and blood pressure will further help guide his cardiopulmonary care. Laboratory assessment of the complete blood count, electrolytes, and standard blood chemistry are indicated. Assessment of his cardiac enzymes (creatinine kinase [CK]) and digitalis levels would help rule out an MI and help guide digitalis therapy.

Bedside and Laboratory Evaluations

ECG: Supraventricular tachycardia of 158/minute, normal axis, first-degree atrioventricular (AV) block, and left bundle branch block

Chest Radiograph: See Figure 10–3

ABGs: pH = 7.24, $Paco_2$ = 51 mm Hg, Pao_2 = 38 mm Hg, HCO_3^- = 22 mEq/liter while breathing oxygen via nasal cannula at 4 liters/minute

Hematology: Hct = 45 percent, Hb = 15 g/dL, RBC = 5.2×10^6/mm³, white blood cell (WBC) count = 15.2×10^3, platelets = 262×10^3

Chemistry: Results pending

QUESTIONS

8. What does the ECG indicate?

9. What does the chest radiograph indicate?

10. How would you interpret the ABG data?

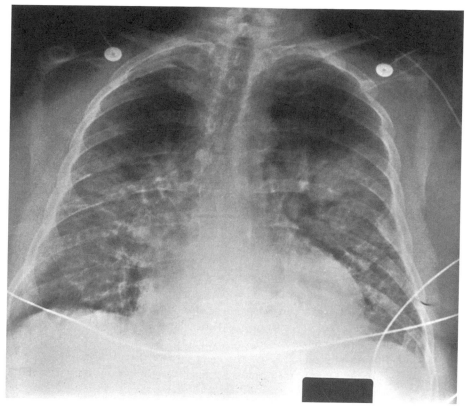

FIGURE 10-3   Portable AP chest radiograph taken at admission in the emergency department.

11. What do the hematologic data indicate?

12. What respiratory care is indicated at this time?

13. What cardiac care is indicated at this time?

ANSWERS

8. The ECG indicates severe tachycardia as well as other cardiac conduction disturbances. This rate is out of proportion with the resulting blood pressure and is probably contributing to or causing acute CHF.

9. The chest radiograph reveals cardiomegaly, bilateral pulmonary vascular engorgement, interstitial and alveolar edema, and atelectasis bilaterally; some Kerley's B lines in both bases; and no signs of pleural effusion or hemopneumothorax. The trachea is seen in the midline. Some scoliosis is seen in the cervical and thoracic vertebral column, but the rib cage looks normal. No mediastinal masses are noted.

10. The ABG shows severe hypoxemia due to one or more of the following: hypoventilation, diffusion defect, shunting, and $\dot{V}/\dot{Q}$ mismatching. Hypoventilation, despite significant tachypnea, indicates a ventilatory decompensation that is producing uncompensated respiratory acidosis. Considering this patient's history of COPD, one should consider applying an alternate acid-base classification: an acute-on-chronic respiratory

acidosis accompanying a loss of accumulated base due to a metabolic acidosis; however, there no other data presented to support such a classification. These findings are consistent with severe cardiogenic pulmonary edema.

11. The hematologic data are relatively normal with the exception of the slight-to-moderate elevation of the WBC count, which may be caused by an infection or induced by stress.

12. The oxygen therapy currently in use is inadequate to support oxygenation. Although the patient has been found to have significant hypoxemia and moderate ventilatory failure, intubation and ventilatory support is not indicated at this time because of the strength of the respiratory efforts and the lucid state of the patient. Mask CPAP may be attempted to improve ventilatory mechanics and improve oxygenation. If the patient's clinical status or the ABGs were to deteriorate, intubation and mechanical ventilatory support would be necessary. Aerosolized bronchodilator therapy (e.g., albuterol) should be continued to optimize airway resistance, given the clinical findings of wheezes and the history of COPD.

13. Supraventricular tachycardia of this magnitude is a dangerous condition requiring immediate treatment and continuous ECG and blood pressure monitoring. Intravenous (IV) lines should be placed in the event that there is an emergent need to give resuscitative drugs. Electrical cardioversion should be attempted to "reset" the heart rate, or drug therapy (e.g., verapamil) should be administered to induce rapid reduction of the heart rate. Fluid retention should be relieved with high-dose diuretics (e.g., furosemide). Reduction of afterload and improvement of myocardial contractility should be carried out carefully with vasodilators (e.g., hydralazine, captopril) and inotropic agents (e.g., digitalis).

CASE STUDY—continued

In the emergency room, continuous ECG and pulse oximetry were started, two peripheral IV lines were placed, and oxygen therapy was switched to a non-rebreathing mask supplied with oxygen at a rate of 15 liters/minute. Two cardioversion attempts were made (100 watt-sec followed by 150 watt-sec), but were both unsuccessful. A single dose of slowly administered verapamil was given with a prompt decline in heart rate to 130/minute. Furosemide, isosorbide, captopril, digitalis, morphine sulfate, and erythromycin were started. He was then transferred to the coronary care unit (CCU) with the diagnosis of CHF secondary to one or more of the following: supraventricular tachycardia, possible MI, possible dietary indiscretion, possible noncompliance in taking his medication, and possible underlying pulmonary infection. Upon admission to the unit, an arterial line was placed and continuous ECG and pulse oximetry monitoring were continued.

Bedside Findings

Mr. N is alert, sitting up in bed, in obvious respiratory distress despite receiving high-concentration oxygen via non-rebreathing mask, and somewhat anxious. Occasionally he coughs up thick, brown sputum. He stated "I'm afraid to be taken off the oxygen." He is being given 2.5 mg of aerosolized albuterol diluted in 3 mL of saline every 2 hours, and he indicates that these treatments help to reduce his dyspnea.

Laboratory Evaluation

Vital Signs, Hemodynamics, and Urine Output:

Rectal temperature 37.2°C (99.0°F)

Respiratory rate 33/minute

Heart rate 132/minute

Systemic arterial blood pressure 143/97 mm Hg

SpO_2 81 percent

Breath sounds: bilateral inspiratory crackles, expiratory wheezes, and occasional expiratory rhonchi

Urine output brisk at 500 mL over the past hour since hospital admission and furosemide administration

ECG Findings: Sinus tachycardia of 130/minute, first-degree AV block, and left bundle branch block

ABGs: pH = 7.26, $PaCO_2$ = 51 mm Hg, PaO_2 = 49 mm Hg, HCO_3^- = 24 mEq/liter, $P(A - a)O_2$ = 660 mm Hg, PaO_2/FIO_2 = 49 (assumes FIO_2 = 100 percent), SaO_2 = 79 percent (calculated), SpO_2 81 percent (pulse oximeter)

Electrolytes and Chemistry: Na^+ = 137 mEq/liter, K^+ = 3.7 mEq/liter, Ca^{++} (ionized) 8.2 mg/dL, Cl^- = 101 mEq/liter, glucose = 239 mg/dL, blood urea nitrogen = 13 mg/dL, creatinine = 1.3 mg/dL

Cardiac Enzymes: Pending

Microbiology: Sputum smear and cultures pending

QUESTIONS

14. What do the bedside findings and vital signs indicate about Mr. N's response to treatment?

15. What do the laboratory findings indicate about Mr. N's status?

16. What changes, if any, in his respiratory care would you recommend?

ANSWERS

14. His bedside findings indicate that his heart rate, blood pressure, and urine output have responded, but that his respiratory status has not improved.

15. The ECG changes are very encouraging, and his chemistry panel is acceptable; however, the ABG and acid-base balance shows severe hypoxemia despite very high concentrations of oxygen and continued hypoventilation with respiratory acidosis in the face of significant tachypnea.

16. Mr. N is now a candidate for a mask-CPAP trial or intubation; clinicians who take a more aggressive approach may consider mechanical ventilation. Continuation of aerosolized bronchodilators to help reduce his work of breathing is appropriate. Leaving him in a state of significant dyspnea and in respiratory failure while waiting for the diuresis to reduce the pulmonary edema borders on cruelty, besides rendering the clinician liable for medical malpractice.

CASE STUDY—continued

Following assessment of Mr. N's condition, he was placed on a continuous high-flow mask-CPAP system (Fig. 10–4), and a nasogastric tube to suction was placed. The initial settings were as follows: flow 60 liters/minute, FIO_2 100 percent, and CPAP 5 cm H_2O. He was initially apprehensive but then became less dyspneic as his respiratory rate decreased to 28/minute, heart rate decreased to 103/minute, blood pressure remained stable at 140/96, and SpO_2 increased to 89 percent after 30 minutes of CPAP and continued diuresis. CPAP was then increased to 7.5 cm H_2O to achieve further improvement in gas exchange and respiratory mechanics and to attempt some reduction of his FIO_2. After another 30 minutes of treatment, the following observations and data were collected.

Bedside Findings

Mr. N is sitting up in bed, wearing a clear plastic CPAP mask. He is alert, communicative, and appearing more comfortable with less dyspnea. He continues to use his accessory muscles with some thoracoabdominal asynchrony. The FIO_2 has been reduced to 80 percent with orders to keep his SpO_2 greater than 92 percent. Chest auscultation reveals improved aeration throughout the lower lung zones with scattered inspiratory crackles and occasional expiratory wheezes and rhonchi.

Laboratory Evaluation

Vital Signs, Hemodynamics, and Urine Output:

Temperature 37.3°C (99.1°F)

Respiratory rate 23/minute

Heart rate 98/minute

Systemic arterial blood pressure 138/98 mm Hg

SpO_2 96 percent

Urine output total of 1.9 liters over the past 4 hours since admission

ECG Findings: sinus tachycardia, first-degree AV block, and left bundle branch block

ABGs (FIO_2 = 0.80): pH = 7.39, $PaCO_2$ = 50 mm Hg, PaO_2 = 96 mm Hg, HCO_3^- = 30 mEq/liter, $P(A - a)O_2$ = 465 mm Hg, PaO_2/FIO_2 = 120, SaO_2 = 97 percent (calculated), SpO_2 = 96 percent (pulse oximeter)

QUESTIONS

17. How would you interpret his bedside findings and vital signs?

18. What do the ABGs indicate?

19. What respiratory care would you recommend at this time?

ANSWERS

17. Mr. N's bedside findings and vital signs indicate mild-to-moderate respiratory distress, reduced work of breathing, enhanced oxygenation, an improving cardiovascular response, and a continued brisk diuresis.

18. ABGs reveal improving oxygenation, although his FIO_2 requirement remains

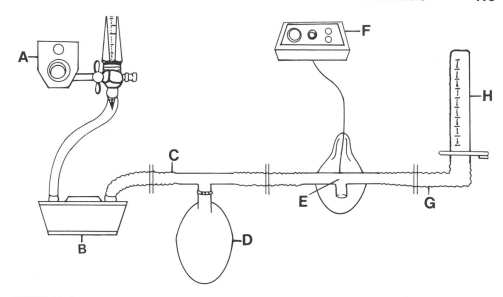

FIGURE 10–4   Continuous high-flow mask-continuous positive airway pressure (CPAP) system. *(A)* High-flow blender and flow meter. *(B)* Low-resistance and high-efficiency humidifier. *(C)* Inspiratory limb and water traps. *(D)* Five-liter reservoir bag. *(E)* Clear plastic soft-seal patient mask. *(F)* Manometer and high-low pressure alarm. *(G)* Expiratory limb and water traps. *(H)* Threshold resistor for CPAP generation. (From Branson, RD, Hurst, JM, and DeHaven, CB: Mask CPAP: State of the art. Respir Care 30:846, 1985, with permission.)

elevated with a declining $P(A - a)O_2$. Hypoventilation and a compensated respiratory acidosis persist, which are common in patients with a history of COPD (see Chapters 5 and 6).

19. Mr. N is having a very good response to the mask CPAP, diuretic, vasodilators, and inotropic therapy. His treatment is on the right course and should allow continued reduction of the FIO_2 by 10 percent increments until 40 percent is reached. If his respiratory and cardiovascular status are stable or improving at that point for 1 hour or more and the tachypnea tapers down to less than 22/minute, the CPAP levels can be reduced to 5 and then 0 cm H_2O. He could then be placed on oxygen therapy via nasal cannula. Continued cardiopulmonary monitoring remains necessary.

CASE STUDY—continued

Mr. N's respiratory status continued to improve over the next 8 hours as the FIO_2 was gradually reduced to 40 percent. His respiratory rate remained less than 20/minute, heart rate was in the 85 to 95 range, blood pressure dropped to 125/75 mm Hg, and SpO_2 was maintained at greater than 95 percent. Breath sounds revealed better aeration with scattered expiratory rhonchi. A chest radiograph (see Fig. 10–5) at this time showed almost complete interval clearing with some scattered atelectasis in the right perihilar region and basal zones of the right and left lungs. Heart size is reduced, and all other anatomic structures appear to be unchanged. Digitalis levels were found to be in the therapeutic range. The ABG results were as follows: pH = 7.37, $PacO_2$ = 49 mm Hg, PaO_2 = 105 mm Hg, and HCO_3^- = 29 mEq/liter. The CPAP level was gradually reduced to 0 cm H_2O over the next hour. Mr. N tolerated this change and exhibited no noticeable changes in clinical state or pulse oximetry. He was then placed on a nasal cannula at 4 liters/minute, which was later reduced to 2 liters/minute. Cardiac enzyme levels (CK and lactate dehydrogenase) were found to be in the high-normal range, suggesting that he did not have a MI. Therapy with diuretics, vasodilators, inotropic agents, aerosolized bronchodilators, and oxygen were continued upon Mr. N's transfer to the post-CCU, and he began to ambulate. He was discharged 2 days later in stable condition with an assortment of medications to support him at home.

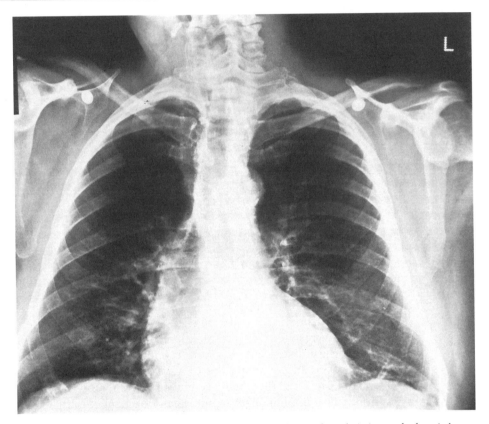

FIGURE 10-5 Portable AP chest radiograph taken 12 hours after admission to the hospital.

REFERENCES

1. Gorlin, R: Incidence, etiology and prognosis of heart failure. Cardiovasc Rev Rep 4:765-770, 1983.
2. Williams, RS: Boosting cardiac contractility with genes. N Engl J Med 332:817-818, 1995.
3. Smith, WM: Epidemiology of congestive heart failure. Am J Cardiol 55:3A, 1985.
4. Alexander, M, et al: Hospitalization for congestive heart failure: Explaining racial differences. JAMA 274:1037-42, 1995.
5. Kannel, WB, et al: Cardiac failure in the Framingham Study: Twenty-year follow-up. In Braunwald, E, et al (eds): Congestive Heart Failure:
Current Research and Clinical Applications. Grune & Stratton, New York, pp 15-30, 1982.
6. Killip, T: Epidemiology of congestive heart failure. Am J Cardiol 56:2A, 1985.
7. Horn, MJ: Pulmonary heart disease (cor pulmonale). In Bordow, RA, and Moser, KM (eds): Manual of Clinical Problems in Pulmonary Medicine. Little, Brown & Co, Boston, pp 262-268, 1985.
8. Smith, JJ, and Kampine, JP: Circulatory Physiology: The Essentials, ed 2. Williams & Wilkins, Baltimore, pp 274-300, 1990.
9. Chesebro, JH, and Burnett, JC: Cardiac failure:

Characteristics and clinical manifestations. In Brandenburg, RO, et al (eds): Cardiology: Fundamentals and Practice. Year Book, Chicago, pp 645-665, 1987.

10. Rushmer, RF: Cardiovascular Dynamics, ed 4. WB Saunders, Philadelphia, pp 532-567, 1976.

11. Braunwald, E: The Myocardium: Failure and Infarction. HP Publishing Co, New York, 1974.

12. Bove, AA, and Santamore, WP: Mechanical performance of the heart. In Brandenburg, RO, et al (eds): Cardiology: Fundamentals and Practice. Year Book, Chicago, pp 149-163, 1987.

13. Zelis, R, and Longhurst, J: The circulation in congestive heart failure. In Zelis, R (ed): The Peripheral Circulation. Grune & Stratton, New York, 1975.

14. Burnett, JC, and Knox, FG: Renal interstitial pressure and sodium excretion during renal vein constriction. Am J Physiol 238:F279-282, 1980.

15. Dzau, VJ, et al: Relation of the renin-angiotensin-aldosterone system to clinical state in congestive heart failure. Circulation 63:645-651, 1981.

16. Lerman, A, et al: Circulating N-terminal atrial natriuretic peptide as a marker for symptomless left-ventricular dysfunction. Lancet 341:1105-1109, 1993.

17. Murray, JF: The lungs and heart failure. Hosp Pract 20:55-63, 1985.

18. Pastore, JO: Cardiac disease in respiratory patients in the intensive care unit. In MacDonnell, KF, et al (eds): Respiratory Intensive Care. Little, Brown & Co, Boston, pp 370-384, 1987.

19. Amsterdam, EA, et al: Today's workup for heart failure. Patient Care 29:58-71, 1995.

20. Kaymakcalan, H, et al: Congestive heart failure as cause of fulminant hepatic failure. Am J Med 65:384-388, 1978.

21. Abelmann, WH, and Gilbert, EM: QT dispersion and sudden unexpected death in chronic heart failure. Lancet 343:327-329, 1994.

22. Forrester, JS, et al: Medical therapy of acute myocardial infarction by application of hemodynamic subsets. N Engl J Med 295:1356-1361, 1976.

23. Weber, KT, et al: Oxygen utilization and ventilation during exercise in patients with chronic cardiac failure. Circulation 65:1213-1223, 1982.

24. Zelis, R, et al: A comparison of regional blood flow and oxygen utilization during dynamic forearm exercise in normal subjects and patients with congestive heart failure. Circulation 50:137-143, 1974.

25. Litchfield, RL, et al: Normal exercise capacity in patients with severe left ventricular dysfunction: Compensatory mechanisms. Circulation 66:129-134, 1982.

26. Bittner, V, et al: Prediction of mortality and morbidity with a 6-minute walk test in patients with left ventricular dysfunction. JAMA 270:1702-1707, 1993.

27. Chesebro, JH: Cardiac failure: Medical management. In Brandenburg, RO, et al (eds): Cardiology: Fundamentals and Practice. Year Book, Chicago, pp 666-688, 1987.

28. Psaty, BM, et al: The risk of myocardial infarction associated with antihypertensive drug therapies. JAMA 274:620-625, 1995.

29. Beller, GA, et al: Digitalis intoxication: a prospective clinical study with serum level correlations. N Engl J Med 284:989-997, 1971.

30. Fuster, V, et al: The natural history of idiopathic dilated cardiomyopathy. Am J Cardiol 47:525-531, 1981.

31. Manley, JC, et al: The "bad" left ventricle: Results of coronary surgery and effects on late survival. J Thorac Cardiovasc Surg 72:841-848, 1976.

32. Branson, RD, et al: Mask CPAP: State of the art. Respir Care 30:846-857, 1985.

33. Rasanen, J, et al: Continuous positive pressure by face mask in acute cardiogenic pulmonary edema: A randomized study. Crit Care Med 12:A325, 1984.

34. Perel, A, et al: Effectiveness of CPAP via face mask for pulmonary edema associated with hypercarbia. Intensive Care Med 9:17-19, 1983.

CHAPTER 11

Smoke Inhalation and Burns

George H. Hicks, MS, RRT

Key Terms

anaerobic metabolism	catabolic hypermetabolism	hydrogen cyanide (HCN)
carbon monoxide (CO) poisoning	escharotomy	pneumonia
carboxyhemoglobin (Hbco)	flash over	

Introduction

Fire continues to be a major source of injury, death, and economic loss. More than 23 million fires are reported annually in the United States and are responsible for more than 28,000 injuries, 5000 deaths, and economic losses that exceeded $12 billion.[1] Residential fires are the most common setting of burn-related injuries and are responsible for more than 80 percent of the deaths.[1] The overall mortality rate for the general burn population is approximately 15 percent, but the rates are significantly higher in the very young (less than 4 years of age) and the elderly (older than 65).[2] According to these statistics, fire-related death is the third most common cause of accidental death in this country behind motor vehicle accidents and accidental falls[1]; however, fire-related morbidity and mortality rates (per 100,000 population) have continued to decline over the past two decades.[1] These changes are probably the result of public education, use of fire detection equipment, improved fire rescue, and better established burn care.

Respiratory tract injury and systemic poisoning from smoke inhalation cause 50 to 90 percent of deaths in burn victims.[2-6] The prevalence of smoke-inhalation injury among burn victims admitted to various burn centers was found to be between 10 and 35 percent.[6-9] There is a dramatically higher mortality rate among burn victims with significant smoke-inhalation injury (Fig. 11-1). For example, the mortality rate among persons with burns covering 50 percent of their body surface area (BSA) approaches 50 percent, whereas the rate can exceed 80 percent in burns of similar size accompanied by significant smoke-inhalation injury.[2,10]

BURN INJURY MORTALITY

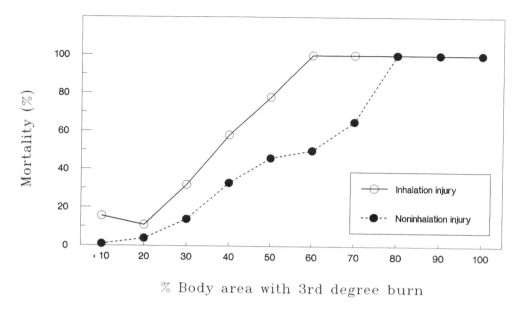

FIGURE 11-1   The distribution of mortality in 914 burn victims, as influenced by the size of the burn and the presence or absence of an inhalation injury. (Adapted from data presented in Venus, B, et al: Prophylactic intubation and continuous positive airway pressure in the management of inhalation injury in burn victims. Crit Care Med 9:519, 1981.)

Burn injuries are highly complex. They are not confined to the integumentary (skin) and respiratory systems. Although it is convenient to categorize postburn problems into various periods or phases, in reality they often present in an overlapping pattern. Pulmonary complications are frequently associated with the burn victim and are found in various time frames after the burn.[6,11-13] The early or resuscitative phase (first 24 hours) is usually associated with complications arising from inhalation of toxic or hot gases, or both. In the intermediate or postresuscitative phase (1 to 5 days), pulmonary edema, secretion retention, atelectasis, adult respiratory distress syndrome (ARDS), and hypermetabolic induced ventilatory failure can occur. During the late phase (beyond 5 days), infectious **pneumonia,** sepsis syndrome, pulmonary embolism, and chronic pulmonary disease are the more frequent types of respiratory dysfunction.

The pulmonary problems listed above, coupled with the other pathophysiological changes, make the burn victim one of the more challenging patients to treat. These problems are complex but predictable, potentially allowing a more successful approach through the principles of prevention. This chapter focuses on the pulmonary changes and required treatment for smoke-inhalation and burn injuries.

Etiology

Analysis of the fire environment is highly complex. Variability in heat production and the chemical and physical nature of the smoke produced must be taken into account. This variability is a factor of the types of fuels being burned and the availability of fresh

TABLE 11–1   **Toxic Gases Found in House Fire Smoke**

Substance	Source	Effect
Ammonia	Melamine resins	Inflammation
Aldehydes (acrolein, acetaldehyde, formaldehyde)	Wood, cotton, paper	Inflammation
Benzene	Petroleum products	Irritation & coma
Carbon dioxide	Organic materials	Asphyxiation & coma
Carbon monoxide	Organic materials	Asphyxiation & coma
Hydrogen chloride	Polyvinyl chloride	Inflammation
Hydrogen cyanide	Polyurethanes	Cellular asphyxia
Isocyanate	Polyurethanes	Inflammation & bronchospasm
Organic acids (acetic & formic acid)	Wood, cotton, paper	Inflammation
Oxides of nitrogen & sulfur	Nitrocellulose film	Pulmonary edema
Phosgene	Polyvinyl chloride	Inflammation

air. The nature and extent of injuries are a product of exposure to heat and the complex chemistry of the fire environment.

Air temperatures can rapidly climb to 1000°F in less than 10 minutes in a fuel-rich environment such as the home or office.[3] As the heat builds, spontaneous combustion of other fuel sources (e.g., carpet, furniture, wall coverings, appliances) can occur, developing into a **flash over** condition. Flash over is usually seen as a wall of fire extending down from the ceiling and billowing out of openings in doors or windows. Industrial or shipboard fires can produce much higher temperatures as well as steam. Steam has a much higher heat energy content than dry gases at the same temperature and can scald greater areas of skin and cause a deeper respiratory tract thermal injury if inhaled.

The burning of various fuels found in modern residential, office, and industrial settings produces a large number of combustion products. Some of the more common toxic gases produced are listed in Table 11–1. A variety of aldehydes (e.g., acrolein) and organic acids (e.g., acetic acid), which are potent respiratory tract irritants, are produced from burning wood, cotton, paper, and many acrylics.[14] As the fire continues, carbon dioxide is produced and can increase beyond 5 percent while the oxygen concentration can drop below 10 percent.[15] With the decreased oxygen availability, incomplete combustion results in the production of carbon monoxide (CO).[3,4] When polyvinyl chloride is burned, it produces more than 75 different toxic chemicals, including hydrogen chloride, phosgene, chlorine, and CO.[16] The burning of polyurethane-rich materials, such as nylon and various types of upholsteries, can produce the very irritating isocyanates and extremely toxic **hydrogen cyanide (HCN).**[17] Inhaled soot particles, which carry toxic chemicals, can penetrate deep into the lung if they have diameters in the range of 0.1 to 5 μm. This deposition of chemically laden soot results in further mucosal injury throughout the respiratory tract.[16,18]

The chemical products of combustion can be divided into two categories: (1) those that produce toxic effects systemically upon absorption; and (2) those that produce local inflammatory changes upon contact with the mucosa. An additional factor that contributes to the severity of smoke-inhalation injuries in enclosed spaces (e.g., closed rooms, cars) is the hypoxic insult that results from the rapid depletion of oxygen during the fire.

In summary, the nature and severity of injury is a function of many factors. The size and depth or degree of the skin burn, heat of the gases inhaled, chemical composition of the smoke, extent and duration of exposure, and the age and preexisting health status of the victim are important factor to assess.[2,10,12,13]

Pathophysiology

Early Pulmonary and Systemic Changes: 24 Hours Postburn

Exposure to the hypoxic and poisonous environment of a fire can cause rapid and severe organ dysfunction. The mechanism of this type of dysfunction centers around reductions in both O_2 transport and its utilization. The tissues of the central nervous system (CNS) and myocardium are particularly at risk. CO is readily produced in the fire environment and is easily absorbed. It rapidly converts oxyhemoglobin (Hbo_2) to **carboxyhemoglobin (Hbco).** This conversion is driven by CO's higher affinity for the ferrous binding sites in hemoglobin (more than 200 times that of O_2). Hbco levels can reach 15 percent in minor smoke inhalation, compared to more than 60 percent in severe smoke inhalation. Conversion of Hbo_2 to Hbco compromises oxygen transport primarily through Hbco's inability to carry O_2. The presence of CO also results in retarding oxygen release from hemoglobin's remaining ferrous binding sites by a chemically induced increase in Hbo_2 affinity. The hemoglobin conversion and inhibition of oxygen release results in a functional form of anemia that causes reduced oxygen transport and hypoxia despite the presence of a normal Pao_2 in the plasma.

Cerebral edema can occur rapidly during severe **carbon monoxide (CO) poisoning** as a result of impaired oxygen transport and hypotension secondary to cardiogenic toxicity.[19] In a small number of victims who appear to recover, latent neurologic dysfunction can occur 3 days to 4 weeks after a significant poisoning.[20] Lethal CO poisoning is generally associated with Hbco concentrations greater than 60 percent. Inhaled HCN has been linked to early and late death in burned patients.[17,21] HCN is easily transported to the tissues through the circulatory system and binds to the cytochrome oxidase enzymes of the mitochondria. This results in inhibition of oxidative cellular metabolism and a shift to an inefficient **anaerobic metabolism.** Fatal exposure to HCN is generally associated with blood levels that exceed 1 mg/liter.[21]

CO is also capable of binding to cytochrome oxidase and causing mitochondrial dysfunction. Some evidence, however, suggests that mitochondrial dysfunction is more often a function of low O_2 delivery to tissues at typical CO exposure levels.[22] Metabolic acidosis, caused by anaerobic metabolism, frequently accompanies CO and HCN exposure and is proportional to the severity of the poisoning. Thus, reduced oxygen transport and cellular metabolic dysfunction rapidly compromise CNS and cardiovascular function. They are the primary causes of death during the immediate period after severe smoke inhalation.[3,6,12]

Thermal injury to the respiratory tract is frequently confined to the face, oral and nasal cavities, pharynx, and rarely into the trachea.[2,6,12] The lower respiratory tract is spared of thermal injury by the upper airway's efficient cooling of hot gases and by reflex laryngospasm and glottic closure.[3,5,6] Thermal injury to the upper airway results in blistering, edema, accumulation of thick saliva, and glottic closure in severe cases.[23] These changes usually develop in the first 2 to 8 hours and can lead to partial or total airway obstruction.

Chemical injury to the respiratory tract, brought about by inhalation of toxic gases and irritant-laden soot particles, extends the injuries further into the lung. This can cause acute tracheobronchitis, bronchospasm, bronchorrhea, and in severe cases pulmonary edema.[24] After chemical exposure, the ciliary transport mechanism of the mucosa is inactivated or destroyed, which potentiates mucus retention and infection.[4] In addition, the following abnormalities have been documented: surfactant dysfunction, increased lung water, decreased lung compliance, increased airway resistance, and increased pulmonary vascular resistance.[6,25,26] These changes result in ventilation-perfusion ($\dot{V}/\dot{Q}$) mismatching and increased ratio of volume of dead space to tidal volume (VD/VT), which decrease Pao_2, increase the alveolar-arterial oxygen tension gradient (P[A − a]O_2), and increase the necessary minute ventilation to normalize the $Paco_2$. The initial arterial blood gas (ABG) changes (Table 11–2) are often associated with hypoxemia and respiratory alkalosis.[27]

Early systemic changes are associated with the extent of inadequate oxygen transport and the degree of the skin burn. Organ dysfunction induced by hypovolemic shock is one of the primary systemic insults in the early period after a major full-thickness skin burn.[13] The early hypovolemia is secondary to massive fluid shifts out of the vascular compartment as a result of a hyperpermeable microvasculature. This massive fluid shift results in a generalized edema that peaks within 8 to 24 hours and is dependent on the magnitude of the burn and the adequacy of the fluid resuscitation.

Burned skin also loses its elasticity and becomes less compliant with the edema formation. In circumferential burns of the extremities and trunk, the tightening skin can further impair circulation and cause increased edema, distal tissue necrosis, and reduced chest wall compliance.[3,12,13] This reduction in chest wall compliance results in an increase in the work of breathing and may lead to severe ventilatory compromise.

Cardiovascular and hematologic instability occurs from the loss of fluid volume, which can exceed 4 mL/kg of body weight per hour in major burns (Table 11–3).[27,28] Cardiac output is decreased as a result of hypovolemia, hypoxia, and increased systemic vascular resistance.[28,29] Blood pressure (BP) may be normal or low, and heart

TABLE 11–2 **Changes in Arterial Blood Gases, Oxygen Consumption, and Acid-Base Balance After Severe Burns**

	PERIOD		
	Early	*Intermediate*	*Late*
Pao_2	−20%	+7%	−60%
Sao_2	−5%	−3%	−40%
Hematocrit	+3%	−30%	−30%
Oxygen transport	−15%	+25%	−60%
Oxygen consumption	+35%	+70%	−40%
$Paco_2$	−40%	−30%	+18%
pH	Normal	7.39–7.30	7.35–7.25

*From six patients (35–60% of BSA third-degree burns). The early period was the first 25% of their course, the late period was the last 25% of their course, and the intermediate period was the time between early and late periods. Values are expressed as percent change from data taken from 17 healthy control subjects.

SOURCE: Adapted from Shoemaker, WC, et al: Burn pathophysiology in man: I. Sequential hemodynamic alterations. J Surg Res 14:64, 1973.

TABLE 11-3   **Changes in Systemic Hemodynamics
and Blood Volume after Severe Burns**

	PERIOD		
	Early	*Intermediate*	*Late*
Heart rate	+50%	+75%	+25%
Blood pressure (mean)	Normal	+10%	−30%
Cardiac index	−15%	+65%	−15%
Left ventricular stroke work	−50%	Normal	−55%
Vascular resistance	+30%	−30%	−20%
Blood volume	−20%	+15%	−30%

*From six patients (35–60% of BSA third-degree burns). The early period was the first 25% of their course, the late period was the last 25% of their course, and the intermediate period was the time between early and late periods. Values are expressed as percent change from data taken from 17 healthy control subjects.

SOURCE: Adapted from Shoemaker, WC, et al: Burn pathophysiology in man: I. Sequential hemodynamic alterations. J Surg Res 14:64, 1973.

rate is usually increased.[27] Older patients may not tolerate the massive fluid resuscitation and are at risk for congestive heart failure. Immune suppression and alterations in leukocyte and macrophage function have been noted.[6,12,13] Hemolysis and the development of disseminated intravascular coagulation can occur and further compromise the microcirculation.[12]

The metabolic rate is often depressed very early as a result of the severe hypoxia and abnormal circulation. After a massive release of catecholamines in response to the stress, metabolism increases and may result in an imbalance between oxygen demand and delivery. Anaerobic metabolism may result and produce metabolic acidosis if the oxygen demand exceeds the delivery rates. These metabolic changes can extend the injury to nonburned tissues.

Intermediate Pulmonary and Systemic Changes: 2 to 5 Days Postburn

Signs of respiratory distress are more often seen in burn victims after 36 to 72 hours. In those with severe burns (greater than 30 percent of total BSA) but no inhalation injury, lung function is often stable but can be complicated by fluid resuscitation-induced pulmonary edema and reduced chest wall compliance. The early increase in pulmonary vascular resistance often returns to normal during this period. The hypermetabolic state (Table 11-2) that results in increased CO_2 production and O_2 consumption, which often begins by the 3rd to 5th day, can result in respiratory failure.

In patients with inhalation injury, the upper airway edema usually begins to resolve between days 2 and 4. Mucosal inflammation secondary to chemical injury results in increased mucus production and decreased clearance secondary to ciliary dysfunction. Smaller airway injury, manifested as a lingering bronchitis with or without bronchospasm, usually peaks on day 2 or 3. With more severe mucosal injury, the mucosal tissue often becomes necrotic and sloughs, usually on day 3 or 4. The necrotic debris and mucus retention often result in airway plugging and atelectasis. The atelectasis is further promoted by the victim's inability to breathe deeply and cough effectively as a result of reduced chest and lung compliance, increased airway resistance, pain, use of narcotics, immobility, and inadequate airway care. The impaired secretion clearance, atelectasis, and burn-induced immune suppression set the stage for bacterial colonization, infectious bronchitis, and pneumonia.

During the intermediate period, major pulmonary complications (primarily atelectasis, increased extravascular lung water, and ARDS) develop in approximately 30 percent of these patients.[6,10,30,31] The risk of ARDS increases when the burn victim becomes septic.[32] In these patients, ARDS is thought to be caused by a complex array of insults, including surfactant dysfunction; microvascular hyperpermeability induced by mediator release (e.g., lipid peroxidants) from the airway or cutaneous burn site, or both; activated leukocytes that migrate to the lung and release toxins (e.g., proteolytic enzymes, free radicals); and coagulation defects.[33-37]

Patients who have had careful fluid resuscitation are usually hemodynamically stable. Cardiac output increases during this period along with a persistent tachycardia secondary to the elevated catecholamines being released by the sympathetic nervous system (Table 11-3). Cardiac failure causes 10 percent of the deaths in this phase.[10] Systemic vascular resistance begins to drop, and the urine output continues to reflect the vascular fluid volume status. The erythrocyte damage secondary to the cutaneous thermal injury is usually seen during this intermediate period as a decline in the hematocrit (Hct) that levels off by day 4 or 5 (Table 11-2).

The metabolic rate during the intermediate phase is characterized by **catabolic hypermetabolism.**[13] A negative nitrogen balance is often seen and signifies the catabolism of blood and muscle proteins. A stress induced diabetes can result in hyperglycemia that frequently resolves during this period.[13]

The use of a mafenide acetate–based cream (Sulfamylon Cream), a potent and painful topical antibiotic, may complicate the patient's cardiorespiratory and metabolic status through its carbonic anhydrase inhibition and subsequent production of metabolic acidosis.[38] This acidosis can be compensated for via reflex respiratory alkalosis; however, in patients with significant pulmonary complications this may not be possible. An alternative topical antibiotic, such as silver sulfadiazine (Silvadene) may prove useful.

Late Pulmonary and Systemic Changes: Beyond 5 Days Postburn

In the late period, one of the pulmonary complications is a continued hypermetabolic state, which may persist for 1 to 3 weeks. The resting CO_2 production rates can frequently exceed 400 mL/minute during this state as the metabolic rate significantly increases.[13] This added load on the respiratory system significantly increases the work of breathing and, compounded by a possible muscle catabolism, can result in respiratory muscle fatigue and ventilatory failure.

Pneumonia occurs in about 35 percent of these patients and continues to be a major complication in the late stage. It remains an important cause of death in burn patients with and without inhalation injury. Increased control of burn wound sepsis through topical antibiotics and skin grafting has decreased the overall mortality rate.

Pulmonary embolism develops in 5 to 30 percent of burned patients, generally within 2 weeks of the burn injury; however, it may develop months after the injury.[39] Tachypnea, increasing minute ventilation, and a marked increase in $P(A - a)O_2$, V_D/V_T, or the difference between arterial and end-tidal PCO_2 $[P(a - ET)CO_2]$ indicate significant embolization.

In the long term, severe inhalation injury can result in mixed restrictive and obstructive lung disease. This is thought to be due to the formation of alveolar fibrosis,

TABLE 11-4   **Clinical Manifestations of Carbon Monoxide Poisoning**

Blood HbCO Concentration (%)	Signs and Symptoms
0-10	None; angina in patients with coronary artery disease
10-20	Mild headache, exercise-induced angina, and dyspnea
20-40	Headache, dyspnea, vomiting, muscular weakness, dizziness, visual disturbance, impaired judgment
40-60	Syncope, increasing tachypnea and tachycardia, coma, convulsion, irregular breathing pattern
>60	Coma, shock, apnea, death

HbCO = carboxyhemoglobin

pleural adhesions, squamous metaplasia of the respiratory mucosa, bronchial stenosis, bronchiectasis, and chronic lobar atelectasis.[40]

The burn wound is a frequent site of infection and is the primary cause of death as a result of sepsis-induced multiorgan failure during the late period.[6,10] Sepsis will compound the pulmonary injuries, drive up the metabolic rate, and promote the hyperdynamic circulatory status.

Clinical Features and Laboratory Findings

The increased morbidity and mortality associated with inhalation injury in the burn victim necessitates early recognition and treatment. Few details taken from the history of a smoke-inhalation victim can help in his or her emergent care. When a patient presents with a history of exposure to a smoke-filled, enclosed environment, despite the absence of clinical findings, there is a high index of suspicion for potential injury. When the patient is unconscious, however, there is a high probability that he or she was exposed to asphyxiating conditions or poisoning by toxic gases (e.g., CO, HCN), or both. This requires the immediate aggressive treatment. Tables 11-4 and 11-5 list the major signs and symptoms associated with various levels of CO and HCN poisoning. The classic description of CO poisoning, a cherry-red skin color, is an unreliable sign, especially in the hypotensive victim. Electrocardiograms (ECGs) often

TABLE 11-5   **Clinical Manifestations of Hydrogen Cyanide (HCN) Poisoning**

Blood HCN Concentrations (mg/liter)	Signs and Symptoms
0.2-0.3	Tachycardia Tachypnea Dizziness Stupor
0.3-1.0	Progressive stupor Cardiac arrhythmias Apnea Seizures
>1.0	Death

show tachycardia and signs of ischemic heart disease. In fact, CO poisoning can resemble the classic clinical and ECG findings of heart attack.[41] The sampling of arterial blood for direct determination of Hbco content is the most important diagnostic indicator of CO poisoning. Hbco content is also a potential indicator of the dose of smoke inhaled.[11] Low levels of Hbco, however, do not rule out significant pulmonary injury in the intermediate or later postburn periods.

Pulse oximetry should not be used to indicate the level of HbO_2 concentration in the patient who is known or suspected to have been poisoned by CO. Oxyhemoglobin and Hbco have similar light-absorption spectra. Thus, pulse oximeters can give a falsely high value for the true HbO_2 concentration when Hbco concentrations are elevated.[42]

Facial burns, singed nasal hair, oral and laryngeal edema, and carbonaceous deposits in the airway and sputum suggest inhalation injury; however, the presence or absence of these findings is not considered a reliable indication of inhalation injury.[6,9,10] Carbonaceous sputum, while considered to be a very sensitive sign of smoke inhalation, may not be seen for 8 to 24 hours and may occur only in about 40 percent of victims with significant pulmonary injury.[43] Stridor, hoarseness, difficulty speaking, and chest retractions suggest upper airway injury and the need for careful evaluation. Fiberoptic laryngoscopy and bronchoscopy have been found very useful in both evaluating the presence of upper airway injury and removing excess saliva and debris.[44,45] Cough, dyspnea, tachypnea, cyanosis, wheezing, crackles, and rhonchi are indicators of a more severe form of inhalation injury.

Chest radiographs frequently do not show signs of inhalation injury in the early period and lag behind the pulmonary changes. The chest x-ray is useful in the initial assessment of the burn victim to determine the position of the endotracheal tube after intubation.

Spirometry has been found useful in detecting small and upper airway injury. Peak expiratory flow and forced expiratory flow rates at 50 percent of the forced vital capacity (FVC) are both markedly decreased and correlate well with xenon-133 scan results in victims of smoke inhalation.[46] The utility of spirometry, however, is limited to those patients who can follow commands and make an acceptable FVC effort.

ABG analysis is useful in diagnosing and trending the patient's pulmonary insult. Reduced PaO_2 and an increased $P(A - a)O_2$ (greater than 300 mm Hg) or a reduced ratio of PaO_2 to fraction of inspired oxygen (PaO_2/FIO_2 less than 350) may be the most practical and sensitive signs of respiratory impairment secondary to $\dot{V}/\dot{Q}$ mismatching.[6,46] Respiratory alkalosis may also be found in the early postburn period and often continues with the hypermetabolic phase. Metabolic acidosis and ventilatory failure due to respiratory acidosis are signs of life-threatening injuries.

ECG and hemodynamic monitoring are essential in patients with third-degree burns greater than 10 percent of their BSA, regardless of whether or not they have concomitant smoke-inhalation injury. Pulmonary artery pressure, cardiac output, and other hemodynamic variables must be monitored to optimize fluid resuscitation in order to avoid hypotension, renal failure, and fluid overload in the severely burned patient.

Physical assessment, fiberoptic bronchoscopy, chest radiography, ABG analysis, ECG, and hemodynamic monitoring form the core of early assessment. Repeated evaluation of the burn victim with these techniques will enable the clinician to detect early cardiopulmonary changes and intervene appropriately.

To assess the cutaneous injury, a complete physical examination, weight determination (for trending fluid balance), and calculation of total BSA burned are performed. The *rule of nines* (Fig. 11-2) can be used to estimate the total size of the injured area by determining the amount of injury to each extremity, the head, and the anterior and

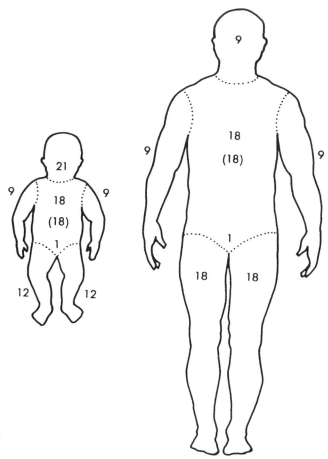

FIGURE 11-2 The percentage of surface area covered by skin in various body regions of the infant and adult.

posterior trunk. Each of these anatomic areas represents approximately 9 to 18 percent of the BSA in adults. The burn depth is determined by its clinical appearance:

First degree: A burn to the epithelium that is manifested by erythema and pain

Second degree: A burn of the epithelium and dermis that is manifested by erythema, blisters, and pain

Third degree: A burn that destroys the skin through or into the hypodermis, manifested by pale or gray-brown, leatherlike skin. There is no pain in this area because all sensory organs in the skin are completely destroyed.

Fourth degree: A full-thickness burn that appears black or charred. This burn may result in exposed bone and lacks pain sensation.

Treatment

The goals of respiratory care for the burn patient are achievement of a patent airway, effective ventilation, adequate oxygenation, maintenance of acid-base balance, cardiovascular stability, maintenance of lung volume, reduction of pulmonary vascular permeability, suppression of infection, and appropriate monitoring.[47]

As stated earlier, the immediate signs of minor or moderate inhalation injury are characterized by partial airway obstruction. Burn victims with minor upper airway injury should be closely monitored for airway closure or other signs of pulmonary involvement, given supplementary oxygen via nasal cannula, and placed in a high Fowler's position to reduce the work of breathing. Bronchospasm should be treated aggressively with aerosolized β-agonists (e.g., metaproterenol [Alupent], albuterol [Ventolin]).

Airway maintenance with an endotracheal tube of appropriate size is needed in cases where upper airway closure is anticipated or clinically significant inhalation injury is found. Early tracheostomy in this setting is not recommended because of its higher mortality and infection rates, but it may become necessary in patients who require long-term airway care.[10,12,13] Early intubation has been found to precipitate transient pulmonary edema in some patients in the early stages after inhalation injury.[48] The addition of 5 to 10 cm H_2O of continuous positive airway pressure (CPAP) can maintain lung volume, support edematous airways, and optimize $\dot{V}/\dot{Q}$ matching.[10,47] The use of systemic corticosteroids to treat edema formation is generally not recommended.[49-51]

The burn victim who is found in a coma must be assumed to have sustained severe asphyxia or CO poisoning. Basic and advanced life support are needed immediately to provide a patent airway and cardiorespiratory support. Oxygen therapy forms the cornerstone for the treatment of hypoxia and CO poisoning. Elimination of CO is accelerated when supplemental O_2 is administered (Table 11-6). Burn victims in whom smoke inhalation is suspected have moderately elevated Hbco (less than 30 percent) and have stable cardiopulmonary function; a tight-fitting non-rebreathing mask delivering 100 percent O_2 at a rate of 10 or 15 liters/minute is the method of choice. Oxygen therapy should continue until the Hbco is reduced to less than 10 percent. Mask CPAP with 70 to 100 percent O_2 may be useful in patients who have minimal thermal injuries to the face and upper airway and have increasing dyspnea and hypoxemia despite the use of a non-rebreathing mask. For those with a more severe form of CO poisoning (Hbco greater than 30 percent) that results in coma, intubation and ventilatory support with 100 percent O_2 is needed. Rapid referral for hyperbaric O_2 therapy at 3 atm for 30 minutes to 1 hour is useful to improve patient outcomes.[52]

Ventilatory support with positive end-expiratory pressure (PEEP) is often needed in patients with early development of pulmonary edema, ARDS, and pneumonia. Ventilatory support is needed when the patient's ABGs indicate respiratory failure (Pao_2 less than 60 mm Hg, $Paco_2$ greater than 50 mm Hg, and pH less than 7.25) or the clinical picture indicates impending respiratory failure (respiratory rate greater than 35/minute and significant use of accessory muscles). The use of PEEP in the range of 5 to 20 cm H_2O is indicated when the patient's Pao_2 falls to less than 60 mm Hg and the Fio_2 requirement climbs above 50 percent. As the pulmonary insult resolves, the

TABLE 11-6 **Half-Life of Carboxyhemoglobin (Hbco) at Different Oxygen Exposures**

Hbco Half-Life (min)	Inhaled O_2 Partial Pressure
280–320	Air (21% @ 1 atm)
80–90	100% @ 1 atm
20–30	100% @ 3 atm

need for ventilatory support may continue in patients who maintain high metabolic rates and minute volume requirements.

Because of the spectrum of pulmonary dysfunctions that may be encountered, the ventilators of choice should be able to provide tidal ventilation that is volume or pressure limited, time or patient cycled on, and capable of pressure support to facilitate spontaneous breathing. In addition, they should be capable of delivering high minute ventilation (up to 50 liters/minute) in the face of high peak airway pressures (often greater than 40 cm H_2O). Burn patients are difficult to ventilate because the use of large VTs (greater than 7 mL/kg) and elevated airway pressures can cause more lung injury. In cases where there is an increased risk of further lung damage and barotrauma, the use of pressure-controlled ventilation and permissive hypercapnia may be an option.[53]

Vigorous attention to airway clearance is necessary as mucosa sloughs and sputum production increases. Chest physical therapy promotes secretion mobilization and prevents airway plugging and atelectasis; however, percussion and vibration should not be done on areas of recent skin grafting.

Careful maintenance of fluid balance is necessary to minimize the development of shock, renal failure, and pulmonary edema. Hemodynamic stability can often be maintained through resuscitation of the patient's fluid balance (Parkland formula: 4 mL isotonic crystalloids per kilogram per percentage burn given over a 24-hour period) and induction of a standard urine output target (e.g., 30 to 50 mL/hour); however, maintenance of hemodynamic stability can result in the development of pulmonary edema.[12] Patients with inhalation injury have an increased fluid requirement. Monitoring pulmonary artery pressures in addition to urine output is needed to guide the adequacy of fluid replacement.[54] Fluid replacement and any needed cardiovascular agents (e.g., dopamine) are then tapered off after 24 to 48 hours. Frequent analysis of the electrolyte panel and acid-base status is required to avoid potential imbalances.

Because a hypermetabolic state often develops in burned patients, careful evaluation is needed for appropriate feeding in order to avoid catabolic wasting of muscle tissue. Predictive formulas (e.g., Harris-Benedict, Curreri) have been used to estimate the metabolic rate of the burn patient; however, the use of commercially developed portable analyzers for serial measurements of indirect calorimetry have been found to be more accurate.[55,56] In very large burns (greater than 50 percent of BSA), the patient is often given a diet with caloric content that is 150 percent of their resting energy expenditure to facilitate wound healing and avoid catabolism. As the wounds are closed and heal, feedings are tapered back to 130 percent of the patient's resting energy expenditure to avoid overfeeding.

In cases where circumferential burns of the thorax occur, the burned skin will need to be cut (**escharotomy**). This is done by making lateral incisions in the anterior axillary line extending from 2 cm below the clavicle to the ninth or tenth rib and transverse incisions across the chest at the top and bottom to form a square. Escharotomy of the chest should improve the elasticity of the chest wall and relieve the compressive effect of the burned skin.

Infections in these patients are often caused by coagulase-positive *Staphylococcus aureus* and gram-negative organisms such as *Klebsiella, Enterobacter, Escherichia coli,* and *Pseudomonas.* Isolation technique, room pressurization, air filtration, and wound covering form the front lines of infection defense. Infections should be treated with specific antibiotics. The appropriate antibiotics are found through serial wound, blood, urine, and sputum cultures. Prophylactic antibiotics are not commonly used in these patients because resistant bacterial strains can develop and produce a pneumonia that is more refractory to treatment.[3,6,12,13]

To prevent disseminated intravascular coagulation and pulmonary embolism, heparin therapy may be needed, especially in patients who remain immobile. Clearly, the prevention and early detection of fires remains the most important actions to be taken to reduce the morbidity and mortality rates associated with the burn victim.

CASE STUDY

History

Mr. A, a 33-year-old man, was in good health before his accident. While he was working above a vat of molten nickel in a foundry, a large tool was accidentally dropped into the vat and broke through the semisolid surface crust and opened it. A tremendous amount of heat was released from the molten nickel upon contact with the air and caused spontaneous combustion of Mr. A's clothes. He jumped off the scaffolding and ran some distance completely engulfed in flames before the fire was put out by fellow workers. His clothes were completely burned off, and the only unburned sites appeared to be his head and feet, which were protected by his helmet and work boots. He was initially taken to a nearby community hospital, where he was assessed and treatment begun.

QUESTIONS

1. What signs and symptoms should be evaluated immediately upon his arrival?
2. What facts should be gathered to help determine the severity of his injuries?
3. What therapeutic techniques should be readily available upon his arrival?

ANSWERS

1. The following signs should be evaluated: patency of the airway, breathing status (e.g., spontaneous), quality of breath sounds and their symmetry, pulse rate, BP, and level of consciousness (Glasgow coma scale). Symptoms of respiratory distress, shock, and mental impairment should be noted.
2. The severity of his injuries can be evaluated by determining whether he was burned in an enclosed space, whether there is evidence of inhalation injury, how long he was exposed to flame and smoke, the percentage of BSA burned and the degree or thickness of the burn, the length of time since his injury, his age, and any underlying medical conditions that may complicate his injuries.
3. Oxygen therapy (cannula or non-rebreathing mask), intubation equipment, manual resuscitation bag with proper mask, oxygen reservoir and a PEEP capability, venous and arterial line placement equipment, crystalloid fluids for vascular support, appropriate resuscitation drugs, and medications for pain and agitation should be ready upon his arrival.

Physical Examination

General: An average-sized man of approximately 80 kg who is obviously burned over approximately 80 percent of his body; lying prone, restless, moaning, poorly responsive to questions with a hoarse voice, and in apparent respiratory distress while breathing with the aid of supplementary oxygen from a non-rebreathing mask and reservoir; Glasgow coma scale 13

Vital Signs: Temperature 38.6°C(101.5°F), respiratory rate 39/minute, BP 121/76 mm Hg, heart rate 147/minute, nail-bed refill 2 seconds

HEENT: Most of his head unburned; pupils equal and reactive to light; nasal flaring, nasal hairs singed; some sign of first- and second-degree burns on face and erythema in the oral cavity

Neck: Third-degree burns start at base of neck; trachea in midline; mild inspiratory stridor; carotid pulses + + + bilaterally without bruit; no signs of lymphadenopathy, thyroidomegaly, or jugular venous distention; obvious tensing of sternocleidomastoid and scalene muscles during inspiration

Chest: Obvious circumferential third-degree burn; some scattered expiratory wheezes but otherwise clear bilaterally; some thoracoabdominal paradoxical motion

Heart: Regular rhythm at 145 to 150/minute; normal first and second heart sounds without murmurs, gallops, or rubs

Abdomen: Obvious circumferential third-degree burn with exception of band around waste, possibly due to protection from belt; soft, nontender; bowel sounds indistinct; no masses or organomegaly

Extremities: Moving all extremities; circumferential third-degree burns on all extremities with exception of feet, right elbow, and axillary areas; no digital clubbing; no obvious cyanosis; some generalized swelling

QUESTIONS

4. Which of Mr. A's signs and symptoms indicate inhalation injury?
5. How will the circumferential burns of his thorax influence respiratory function?
6. What are the possible causes of his respiratory distress?
7. What diagnostic techniques should be used to evaluate his respiratory distress?
8. What laboratory tests and other determinations are now needed to make a more complete evaluation?
9. What techniques are needed to monitor his cardiovascular status?

ANSWERS

4. Inhalation injury is indicated by the presence of tachypnea, stridor, voice changes, accessory muscle tensing, erythema about the face and in the mouth, nasal flaring, singed nasal hair, wheezing, and thoracoabdominal wall paradoxical motion.

5. Circumferential burns of the thorax result in decreased thoracic compliance and increased work of breathing.

6. His respiratory distress is probably due to some inhalation of hot gas and smoke, which has caused upper airway edema, bronchospasm, and possibly chemically induced acute tracheobronchitis. Increasing lung water, secondary to the inhalation injury and very large cutaneous burn, may be accumulating and inducing increased airway resistance, decreased pulmonary compliance, $\dot{V}/\dot{Q}$ mismatching, and hypoxemia. The circumferential burn is also complicating his ease of breathing.

7. To evaluate his respiratory distress further, the following tests may be useful: spirometry (only if he can follow commands); fiberoptic laryngoscopy and bronchoscopy; and a chest radiograph, but only as a baseline. A xenon-133 lung scan would be helpful in making the diagnosis of inhalation injury, but it may not be practical in this setting.

8. Laboratory assessment should include a complete blood count, electrolytes, ABG, HbCO, standard blood chemistry, and a screening for alcohol and illegal drugs. A more precise estimation of the burn size should be determined through careful physical examination and the use of a Lund-Browder burn chart to help guide therapy.

9. ECG monitoring and placement of peripheral venous, central venous, and arterial lines are needed to guide the maintenance of hemodynamic stability.

Bedside and Laboratory Evaluations

Burn Size: 85 percent of total BSA

ECG: Sinus tachycardia of 148/minute without any other abnormalities

Arterial BP and Central Venous Pressure (CVP): BP 130/81 mm Hg, CVP 3 mm Hg

Bronchoscopy: Patchy erythema and some soot deposits on mucosa of nasal pharynx; epiglottic and laryngeal erythema and edema with some soot-streaked mucous membranes; bronchoscope not advanced further

Chest Radiograph: Normal thoracic, diaphragmatic, cardiac, and pulmonary anatomy; no signs of infiltrate, atelectasis, pulmonary edema, masses, or foreign bodies

ABGs: pH 7.33, $PaCO_2$ 32 mm Hg, PaO_2 94 mm Hg, arterial oxygen saturation (SaO_2) 91 percent, HbCO 8 percent, HCO_3^- 18 mEq/liter on 100 percent O_2 from a non-rebreathing mask

Hematology: Hct 45 percent, red blood cells (RBCs) $4.7 \times 10^6/mm^3$, white blood cells (WBCs) 9.2×10^3, platelets 270×10^3

Chemistry and Toxicology: Results pending

QUESTIONS

10. How would you evaluate the ECG and hemodynamic findings?

11. What do the bronchoscopy and chest radiograph indicate?

12. How would you interpret the ABG data?

13. What do the hematologic data indicate?

14. What respiratory care is indicated at this time, and how should it be evaluated?

15. What hemodynamic support is indicated at this time, and how should it be evaluated?

16. What complications may occur in the next 24 to 48 hours?

ANSWERS

10. The ECG and hemodynamic measurements indicate an acceptable status, given the extent of injuries. Placement of a pulmonary artery catheter is

necessary to achieve better guidance for fluid replacement and administration of cardiovascular agents.

11. The bronchoscopy reveals thermal injury to the upper airway and probable smoke inhalation. The bronchoscope was not advanced further for fear of inducing more upper airway edema and closure. The chest radiograph shows no evidence of pathology.

12. The ABG shows maximal compensated metabolic acidosis; hyperventilation; hypoxemia; minor CO poisoning; a $P(A - a)O_2$ of 585 mm Hg and PaO_2/FIO_2 of 94, which indicate $\dot{V}/\dot{Q}$ abnormality; and a diffusion defect or venous-to-arterial intrapulmonary shunting, or both.

13. The hematologic data are normal and do not indicate loss of blood.

14. The patient needs to be intubated with a cuffed endotracheal tube (8.0 or 8.5 mm internal diameter) with the aid of the bronchoscope. After intubation, visual inspection of chest motion and breath sounds is needed for initial determination of proper tube placement. Mr. A will need mechanical ventilatory support to help avoid and manage further gas exchange derangement. Initial ventilator settings should be as follows: assist/control mode, set V_T at 800 mL, set rate at 20/minute, adequate inspiratory flow to maintain an inspiratory-expiratory ratio (I:E) greater than 1:2, set PEEP at 5, and 100 percent FIO_2. Oxygen therapy is primarily directed toward support of the poor lung function, rather than the minor CO poisoning. In-line aerosolized bronchodilator treatment (e.g., 10 puffs of albuterol metered dose inhaler) is needed for the apparent bronchospasm. Physical examination of the chest, vital signs, ABG, and chest radiograph should be done to determine Mr. A's response. Escharotomy of his chest is needed to prevent constriction of the chest cavity.

15. Fluid resuscitation with crystalloid intravenous (IV) infusion according to the Parkland formula (i.e., 4 mL per kilogram per percentage burn over 24 hours) must be started. Evaluation of CVP, pulmonary artery wedge pressure (PAWP), cardiac output, and renal output must be monitored to avoid hypotension and fluid overload.

16. Considering the size of the burn and the presence of inhalation injury, intensive care in a burn unit is required over the next 24 to 48 hours and beyond for continued fluid resuscitation, ventilatory support, wound management, and monitoring of cardiovascular, pulmonary, and renal function. Mr. A is at risk for the development of circulatory failure, renal failure, pulmonary edema, acid-base and electrolyte imbalance, disseminated intravascular coagulation, and sepsis.

CASE STUDY—continued

In the emergency room, Mr. A was orally intubated and placed on mechanical ventilation with 100 percent O_2. IV and arterial lines were placed and fluid resuscitation started. A nasogastric tube was inserted, along with a urinary catheter with a closed-collection system. Mr. A was stabilized at the community hospital and then transferred by air ambulance to a metropolitan burn center for intensive burn care. Upon arrival at the burn center, approximately 3 hours after the accident, he was evaluated and found to have received full-thickness burns over 88 percent of his body and probable inhalation injury.

His initial treatment concentrated on fluid resuscitation, escharotomies of the chest and extremities, wound care with silver sulfadiazine cream and dressings, and ventilator support with 100 percent O_2 was continued with a PEEP of 5 cm H_2O. Shortly after admission, a chest radiograph was taken (Fig. 11–3). A fiberoptic-equipped Swan-Ganz–type pulmonary artery catheter was placed for fluid administration and monitoring of right atrial pressure, PAWP, cardiac output, and continuous mixed venous HbO_2 saturation.

Over the next 2 days, his aggressive fluid resuscitation was continued and FIO_2 adjusted down to 70 percent while ABGs, pulse oximetry, and mixed venous HbO_2 saturation were monitored. During this time, his oxygenation began to deteriorate and he required higher FIO_2 and PEEP levels. At approximately 40 hours after injury, his bedside findings, vital signs, chest radiograph, ventilator settings, and laboratory data were as follows.

Bedside Findings

Mr. A is lying supine with silver sulfadiazine cream and bandages covering all burned areas. Generalized edema is developing throughout the burned areas. He is responsive and follows commands. He is spontaneously initiating each breath from the Siemens Servo 900c ventilator through an oral endotracheal tube (8.0 mm internal diameter). The airway has 25 cm H_2O pressure in the cuff, and no gas leakage is heard over the cuff site. The airway is secured to the upper lip with waterproof tape and shows the 24-cm mark at the lip. His breath sounds reveal scattered inspiratory crackles and expiratory wheezes and rhonchi with diminished air movement symmetrically. On suctioning his airway, small amounts of mucoid sputum flecked with soot are removed. In-line ventilator circuit delivery of 2.5 mg albuterol diluted in 3 mL of saline is being given every 4 hours and as needed. He is also receiving morphine sulfate and midazolam (Versed) for analgesia and sedation. His total fluid intake since the accident has been 61.3 liters with a total urine output of 4.2 liters.

Physical Examination

Vital Signs, Hemodynamics, and Urine Output:

Temperature 37.6°C (99.7°F)

Respiratory rate 30/minute

Heart rate 100/minute

Systemic arterial BP 110/53 mm Hg

CVP 9 mm Hg

Pulmonary artery BP 34/19 mm Hg

Pulmonary artery wedge pressure (PAWP) 18 mm Hg

Cardiac output 7.7 liters/minute

Urine output averaging 55 to 65 mL/hour since admission

Chest Radiograph: See Figure 11–4

Ventilator Settings and Findings

Assist/control mode

V_T set at 1.0 liter

Rate set at 20/minute

Total respiratory rate 30/minute

FIO_2 0.85

Inspiratory flow 80 liters/minute

$\dot{V}E$ 30.4 liters/minute

Peak inspiratory pressure 55 cm H_2O

Plateau pressure 38 cm H_2O

PEEP set at 10 cm H_2O

Auto-PEEP at 15 cm H_2O

Static compliance (Cs) 40 mL/cm H_2O

Effective airway resistance (R_{AW}) 13 cm H_2O/liter per second

Laboratory Evaluation

ABGs: pH 7.43, $PaCO_2$ 34 mm Hg, PaO_2 65 mm Hg, HCO_3^- 22 mEq/liter, $P(A - a)O_2$ 498 mm Hg, PaO_2/FIO_2 76, SaO_2 92 percent (co-oximeter), SpO_2 91 percent (pulse oximeter), oxygen saturation in mixed venous blood ($S\bar{v}O_2$) 66 percent

Hematology: Hct 43 percent, RBC $4.7 \times 10^6/mm^3$, WBC 11.1×10^3, platelets 253×10^3

Electrolytes and Chemistry: Na^+ 139 mEq/liter, K^+ 3.5 mEq/liter, Cl^- 101 mEq/liter, glucose 153 mg/dL, BUN 20 mg/dL, creatinine 1.0 mg/dL

Microbiology: Blood, sputum, and wound smear cultures pending

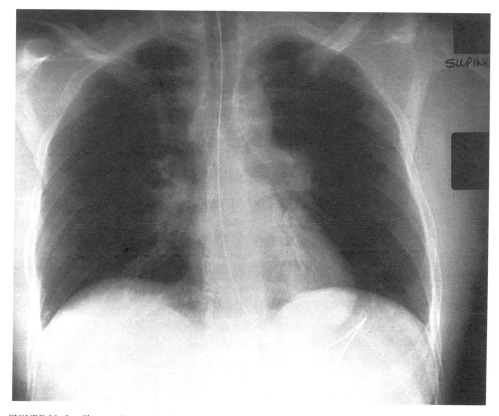

FIGURE 11-3   Chest radiograph taken approximately 5 hours after the burn and shortly after admission to the burn intensive care unit.

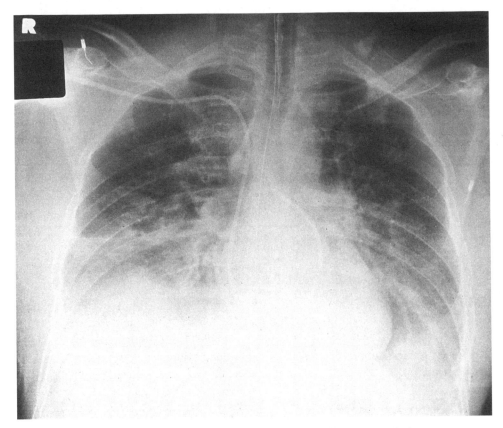

FIGURE 11-4   Chest radiograph taken approximately 40 hours after the burn.

QUESTIONS

17. What do Mr. A's airway care and breath sounds indicate? What would you recommend at this time?

18. How would you describe his hemodynamics? What effects could these hemodynamics have on lung function?

19. How would you describe the radiographic changes since the initial chest film taken shortly after admission to the burn center?

20. How would you describe the ventilator settings, breathing pattern, pulmonary mechanics, and ABG findings? What would you recommended at this time?

21. What do his other laboratory findings indicate?

ANSWERS

17. His airway is of an appropriate size, although use of the nasal route would be preferred. Tube position and breath sounds indicate proper placement. Cuff pressure is effectively sealing the trachea at a safe pressure that is high enough to help avoid silent aspiration of saliva around the cuff. Placement of a tracheostomy tube is not indicated at this time. His breath sounds indicate pulmonary edema, retained secretions, continuing bronchospasms, and decreased aeration. The in-line aerosolization of albuterol is appropriate, but its dosage should be doubled; an in-line metered dose inhaler with 10 to 20

"puffs" may be more efficacious. The sooty sputum removed from the airway indicates inhalation injury and does not appear to be grossly consistent with airway plugging, hemorrhage, or infection at this time. Special attention to the airway, its maintenance, and sterile technique is necessary to help avoid complications.

18. The hemodynamics are consistent with a moderate hyperdynamic state, which is often seen after aggressive fluid resuscitation of a large burn complicated by inhalation injury. The filling pressures (CVP and PAWP) indicate that Mr. A is adequately hydrated and may need the infusion rate tapered. His moderately high cardiac output is typical of a burn victim's response to stress. The possible pulmonary consequence of the high pulmonary artery pressure is pulmonary edema. If fluids are tapered too much, however, renal function and other organ function could be jeopardized as a result of hypovolemic shock.

19. The portable anteroposterior chest radiograph taken shortly after admission (Fig. 11–3) shows normal bony structures, normal heart size, normal lung volume, and sharp costophrenic angles with small areas of atelectasis in the mid and upper zones of the right lung. No signs of a pneumothorax are seen. An endotracheal tube is in good position. Its tip is approximately 4 cm above the carina, and there is no tracheal bulging. A nasogastric tube is present and terminates in the midstomach.

    The portable anteroposterior chest radiograph taken approximately 40 hours after injury (Fig. 11–4) shows the endotracheal tube in the same position, a nasogastric tube that extends down into the stomach, and a pulmonary artery catheter that ends in the right pulmonary outflow tract. Pleural effusion, pulmonary edema, atelectasis, and air bronchograms are seen in the right middle and lower lobes. Some atelectasis is noted in the right upper lobe. Atelectasis and pulmonary edema are also seen in the left lung base. Lung volume has diminished, and no signs of pneumothorax are present.

20. Mr. A's ventilator settings indicate that he is on a high level of support. The V_T setting (10 mL/kg) may increase his risk of further lung injury through overexpansion. Consider reducing it to 7 or 8 mL/kg. He is receiving very high Fio_2 and is triggering all breaths beyond the set rate of 20/minute, resulting in a very high minute ventilation. It is important to point out that he is generating occult or auto-PEEP as a result of gas trapping. His respiratory pattern combined with the increased effective airway resistance is producing the gas trapping. It is important to track the auto-PEEP in order to evaluate its effects on lung distention, lung mechanics, and hemodynamics. The auto-PEEP can be reduced by lowering the respiratory rate, increasing the inspiratory flow rate, continuing the bronchodilator treatments and airway care, and sedating the patient. The compliance and resistance measurements are consistent with the chest radiographic and bedside findings of pulmonary edema, atelectasis, and increased airway resistance. His oxygenation is adequate, but the measures to maintain it are dangerously excessive and need reevaluation and adjustment. The $S\bar{v}o_2$ indicates tissue hypoxia and may be one of the reasons for his ventilatory pattern and poor arterial oxygenation. The very high minute ventilation and moderate respiratory alkalosis indicate increased V_D or increased metabolic

rate, or both. The respiratory alkalosis could be resolved by normalizing the $PaCO_2$ with care to avoid a further deterioration of oxygenation. At this point it would be appropriate to control Mr. A's respiratory pattern through paralysis and sedation, perform an optimal PEEP study, reduce the respiratory rate, taper off the fluid administration, and continue monitoring.

21. The hematologic data indicate an acceptable RBC mass and count. The mildly elevated WBC and increased band cell counts are consistent with this type of trauma or early sepsis, or both. The electrolytes, hemodynamics, and renal function are remarkably normal, considering the amount of fluid that he has received. A slight hyperglycemia is noted and may be a result of glucocorticoid and catecholamine release secondary to the trauma or the IV fluids being given, or both.

CASE STUDY—continued

After Mr. A's cardiopulmonary status was assessed, he was paralyzed with IV pancuronium bromide (Pavulon) and his fluid administration was tapered down. An optimal PEEP study was then done, which yielded the following results:

$S\bar{v}O_2$ (%)	SpO_2 (%)	BP (mm Hg)	Cs (mL/cm H_2O)	PEEP (cm H_2O)
66	90	108/53	42	5
64	90	111/54	41	8
62	89	109/53	41	10
64	90	109/52	42	12
65	91	106/54	44	14
61	88	99/48	37	16

The PEEP of 14 cm H_2O was selected as the optimal setting, and an ABG was taken with the ventilator on the same settings as noted above. The following results were found: pH 7.40, $PaCO_2$ 38 mm Hg, PaO_2 92 mm Hg, HCO_3^- 24 mEq/liter on an FIO_2 of 85 percent.

Improved oxygenation is noted by the increase in the PaO_2, which continued through the next day. Mr. A's chest radiograph began to improve with signs of reduced atelectasis and reduction in pulmonary infiltrates. The pancuronium bromide was discontinued, and he was switched to synchronized intermittent mandatory ventilation with pressure-support ventilation (SIMV + PS), which was tolerated well despite a persistent tachypnea of 20 to 25/minute.

Mr. A's pulmonary status continued to improve over the next 5 days, with toleration of reductions in FIO_2, PEEP, and SIMV rate. His minute ventilation continued to remain elevated in the range of 18 to 25 liters/minute. During this period, he began the first of many surgical excisions of burned tissue and grafting. After these procedures, his minute ventilation requirements would increase and necessitate increasing his SIMV and FIO_2 settings. His breath sounds were found to be consistent with coarse expiratory rhonchi in both lung fields, and large amounts of tan-colored sputum were suctioned from his airway. His cultures revealed *E. coli* in areas of the wound, *Streptococcus pneumoniae* and yeast in his sputum, and negative blood cultures. He was started on appropriate antibiotics with repeat cultures planned.

Nine days after his burn, weaning studies were found to be acceptable, with a

PaO_2/FIO_2 of 332 on an FIO_2 of 40 percent. He was placed on a PS ventilation of 10 cm H_2O, a PEEP of 5 cm H_2O, and 40 percent FIO_2. He tolerated this for 2 days and then became increasingly tachypneic with respiratory rates of up to 40/minute. Large amounts of foul-smelling, tan-colored sputum were suctioned from his airway. He was returned to SIMV + PS, and the decision was made to place a tracheostomy tube for better airway clearance. Sputum cultures from this period were positive for *S. aureus,* and his antibiotic coverage was adjusted. His clinical picture and chest radiograph did not indicate pneumonia.

Thirteen days postburn, he increased his minute ventilation to 38 liters/minute while being supported in the SIMV + PS. His CO_2 production rate was found to be 505 mL/minute with a resting energy expenditure of 3813 kcal. This excessive minute ventilation was being driven by his very high metabolic rate, and the decision was made to paralyze him in order to reduce both his metabolic rate and the required ventilatory support. He remained paralyzed for the next 10 days, continued to have weekly metabolic rate determinations, and had additional burn excisions and grafting. During this period, his chest radiograph remained relatively clear despite continued suctioning of tan-colored sputum from his airway and sputum cultures occasionally showing gram-positive cocci.

On the 24th day postburn, the pancuronium bromide was discontinued, and he was gradually weaned to T-tube on an FIO_2 of 40 percent 10 days later. During this period, his metabolic rate decreased by 20 percent, and his feedings were tapered accordingly. A fenestrated tracheostomy tube was placed to enable him to communicate with his family and to alleviate some of his anxiety.

Sixty-five days after his admission to the burn unit, he continued to require the tracheostomy tube for secretion management, and wound care was continued. At this point, his effective wound size had been reduced to approximately 35 percent of his total BSA. Pneumonia, wound sepsis, pulmonary emboli, and chronic pulmonary complications had not developed. Tracheostomy removal was planned contingent upon his ability to clear his secretions spontaneously, protect his airway, and tolerate the next set of surgeries with the use of short-term endotracheal intubation.

Up to this point, his recovery remained quite remarkable considering his risks for major pulmonary and cardiovascular complications.

REFERENCES

1. Statistical Abstracts of the United States, National Data Book, ed 114. US Department of Commerce, 1994.
2. Herndon, DN, et al: Incidence, mortality, pathogenesis and treatment of pulmonary injury. J Burn Care Rehabil 7:184, 1986.
3. Trunkey, DD: Inhalation injury. Surg Clin North Am 56:1133, 1978.
4. Cohen, MA, and Guzzardi, LJ: Inhalation of products of combustion. Ann Emerg Med 12:628, 1983.
5. Coleman, DL: Smoke inhalation. West J Med 135:300, 1981.
6. Strongin, J, and Hales, C: Pulmonary disorders in the burn patient. In Martyn, JAJ (ed): Acute Management of the Burned Patient. WB Saunders, Philadelphia, 1990.
7. Moylan, JA: Inhalation injury. J Trauma (suppl) 21:720, 1981.
8. Nishimura, N, and Hiranuma, N: Respiratory changes after major burn injury. Crit Care Med 10:25, 1982.
9. Cahalane, M, and Demling, RH: Early respiratory abnormalities from smoke inhalation. JAMA 251:771, 1984.
10. Venus, B, et al: Prophylactic intubation and continuous positive airway pressure in the management of inhalation injury in burn victims. Crit Care Med 9:519, 1981.
11. Zawacki, B, et al: Smoke, burns and the natural history of inhalation injury in fire victims. Ann Surg 185:100, 1977.
12. Demling, RH, and LaLonde, C: Burn Trauma. New York. Thieme Medical Publishers, Inc., 1989.
13. Demling, RH: Management of the burn patient. In Shoemaker, WC, et al (eds): Textbook of Critical Care, ed 2. WB Saunders, Philadelphia, 1989.

14. Terrill, JB, et al: Toxic gases from fires. Science 200:1343, 1978.
15. Crapo, RO: Smoke-inhalation injuries. JAMA 246:1694, 1981.
16. Dyer, RF, and Esch, VH: Polyvinyl chloride toxicity in fires. JAMA 235:393, 1975.
17. Symington, IS, et al: Cyanide exposure in fires. Lancet 1:91, 1978.
18. Stone, JP, et al: The transport of hydrogen chloride by soot from burning polyvinyl chloride. J Fire Flamm 4:42, 1973.
19. Okeda, R, et al: The pathogenesis of carbon monoxide encephalopathy in the acute phase: Physiological and morphological condition. Acta Neuropathol 54:1, 1981.
20. Myers, RAM, et al: Subacute sequela of carbon monoxide poisoning. Ann Emerg Med 14:1163, 1985.
21. Baud, FJ, et al: Elevated blood cyanide concentrations in victims of smoke inhalation. N Engl J Med 325:1761, 1991.
22. Halebein, P, et al: Whole body oxygen utilization during acute carbon monoxide poisoning and isocapneic nitrogen hypoxia. J Trauma 26:110, 1986.
23. Haponik, EF, and Lykens, MG: Acute upper airway obstruction in burned patients. Crit Care Report 2:28, 1990.
24. Chu, C: New concepts of pulmonary burn injury. J Trauma 21:958, 1981.
25. Robinson, NB, et al: Ventilation and perfusion alterations after smoke inhalation injury. Surgery 90:352, 1980.
26. Loke, J, et al: Acute and chronic effects of fire fighting on pulmonary function. Chest 77:369, 1980.
27. Shoemaker, WC, et al: Burn pathophysiology in man: I. Sequential hemodynamic alterations. J Surg Res 14:64, 1973.
28. Mason, AD, et al: Hemodynamic changes in the early post-burn period: The influence of fluid administration and a vasodilator. J Trauma 11:36, 1971.
29. Petroff, P, and Pruitt, BA: Pulmonary disease in the burn patient. In Artz, C, et al (eds): Burns: A Team Approach. WB Saunders, Philadelphia, 1979.
30. McArdle, CS, and Finlay, WEI: Pulmonary complications following smoke inhalation. Br J Anaesth 47:618, 1975.
31. Pruitt, BA, et al: Progressive pulmonary insufficiency and other pulmonary complications of thermal injury. J Trauma 15:369, 1975.
32. Hudson, LD, et al: Clinical risks for development of the acute respiratory distress syndrome. Am J Respir Crit Care Med 151:293, 1995.
33. Till, GO, et al: Oxygen radical dependent lung damage following thermal injury of rat skin. J Trauma 23:269, 1983.
34. Jin, LJ, et al: Lung dysfunction after thermal injury in relation to prostanoid and oxygen radical release. J Appl Physiol 6:103, 1986.
35. Oldham, KT, et al: Activation of complement by hydroxyl radicals in thermal injury. Surgery 104:272, 1988.
36. Deming, R, et al: Relationship of burn-induced lung lipid peroxidation on the degree of injury after smoke inhalation and body burn. Crit Care Med 21:1935, 1993.
37. Clark, WR, and Nieman, GF: Smoke inhalation. Burns 14:473, 1988.
38. Asch, MJ, et al: Acid base changes associated with topical Sulfamylon therapy: Retrospective study of 100 burn patients. Ann Surg 172:946, 1970.
39. Coleman, JB, and Chang, FC: Pulmonary embolism: An unrecognized event in severely burned patients. Am J Surg 130:697, 1975.
40. Chu, C: Early and late pathological changes in severe chemical burns to the respiratory tract complicated with acute respiratory failure. Burns 8:387, 1982.
41. Mevorach, D, and Heyman, SN: Pain in the marriage (husband and wife have heart-attack symptoms caused by carbon monoxide poisoning). N Engl J Med 332:48, 1995.
42. Craig, KC: Clinical application of pulse oximetry. In Hicks, GH (ed): Problems in Respiratory Care: Applied Noninvasive Respiratory Monitoring, Vol 2. Lippincott, Philadelphia, 1989, p 255
43. DiVencenti, FC, et al: Inhalation injuries. J Trauma 11:109, 1971.
44. Hunt, JL, et al: Fiberoptic bronchoscopy in acute inhalation injury. J Trauma 15:641, 1975.
45. Horovitz, JA: Diagnostic tools for use in smoke inhalation. J Trauma (suppl)21:717, 1981.
46. Petroff, PA, et al: Pulmonary function studies after smoke inhalation. Am J Surg 132:346, 1976.
47. Haponik, EF: Smoke inhalation injury: Some priorities for the respiratory care professional. Respir Care 37:609, 1992.
48. Mathru, M, et al: Noncardiac pulmonary edema precipitated by tracheal intubation in patients with inhalation injury. Crit Care Med 11:804, 1983.
49. Skornik, WA, and Dressler, DP: The effects of short-term steroid therapy on lung clearance and survival in rats. Ann Surg 719:415, 1974.
50. Welch, GW, et al: The use of steroids in inhalation injury. Surg Gynecol Obstet 145:539, 1977.
51. Robinson, NB, et al: Steroid therapy following isolated smoke inhalation injury. J Trauma 22:876, 1982.
52. Thom, SR, and Keim, LW: Carbon monoxide poisoning: A review of epidemiology, pathophysiology, clinical findings, and treatment options including hyperbaric oxygen therapy. Clin Toxicol 27:141, 1989.
53. Reynolds, EM, et al: Permissive hypercapnia and pressure-controlled ventilation as treatment of severe adult respiratory distress syndrome in a pediatric burn patient. Crit Care Med 21:944, 1993.
54. Scheulenm, JJ, and Munster, AM: The Parkland formula in patients with burns and inhalation injury. J Trauma 22:869–871, 1982.
55. Turner, WW, et al: Predicting energy expenditures in burned patients. J Trauma 25:11, 1985.
56. Saffle, JR, et al: Use of indirect calorimetry in the nutritional management of burned patients. J Trauma 25:32, 1985.

CHAPTER **12**

Near Drowning

David M. Stanton, MS, RRT, CPFT, RCP

Key Terms

aerobic	hyperventilation-	persistent vegetative state
anaerobic	submersion syndrome	postimmersion syndrome
anoxia	hypoxia	postresuscitation
aspiration	immersion syndrome	neurological
decerebrate posturing	intrapulmonary shunting	classification
decorticate posturing	($\dot{Q}_S/\dot{Q}_T$)	refractory hypoxemia
drowning	ischemia	tricarboxylic acid cycle
dry drowning	lactic acid	universal precautions
Glasgow coma scale	near drowning	ventilation-perfusion ($\dot{V}/\dot{Q}$)
(GCS)	Orlowski score	mismatch
glycolysis	oxidative phosphorylation	wet drowning

Introduction

Drowning is defined as death by suffocation resulting from submersion.[1-7] Drowning in fresh water is most frequent, but it can occur in salt water (sea, brackish) or in any fluid. The majority (85 to 90 percent) of drowning victims aspirate fluid into their lungs (**wet drowning**). The volume aspirated is usually small (less than 22 mL/kg) and often may include vomit, bacteria, and other debris present in the fluid. Victims usually swallow large amounts of water (liquid) during their struggle to remain afloat, and vomiting with aspiration is a frequent occurrence, especially during resuscitation. Approximately 10 to 15 percent of drowning victims do not aspirate fluid into their lungs (**dry drowning**). Death without aspiration results from acute asphyxia thought to be brought about by laryngospasm or prolonged breath-holding. Laryngospasm can result when a small amount of fluid enters the region of the larynx as the victim gasps for air while fully or partially submerged.

    Near drowning is a term applied to those who are successfully resuscitated and survive at least 24 hours.[1-4,6] If death occurs within the first 24 hours, drowning will be listed as the primary cause. Should the victim survive the initial 24 hours but die later of complications, the primary cause of death is attributed to the complications (e.g., brain death, renal failure, sepsis, adult respiratory distress syndrome [ARDS]), and the secondary cause is listed as near drowning. Wet or dry near-drowning terminology can be applied to near-drowning victims based on whether or not the patient has aspirated.

The following are other pertinent nomenclature:

Immersion syndrome: The development of asystole or ventricular fibrillation resulting from sudden immersion in very cold water[1,4-7]

Postimmersion syndrome (secondary drowning): The development of ARDS after a near-drowning incident[1,4,6-8]

Hyperventilation-submersion syndrome (shallow water blackout): Unconsciousness brought about by brain hypoxia.[4,5,9] In normal individuals, elevated carbon dioxide levels in the blood cross the blood-brain barrier to stimulate respiration; when we hyperventilate before diving or swimming underwater, we remove carbon dioxide from the blood. In hyperventilation-submersion syndrome, however, hypoxia-induced unconsciousness may occur before blood carbon dioxide levels increase sufficiently to stimulate respiration, forcing the swimmer to the surface.

Drownings are responsible for 150,000 deaths worldwide each year,[4,10] with between 6000 and 8000[1,2,4-6,8-10] occurring in the United States. An estimated 80,000 near-drowning incidents occur annually in the United States.[9] A high incidence occurs in males between 10 and 19 years of age,[1-3,7,8,11,12] and in children less than 5 years of age.[4,6,8,11,12] Drowning is the third most common cause of mortality in children[2,6,10] and the fourth most common cause of accidental death overall.[6,10] Alcohol is a related factor in 38 to 50 percent of teenage drownings.[2,4,6,9] Poor judgment and lack of supervision[3,8] are also major contributing factors in drownings.

Pathology and Pathophysiology

Neurological Insult

Hypoxia and ischemia are important concepts that require clarification. **Hypoxia** is an insufficient oxygen supply to a particular tissue of the body. **Ischemia** results when blood flow to a tissue or organ system is diminished or when the blood oxygen content is markedly diminished. In near-drowning incidents, the brain may become hypoxic before cardiac arrest occurs. Blood flow may continue under **anaerobic** conditions for a period even after the oxygen supply has been depleted. Most people lose consciousness after 2 minutes of **anoxia,** and brain damage may occur after 4 to 6 minutes.[8]

Submersion times as long as 40 minutes[13] have been reported with full recovery. These unique incidents are more common in frigid water. The brain-protective effects of a rapidly induced hypothermia are more likely to occur in children less than 5 years of age because they have a greater body surface area to body weight (mass) ratio than adults and can lose body heat more rapidly. This, combined with ingestion of frigid water, may protect the brain by decreasing brain metabolism and reducing oxygen requirements before cardiac arrest. An intact diving reflex[1,4,5] (i.e., breath holding, bradycardia, and peripheral vasoconstriction when the face is immersed in cold water) is another possible explanation contributing to full recovery.

Energy in the form of adenosine triphosphate (ATP) is produced by metabolic pathways including glycolysis, the **tricarboxylic acid (TCA) cycle,** and oxidative phosphorylation[14] under **aerobic** conditions (Fig. 12-1). **Glycolysis** occurs in the cell cytoplasm, whereas the TCA cycle and **oxidative phosphorylation** take place in the mitochondria of the cell. ATP provides energy for many active transport mechanisms that maintain homeostasis (e.g., sodium-potassium pumps, calcium pumps),

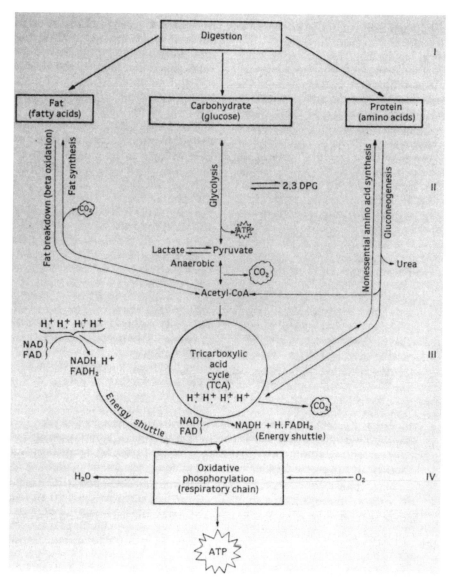

FIGURE 12-1   Four major phases of metabolism are schematically illustrated. *Phase I:* Digestion and nutrient absorption of fat, carbohydrate, and protein. *Phase II:* Breakdown of fatty acids, glucose, and amino acids to acetylcoenzyme A (acetyl = CoA), which can either synthesize—directly or indirectly—fat, carbohydrate, or amino acids as needed or go on to have more energy extracted from it in phases III and IV. *Phase III:* Tricarboxylic acid cycle, where most of the body's carbon dioxide (CO_2) is produced, as well as where most of the molecular energy shuttles (nicotinamide-adenine dinucleotide [NAD], flavin adenine dinucleotide [FAD]) receive their energy supply (in the form of hydrogen atoms). Shuttles transport energy to the respiratory chain. *Phase IV:* Inner mitochondrial membrane, where oxidative phosphorylation occurs (production of adenosine triphosphate [ATP] in the presence of oxygen) and oxygen is the final acceptor of the now energy-depleted electrons and hydrogen ions.

which are found in cellular membranes.[15] Under anaerobic conditions (inadequate oxygenation), the TCA cycle and oxidative phosphorylation no longer function, leaving glycolysis as the major ATP producer.[14] Glycolysis under anaerobic conditions is rapid; however, for a new supply of glucose to be provided, tissue perfusion must continue. The anaerobic metabolism of each glucose molecule produces a net of 2 ATP compared to 36 ATP produced when aerobic conditions exist.

Brain cells are strictly aerobic, and during hypoxic conditions, injury can rapidly occur as oxygen and energy supplies diminish. Active transport mechanisms begin to slow down or quit working altogether as a result of the diminished supply of energy. Cellular integrity becomes jeopardized as potassium is lost from within the cell and sodium and calcium flood into it.

Mitochondria and the endoplasmic reticulum are cellular organelles that assist in intracellular calcium regulation by absorbing it when it is in excess.[15] As the cellular integrity becomes compromised during hypoxic events, calcium absorption may ultimately cause the uncoupling of oxidative phosphorylation, which greatly reduces energy production and further compromises cellular metabolism. Water follows sodium and calcium into the cell, causing swelling and resulting in cerebral edema.[16,17]

Pulmonary Insult

The endpoint of the glycolytic pathway under aerobic conditions is pyruvate, but when anaerobic conditions exist, lactate (**lactic acid**) is produced. Accumulation of lactate decreases pH and may alter enzyme function, leading to cell death if oxygenation and perfusion are not restored.

Aspiration occurs in 85 to 90 percent of near drowning patients. Pulmonary injury is more frequent in this group than in those who do not aspirate. The volume, type of fluid aspirated, and components found in the aspirated fluid (e.g., bacteria, emesis) determine the extent of pulmonary injury.

Fresh water is hypotonic to the blood and is rapidly absorbed into the blood stream when aspirated. It destroys pulmonary surfactant, thereby increasing surface tension properties within the lung, which results in atelectasis or flooding, or both.[18-22] Sea water is hypertonic to the blood (approximately 3 percent saline), and upon aspiration, causes fluid from the blood to flood into the alveoli. Alveolar collapse occurs as surfactant is washed out and surface tension forces increase. In either fresh or salt water aspiration, the end result is usually a combination of pulmonary edema and atelectasis.

Pulmonary edema and atelectasis both result in **ventilation-perfusion ($\dot{V}/\dot{Q}$) mismatch, intrapulmonary shunting** ($\dot{Q}s/\dot{Q}\text{T}$), a decrease in functional residual capacity, and a decrease in lung compliance. These abnormalities often lead to **refractory hypoxemia** (Fig. 12-1).[23]

Aspirated substances may include mud, sand, bacteria, and gastric contents. Such substances create inflammatory processes throughout the respiratory tract, resulting in alveolitis, bronchitis, and pneumonitis when aspirated.

ARDS is a common complication of near drowning and probably results from pulmonary and microvascular injury associated with aspiration or an inflammatory response, or both. Activated granulocytes can cause alveolar-capillary membrane injury by releasing lysosomal enzymes and oxygen free radicals. As the alveolar-capillary membrane is damaged, protein-rich fluid can flood the interstitial space, overwhelming the ability of the pulmonary lymphatics to remove it. If not removed, protein attachment to the alveolar walls can form hyaline membranes, producing the "white-out" appearance on chest radiograph, which is consistent with ARDS (see Chapter 13).

Hemodynamic and Electrolyte Effects

Evaluations of near-drowning patients have not demonstrated severe electrolyte or hemoglobin abnormalities either with salt or fresh water aspiration. This suggests that victims do not swallow or aspirate volumes sufficient to cause death through altered electrolyte or hemoglobin concentrations. Neither hemoglobin nor hematocrit can be used to determine whether fresh or sea water has been aspirated.[24] Animal studies have found that the type of fluid aspirated (hypotonic, isotonic, or hypertonic) is not important in determining the hemodynamic response to near drowning. Pulmonary vascular resistance increases and cardiac output decreases, regardless of the tonicity of the fluid aspirated.[25]

Renal Function

Most near-drowning patients do not exhibit renal dysfunction. Acute tubular necrosis, however may result from myoglobinuria and diminished renal blood flow. Maintenance of adequate cardiac output usually prevents renal insufficiency.[1,12,24]

Clinical Features

The initial assessment of drowning victims should be rapid and directed toward the victim's level of consciousness, as well as the presence of pulse and respiration. Information from onlookers can also be very helpful in determining the extent of injury.

If possible, the history should include information regarding the approximate length of time the patient was submerged; the type of fluid or water in which the victim was submerged; whether vital signs were present upon removal of the victim from the water; the approximate length of time that transpired between submersion and the initiation of cardiopulmonary resuscitation (CPR); whether CPR was performed immediately after removal of the victim from the water; how long CPR was performed before vital signs returned; the approximate temperature of the water; the victim's age; and any other circumstances related to the near-drowning incident (e.g., diving or other accident, alcohol ingestion).

Vital signs may be highly variable in near-drowning victims. Patients may be in a full arrest state, whereas others may have a pulse and respirations within normal limits. Their temperature is variable depending on the water temperature in which they were submerged, the patient's body surface area, and the duration of exposure. Hypothermia (less than 33°C [91.4°F]) can occur within a few minutes of exposure to frigid water, and although it may improve survival, careful rewarming of the patient is required. The cardiac effect of near drowning is usually bradycardia, which may be followed by asystole.[26] Hypothermia resulting from a near-drowning incident in more temperate regions (with warmer water temperatures) may indicate a longer submersion time and probably will not have a positive patient prognosis.

Neurological impairment from hypoxia results in (1) dilated pupils that respond slowly, or not at all, to light; and (2) an impaired sensorium.

The head and neck should be carefully inspected for possible trauma. Some near-drowning victims may have neck injuries due to diving into shallow waters. Suspected spinal cord injuries require immobilization before transport.

Auscultation over the chest may reveal one or both of the following: wheezing due to bronchospasm or foreign-body aspiration, and late-inspiratory crackles associated with atelectasis or pulmonary edema.[23] The presence of adventitious lung sounds (e.g., coarse crackles) suggests that the patient has aspirated and is at risk for pneumonia and ARDS.

The extremities of the near-drowning patient are often cool to the touch as a result of hypothermia and peripheral vasoconstriction in response to hypotension, or sympathetic outflow stimulated by brain hypoxia. A slow capillary refill is present when peripheral circulation is reduced.

Arterial blood gas (ABG) studies often reveal hypoxemia (especially when aspiration has occurred) and metabolic acidosis. The severity of the metabolic acidosis is usually related to the severity of the tissue hypoxia. Hemoglobin, hematocrit, and electrolyte concentrations may decrease when large volumes of fresh water are swallowed or aspirated. This is the result of the dilution effects of the water when it enters the circulating blood volume.

Initial Assessment and Prognosis

Several scoring systems have been devised for the initial assessment of near-drowning victims. No system can predict outcome with 100 percent accuracy. Three commonly used systems are the Glasgow coma scale, the Orlowski score,[2,27-29] and the postsubmersion neurological classification system published independently by Modell and associates[30] and Conn and colleagues.[31]

The **Glasgow coma scale (GCS)**[2,27-29] has three categories; the best response from each category is determined and given the numeric value assigned to that response (Table 12-1). Scores from each category are then added for a total score. A score of 3 is the lowest possible, a score of 7 or less indicates coma, and a score of 14 indicates full consciousness. Prognosis is then based on the initial GCS examination.

TABLE 12-1   **Glascow Coma Scale***

Eye opening
  1. None
  2. To pain
  3. To speech
  4. Spontaneous
Best verbal response
  1. None
  2. Incomprehensible
  3. Inappropriate
  4. Confused
  5. Oriented
Best motor response
  1. None
  2. Extension (decerebrate)
  3. Flexion (decorticate)
  4. Localizing pain
  5. Obeying commands

*The Glasgow coma scale scores the patient's best response from each category. The numeric value to the left of each chosen response is then added together for all three categories for a total value. A total score less than 7 indicates presence of coma, whereas 14 signifies full consciousness.
SOURCE: From Orlowski, J: Drowning, near-drowning, and ice-water submersions. Pediatr Clin North Am 34(1):75, 1987, with permission.

TABLE 12-2   **Orlowski Score***

UNFAVORABLE PROGNOSTIC FACTORS
1. Age $\leq$3 years
2. Estimated submersion time longer than 5 minutes
3. No resuscitative measure attempted for at least 10 minutes
4. Patient comatose upon arrival at the emergency room
5. Arterial blood gas pH $\leq$7.10

*The Orlowski score is determined by the number of unfavorable factors listed that apply to the near-drowning victim. Lower scores are prognostic of a more favorable outcome.
SOURCE: From Orlowski, J: Drowning, near-drowning, and ice-water submersions. Pediatr Clin North Am 34(1):75, 1987, with permission.

Near-drowning patients with an initial GCS of 4 or less have an 80 percent chance of dying or having permanent neurological sequelae.[27] Patients with a GCS 6 or higher have a very low risk for permanent neurological sequelae or mortality.

The **Orlowski score**[2,27-29] is based on evidence of unfavorable factors related to the patient's recovery (Table 12-2). Patients with two or fewer unfavorable prognostic factors have a 90 percent chance for a good recovery, compared to a 5 percent chance in patients with three or more unfavorable factor.

In 1980, Modell and associates[30] and Conn and colleagues[31] independently published a **postsubmersion neurological classification** system based on the near-drowning patient's initial level of consciousness (Table 12-3). Conn and colleagues subcategorized the coma group, whereas Modell did not. Cerebral damage may cause **decorticate posturing** upon (painful) stimulation, in which the arms, wrists, and fingers are bent upon themselves (flexed) and pulled inward toward the body (adducted). The legs are rigidly kept in a straight position (extension) and feet are rotated inward. Damage to the brain stem may result in **decerebrate posturing** upon stimulation, in which the arms are extended and rotated inward, while the spine, legs, and feet are rigid and hyperextended.

All patients in one retrospective study with an admission assessment of category A (Table 12-3) survived without complications.[30] Ninety percent of category B patients survived with complete recovery, but 10 percent died. Fifty-five percent of category C patients completely recovered, but 34 percent died and 10 percent had permanent neurological sequelae.

Except for those recovered from frigid waters, near-drowning victims with submersion times greater than 10 minutes and an initial resuscitation lasting longer than

TABLE 12-3   **Postsubmersion Neurological Classification System***

Category	Description
A. Awake	Alert, fully conscious and oriented
B. Blunted	Blunted consciousness, lethargic but rousable, purposeful response to pain
C. Comatose	Not arousable, abnormal response to pain
C_1	Decorticate flexion in response to pain
C_2	Decerebrate extension in response to pain
C_3	Flaccid or no pain response

*By Modell and Conn. Prognosis is determined by category, with those in categories A and B having an excellent prognosis. Prognosis worsens in category C according to the depth of coma.
SOURCE: From Conn A, et al: Cerebral salvage in near-drowning following neurological classification by triage. Can Anaesth Soc J 27(3):201, 1980, with permission.

25 minutes are predicted to have a poor prognosis (**persistent vegetative state** or death).[32] One group predicted a poor outcome in patients with nonreactive pupils in the emergency room and a GCS of 5 or less upon arrival to the intensive care unit (ICU).[33] Another group reported poor outcome in comatose patients with absent pupillary light reflex, patients with an increase in initial blood glucose, and male patients.[34] One report recommended that a neurological examination be performed 24 hours after the submersion to predict satisfactory versus unsatisfactory outcome. They found that all survivors who were awake and making purposeful movements 24 hours postimmersion had normal neurological function or mild deficits, whereas those who remained comatose died or had severe neurological deficits.[35] Another report suggested that prolonged in-hospital resuscitation and aggressive treatment of victims who lack vital signs and who are not hypothermic (less than 33°C [91.4°F]) is usually unsuccessful.[36]

Treatment

Basic life support[37] and activation of the emergency medical services (EMS) system should begin as soon as possible. The rescuer should carefully open the victim's airway and, if there is no breathing, perform mouth-to-mouth resuscitation, initially giving two slow breaths. If the apneic victim cannot be rapidly removed from the water, mouth to mouth resuscitation should be attempted in the water. Assessment for a heartbeat should be done when the victim is either brought to shore or placed on a flotation device large enough for both rescuer and the victim. Chest compressions performed in the water will not restore brain perfusion and should not be attempted until the victim is ashore or placed on a flotation device. If the victim is recovered from cold water, the recommended pulse check should take up to 1 minute[2,38] to rule out bradycardia or a faint heartbeat. Chest compressions started in haste can result in ventricular fibrillation and can actually decrease cerebral perfusion. The victim should be transported to a medical center as soon as possible.

The Heimlich maneuver should not be performed unless an airway obstruction is present.[3,39] A drowning victim may swallow a large amount of water, and the Heimlich maneuver can result in vomiting and aspiration of the stomach contents.

Health care practitioners at the hospital should prepare appropriate equipment in anticipation of the near-drowning victim's arrival. Equipment for intubation—including laryngoscope, an assortment of blades, various tube sizes, stylets, Magill forceps, syringe to check cuff patency and for cuff inflation, equipment for suctioning, tape to secure the endotracheal tube, and an appropriate bag-valve-mask device—needs to be present. An ABG kit should be available, as well as appropriate gowning provisions for **universal precautions.**

Treatment for near-drowning patients is based on initial assessment and categorization. The following summary is based on the postsubmersion neurological classification system.

Category A (Awake)

The neurological status of these patients is alert and awake with a GCS of 14, indicating minimal hypoxic injury. These patients should be hospitalized and placed under continuous observation for 12 to 24 hours to allow early intervention should pulmonary or neurological deterioration occur. Laboratory evaluation should include a complete blood count (CBC), serum electrolytes, chest radiograph, ABG, sputum cultures, blood glucose levels, and clotting times.[26,31] A drug toxicological screen may also be necessary. A radiograph of the cervical spine should be obtained if there is a possibility of neck injury.

Treatment for this group is primarily symptomatic. Oxygen can be delivered via cannula or mask to maintain a PaO_2 above 60 mm Hg. An incentive spirometry device (volume type) may be helpful. Foreign-body aspiration can be evaluated by chest radiograph. Bronchospasm can be treated with aerosolized β_2-adrenergic agents. Intravenous (IV) access is important for fluid and electrolyte management and allows rapid intervention should deterioration occur.

Neurological deterioration may result from:

Hypoxemia due to worsening pulmonary condition
An increase in intracranial pressure (ICP) caused by hypoxic injury
Drug ingestion before the event

If the patient is stable and no neurological or pulmonary deterioration has occurred within 12 to 24 hours, the patient may be discharged. Physician follow-up within 2 to 3 days after discharge is strongly recommended to evaluate the patient for a potential pulmonary infection.

Category B (Blunted)

The neurological status of these patients is obtunded, or semiconscious but rousable. GCS is usually 10 to 13, indicating a more serious and prolonged episode of asphyxia. They have purposeful pain responses, normal respirations, and normal pupillary reactions. They may be irritable and combative. After resuscitation and initial evaluation in the emergency room, these patients should be placed in the ICU with close attention paid to any changes in neurological, pulmonary, or cardiovascular status. The hospital stay for category B patients is usually longer than that for category A patients. All testing and treatment mentioned earlier for category A patients should be implemented for category B patients. Blood, sputum, and possibly urine cultures should be performed daily. Vitamin K administration may improve clotting times. Antibiotics should be implemented only when culture specimens show bacterial growth other than normal flora. Changes in the patient's neurological status can rapidly occur, and a normal routine for head injury should be followed. Pulmonary edema, intractable metabolic acidosis, and a prolonged resuscitation period generally indicate severe hypoxia (except in patients found in cold water). Hypoxemia may become refractory to increased inspired oxygen concentrations. Continuous positive airway pressure (CPAP) delivered via mask or mechanical ventilator may be necessary to maintain a PaO_2 of greater than 60 mm Hg or an SpO_2 of greater than 90 percent. Fluid restriction may be necessary, but serum osmolality should not exceed 320 mOsm/liter.

Category C (Comatose)

The neurological status of these severely ill patients is unarousable. The GCS is less than 7. Treatment should ultimately be directed toward maintaining normal oxygenation, ventilation, perfusion, blood pressure, blood sugar, and electrolyte levels.

Limited animal studies on brain resuscitation brought new hope for salvaging comatose patients who had suffered severe anoxic episodes.[40-53] The goals of brain resuscitation are to prevent increases in ICP and to preserve brain cells that are viable but nonfunctional. Treatment might include use of hypothermia, hyperventilation, calcium channel blockers, barbiturates, muscle relaxation or paralysis, etomidate, and fluorocarbon infusions. Unfortunately the results of brain resuscitation have been mixed, and the therapies remain controversial.[5] Some of these offer brain protection when applied before the hypoxic event but not after, as in the near-drowning patient. A serious ethical issue is whether brain resuscitation improves postresuscitation quality of life or merely prolongs the dying process by creating a greater population of patients in a persistent vegetative state.

The following sections are based on Conn and colleagues' brain resuscitation recommendations.[31] They used the term "hyper" because seriously brain-injured patients are frequently hyperhydrated, hyperventilating, hyperpyrexic, hyperexcitable, and hyper-rigid.

Hyperhydration. The hyperhydrated state may contribute to an increase in both ICP and pulmonary edema. In an attempt to control both, diuretics are usually implemented. Hemodynamic monitoring is used to avoid excessive fluid restriction that may lead to renal insufficiency and failure. Small doses of dopamine (less than 5 µg/kg per minute) act on dopaminergic receptors in the kidneys to increase renal perfusion and possibly urine output. Diuresis should not drive the serum osmolality above 320 mOsm/liter. Invasive hemodynamic monitoring requires use of a pulmonary artery catheter for monitoring central venous, pulmonary artery, and wedge pressures. Arterial lines may also be necessary if blood pressure is unstable or frequent ABG measurements are needed.

ICP monitoring was widely used during the 1980s to control or prevent increases in ICP. It is now most commonly used for patients in categories A or B who show signs of mental and neurological deterioration. It is hoped that hyperventilation, osmotic diuretics, and thiopental will reverse the cerebral edema resulting from ischemia. Unfortunately, successful control of ICP does not ensure survival with normal brain function.[54-57]

Hyperventilation. Patients requiring mechanical ventilation should be hyperventilated and $Paco_2$ kept between 25 and 30 mm Hg. Cerebral vascular resistance is controlled by the arterioles, which respond to changes in $Paco_2$. Hyperventilation causes cerebral vasoconstriction and can lower ICP. A patient's tidal volume (VT) can be set in the range of 10 to 15 mL/kg at a rate necessary to achieve the appropriate reduction in $Paco_2$. ICP can also be somewhat relieved by elevating the head of the patient's bed by 30° and keeping the patients head midline.

Oxygen delivery to the tissues is an important goal in patients with more extensive lung involvement. Maintaining an arterial oxygen saturation (Sao_2) of greater than 96 percent (Pao_2 of 100 mm Hg) is ideal, but not always possible. Positive end-expiratory pressure (PEEP) is a valuable adjunct for achieving adequate oxygenation (Pao_2 greater than 60 mm Hg). In adults and older pediatric patients, PEEP levels should be increased by increments of 5 cm H_2O until acceptable oxygenation is achieved. Smaller changes in PEEP should be made in younger patients.

Hyperpyrexia. Hypothermia (body temperature 29°C to 31°C [86°F to 88°F] or less) is known to protect the brain when induced before cerebral hypoxia. However, it has not improved neurological outcome in patients who have already suffered cerebral hypoxia and can induce other complications, such as suppression of normal immune response, a left shift in the oxyhemoglobin dissociation curve, and cardiac arrhythmias. Normothermia should be maintained via antipyretics and a cooling mattress when fever is present, since fever increases oxygen consumption.

Hyperexcitability. Barbiturates are thought to bring about reduction of ICP via cerebral vasoconstriction, suppression of seizure activity, and reduction of cerebral metabolic rate. Thiopental is probably the only barbiturate that may remove oxygen free radicals. Induction of a barbiturate coma has not been shown to improve survival or neurological outcome in near-drowning patients with severe deficit and may enhance cardiovascular instability. Barbiturate coma is no longer a part of the recommended treatment because of these problems.[56-58] Barbiturates are used, however, to control seizure activity. Steroid use was also advocated in near-drowning treatment in the hope of controlling ICP. Subsequent studies have shown steroids to be an ineffective treatment for postanoxic near-drowning patients. Steroid use may also inhibit normal immune responses to bacterial infection, resulting in a higher risk of sepsis.[5,58]

Hyper-rigidity. Decerebrate and decorticate rigid posturing are signs of raised ICP (cerebral or brain stem damage, or both). ICP may be elevated as a result of brain swelling caused by hypoxia; mechanical ventilation and PEEP; coughing; and Trendelenburg's positioning. Suctioning procedures may elevate ICP for as long as 30 minutes. ICP might be reduced in patients requiring mechanical ventilation with sedation and use of paralytic agents.

CASE STUDY NO. 1

History

JR is a 1-year-old white male infant found floating face down in his grandparents' swimming pool after having been missed for approximately 5 minutes. The patient's mother immediately began mouth-to-mouth resuscitation and he responded after four to five breaths. He began breathing spontaneously, cried, and vomited a large amount of water. He was taken to the local emergency medical services facility, where he was alert, active, and crying. His initial ABG analysis on room air was pH 7.34, $Paco_2$ 34 mm Hg, Pao_2 51 mm Hg, Sao_2 84 percent, HCO_3^- 19 mEq/liter, and base excess (BF) −5.6 mEq/liter. I lis temperature at that time was 38.8°C (96.4°F) (rectally), and chest auscultation revealed bilateral coarse crackles.

The patient was given oxygen by cannula and was warmed with blankets.

QUESTIONS

1. Interpret the acid-base and oxygenation status of this patient's initial ABG. What accounts for the acid-base abnormality?

2. What could be the cause of the coarse crackles?

ANSWERS

1. His acid-base status is consistent with a partially compensated metabolic acidemia. The metabolic acidosis is probably the result of lactic acidosis from anaerobic metabolism. He is moderately hypoxemic on room air.

2. The coarse crackles are most likely due to aspiration.

Physical Examination

General: Height 88 cm, weight 10.87 kg; patient alert, cooperative, oriented, and in no acute respiratory distress

Vital Signs: Rectal temperature 35.8°C (96.4°F), pulse 156/minute, respiratory rate 46/minute, blood pressure 98/58 mm Hg, mean arterial pressure 72 mm Hg

HEENT: Normocephalic; atraumatic; pupils equal, round, reactive to light and accommodation (PERRLA); sclera and conjunctiva nonicteric; nasopharynx showing nasal crusting, no nasal flaring; oropharynx clear; tympanic membranes showing erythema on left with a decreased light reflex on the right with some cerumen; head circumference 47.4 cm

Neck: Supple, full range of motion without rigidity or tenderness

Lungs: Coarse crackles anteriorly and posteriorly on auscultation of the lower lung fields

Heart: Regular rhythm and normal S_1 and S_2; no murmurs, gallops, or rubs

Back: Straight, without presacral edema or gross abnormalities

Extremities: Full range of motion with ++ pulses, and normal reflexes

Skin: Warm and pink

Neurological: Patient is alert and oriented; cranial nerves II through XII fully intact; motor and sensory examination within normal limits.

QUESTIONS

3. Based on his initial evaluation, what GCS would you give JR? What Orlowski score would you give him? Under what category would he be placed according to the Conn-Modell postsubmersion neurological classification system?

4. Based on these evaluation methods, what is his prognosis?

ANSWERS

3. His GCS score is 14; his Orlowski score shows only one unfavorable prognostic factor (age ≤ 3 years); and his postsubmersion neurological classification is category A.

4. His prognosis is 100 percent full recovery without neurological deficit, although pneumonia and sepsis are possible and could be life threatening.

Laboratory Evaluation

CBC: White blood cell (WBC) count 14.9 $\times$ $10^3/\mu L$, red blood cell (RBC) count 4.41 $\times$ $10^6/\mu L$, hemoglobin (Hb) 12.0 g/dL, hematocrit (Hct) 34.7 percent, platelets 480 $\times$ $10^3/\mu L$, and differential as follows: segmented neutrophils 33 percent, bands 47 percent, lymphocytes 19 percent, monocytes 1 percent

Electrolytes: Na^+ 133 mEq/liter, K^+ 3.6 mEg/liter, Cl^- 106 mEq/liter, total CO_2 18 mmol/liter, blood urea nitrogen (BUN) 6 mg/dL, creatinine 0.4 mg/dL

ABGs on 2 liters/minute: pH 7.37, $PaCO_2$ 33 mm Hg, PaO_2 73 mm Hg, SaO_2 94 percent, CaO_2 13.7 vol%, HCO_3^- 19 mEq/liter, BE −5 mEq/liter, Hb 10.7 g/dL

Chest Radiograph: Patchy opacifications in both lower lobes with the left clearer than the right, consistent with bibasalar subsegmental atelectasis

Mild central pulmonary congestion and interstitial edema consistent with noncardiogenic interstitial pulmonary edema (Fig. 12–2).

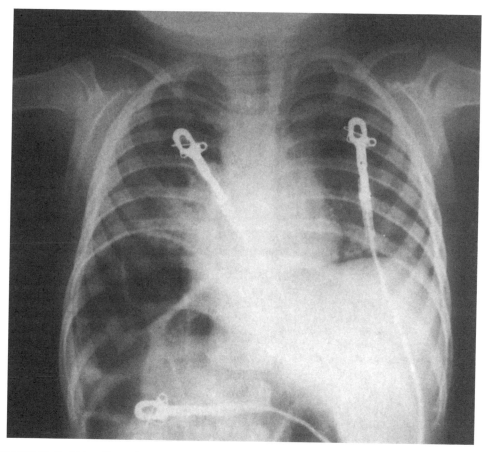

FIGURE 12–2   This radiograph is consistent with mild noncardiogenic interstitial pulmonary edema. Note the elevation of the left hemidiaphragm resulting from subsegmental atelectasis.

QUESTIONS

5. Interpret the ABG analysis.

6. Electrolytes show a diminished Na$^+$. What might be the cause?

7. What pathophysiology might account for hypoxemia in this patient?

8. How soon could the child return home, and what follow-up is necessary?

ANSWERS

5. The acid-base status is consistent with a completely compensated metabolic acidosis. There is mild hypoxemia on 2 liters/minute.

6. The drop in Na$^+$ is most likely due to dilutional hypervolemia resulting from

swallowing large amounts of water. Dilution may also occur from aspiration and absorption of water through the lungs.

7. The Pa_{CO_2} is low, ruling out hypoventilation as a source of hypoxemia. The Pa_{O_2} response to supplemental oxygen would help determine whether the hypoxemia is due to $\dot{V}/\dot{Q}$ mismatching (which is associated with an improved Pa_{O_2}, as in this case) or shunt (which would not be associated with an improved Pa_{O_2}).

8. The patient is stable and can be discharged after 12 to 24 hours of observation if he continues to improve and shows no signs of lung complications. He should be reevaluated after 2 to 3 days in the outpatient clinic.

CASE STUDY NO. 2

History

JM is a 2-year-old Latino boy who had been missing for 10 to 15 minutes and was found floating face down under the solar cover of the family's backyard swimming pool. He was unresponsive upon removal from the pool.

QUESTIONS

1. What treatment is indicated, and when should it be implemented?
2. Should the Heimlich maneuver be implemented? Why or why not?

ANSWERS

1. The ABCs of CPR should be started immediately, as follows:
   a. Determine unresponsiveness by shaking and shouting. Call for help! Open the *airway.*
   b. Evaluate whether *breathing* is present by looking, listening, and feeling for breathing. Give two full breaths if the victim is apneic.
   c. Assess whether *circulation* is present by monitoring pulse for 5 to 10 seconds; if there is no pulse during this interval, begin chest compressions. Continue CPR at a ratio of chest compressions to ventilations of 5:1. If this had been an adult victim, the ratio of chest compressions to ventilations would have been 15:2 in one-rescuer CPR and 5:1 for two-rescuer CPR. Activate the EMS system as soon as possible!

2. The Heimlich maneuver should not be implemented at this time. It is used only when complete airway obstruction is present. Near-drowning patients frequently swallow large quantities of water, and the likelihood of vomiting and aspiration is increased when the Heimlich maneuver is performed.

CASE STUDY—continued

One family member started CPR while another activated the EMS system. The paramedics arrived shortly thereafter and took over CPR performance. JM was transported to the nearest EMS facility, arriving there within 20 minutes from the time of initial discovery.

QUESTION

3. What airway preparations should you make before the patient arrives?

ANSWER

3. Make the following preparations:
   a. Ensure that the appropriate intubation equipment—laryngoscope with various blade sizes (straight and curved), endotracheal tubes (cuffed and uncuffed), batteries, replacement bulbs for the blades, stylet, tape, Magill forceps, syringe for cuff inflation, nonpetroleum base lubricating gel—is in good working condition. Once the tube size is determined, if there is a cuff, determine cuff patency by inflating and then removing the air. Insert stylet and lubricate the distal end of the tube.
   b. Ensure that appropriate suctioning equipment is present (wall or portable suction device, reservoir, tubing, suction catheters, Yankauer's suctioning device) and is in good working condition.
   c. Ensure that an appropriate bag-valve-mask device with a face mask assortment and an adequate 100 percent oxygen source is available and working.
   d. Ensure that appropriate equipment is available for drawing arterial blood for ABG analysis.
   e. Gown as appropriate for universal precautions.

CASE STUDY—continued

JM remained in a full arrest upon arrival to the EMS facility. The initial ABG with CPR in progress and the patient on 100 percent oxygen by bag-valve device showed the following: pH 6.69, $Paco_2$ 55 mm Hg, Pao_2 70 mm Hg, BE −30 mEq/liter, and plasma HCO_3^- 7 mEq/liter. He was orally intubated with a 4.5-mm-diameter endotracheal tube and given one dose (0.2 mg IV) of epinephrine and 2 mEq of sodium bicarbonate ($NaHCO_3$). CPR continued, and after 10 minutes, a second round of drug therapy was administered.

QUESTIONS

4. Interpret the initial ABG analysis.

5. What treatment is indicated by the ABG results?

6. After intubation, what should be done to determine endotracheal tube placement?

ANSWERS

4. The acid-base status is consistent with a severe combined respiratory and metabolic acidemia. The oxygenation status is consistent with mild hypoxemia despite manual ventilation with 100 percent oxygen.

5. The extreme acidemia indicates the need for $NaHCO_3$ administration. The elevation of the $Paco_2$ indicates the need to increase alveolar ventilation.

6. Assessment of endotracheal tube position can be done by auscultating the lungs for equal, bilateral breath sounds; by checking the linear measurement

of the tube at the lip to determine how far it was inserted; and by reviewing the chest radiograph to assess proper tube placement. The right mainstem bronchus is shorter, wider, and straighter than the left mainstem bronchus so that the endotracheal tube will usually enter the right side if it is inserted too far. Intubation of the right mainstem bronchus usually leaves the left lung without ventilation and breath sounds.

CASE STUDY—continued

JM remained asystolic in the emergency room for about 1 hour. He required several dosages of epinephrine, $NaHCO_3$, and atropine. A nasogastric tube was inserted and 15 mL of clear fluid removed. The advanced cardiac life support measures restored JM's heartbeat. An ABG analysis was performed while JM was receiving 100 percent oxygen via manual resuscitator. Results were as follows: pH 7.02, $Paco_2$ 11 mm Hg, Pao_2 464 mm Hg, BE -26 mEq/liter, and HCO_3^- 3 mEq/liter.

After resuscitation, JM's initial temperature was 34.4°C (94.0°F) rectally; respirations were sporadic, requiring assistance; pulses ranged from 80 to 130/minute; blood pressure varied from 99/25 to 134/69 mm Hg; and pupils were 4 mm and reacted sluggishly to light. JM was unresponsive to stimuli (i.e., without eye opening, without verbal response) and exhibited decorticate posturing. His initial glucose level was 744 mg/dL. Initial electrolytes revealed the following: Na^+ 118 mEq/liter, K^+ 3.6 mEq/liter, Cl^- 92 mEq/liter, total CO_2 less than 5 mmol/liter, BUN 18 mg/dL, and creatinine 0.9 mg/dL. His initial CBC revealed the following: WBCs $7.2 \times 10^3/\mu L$, RBCs $4.5 \times 10^6/\mu L$, Hb 12.2 g/dL, Hct 35.6 percent, and a differential morphology showing segmented neutrophils 22 percent and lymphocytes 78 percent. Warming measures were started, and JM was transported to a tertiary care facility. The initial chest radiograph showed proper endotracheal tube placement; bilateral fluffy infiltrates, more extensive on the left, consistent with noncardiogenic pulmonary edema; and a right-sided pleural effusion. The heart was normal in size, and the tip of the nasogastric tube was seen in the fundus of the stomach (Fig. 12–3).

QUESTIONS

7. What GCS score would you give the patient? What Orlowski score would you give him? Under what category would you place him according to the Conn-Modell postsubmersion neurological classification system?

8. What is his prognosis?

9. What do his initial electrolytes and CBC reveal, and what is the most likely cause of these results?

10. What is indicated by the bilateral fluffy infiltrates and normal heart size on his chest radiograph?

11. Should life support efforts be continued?

ANSWERS

7. His GCS is 5; his Orlowski score shows four unfavorable prognostic factors (see Table 12–2); and his postsubmersion neurological classification category is C_1.

8. The Orlowski score indicates a 5 percent chance of a good recovery. The

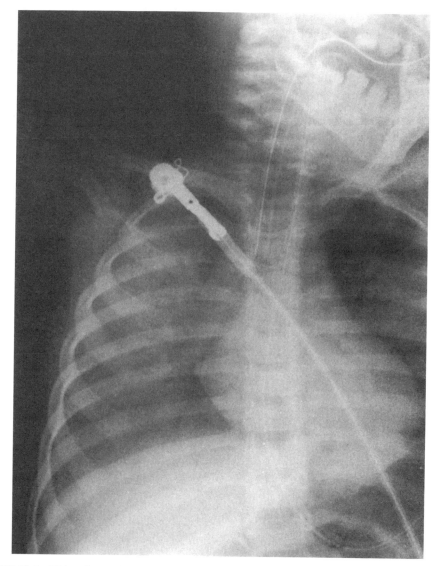

FIGURE 12-3   This radiograph is consistent with noncardiogenic pulmonary edema with probable right-sided pleural effusion.

GCS indicates an 80 percent chance of mortality or permanent neurological sequelae. According to the Conn Model system, there is an approximately 33 percent chance of mortality, a 10 to 23 percent chance of permanent neurological sequelae, and a 44 to 55 percent chance of full recovery.

9. His electrolytes reveal hyponatremia and hypochloremia, which are likely caused by hypervolemia resulting from swallowing and aspirating water. The diminished total CO_2 is consistent with marked acidemia. His CBC reveals mild anemia, again consistent with hypervolemia.

10. The radiography results are consistent with aspiration or noncardiogenic pulmonary edema.

11. Yes, resuscitation should continue because there is a chance of full recovery.

Physical Examination

General: Weight 35 pounds; patient responsive to deep pain only; difficult to assess secondary to decorticate movements involving all extremities, head, and trunk

Vital Signs: Temperature 36.7°C (98.1°F), heart rate 169/minute, respiratory rate 28/minute by manual resuscitation, blood pressure 140/90 mm Hg

HEENT: Head normocephalic, atraumatic; patient unable to focus; pupils sluggishly reactive, 4 mm, sclerae not icteric or injected; ears showing normally shaped pinna, auditory canals patent, tympanic membranes clear, without sign of infection; nose without nasal discharge; patient intubated

Neck: No adenopathy or thyromegaly

Heart: Regular rate and rhythm; normal S_1, S_2, without gallop

Lungs: Coarse crackles heard throughout chest

Abdomen: Soft, nondistended; no spleen tip or other masses palpated

Back: Intact; no spina bifida, hair tuft, or sacral dimple

Extremities: Pulses barely palpable in axillae, carotids, and femoral arteries; nail beds dusky

Skin: Very poor perfusion, cool to the touch; no rashes noted on examination; no signs of trauma

Neurological: Responds to deep pain only; hyper-reflexic deep tendon reflexes; decorticate posturing

QUESTIONS

12. What is the significance of the sluggish pupils?

13. What is the significance of dusky nail beds?

ANSWERS

12. The sluggish pupils indicate an impaired neurological function that may be due to the hypoxic event. The atropine given during the resuscitation may also be contributing to the sluggish pupils.

13. The dusky nail beds indicate poor cardiac output, poor peripheral perfusion, or hypothermia. In this case, shock and poor cardiac output are the most likely causes.

CASE STUDY—continued

Ventilator settings were intermittent mandatory ventilation (IMV) at a rate of 20/minute, F_{IO_2} 0.70, V_T 170 mL, and PEEP 5 cm H_2O. ABG analysis on these parameters revealed pH 7.42, $PaCO_2$ 30 mm Hg, PaO_2 75 mm Hg, BE −4 mEq/liter, HCO_3^- 19 mEq/liter.

During the first 8 hours, JM's intake was 282 mL and output 497 mL. After 12 hours, his neurological status improved, showing some purposeful movements, pupils 4 mm bilaterally and reactive, purposeful response to pain, and occasional back arching. Breath sounds were improved. An electrocardiogram showed a regular rate and rhythm. A foul-smelling, bloody discharge from his rectum was thought to be consistent with a compromised gastrointestinal tract caused by severe ischemia.

Laboratory Evaluation

Electrolyte Evaluation:

Na^+ 133 mEq/liter

K^+ 3.3 mEq/liter

Cl^- 105 mEq/liter

Total CO_2 19 mmol/liter

BUN 20 mg/dL

Creatinine 0.5 mg/dL

Glucose 181 mg/dL

Serum osmolality 273 mOsm/liter

CBC:

WBC $5.6 \times 10^3/\mu L$

RBC within normal limits

Hb 14.7 g/dL

Hct 42.8 percent

His platelet count $368 \times 10^3/\mu L$

Prothrombin time 13.3 seconds

Partial thromboplastin time 32 seconds

QUESTIONS

14. Which data indicate persistent metabolic acidosis?
15. How would you interpret the ABG?
16. Why is the serum Na^+ rising?
17. What changes in ventilator parameters would you make, if any?

ANSWERS

14. The parameters that indicate persistent metabolic acidosis include BE -4 mEq/liter, HCO_3^- 19 mEq/liter, and total CO_2 19 mmol/liter.
15. The acid-base status is consistent with a completely compensated metabolic acidosis. There is mild hypoxemia on an FIO_2 of 0.70 and a PEEP of 5 cm H_2O. The calculated CaO_2 is 18.5 vol%, which is within normal limits.
16. The hyponatremia is resolving as diuresis occurs, ridding the body of the excess fluids.
17. If tolerated, a PEEP increase might improve his PaO_2 and allow the FIO_2 to be diminished below 0.50. This would reduce the risk of oxygen toxicity.

CASE STUDY—continued

On the 14th hour of hospitalization, there was a sudden drop in the pulse oximeter saturation accompanied by an increase in both pulse and respiratory rate. The patient began fighting the ventilator and was paralyzed. Auscultation revealed his breath sounds to be markedly diminished on the left side.

QUESTIONS

18. What are possible causes of the sudden fall in the pulse oximeter saturation, increase in pulse and respiratory rate, and decreased breath sounds on the left side?

19. What should be done to confirm the cause and treat it?

ANSWERS

18. Causes of the sudden deterioration might include advancement of the endotracheal tube into the right mainstem bronchus, pneumothorax, or obstruction of the left mainstem bronchus by mucus and debris.

19. Check the position of the endotracheal tube to determine if it has slipped. If so, reposition it and auscultate for equal bilateral breath sounds. Obtain a chest radiograph immediately to confirm endotracheal tube position and rule out pneumothorax and atelectasis. Pneumothorax may be corrected by chest tube placement. Mucus plugging can usually be corrected by chest physical therapy and postural drainage. Bronchoscopy may be used if these techniques fail to reverse the atelectasis.

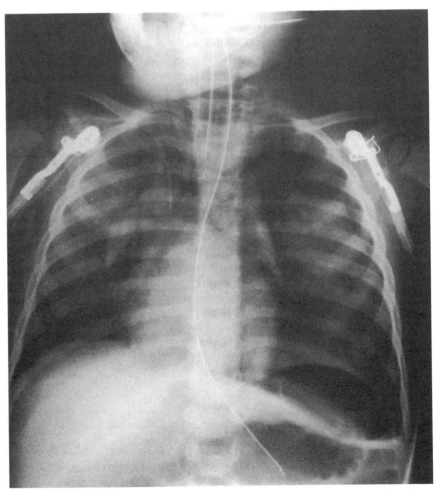

FIGURE 12-4   This radiograph is consistent with pneumomediastinum and a fairly large left pneumothorax. Also, there is persistent bilateral diffuse pulmonary edema, and subcutaneous emphysema extends into the soft tissue of the neck.

CASE STUDY—continued

His chest radiograph revealed a moderate-sized pneumothorax on the left side with pneumomediastinum. The bilateral diffuse pulmonary edema was essentially unchanged from the previous chest radiograph. Also, the endotracheal tube had been retracted to the level of the thoracic inlet; a central venous line was present with the tip in the right atrium, and the nasogastric tube tip remained in the fundus of the stomach (Fig. 12–4). A chest tube was placed on the left side, and the follow-up radiograph showed marked decreases of the pneumomediastinum and left pneumothorax. The left hemidiaphragm was elevated, which is associated with atelectasis in the left lower lobe. The bilateral pulmonary edema appeared to be worsening, as evidenced by the increased hazy opacification of the lungs (Fig. 12–5). The ventilator parameters were changed to FIO_2 1.00 and PEEP 12 cm H_2O, which resulted in a PaO_2 of 77 mm Hg.

JM never regained consciousness, and after 6 weeks he died of respiratory complications.

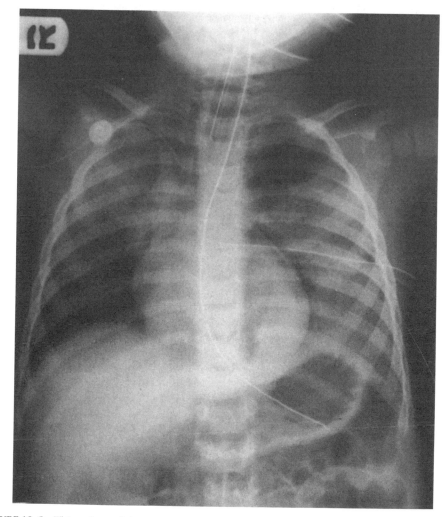

FIGURE 12-5   This radiograph is consistent with the presence of chest tube placement on the left, with reinflation of the left lung. Pneumomediastinum is present, and the bilateral pulmonary edema is worsening. Also, left lower lobe subsegmental atelectasis is present.

REFERENCES

1. Levin D, et al: Drowning and near-drowning. Pediatr Clin North Am 40(2):321, 1993.
2. Orlowski, J: Drowning, near-drowning, and ice-water submersions. Pediatr Clin North Am 34(1):75, 1987.
3. Ornato, J: The resuscitation of near-drowning victims. JAMA 256(1):75, 1986.
4. Neal, J: Near-drowning. J Emerg Med 3(1):41, 1985.
5. Gonzalez-Rothi, R: Near drowning: Consensus and controversies in pulmonary and cerebral resuscitation. Heart Lung 16(5):474, 1987.
6. Martin, T: Near drowning and cold water immersion. Ann Emerg Med 13:263, 1984.
7. Spyker, D: Submersion injury: Epidemiology, prevention, and management. Pediatr Clin North Am 32(1):113, 1985.
8. Olshaker, J: Near drowning. Emerg Med Clin North Am 10:339, 1992.
9. Layon, J, and Modell, J: Treatment of near drowning. J Fla Med Assoc 79:625, 1992.
10. Shepherd, S: Immersion injury: Drowning and near drowning. Postgrad Med 85:183, 1989.
11. Wintemute, G: Childhood drowning and near-drowning in the United States. Am J Dis Child 144:663, 1990.
12. Fields, A: Near-drowning in the pediatric population. Crit Care Clin 8:113, 1992.
13. Siebke, H, et al: Survival after 40 minutes' submersion without cerebral sequelae. Lancet 1:1275, 1975.
14. Stryer, L: Biochemistry, ed 3. WH Freeman, New York, 1988.
15. Darnell, J, et al: Molecular cell biology. Sci Am 15:617, 1986.
16. Brierley, J, et al: The threshold and neuropathology of cerebral anoxic-ischemic cell change. Arch Neurol 29:367, 1973.
17. Brown, A, and Brierley, J: The earliest alterations in rat neurones and astrocytes after anoxia-ischemia. Acta Neuropathol (Berl) 23:9, 1973.
18. Modell, J, et al: Serum electrolyte concentrations after fresh-water aspiration. Anesthesiology 30(4):421, 1969.
19. Modell J, et al: The effects of fluid volume in seawater drowning. Ann Intern Med 67(1):68, 1967.
20. Giammona, S, and Modell, J: Drowning by total immersion: Effects on pulmonary surfactant of distilled water, isotonic saline, and sea water. Am J Dis Child 114:612, 1967.
21. Halmagyi, D: Lung changes and incidence of respiratory arrest in rats after aspiration of sea and fresh water. J Appl Physiol 16:41, 1961.
22. Reidbord, H, and Spitz, W: Ultrastructural alterations in rat lungs: Changes after intratracheal perfusion with freshwater and seawater. Arch Pathol 81:103, 1966.
23. Nichols, D, and Rogers, M: Adult respiratory distress syndrome. In Rogers, M (ed): Textbook of Pediatric Intensive Care. Williams & Wilkins, Baltimore, 1987.
24. Modell, J, et al: Clinical course of 91 consecutive near-drowning victims. Chest 70:231, 1976.
25. Orlowski, J, et al: The hemodynamic and cardiovascular effects of near-drowning in hypotonic, isotonic, or hypertonic solutions. Ann Emerg Med 18:1044, 1989.
26. Gilbert, J, et al: Near drowning: Current concepts of management. Respir Care 30(2):108, 1985.
27. Dean, J, and Kaufman, N: Prognostic indicators in pediatric near-drowning: The Glasgow coma scale. Crit Care Med 9(7):536, 1981.
28. Frewen, T, et al: Cerebral resuscitation therapy in pediatric near-drowning. J Pediatr 106(4):615, 1985.
29. Allman, F, et al: Outcome following cardiopulmonary resuscitation in severe pediatric near-drowning. Am J Dis Child 140:571, 1986.
30. Modell, J, et al: Near-drowning: Correlation of level of consciousness and survival. Can Anaesth Soc J 27(3):211, 1980.
31. Conn, A, et al: Cerebral salvage in near-drowning following neurological classification by triage. Can Anaesth Soc J 27(3):201, 1980.
32. Quan, L, and Kinder, D: Pediatric submersions: Prehospital predictors of outcome. Pediatrics 90:909, 1992.
33. Lavelle, J, and Shaw, K: Near drowning: Is emergency department cardiopulmonary resuscitation or intensive care unit cerebral resuscitation indicated? Crit Care Med 21(3):368, 1993.
34. Graf, W, et al: Predicting outcome in pediatric submersion victims. Ann Emerg Med 26:312, 1995.
35. Bratton, S, et al: Serial neurological examinations after near drowning and outcome. Arch Pediatr Adolesc Med 148:167, 1994.
36. Biggart, M, and Bohn, D: Effect of hypothermia and cardiac arrest on outcome of near-drowning accidents in children. J Pediatr 117:179, 1990.
37. Textbook of basic life support for healthcare providers. American Heart Association, Dallas, 1994.
38. Steinman, A: Cardiopulmonary resuscitation and hypothermia. Circulation (suppl IV)74:29, 1986.
39. Modell, J: Near drowning. Circulation (suppl IV)74:27, 1986.
40. Steen, P, and Michenfelder, J: Barbiturate protection in tolerant and non-tolerant hypoxic mice: Comparison with hypothermic protection. Anesthesiology 50:404, 1979.
41. Carlsson, C, et al: Protective effect of hypothermia in cerebral oxygen deficiency caused by arterial hypoxia. Anesthesiology 44:27, 1976.
42. Hagerdal, M, et al: Protective effects of combination of hypothermia and barbiturates in cerebral hypoxia in the rat. Anesthesiology 49:165, 1978.
43. Bleyaert, A, et al: Thiopental amelioration of brain damage after global ischemia in monkeys. Anesthesiology 49:390, 1978.
44. Lafferty, J, et al: Cerebral hypometabolism obtained with deep pentobarbital anesthesia and hypothermia (30 C). Anesthesiology 49:159, 1978.

45. Michenfelder, J, et al: Cerebral protection by barbiturate anesthesia: Use after middle cerebral artery occlusion in Java monkeys. Arch Neurol 33:345, 1976.
46. Hoff, J, et al: Barbiturate protection from cerebral infarction in primates. Stroke 6:28, 1975.
47. Hankinson, J, et al: Effect of thiopental on focal cerebral ischemia in dogs. Surg Forum 25:445, 1974.
48. Bleyaert, A, et al: Amelioration of post ischemic brain damage in the monkey by immobilization and controlled ventilation. Crit Care Med 6:112, 1978.
49. Soloway, M, et al: The effect of hyperventilation on subsequent cerebral infarction. Anesthesiology 29:975, 1968.
50. Safar, P, et al: Resuscitation after global brain ischemia-anoxia. Crit Care Med 6:215, 1978.
51. Pappius, H, and McCann, W: Effects of steroids on cerebral edema in cats. Arch Neurol 20:207, 1969.
52. Rovit, R, and Hagan, R: Steroids and cerebral edema: The effect of glucocorticoids on abnormal capillary permeability following cerebral injury in cats. J Neuropathol Exp Neurol 27:277, 1968.
53. Wilkinson, H, et al: Diuretic synergy in the treatment of acute experimental cerebral edema. J Neurosurg 34:203, 1971.
54. Sarnaik, A, et al: Intracranial pressure and cerebral perfusion pressure in near-drowning. Crit Care Med 13(4):224, 1985.
55. Nussbaum, E, and Galant, S: Intracranial pressure monitoring as a guide to prognosis in the nearly-drowned, severely comatose child. J Pediatr 102:215, 1983.
56. Dean, J, and McComb, J: Intracranial pressure monitoring in severe pediatric near-drowning. Neurosurgery 9:627, 1981.
57. Bohn, D, et al: Influence of hypothermia, barbiturate therapy, and intracranial pressure monitoring on morbidity and mortality after near-drowning. Crit Care Med 14(6):529, 1986.
58. Conn, A, and Barker, G: Fresh water drowning and near-drowning: An update. Can Anaesth Soc J 31(3):S38, 1984.

CHAPTER **13**

Adult Respiratory Distress Syndrome

Kenneth D. McCarty, MS, RRT

Key Terms

adult respiratory distress
    syndrome (ARDS)
optimal PEEP
partial pressure of mixed
    venous oxygen ($P\bar{v}o_2$)

permissive hypercapnia
positive end-expiratory
    pressure (PEEP)
refractory hypoxemia
shunt

static compliance

Introduction

Adult respiratory distress syndrome (ARDS) was first described by Ashbaugh and Petty in 1967.[1] It is characterized by hypoxemic respiratory failure from damage to the alveolar-capillary membrane, which increases pulmonary vascular permeability and leads to pulmonary edema. The syndrome may occur after injury or illness in previously healthy people at any age. Many synonyms have been used to describe ARDS, including noncardiogenic pulmonary edema and shock lung (Table 13–1).

ARDS is often accompanied by multiple organ system failure, sepsis being a major contributing factor.[2,3] The most commonly affected organ systems include the cardiovascular, renal, hepatic, central nervous, and bone marrow systems (Table 13–2).[2,4-6]

TABLE 13–1   **Synonyms for ARDS**

Capillary leak syndrome
Da Nang lung
Hemorrhagic atelectasis
Increased permeability pulmonary edema
Noncardiogenic pulmonary edema
Post-traumatic pulmonary insufficiency
Shock lung
Wet lung syndrome
White lung syndrome

TABLE 13-2   **Frequency of Nonpulmonary Organ Failure in ARDS**

Cardiovascular	10–23%
Renal	40–55%
Hepatic	12–95%
Gastrointestinal	7–30%
Central nervous system	7–30%

SOURCE: From Dorinsky, PM, and Gadek, JE: Mechanisms of multiple nonpulmonary organ failure in ARDS. Chest 96:885, 1989, with permission.

When ARDS was first described, its mortality rate was approximately 95 percent and the majority of deaths were due to respiratory failure.[7] Currently, the mortality rate is between 50 percent and 70 percent and is due most often to nonpulmonary multiple organ system failure.[5] As the number of organ systems in failure increases, so does the mortality rate.

Etiology

Many disorders are associated with ARDS (Table 13-3); however, shock (see Chapter 8), infection, and trauma (see Chapter 14) are most common. Although the potential causes of ARDS are varied, each disorder ultimately results in serious damage to the alveolar-capillary membrane. Exactly how this damage to the lung parenchyma occurs is still under investigation, mainly via the use of experimental animal models. Lung injury appears to involve direct and indirect mechanisms. Numerous humoral and cellular agents are probably involved (Table 13-4). Chemical mediators released by neutrophils are known to accumulate in the pulmonary capillary bed of the patient with acute lung injury.[2,8,9] Capillary injury results in pulmonary edema, which is generally evident within 24 hours after the precipitating event.

Pathology

The predominant pathologic abnormalities of ARDS change as the syndrome progresses and are often described as the exudative, proliferative, and fibrotic phases.[9]

TABLE 13-3   **Disorders Associated with ARDS**

Aspiration (GI fluid, near-drowning)
Drug toxicity (overdose or toxic effects)
Hematologic disorders (DIC, multiple transfusions)
Hemodynamic disorders (shock, embolization)
Infection (pneumonia, sepsis)*
Inhalation injury (oxygen toxicity, smoke inhalation, caustic chemicals)
Metabolic disorders (pancreatitis, uremia)
Neurological disorders (head trauma, brain tumor)
Obstetric/gynecologic disorders (preeclampsia, eclampsia)
Shock (any cause)*
Trauma (thoracic and nonthoracic)*

*Most common causes.
DIC = disseminated intravascular coagulation; GI = gastrointestinal.

TABLE 13-4   **Possible Inflammatory Mediators of Organ Damage in ARDS**

Arachidonic acid metabolites (leukotrienes B_4, C_4, D_4, and E_4; prostaglandins $F_{2\alpha}$ and thromboxane)
Clotting factors
Complement
Interleukin 1
Oxygen metabolites (superoxide anion, hydroxyl radical, hydrogen peroxide)
Proteases
Tumor necrosis factor (TNFα)

The *exudative phase* begins within 24 hours of the precipitating event and lasts for up to 1 week. This phase is characterized by endothelial cell swelling, widening of the intercellular junctions, and widespread type I pneumocyte damage. As a result, interstitial and alveolar edema occur, and dense eosinophilic hyaline membranes are formed.[2,9] Lungs from patients who die of ARDS during this stage are edematous, hemorrhagic, heavy, and relatively airless. The *proliferative phase* is characterized by regeneration of alveolar epithelial cells over a period of about 2 weeks. The *fibrotic phase* occurs 3 to 4 weeks after the onset of the syndrome and is characterized by widespread formation of collagenous tissue causing thickened alveolar septa.[9,10] Oxygen diffusion across the alveolar-capillary (A-C) membrane is impaired during this phase. Eventually the A-C membrane returns to normal in most patients.

Alterations of the pulmonary vasculature also occur in acute ARDS. The exudative phase is associated with hypoxemia-induced pulmonary vasoconstriction, formation of thrombi, and interstitial edema, which all contribute to an increase in pulmonary artery pressure (PAP). The fibrotic phase is associated with fibrous obliteration of the pulmonary microvasculature and increased arteriolar muscularization and may produce prolonged pulmonary hypertension.[11]

Pathophysiology

ARDS affects lung mechanics, gas exchange, and the pulmonary vasculature. Intravascular fluid leaks from the pulmonary capillaries, overwhelms lymphatic drainage, and floods the alveoli, thus diluting surfactant. Injury of type II pneumocytes decreases the production of surfactant. As a result, microatelectasis occurs and lung compliance decreases.[2,9] These changes in lung mechanics increase the patient's work of breathing.

Alveolar flooding and atelectasis produce uneven pathologic changes in the lung and areas of perfusion without ventilation (**shunt**). Ventilation-perfusion ($\dot{V}/\dot{Q}$) mismatch is present throughout both lungs.[9] These abnormalities cause hypoxemia that responds poorly to supplemental oxygen administration (**refractory hypoxemia**).

Hypoxemia, microemboli, and capillary compression increase the pulmonary vascular resistance (PVR). This alters the distribution of blood flow through the lungs, contributes to the $\dot{V}/\dot{Q}$ mismatch, and produces pulmonary hypertension.[12,13] Right ventricular pressure, size, and work increase in order to maintain cardiac output.[14] Right ventricular failure may develop if the increased work placed on the heart exceeds its capabilities.

Clinical Features

Regardless of the etiology, the clinical course of ARDS usually follows a specific pattern[15]:

1. Initial injury or acute illness
2. Apparent respiratory stability
3. Respiratory deterioration and insufficiency
4. Terminal stage

The initial indication of ARDS comes from the patient's history of a recent accident or illness, such as chest trauma from an automobile accident. After the initial insult, a period of time occurs in which the patient does not appear to have pulmonary abnormalities. This lasts from a few hours to about 1 day after injury. Respiratory deterioration is accompanied by dyspnea, an apparent increase in work of breathing, tachypnea, tachycardia, and possibly cough. Chest radiographs and auscultation are often normal at this stage. Arterial blood gases (ABGs) reveal an uncompensated respiratory alkalosis with moderate hypoxemia and an increased $P(A-a)O_2$.[9]

As intravascular fluid leaks into the interstitial and alveolar spaces, respiratory dysfunction becomes increasingly severe. Physical examination of the ARDS patient in this stage often reveals tachypnea, labored breathing, retractions, and cyanosis. Auscultation typically reveals inspiratory crackles due to pulmonary edema and atelectasis. Severe hypoxemia is usually present at this point.

Respiratory acidosis may occur late in the course of ARDS as the increased work of breathing causes respiratory muscle fatigue. Severe hypoxemia and high metabolic rate combined with a poor cardiac output can result in metabolic acidosis from anaerobic metabolism and lactic acid production. Results of other diagnostic tests, including electrocardiogram (ECG), complete blood count (CBC), and chemistry profile, are usually abnormal as well.

The chest radiographic findings, which may lag behind the pathology and symptoms of ARDS, can be divided into three stages according to the extent of lung injury.[16] In stage I (radiographically latent), pathophysiologic changes are occurring, but the radiograph shows minimal abnormalities.[17] Stage II (acute) usually develops about 24 hours after the initial injury and is characterized by bilateral, diffuse, "fluffy" interstitial and alveolar infiltrates that are the hallmark of ARDS.[17,18] In contrast to "cardiogenic" pulmonary edema, the heart size is normal in ARDS.[18] Fluid in the lung tissue highlights air in the airways and produces "air bronchograms." Stage III begins late in the first week after lung injury. Alveolar fluid diminishes, leaving interstitial edema. Pulmonary interstitial emphysema may also be seen.[17] Most patients who survive ARDS eventually return to nearly normal gas exchange and chest radiograph findings.[9]

Pulmonary capillary wedge pressure (PCWP) is usually normal or low in ARDS. In contrast, the patient with "cardiogenic" pulmonary edema has markedly elevated PCWP measurements.

The diagnostic criteria for ARDS are listed in Table 13-5.

Treatment

The treatment of ARDS is primarily supportive. Care for the patient with ARDS includes the following:

1. Treatment of the precipitating problem

TABLE 13-5   **Criteria for Diagnosis of ARDS**

Clinical presentation
Tachypnea and dyspnea
Crackles on auscultation
Clinical setting
Direct lung insult (e.g., aspiration) or systemic process with potential for lung injury (e.g.
  sepsis)
Radiographic appearance
Three or four quadrant filling
Lung mechanics
Diminished compliance (<40 mL/cm H_2O)
Gas exchange
Severe hypoxemia refractory to oxygen therapy (Pao_2 / Fio_2 <150)
Normal pulmonary vascular pressures
PCWP $<$ 16 mm Hg

SOURCE: From Hall, JB, Schmidt, GA, and Wood, LDW: WB Saunders, Philadelphia, 1994, p 2595, with permission.

2. Ensuring adequate tissue oxygenation (ventilation plus cardiovascular support)
3. Nutritional support

ARDS is a syndrome in which each of a number of precipitating factors results in similar pulmonary damage. Early treatment of the precipitating problem is crucial in limiting the severity of the ARDS when possible. Aggressive treatment of shock or sepsis when present is essential to improving outcome.

Pharmacologic treatment of ARDS is aimed primarily at correcting the underlying disorder and providing cardiovascular support. Examples of this include antibiotics to treat infection and vasopressors to treat hypotension, when present. Administration of corticosteroids in all cases of ARDS is not justifiable according to on current research.[2,9] The use of prostaglandins (e.g., PGE_1) to inhibit platelet aggregation and neutrophil chemotaxis in ARDS is likewise of unproved benefit.[9] Inhaled pulmonary vasodilators such as nitric oxide may be of value to increase pulmonary perfusion and oxygenation in ARDS, but further research is required.[9,19] Aerosolized surfactant replacement therapy is currently being investigated to determine its effectiveness in ARDS.[2,9,20]

Tissue oxygenation is dependent upon adequate oxygen delivery (O_{2del}), which is a function of arterial oxygen content and cardiac output. This means that both ventilation and cardiac function are vital to the patient's survival. Mechanical ventilation is often needed to ensure adequate oxygenation of the arterial blood in patients with ARDS. Positive pressure ventilation, however, may decrease cardiac output while improving arterial blood oxygenation (see later discussion). Increases in arterial oxygenation from positive pressure ventilation are of little or no value if the cardiac output is correspondingly reduced by the increased intrathoracic pressure. As a result, the maximum level of airway pressure tolerated by the patient is usually determined by cardiac function. Severe ARDS may cause death due to tissue hypoxia when maximum fluid and vasopressor support for circulation do not provide adequate cardiac output and perfusion of vital organs.

Malnutrition often occurs in patients who are severely ill, particularly in those receiving mechanical ventilation.[21,22] The effects of malnutrition on the pulmonary system include immunosuppression (specifically decreased macrophage and T-lymphocyte activity), decreased hypoxic and hypercapnic drive, abnormal surfactant function, decreased intercostal and diaphragmatic muscle mass, and decreased strength due to catabolism of respiratory muscles.[23] Malnutrition, therefore, can affect many factors, including the ability to wean from the mechanical ventilator. Basic assessment of nutritional status involves evaluation of the patient's history (e.g., food intake, weight loss, caloric requirements, catabolic drugs, absorption impairment); physical examination (e.g., edema, muscle wasting, fat loss, dry skin, bleeding abnormalities, glossitis, cheilosis); and laboratory tests (e.g., serum albumin, transferrin, nitrogen balance). Enteral alimentation (i.e., food supplement via the nasogastric tube) is preferable whenever possible; however, if the bowel is not functional, parenteral (intravenous [IV]) feeding is mandatory for providing adequate protein, fat, and carbohydrate, along with minerals and vitamins. Although preventing malnutrition is mandatory for ensuring adequate patient care, overfeeding also can cause some adverse effects, such as increased carbon dioxide and glucose production with excess dietary carbohydrates.[24]

Mechanical Ventilation

Mechanical ventilation of the patient with ARDS is needed in most cases to maintain adequate oxygenation. Mechanical ventilators neither prevent nor directly treat ARDS, but rather keep the patient alive until the underlying problem resolves and the lungs heal enough to support the patient again. The most recent attempts at determining a better method of ventilation in ARDS involve pressure-targeted strategies. The goal of these strategies is adequate oxygenation without the hemodynamic and pulmonary complications associated with high mean airway pressure that frequently occur with conventional volume-targeted strategies (Table 13–6).[25,26]

Continuous mechanical ventilation (CMV) in ARDS is best administered using a tidal volume (VT) range of 5 to 8 mL/kg and respiratory rates of 15 to 25/minute, with the goal of maintaining peak airway pressures of less than 35 to 45 cm H_2O.[9,27] The patient should initially be sedated and paralyzed to minimize discomfort.

An approach to ventilating ARDS patients that has recently gained popularity is the use of **permissive hypercapnia.**[27,29] This strategy calls for the use of a small VT to keep the peak airway low enough to minimize adverse pressure effects. The patient's $PaCO_2$ is allowed to increase slowly (hence the term permissive hypercapnia) above the normal range so that the kidney can compensate. Oxygenation is maintained by the adjustment of **positive end-expiratory pressure** (PEEP) to keep the arterial oxygen saturation (SaO_2) greater than 90 percent, with a fraction of inspired oxygen (FIO_2)of less than 0.60. Arterial pH is generally not allowed to fall below 7.25. Further randomized and controlled studies are required to determine the absolute ef-

---

TABLE 13–6　**Guidelines for Provision of Mechanical Ventilation**

VT appropriate to maintain PAP, frequently 5–7 mL/kg in ARDS
PEEP 10–15 cm H_2O
Eliminate inflection point on P-V curve
Avoid air trapping and auto-PEEP
Respiratory rate ≤20–25; limit set by development of auto-PEEP
Inspiratory time limit set by development of auto-PEEP
I:E generally ≤1:1; may be greater, but limited by the development of auto-PEEP

I:E = inhalation:exhalation ratio; PAP = peak alveolar pressure; PEEP = positive end-expiratory pressure.
SOURCE: From Kacmarek, RM, and Hickling, KG: Permissive hypercapnia. Respir Care 38(4):380, 1993, with permission.

fectiveness of this mode of ventilation, although initial studies have demonstrated good results.[29]

Atelectatic regions may be reopened by application of PEEP to the mechanical ventilation. PEEP converts areas of shunt to functional gas exchange units, resulting in increased arterial oxygenation at a lower FIO_2. Recruitment of atelectatic alveoli also increases functional residual capacity (FRC) and pulmonary compliance.[9] Generally, the goal of CMV with PEEP is to obtain a PaO_2 of greater than 60 mm Hg on an FIO_2 of less than 0.60.

Although PEEP is an important part of maintaining adequate gas exchange in the lungs of the ARDS patient, side effects are possible. Decreased pulmonary compliance from overdistended alveoli, decreased venous return and cardiac output, increased PVR, increased right ventricular afterload, and barotrauma may occur.[9] For these reasons, the use of **optimal PEEP** is suggested,[30] which is generally defined as the level of PEEP whereby the best O_{2del} is achieved at an FIO_2 of less than 0.60.[31] PEEP levels that improve arterial oxygenation but significantly reduce cardiac output are not optimal because this causes O_{2del} to be reduced.

The **partial pressure of mixed venous oxygen** ($P\bar{v}O_2$) provides information related to tissue oxygenation. A $P\bar{v}O_2$ of less than 35 mm Hg indicates that tissue oxygenation is not optimal. Reductions in cardiac output (as may occur with the application of PEEP) typically result in a low $P\bar{v}O_2$. For this reason, $P\bar{v}O_2$ can also be used to monitor optimal PEEP.

Failure of PEEP to maintain adequate oxygenation is the most common reason for switching to ventilation with inverse inspiratory:expiratory (I:E) ratio ventilation (IRV). Several studies have reported the usefulness of IRV as a "salvage strategy" in ventilating ARDS patients.[32-35] It works best when the patient is pharmacologically paralyzed and the ventilator is set (in a time-cycled mode) to a rate that allows each breath to start when exhalation from the previous breath has just reached the desired PEEP level.[9] Respiratory rate can be lowered by adding inspiratory hold. This often results in lower average intrathoracic pressures despite higher PEEP and thus provides better O_{2del} as a result of improved cardiac output. The mechanism of action of IRV may be the production of auto-PEEP; however, some suggest a different mechanism of action.[36,37] Regardless of the mechanism of action, IRV is probably best used as a second-line mode of ventilation when more conventional modes of mechanical ventilation fail.

High-frequency positive pressure ventilation, high-frequency oscillation, and high-frequency jet ventilation (HFJV) can provide adequate ventilation and oxygenation without the use of high lung volumes and high pressures. Only HFJV has been widely evaluated for the treatment of ARDS. No conclusive benefits, however, have yet been shown for HFJV over conventional CMV with PEEP.[9,31]

Extracorporeal membrane oxygenation (ECMO) and extracorporeal carbon dioxide removal with low-frequency positive pressure ventilation, though initially offering promising advantages in terms of oxygenation without pressure-induced lung injury in the management of ARDS, have not been shown to have any advantages over conventional mechanical ventilation.[9,31]

Weaning from Mechanical Ventilation

Assurance of the patient's ability to survive without ventilator support is required prior to weaning the patient from the ventilator. The minimum criteria for these weaning parameters or "respiratory mechanics" are listed in Chapter 3. Mechanical indices such as maximum inspiratory pressure (MIP), vital capacity (VC), and spontaneous V_T measure respiratory muscle strength and the patient's ability to move air in and out of the chest. None of these measurements, however, reflects the endurance capabilities of the respiratory muscles. Physiologic indices such as pH, dead space–V_T ratio (V_{DS}:V_T), $P(A-a)O_2$, nutritional status, cardiovascular stability, and metabolic acid-base status reflect the patient's general reserve and ability to tolerate the stress of weaning.

Weaning from mechanical ventilation is done in a stepwise fashion to ensure that the patient has recovered to the point where weaning will be successful. Weaning is usually initiated when the patient is medically stable, FIO_2 requirement is less than 0.40, PEEP requirement is 5 cm H_2O or less, and weaning parameters indicate a reasonable chance that the patient will achieve spontaneous ventilation. Synchronized intermittent mandatory ventilation (SIMV) is popular as a weaning mode for patients recovering from ARDS because it allows the use of a small amount of PEEP until the patient is extubated. Thus, SIMV enables the patient to gradually assume the work of breathing required for spontaneous ventilation.

Weaning must be monitored to ensure its success. Significant changes in blood pressure, increases in heart rate and respiratory rate, a drop in pulse oximeter–measured SaO_2, and decreased mental function indicate *weaning failure*. Gradual lengthening of the weaning periods can help prevent weaning failure caused by fatigue while the patient regains independent pulmonary function. The different methods of weaning from mechanical ventilation are described in more detail in Chapter 3.

Monitoring

Pulmonary artery monitoring allows measurement of cardiac output, calculation of O_{2del}, and measurement of $P\bar{v}O_2$. These parameters are essential for the management of hemodynamic complications. Pulmonary artery monitoring also allows measurement of the filling pressures for the right (CVP) and left (PCWP) ventricles of the heart, which is useful in optimizing cardiac output (see Chapter 8).

A pulmonary artery catheter for hemodynamic monitoring becomes important when blood pressure is unstable enough to require vasoactive drugs (e.g., dopamine, norepinephrine [Levophed]) or when pulmonary function deteriorates to the point where a PEEP of greater than 10 cm H_2O is needed. Unstable blood pressure requiring large volumes of fluid in a patient with cardiac or pulmonary instability may also require placement of a pulmonary artery catheter and hemodynamic monitoring even before vasopressors are needed.

Positive pressure ventilation may affect hemodynamic monitoring by falsely increasing the measured PCWP. PEEP may be transmitted to the monitoring catheter and may falsely elevate CVP and PCWP.[38] This is more likely to occur if the tip of the monitoring catheter is near the anterior chest (zone I) while the patient is lying supine. Zone I is the nondependent region of the lungs where blood vessels are minimally distended with blood. If the catheter tip is located in one of these vessels, the pulmonary capillary pressure readings will be greatly affected by alveolar pressures and therefore will be inaccurate. Zone III is the most dependent portion of the lung, where blood vessels are almost always fully distended with blood. If the catheter tip is located in zone III, the catheter measurement is minimally influenced by ventilation pressures. The location of zone III can be assessed with a lateral chest radiograph. When positioned in zone III, the catheter tip will be visualized below the left atrium on the radiograph.

Static compliance (Cst) gives valuable information regarding stiffness of the lungs and chest wall, whereas dynamic compliance (Cdyn) also provides information about airway resistance. Cst is calculated by dividing V_T by static (plateau) pressure (Pstat) less PEEP pressure:

$$Cst = \frac{V_T}{(Pstat - PEEP)}$$

Pstat is measured by obtaining a short inspiratory hold after a volume-limited breath. This hold can be achieved by using the pause control on the ventilator or by manual occlusion of the expiratory limb of the patient circuit. Pstat is monitored on the ventilator manometer during volume hold and should be less than the peak airway pressure (Ppk). Cdyn is similarly calculated, although Ppk is used instead of Pstat, as follows:

$$Cdyn = \frac{V_T}{(Ppk - PEEP)}$$

Normal Cst is from 60 to 100 mL/cm H_2O and may be decreased to around 15 or 20 mL/cm H_2O in severe cases of pneumonia, pulmonary edema, atelectasis, and ARDS.[38] Because pressure is required to overcome airway resistance during ventilation, a portion of the peak airway pressure generated during the mechanical breath represents resistance to flow through the airways and ventilator circuit. Cdyn thus measures total impairment in airway flow due to both compliance and resistance. Normal Cdyn is 35 to 55 mL/cm H_2O. All of the problems that decrease Cst can adversely affect Cdyn, as can factors that affect resistance (e.g., bronchoconstriction, airway edema, retained secretions, and airway compression by tumor).[39]

CASE STUDY

History

Ms. Y is a 23-year-old woman who was feeling fine until the morning of admission, when she began having severe chills, vomiting, diarrhea, headache, and a fever of 40.3°C (104.5°F). The symptoms persisted throughout the day and caused her to seek medical attention at the local emergency room about 6 PM. Ms. Y had a intrauterine device (IUD) inserted at a local family planning clinic 3 days prior to admission.

At the time of admission she denied shortness of breath, wheezing, sputum production, cough, hemoptysis, orthopnea, chest pain; illicit drug use; and exposure to tuberculosis.

Physical Examination

General: Patient well nourished, alert, and oriented to time, place, and person; appears anxious, but has no evidence of respiratory distress

Vital Signs: Temperature 40.3°C (104.5°F), respiratory rate 24/minute; heart rate 104/minute; blood pressure 126/75 mm Hg

HEENT: Sinuses not tender, throat not inflamed

Neck: Supple with full range of motion; trachea midline and mobile; carotid pulses ++ bilaterally with no bruits; no jugular venous distention; no cervical or supraclavicular lymphadenopathy

Chest: Normal configuration and normal expansion with breathing; normal resonance to percussion bilaterally

Heart: Regular rhythm with a rate of 104/minute; no murmurs, heaves, or rubs noted

Lungs: Clear breath sounds bilaterally

Abdomen: Lower abdominal tenderness to palpation; no masses or organomegaly; bowel sounds present

Extremities: No cyanosis, edema, or clubbing; pulses and reflexes ++ and symmetric

---

Laboratory Evaluation

Chest Radiograph: (Fig. 13–1)

CBC:

White blood cells 15,500/mm^3

bands 16 percent

segmented neutrophils 65 percent

Hb 10.2 g/100 mL

Electrolytes:

Na$^+$ 135 mEq/liter

K$^+$ 4.5 mEq/liter

Cl$^-$ 105 mEq/liter

HCO$_3^-$ 15 mEq/liter

QUESTIONS

1. Does the patient appear to have a pulmonary problem at this time?
2. Does the patient's medical problem predispose her to developing ARDS?
3. What are the typical signs and symptoms of ARDS?
4. What is the significance of the lower abdominal tenderness?
5. What is the significance of the CBC and electrolyte findings?

ANSWERS

1. No, the patient does not appear to have a pulmonary problem at this time, although the respiratory rate is slightly elevated.
2. Yes, the patient's problem may predispose her to developing ARDS. Severe chills and fever suggest that an infection may be present, and the most common cause of ARDS in medical intensive care units is infection.
3. Typical signs of ARDS include dyspnea, tachypnea, tachycardia, increased work of breathing, use of accessory muscles of ventilation, and cyanosis. On laboratory evaluation, ABGs may reveal hypoxemia despite a normal chest film early in the course of the disorder.
4. Lower abdominal tenderness 2 to 4 days after placement of an IUD suggests infection in the lining of the uterus.
5. The elevated WBC suggests infection. The increase in bands and segmented neutrophils also suggests acute infection. Bands are immature forms of

neutrophils used in defense against infection only under severe conditions. Electrolytes show a decreased serum HCO_3^-, which is consistent with metabolic acidosis or compensation for respiratory alkalosis.

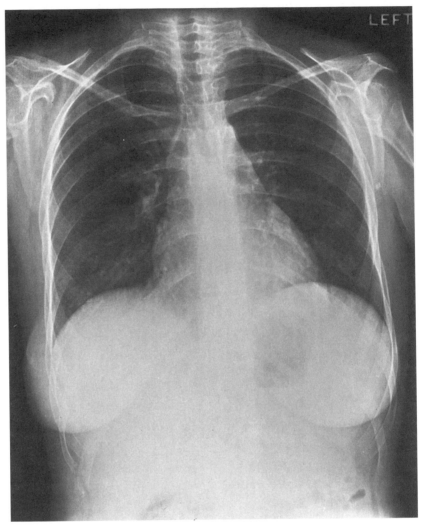

FIGURE 13-1   Chest radiograph illustrating normal appearance during the initial onset of ARDS.

CASE STUDY—continued

Ms. Y was started on IV antibiotic therapy. Results of a uterine swab showed gram-negative diplococci, and a preliminary blood culture also showed gram-negative cocci. Twelve hours later, she began complaining of increased shortness of breath. Respiratory rate was 34/minute, heart rate 120/minute, and temperature 39.6°C (103.3°F). She was using her accessory muscles to breathe, and chest auscultation revealed fine, inspiratory crackles bilaterally.

   An ABG was ordered immediately, with the following results: pH 7.25, $PaCO_2$ 21 mm Hg, PaO_2 62 mm Hg, HCO_3^- 9 mEq/liter, base excess (BE) −17, and SaO_2 88 percent on room air. Based on these ABG results, the patient was placed on nasal cannula at 3 liters/minute.

QUESTIONS

6. What is the patient's acid-base and oxygenation status on the initial ABG?

7. What is the most likely explanation for the sudden onset of dyspnea, tachypnea, and tachycardia?

8. Why is the chest film normal just 4 hours prior to the onset of the respiratory problems?

9. What pathophysiology accounts for the adventitious lungs sounds (fine, inspiratory crackles)?

10. What is the most likely cause of the accessory muscle usage?

ANSWERS

6. The acid-base status of the patient is suggestive of metabolic acidosis, most likely as a result of lactic acidosis. Moderate hypoxemia is present with the patient on room air. The hypoxemia would probably be worse if the patient were not hyperventilating.

7. The sudden onset of dyspnea, tachypnea, and tachycardia is most likely due to the acute onset of noncardiogenic pulmonary edema, also known as ARDS. The leakage of pulmonary edema into the lung causes surfactant dysfunction, atelectasis, hypoxemia, and a subsequent increase in the patient's work of breathing. These changes often occur suddenly and result in acute changes in the clinical condition of the patient. Less likely causes of sudden onset of dyspnea would be pulmonary embolus and pneumothorax.

8. The chest radiograph is not sensitive to the early detection of damage to the alveolar capillary membrane. For this reason, it often lags behind the clinical findings in patients with ARDS.

9. Fine, inspiratory crackles are common in any disease that allows peripheral airways to shut during exhalation and pop open during subsequent inhalation. In ARDS patients, damage to the alveolar capillary membrane allows fluid to leak into the interstitial spaces and peripheral airways. The fluid sticks the small airways shut during exhalation and results in fine, inspiratory crackles over the entire chest.

10. The patient is using her accessory muscles to breathe because the lungs are much less compliant and more difficult to expand as a result of the pulmonary edema and atelectasis associated with ARDS.

CASE STUDY—continued

The patient continued to experience severe respiratory distress, and she was placed on an FIO_2 of 0.60 by entrainment device with the following ABG results: pH 7.26, $Paco_2$ 35 mm Hg, Pao_2 49 mm Hg, and HCO_3^- 16 mEq/liter. Her respiratory rate was now 38/minute and heart rate 134/minute. A portable chest radiograph was obtained (Fig. 13–2).

QUESTIONS

11. Interpret the ABGs.

12. What treatment is needed at this point?

13. What does the chest film demonstrate, and are the findings typical of ARDS?

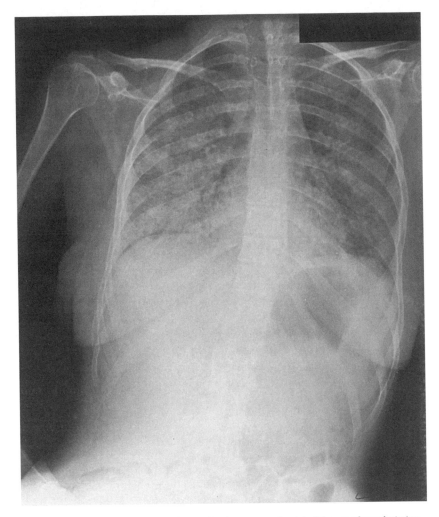

FIGURE 13-2   Portable chest radiograph taken approximately 8 hours after admission.

ANSWERS

11. The ABGs show metabolic acidosis with moderate hypoxemia on 60 percent oxygen. Although the $Paco_2$ is not elevated, it is increased compared to the previous blood gas. This is suggestive of the relative hypoventilation that would accompany respiratory muscle fatigue.

12. Mechanical ventilation with PEEP is required because of the refractory nature of the hypoxemia. Refractory hypoxemia is most often caused by intrapulmonary shunting. PEEP holds the airways open and improves the distribution of ventilation, thereby reducing shunt and increasing Pao_2. PEEP allows adequate oxygenation at a lower Fio_2 and reduces the chance of oxygen toxicity. Mechanical ventilation may not be required initially, as the major problem is hypoxemia, but the patient with stiff lungs will soon tire and need ventilatory support.

13. The chest radiograph now shows bilateral alveolar infiltrates, air bronchograms, and no cardiomegaly, which is typical of ARDS.

CASE STUDY—continued

The patient was sedated, intubated, and placed on a volume ventilator.

QUESTIONS

14. What ventilator settings do you recommend?

15. How should the position of the endotracheal tube be assessed?

ANSWERS

14. The patient can be placed a volume ventilator with a V_T of 6 to 8 mL/kg of ideal body weight. Since she weighs 55 kg, an ideal V_T would be about 330 to 440 mL. The ventilator should be set in the assist-control or IMV mode with a backup rate of 20 to 25/minute. Initially a PEEP of 5 cm H_2O and an F_{IO_2} of 0.60 is reasonable. The patient should be sedated and paralyzed for her comfort, as well as to control her ventilation.

15. The endotracheal tube position should be evaluated by listening to breath sounds bilaterally and by inspecting the chest x-ray. The tip of the tube should be 3 to 5 cm above the carina, as seen on the chest x-ray.

CASE STUDY—continued

After being placed on mechanical ventilation, the patient had the following vital signs: pulse 120/minute, respiratory rate 22/minute, temperature 38.9°C (102°F), and blood pressure 90/60 mm Hg. A pulmonary artery catheter was inserted because of the hypotension, and an ABG showed the following results: pH 7.25, $Paco_2$ 47 mm Hg, Pao_2 55 mm Hg, and HCO_3^- 20 mEq/liter. Chest auscultation revealed bilateral inspiratory crackles. Chest x-ray showed diffuse, bilateral, fluffy infiltrates and normal heart size consistent with noncardiogenic pulmonary edema. It also showed that the endotracheal tube was in good position. During a mechanical breath, the Ppk was 60 cm H_2O and Pstat 45 cm H_2O with an exhaled V_T of 420 mL and a PEEP of 5 cm H_2O.

QUESTIONS

16. What is the patient's Cst and Cdyn and how do you interpret the measurements?

17. What pathophysiology accounts for the Cst measurement?

18. To what hazards does the increased ventilating pressure predispose the patient?

19. What changes in the mechanical ventilator mode of ventilation could be used to reduce the hazards of increased pressure?

ANSWERS

16. Cst is calculated by dividing Pstat minus the PEEP level into the exhaled V_T. In this case, the Cst is calculated as follows:

$$\frac{420 \text{ mL}}{(45 - 5) \text{ cm } H_2O} = 10.5 \text{ mL/cm } H_2O$$

The Cdyn is calculated by dividing the peak pressure minus the PEEP level into the VT. In this case, the Cdyn is calculated as follows:

$$\frac{420 \text{ mL}}{(60 - 5) \text{ cm H}_2\text{O}} = 7.6 \text{ mL/cm H}_2\text{O}$$

Since normal Cst is 60 to 100 mL/cm H_2O and Cdyn is normally 35 to 55 mL/cm H_2O, the above values are well below normal. The measurements indicate that an increased pressure is required to inflate the lungs to a specific volume. This increases the work of breathing during spontaneous breathing and eventually will fatigue the respiratory muscles.

17. Pulmonary compliance is reduced when fluid moves from the injured pulmonary capillaries into the interstitial spaces, airways, and alveoli. Loss of surfactant, atelectasis, and fibrous tissue also reduce lung compliance.

18. Increased airway pressures predispose the patient to barotrauma (e.g., pneumothorax, cardiovascular compromise) and therefore further impairment in ventilation and oxygenation.

19. Further reducing the VT within the range of 5 to 8 mL/kg to limit peak airway pressures to 40 cm H_2O should allow adequate ventilation (although the $Paco_2$ will increase further) while minimizing the side effects of increased pressure. Because the Pao_2 is still less than 60 mm Hg on an Fio_2 greater than 0.60, an increase in PEEP is indicated. In addition, application of appropriate PEEP levels improves compliance by reducing alveolar opening pressures and dincreasing the distribution of ventilation.

CASE STUDY—continued

The patient was placed on a VT of 330 mL and a respiratory rate of 20/minute. A PEEP study was performed, yielding the following results:

PEEP (cm H₂O)	Pao₂ (mm Hg)	Pv̄o₂ (mm Hg)	PAP (mm Hg)	PCWP	Cardiac Output (liters/minute)	Cst (mL/cm H₂O)
5	55	32	28/14	18	4.2	13
10	71	36	27/16	22	4.1	25
15	82	33	32/20	29	3.1	18

QUESTIONS

20. Based on the above data, what is the optimal PEEP? Why?

21. Are the PAP and PCWP readings believable at a PEEP level of 15 cm H_2O? Why or why not?

22. Why did the $P\bar{v}o_2$ drop when the PEEP was increased from 10 to 15 cm H_2O?

23. Why did the Cst drop when the PEEP was increased from 10 to 15 cm H_2O?

24. How can the zone position of the pulmonary artery catheter be assessed?

25. If the $Paco_2$ on the next ABG were found to be 54 mm Hg, what would be the best course of action?

ANSWERS

20. The optimal PEEP level at present is 10 cm H_2O. At a PEEP level of 10 cm

H_2O, the cardiac output and Pao_2 are both at an acceptable level. The cardiac output dropped significantly when the PEEP was increased to 15 cm H_2O, suggesting that tissue oxygenation is not as good as it was when the PEEP was 10 cm H_2O.

21. No, the pulmonary artery measurements are not believable at a PEEP level of 15 cm H_2O. A PCWP that is almost equivalent to the systolic PAP indicates that blood would be flowing backward through most of the cardiac cycle. This is probably impossible and certainly not consistent with life. Pressure from the airways is apparently being transmitted to the pulmonary artery catheter at higher PEEP levels. The catheter may be in a zone I position.

22. The $P\bar{v}o_2$ dropped when the PEEP was increased from 10 to 15 cm H_2O because of the drop in cardiac output and oxygen delivery to the tissues. A lack of adequate tissue oxygenation causes severe desaturation of the blood in the tissues, and venous blood returning to the heart thus has lower-than-normal oxygen levels.

23. Initially PEEP increases pulmonary compliance by increasing alveolar recruitment; however, as PEEP is increased beyond optimal levels, overdistention of alveoli can occur, reducing lung compliance.

24. Since patent blood vessels are present in true zone III conditions, a wedged catheter in zone III shows an undamped waveform with distinct a and v waves. Location of the wedged pulmonary artery catheter can also be assessed via chest radiograph. When positioned in zone III, the catheter tip will appear below the left atrium on a lateral chest radiograph.

25. No changes are absolutely necessary at this point. A gradual rise in $Paco_2$ while allowing the kidneys to compensate is well tolerated and is the definition of permissive hypercapnia. In this mode, eucapnic ventilation is not the goal of therapy; rather, maintaining the patient's airway pressure at a reasonable level, while still achieving adequate oxygenation through changes in PEEP and Fio_2, is desired.

CASE STUDY—continued

A few hours later the patient had a sudden onset of labored breathing, a pulse rate of 140/minute, and a blood pressure of 70/40 mm Hg. A check of the ventilator revealed a significant increase in the peak inspiratory pressure with each mechanical breath and frequent sounding of the pressure limit alarm. The patient's level of consciousness deteriorated, and peripheral cyanosis was present.

QUESTIONS

26. What may be causing the sudden deterioration of the patient?

27. What assessment procedures should be done to identify the cause of the sudden clinical deterioration?

28. What therapeutic procedures should be done in response to each of the most likely causes of the patient's problem?

ANSWERS

26. The most likely causes of the sudden increases in peak pressure and clinical

deterioration of the patient are pneumothorax or mucus plugging or kinking of the endotracheal tube.

27. Auscultation should be done to see if bilateral breath sounds are present. A chest x-ray should be ordered immediately. Attempts to pass a suction catheter should help assess whether the endotracheal tube is blocked.

28. The patient's FIO_2 should be increased to 1.0. If breath sounds are present only on one side and increased resonance to percussion is present on the side with absent breath sounds, a pneumothorax is probably present. A chest radiograph would confirm the pneumothorax, but the patient may not survive the time needed to obtain and develop one. The attending physician should insert a large-bore needle between the ribs on the affected side if a pneumothorax is strongly suggested by the clinical findings and the patient is rapidly deteriorating. Once the patient is stable, a chest x-ray can be ordered and a chest tube inserted if the x-ray confirms the pneumothorax. If the endotracheal tube is blocked, it should be cleared or removed and replaced.

CASE STUDY—continued

A portable chest radiograph was taken immediately and confirmed a right-sided pneumothorax. A chest tube was inserted, which resulted in immediate improvement in pulmonary and cardiovascular function. The patient's condition stabilized within a few hours.

Over the next 5 days, the patient was maintained on mechanical ventilation with a PEEP of 10 to 12 cm H_2O and an FIO_2 of 0.40 to 0.45. Her vital signs remained stable, and body temperature gradually decreased to near normal. Her hemodynamic status stabilized, and on day 6 her cardiac output was 5.2 liter/minute with a PCWP of 14 mm Hg. Her Cst was calculated to be 35 mL/cm H_2O, and her chest x-ray demonstrated minimal improvement in the alveolar infiltrates. Auscultation revealed bilateral inspiratory crackles, especially in the dependent regions. Spontaneous respiratory mechanics demonstrated a VC of 1100 mL, VT of 420 mL, and MIP of −28 cm H_2O.

QUESTIONS

29. Is the patient ready to begin weaning from the mechanical ventilator? Why or why not?

30. What modes of ventilation can be used to wean the patient?

31. How should weaning proceed?

ANSWERS

29. The patient appears to be ready for weaning because the values for respiratory mechanics (VC, VT, MIP) are acceptable; her Cst is much improved; her cardiovascular parameters and vitals (cardiac output, blood pressure, and PCWP) are stable; and the infection appears to be clearing.

30. Weaning can take place by using IMV and slowly decreasing the mechanical rate, by using pressure support, or by using continuous positive airway pressure for increasing periods of time, as tolerated. The ventilatory support

should allow the patient to resume her own work of breathing gradually, without producing undue stress. The weaning can continue as long as the stress of weaning does not produce more than a 20 percent change in blood pressure, respiratory rate, or pulse rate.

31. After the FIO_2 is less than 0.45, the PEEP can be decreased in increments of 3 to 5 cm H_2O, as tolerated, to approximately 5 cm H_2O. Waiting at least 3 to 4 hours to assess the patient's response to each decrease in the PEEP before proceeding is desirable. Mechanical support can then be decreased until the patient is breathing on her own. After 12 to 24 hours of stability, the endotracheal tube can be removed.

CASE STUDY—continued

Over the next 24 hours the patient was weaned from PEEP and mechanical ventilation. She was extubated and placed on a nasal cannula at 3 liters/minute. Over the next several days, the chest radiograph continued to demonstrate improvement of the alveolar infiltrates with no residual fibrotic changes. Auscultation revealed improved breaths sounds, although scattered inspiratory crackles remained. The patient was discharged on the 12th hospital day.

REFERENCES

1. Ashbaugh, DG, et al: Acute respiratory distress in adults. Lancet 2:319, 1967.
2. McCaffree, RD: Adult respiratory distress syndrome. In Dantzker, DR (ed): Cardiopulmonary Critical Care. WB Saunders, Philadelphia, 1991, p 657.
3. Dorinsky, PM, and Gadek, JE: Mechanisms of multiple nonpulmonary organ failure in ARDS. Chest 96:885, 1989.
4. Bell, RC, et al: Multiple organ system failure and infection in adult respiratory distress syndrome. Ann Intern Med 99:293, 1983.
5. Montgomery, AB, et al: Causes of mortality in patients with the adult respiratory distress syndrome. Am Rev Respir Dis 132:485, 1985.
6. Matuschak, GM, et al: Effect of end stage liver failure on the incidence and resolution of adult respiratory distress syndrome. J Crit Care 2:162, 1986.
7. Dorinsky, PM, and Gadek, JE: Multiple organ failure. Clin Chest Med 11(4):581, 1990
8. Mizer, L, et al: Neutrophil accumulation and structural changes in non-pulmonary organs following phorbol myristate acetate-induced acute lung injury. Am Rev Respir Dis 139:1017, 1989.
9. Flick, MR: Pulmonary edema and acute lung injury. In Murray, JF, and Nadel, JA (eds):Textbook of Respiratory Medicine, ed 2. WB Saunders, Philadelphia, 1994, p 1725.
10. Tomashefski, JF: Pulmonary pathology of the adult respiratory distress syndrome. Clin Chest Med 11(4):593, 1990
11. Tomashefski, JF: The pulmonary vascular lesions of the adult respiratory distress syndrome. Am J Pathol 112:112, 1983.
12. Calvin, JE, et al: Ventricular interaction in a canine model of acute pulmonary hypertension and its modulation by vasoactive drugs. J Crit Care 3:43, 1988.
13. Zapol, WM, and Snider, MT: Pulmonary hypertension in severe acute respiratory failure. N Engl J Med 296(9):476, 1977.
14. Stool, EW, et al: Dimensional changes of the left ventricle during acute pulmonary arterial hypertension in dogs. Am J Cardiol 33:868, 1974.
15. Bone, RC: The adult respiratory distress syndrome: Diagnosis and treatment. Proc Cardiol 5:49, 1979.
16. Aberle, DR, and Brown, K: Radiologic considerations in the adult respiratory distress syndrome. Clin Chest Med 11(4):737, 1990.
17. Greene, R: Adult respiratory distress syndrome: Acute alveolar damage. Radiology 163:57, 1987.
18. Milne, EN, et al: The radiologic distinction of cardiogenic and noncardiogenic edema. AJR 144:879, 1985.
19. Gerlach, H, et al: Long-term inhalation with evaluated low doses of nitric oxide for selective improvement of oxygenation in patients with adult respiratory distress syndrome. Int Care Med 19:443, 1993.
20. Heikinhelmo, M, et al: Successful treatment of ARDS with two doses of synthetic surfactant. Chest 105(4):1263, 1994.
21. Driver, AG, and LeBrun, M: Iatrogenic malnutrition in patients receiving ventilator support. JAMA 244:2195, 1980
22. Larca, L, and Greenbaum, DM: Effectiveness of intensive nutritional regimens in patients who fail to wean from mechanical ventilation. Crit Care Med 10:297, 1982.

23. Procter, CD: Nutritional support. In Kirby, RR, and Taylor, RW (eds): Respiratory Failure. Year Book Medical, Chicago, 1986.

24. Mahutte, CK: Metabolism, nutrition, and respiration in critically ill patients. In George, RB, et al (eds): Chest Medicine: Essentials of Pulmonary and Critical Care Medicine. Williams & Wilkins, Baltimore, 1995.

25. MacIntyre, NR: Letter to the Editor. Crit Care Med 22(1):4, 1994.

26. Rappaport, SH, et al: Randomized, prospective trial of pressure-limited versus volume-controlled ventilation in severe respiratory failure. Crit Care Med 22(1):22, 1994.

27. Kacmarek, RM, and Hickling, KG: Permissive hypercapnia. Respir Care 38(4):373, 1993.

28. Bidani, A, et al: Permissive hypercapnia in acute respiratory failure. JAMA 272(12):957, 1994.

29. Hickling, KG, et al: Low mortality rate in adult respiratory distress syndrome using low-volume, pressure limited ventilation with permissive hypercapnia: A prospective study. Crit Care Med 22:1568–1578, 1994.

30. Suter, PM, et al: Optimum end-expiratory airway pressure in patients with acute pulmonary failure. N Engl J Med 292:284, 1975.

31. Stoller, JK, and Kacmarek, RM: Ventilatory strategies in the management of the adult respiratory distress syndrome. Clin Chest Med 11(4):755, 1990.

32. Gurevitch, MJ, et al.: Improved oxygenation and lower peak airway pressure in severe adult respiratory distress syndrome: Treatment with inverse ratio ventilation. Chest 89(2):211, 1986.

33. Lain, DC, et al: Pressure control inverse ratio ventilation as a method to reduce peak inspiratory pressure and provide adequate ventilation and oxygenation. Chest 95:1081, 1989.

34. Tharratt, RS, et al: Pressure controlled inverse ratio ventilation in severe adult respiratory failure. Chest 94:755, 1988.

35. Abraham, E, and Yoshihara, G: Cardiorespiratory effects of pressure-controlled inverse ratio ventilation in severe respiratory failure. Chest 96:1356, 1989.

36. Cole, AGH, et al: Inverse ratio ventilation compared with PEEP in adult respiratory failure. Int Care Med 10:227, 1984.

37. Manthous, CA, and Schmidt, GA: Inverse ratio ventilation in ARDS: Improved oxygenation without auto PEEP. Chest 103:953, 1993.

38. Williams-Colon, S, and Thalken, FR: Management and monitoring of the patient in respiratory failure. In Scanlan, CL, et al (eds): Egan's Fundamentals of Respiratory Care. CV Mosby, St Louis, 1990, p 780.

CHAPTER **14**

Chest Trauma

George H. Hicks, MS, RRT

Key Terms

aortic rupture
bronchopleural fistula
cardiac contusion
cardiac tamponade

flail chest
hemothorax
lung contusion
pneumothorax

pulmonary contusion
subcutaneous
  emphysema

Introduction

Various forms of trauma are responsible for approximately 130,000 deaths, 70 million injuries, and economic losses that exceed 80 billion dollars annually in the United States.[1-3] It is the leading cause of death in persons less than 40 years of age and is the third leading cause of death in the general population behind heart disease and cancer.[1,2] Approximately one fourth of these injuries result in a disabling condition requiring extended care and rehabilitation. Because of the younger age of most victims, trauma causes more disability and loss of productivity than heart disease and cancer combined.[2]

Motor vehicle accidents, suicide, homicide, accidental falls, and burns are the most common causes of trauma.[1] Chest trauma is the third most common injury site (Table 14–1).[4] Approximately 25 percent of all trauma-related deaths per year are attributable to chest injuries.[4] The mortality rate from chest trauma alone is about 15 percent.[3,5] In multiple-trauma patients, the presence of major chest trauma (e.g., **flail**

TABLE 14–1   **Distribution of Various Injuries from Motor Vehicle Accidents**

Extremities	34
Head and neck	32
Chest	25
Abdomen	15

SOURCE: Adapted from LoCicero, J, and Mattox, KL: Epidemiology of chest trauma. Surg Clin North Am 69:15, 1989.

chest or **lung contusion**) increases the overall mortality rate from about 30 percent to as high as 70 percent.[6,7] Different sites within the thorax can be injured. Chest wall injury (e.g., rib fractures) is the most common type, followed by parenchymal injuries (e.g., lung contusion) (Fig. 14–1).

Etiology

Chest trauma injuries are classified as penetrating, blunt, or a combination of these (Table 14–2). Approximately 70 percent of chest trauma is caused by blunt force injuries.[4]

Most penetrating injuries of the chest are the result of homicide, suicide, or their attempts. Penetrating wounds are more commonly produced by knives and high-speed missiles, such as bullets and metal fragments from explosions. The injuries produced by high-speed missiles are proportional to the kinetic energy they impart to the tissues through which they pass. The mass of the missile and its velocity determine the extent of the injury. For example, a rifle bullet traveling 1000 meters/second can induce 36 times more damage than a pistol bullet of similar size traveling 170 meters/second.[3]

Missiles traveling at high speeds and possessing high kinetic energy cause damage to both the organs they pierce and the surrounding tissues. The explosive effects of high-speed bullets not only cause massive tissue and blood vessel destruction along their trajectory, but can also cause cavitational effects that pull external debris deep into the tissue.[3] In contrast, slower bullets often cause minimal soft tissue in-

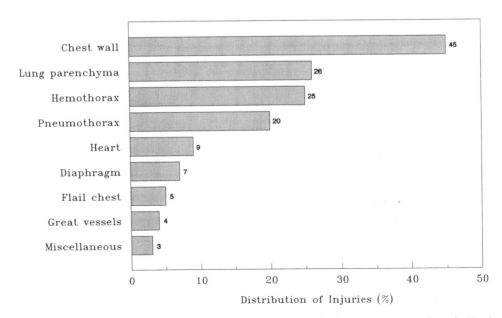

FIGURE 14–1   The distribution of specific types of injuries in 15,047 chest trauma patients from the North American Trauma Outcome Study. (Developed from data presented in LoCicero, J and Mattox, KL: Epidemiology of chest trauma. Surg Clin North Am 69:15–19, 1989.)

TABLE 14- 2   **Mechanisms of Injuries in Chest Trauma**

Mechanism	*Example*
BLUNT TRAUMA	
Acceleration/deceleration	Motor vehicle accidents and falls
Compression	Crushing and blasts
PENETRATION TRAUMA	
High-speed impact/penetration	Gunshot wound
Low-speed penetration	Stab wound

juries to surrounding tissues.[8] The extent of tissue damage is increased when softer bullets (e.g., unjacketed lead or hollow point bullets) break up upon contact with bone. The fragments penetrate and damage the surrounding tissue.

Wounds from close-range shotgun blasts cause severe damage by producing one large entrance wound and extensive underlying tissue damage from numerous pellet penetrations. These wounds are further complicated by the wad, a plastic casing that separates the pellets and the gun powder, which enters the tissue and can cause severe infections.[9] At greater distances, shotgun blast injuries cause numerous small-caliber pellet entrance wounds that cause less deep tissue destruction.[9]

Low-speed penetrating knife wounds cause chest injuries that are largely localized to the tissues that have been pierced and the resulting hemorrhage.

Blunt force trauma to the chest causes severe damage by crushing tissue, fracturing bones, and shearing tissue after rapid acceleration or deceleration.[3,5,10] Sudden and severe deceleration causes violent motion of mobile structures, resulting in shearing forces that cause microscopic and macroscopic tears in the tissues. In this country, blunt chest trauma occurs most frequently during motor vehicle accidents.[4]

Injury Pathophysiology

Chest Wall Injuries

Cutaneous injuries are rarely fatal (with the exception of a major burn injury; see Chapter 11), but they may be the source of considerable morbidity. **Subcutaneous emphysema,** a common manifestation of chest injuries, usually develops secondary to air leakage from a disrupted airway. Air migrates along the great vessels to the mediastinum and then into the soft tissues of the neck and chest. Subcutaneous emphysema is usually only a temporary cosmetic problem because of the skin's distensible behavior; however, it indicates underlying problems that could be life threatening.

Open or "sucking" chest wounds can act as one-way valves that allow air to enter upon inspiration and to be trapped during exhalation. This can lead to a **pneumothorax** that can rapidly escalate to a fatal tension pneumothorax. The loss of lung volume, compromised alveolar ventilation, and ventilation-perfusion ($\dot{V}/\dot{Q}$) mismatching that result from an open chest wound and pneumothorax can lead to respiratory failure and shock.

Clavicular fractures are rarely a clinical problem unless their sharp, bony ends lacerate the underlying blood vessels, brachial plexus, the lung, or a combination of these.

Rib fractures are more common in adults than children because children have a highly elastic costochondral cartilage; the ribs of adults are more brittle and more likely to break on impact. Fractures to ribs 1 and 2 are rare because of the added protection and support provided by the bones and tissues of the shoulder girdle. An impact great enough to fracture ribs 1 and 2 is often associated with severe injuries to the head, neck, lung, great vessels, and tracheobronchial tree.[3,11-13] Ribs 5 through 9 are more often broken with fractures that occur along the posterior aspect and midaxillary line.[13,14] Blunt force trauma to the chest can cause the ribs to break and then force them through the pleural membranes and into the lung. This often results in **hemothorax,** pneumothorax, or a hemopneumothorax. Impacts that fracture ribs 9 through 11 can cause abdominal injuries and have a higher association with intra-abdominal bleeding and shock from liver or splenic laceration.[12,14]

Rib fractures often cause pain, shallow breathing, guarded cough, and atelectasis. Fifty to 70 percent of patients with multiple rib fractures have associated complications, including pneumothorax, hemopneumothorax, flail chest, **pulmonary contusion, cardiac contusion,** and abdominal injuries (Fig. 14–2).[12,14]

Sternal fractures and costochondral separations are often the result of a high-speed deceleration impact to the anterior chest during a motor vehicle accident. Sternal injuries are frequently associated with flail chest, cardiac contusion, great vessel rupture, or tracheobronchial rupture.[3] The most common site of sternal fractures is

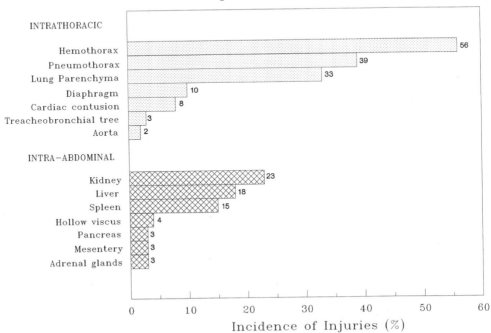

FIGURE 14–2 The incidence of intrathoracic and intra-abdominal injuries associated with multiple rib fractures in chest injury cases. (Developed from data presented in Wilson, JM, et al: Severe chest trauma: Morbidity implication of first and second rib fracture in 120 patients. Arch Surg 113:846, 1978.)

along the junction of the manubrium and sternal body or transversely through the sternal body.

Flail chest is characterized by an unstable chest wall that has an asymmetric or paradoxical motion during the breathing cycle. It is caused by two fractures along the length of the same rib in three or more adjacent ribs (Fig. 14-3).[13-15] A two-point multiple rib fracture produces an unsupported region of the chest wall and can produce a paradoxical or "flail" motion (Fig. 14-4). During the inspiratory phase, the unsupported region is pulled in while the rest of the chest expands; the reverse occurs during exhalation. Hypoxemia and CO_2 retention may occur as a result of both increased work of breathing and underlying pulmonary contusion.[3,14,15] The paradoxical motion associated with a flail chest becomes more apparent over the first 48 hours as lung compliance decreases and the respiratory effort increases. Mortality has been reduced from approximately 50 percent to less than 5 percent through the use of positive pressure ventilation to "splint" the flail segment internally and to support the patient's breathing.[15-17] In very severe cases, the use of surgically placed rib plates or wiring has been successful in stabilizing the chest wall.[14,18,19]

Lung Parenchymal Injuries

Pneumothorax, hemothorax, and hemopneumothorax are frequently associated with blunt force chest trauma (Fig. 14-1) and are characterized by the collection of air, blood, or a mixture of air and blood, respectively, in the pleural cavity. These conditions are commonly caused by broken ribs that penetrate and lacerate the lungs. Bleeding from the lung's low-pressure pulmonary circulation is relatively slow and of-

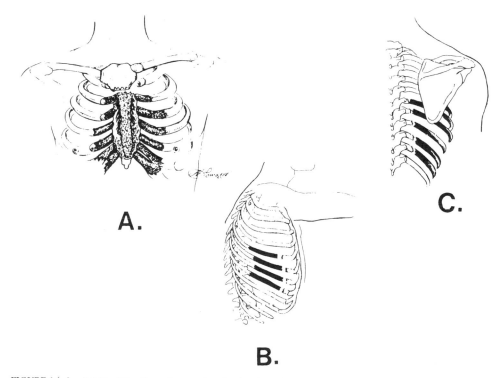

A.

B.

C.

FIGURE 14-3   Areas of the thoracic cage involved in flail chests. *(A)* Anterior sternal flail. *(B)* Lateral flail. *(C)* Posterior flail. (From Pate, JW: Chest wall injuries. Surg Clin North Am 69:59-70, 1989, with permission.)

Inspiration   Expiration

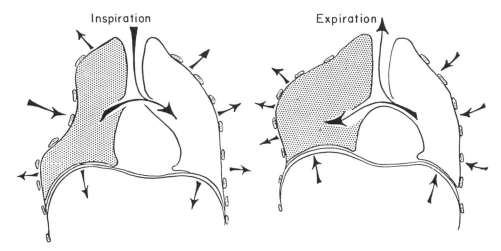

FIGURE 14-4   Paradoxical or flail motion of the chest following multiple rib fractures. The resulting motion produces a very inefficient movement of gas that can lead to respiratory muscle fatigue and respiratory failure. (From Wilkins, EW: Non-cardiovascular thoracic injuries: Chest wall, bronchus, lung, esophagus, and diaphragm. In Burke JF, Boyd, RJ, and McCabe, CJ (eds): Trauma Management. Year Book Medical, Chicago, 1988, with permission.)

ten self-limiting compared to that from higher pressure intercostal arteries, which can produce more brisk bleeding. Air and blood in the pleural cavity decrease lung volume and cause increased $\dot{V}/\dot{Q}$ mismatching.

Pneumothorax is usually not associated with significant physiologic impairment until more than 30 percent of the lung has collapsed. The diagnosis of pneumothorax is suggested by diminished breath sounds on the affected side and confirmed by chest radiographic findings of air or fluid, or both, in the pleural space. Placement of a chest tube is the treatment of choice to evacuate the air and blood and to reexpand the lung.

A **bronchopleural fistula** is characterized by persistent leakage of air into the pleural space despite proper chest tube placement and suction. Its occurrence is rare and is almost always associated with a severe lung laceration or tracheobronchial rupture and the use of positive pressure ventilation. In severe cases, the leakage can exceed 50 percent of a delivered tidal breath during mechanical ventilation and can be further exacerbated by the application of positive end-expiratory pressure (PEEP). As the leakage increases, effective ventilation and oxygenation become more difficult. Multiple chest tubes, independent lung ventilation, high-frequency jet ventilation, and surgical repair or resection have been used successfully.[19,20]

Lung contusion is associated with interstitial edema and hemorrhage, generally localized to the area of lung underlying an impact site.[3] On occasion, contusions can occur on opposite sides of the chest or throughout both lungs as a result of high-impact shock waves from a blast injury. The edema and bleeding in the contused region of the lung cause a progressive decline in local lung compliance and airway inflammation, leading to atelectasis. Hypoxemia and the work of breathing intensify during the first 48 to 72 hours as the pathologic changes evolve.[3] These changes can progress to the development of adult respiratory distress syndrome (ARDS) (see Chapter 13). Small contusions can be managed with supplemental oxygen and monitoring. Use of ventilatory support with PEEP is needed when respiratory failure occurs. Independent lung ventilation may be necessary if severe asymmetric lung injury is present.[19]

Intrabronchial bleeding occurs in many chest trauma victims with penetrating wounds. Massive bleeding can rapidly lead to asphyxiation. Therapeutic efforts are aimed at reducing the bleeding and suctioning the airway.

Aspiration of stomach contents is relatively common in the trauma patient and should always be suspected in the unconscious patient with an elevated alveolar-arterial difference in partial pressure of oxygen (P[A − a]o$_2$). Airway obstruction and aspiration pneumonitis in the gravity-dependent portions of the lungs are the major complications of gastric aspiration. The signs of inflammatory changes in the lung are often delayed for 12 to 24 hours. The combination of chest trauma and aspiration increases a patient's risk of pneumonia and ARDS.[21]

Airway Injuries

Blunt force injury to the larynx may produce sudden airway occlusion secondary to a crushed larynx or cricotracheal dislocation. A more common problem is progressive airway obstruction from edema. Most laryngeal injuries are caused by steering wheel or dashboard impacts in unrestrained drivers involved in motor vehicle accidents. Symptoms of laryngeal and tracheal injury include hoarseness, inability to lay supine, dysphagia, laryngeal tenderness, tracheal deviation, and subcutaneous emphysema.[22] These signs and symptoms produce important clues to tracheal injury. Inspiratory stridor may not be apparent until the airway is 70 to 80 percent occluded.[3] Lateral neck radiographs may be deceptively negative; a computed tomographic (CT) scan can provide a more accurate view of the laryngeal anatomy. Initial laryngoscopy should be done cautiously in the operating room in case sudden airway obstruction occurs and emergent tracheostomy is required. Placement of an endotracheal tube with the aid of a bronchoscope, or emergent tracheostomy if emergent bronchoscopy is impossible, is the treatment of choice for severe laryngeal trauma and airway obstruction.[3,22]

Blunt and penetrating chest injuries can lead to tracheal and bronchial injuries. Sudden compression of the thorax can cause deceleration shearing of the trachea or bronchus.[23] Most of these injuries occur within 2 cm of the carina and result in pneumothorax and subcutaneous emphysema.[23] Almost all victims of transection of the trachea are dead on arrival to the emergency department and frequently have two or more other major injuries.[24] Tracheal and bronchial laceration or rupture requires rapid bronchoscopic evaluation and direct repair by thoracotomy. Emergent surgical repair of a lacerated trachea or bronchus is the treatment of choice. Diagnostic and therapeutic bronchoscopy is an important tool in managing the patient with tracheobronchial injuries.

Heart and Great Vessel Injuries

Chest trauma can lead to a variety of cardiac injuries, including penetration, rupture, **cardiac tamponade,** coronary artery lacerations and occlusion, myocardial contusion, pericardial effusion, septal defects, valvular injuries, and great vessel rupture.[3] These injuries can be rapidly fatal.

Cardiac penetrating injuries are more frequently caused by knife and gunshot wounds and have a mortality rates ranging from 50 to 85 percent.[21] Blunt trauma is more often associated with cardiac rupture injuries (right heart more common than left) and has been found to have a survival rate of approximately 50 percent for those patients who are still alive at the time of admission to the emergency department with vital signs.[25] After rupture of a cardiac chamber or lacerations of the coronary or great vessels, blood will rapidly fill the pericardial sac and result in cardiac tamponade. Collection of only 60 to 100 mL of blood in the pericardial cavity can produce cardiac tamponade, which can result in cardiogenic shock secondary to reduced cardiac filling.[26] Puncture wounds through the pericardial sac and cardiac chamber result in brisk bleeding, which will dominate the clinical picture as a poorly responsive hypotension. Interestingly, the presence of cardiac tamponade after a cardiac gunshot wound is actually associated with a higher survival rate because of its effects of reducing the blood loss and associated hypotension.[27] Cardiac tamponade is often associated with clinical signs of *Beck's triad:* distended neck veins, hypotension, and diminished heart tones.[3] However, Beck's triad may not be seen in patients who are hypovolemic after hemorrhage. A widened mediastinum on the chest radiograph may suggest mediastinal bleeding or cardiac tamponade, or both. Echocardiography is more helpful in establishing the diagnosis of cardiac tamponade. Emergency exploratory thoracotomy with heart-lung bypass circulatory support, surgical repair, and adequate transfusion are the corrective measures of choice for cardiac rupture.

Myocardial contusion after blunt chest trauma is not easily identified. In carefully evaluated patients, the incidence probably approaches 25 percent in general chest trauma and about 80 percent after sternal fractures.[3,12] The pathologic changes in the contused heart include intramyocardial hemorrhage, myocardial edema, coronary artery occlusion, myofibril degeneration, and myocardial cell necrosis.[28] These changes lead to arrhythmias and hemodynamic instability, which are very similar to those found after a myocardial infarction.

Electrocardiographic (ECG) findings often show tachycardia, ST-segment elevation, T-wave changes, and occasional premature ventricular contractions.[3,25,29] Cardiac enzyme levels in plasma (e.g., aspartate aminotransferase [AST], lactate dehydrogenase [LDH], and creatine kinase [CK]) are almost always elevated after blunt chest trauma and are therefore of little diagnostic value. Plasma CPK-MB isoenzyme elevation appears to be more discriminatory and helps confirm the diagnosis of myocardial contusion.[25,29] Pulmonary artery catheterization is often useful in monitoring hemodynamic performance and for treating heart failure. Echocardiography, radionuclide angiography, and serial ECG, hemodynamics, and CPK-MB monitoring form the diagnostic array for detecting and monitoring myocardial contusion. Patients are treated as though they had a myocardial infarction. In those patients with cardiac failure, use of an intra-aortic balloon pump has been found useful in supporting cardiac output.[30] Often there is complete clinical recovery with minimal scarring of the myocardium. The overall mortality in patients with myocardial contusion is approximately 10 percent.[31]

Aortic rupture and exsanguination after blunt chest trauma in a motor vehicle accident leads to rapid death. Approximately 8000 people have aortic ruptures in this country each year and about 80 to 90 percent die in the first few minutes after the event.[31,32] The upper descending thoracic aorta is the most common site of rupture in those who are admitted to the emergency department with vital signs.[31] The patient frequently presents with profound hypotension and often with chest radiographic findings showing a widened mediastinum. Aortic angiography or direct visualization during emergent thoracotomy are the diagnostic methods of choice for detecting a ruptured or lacerated aorta. If the patient presents in shock and with an obviously widened mediastinum, emergent thoracotomy, surgical repair, and transfusion are needed.

Diaphragmatic Injuries

Penetrating trauma is the most frequent cause of diaphragmatic injury. Blunt force trauma to the abdomen causes diaphragmatic rupture in only 5 percent of abdominal injuries, the left diaphragm being injured about 90 percent of the time.[33] Rupture of the diaphragm is frequently associated with splenic rupture; hemothorax; bowel herniation up into the thorax, which reduces lung volume; shock; impaired diaphragmatic motion; ventilatory failure; CO_2 retention; and coma.[3,18,33] The mortality rate of diaphragmatic rupture is reported to be about 30 percent, but it is frequently associated with other injuries.[33] The diagnosis is usually made by evaluation of the chest and abdominal radiographs, by CT scans of the abdomen, or during exploratory laparotomy. Diaphragmatic rupture requires surgical evaluation and closure.

Delayed and Long-Term Complications of Chest Wall Trauma

Chronic pain, recurring atelectasis, dyspnea, and pneumonia are the most common delayed and prolonged chest wall problems after chest injuries.[34,35] In most patients the cause remains unclear, although reduced lung volume probably plays a major role.[35] The chronic pain and dyspnea are usually managed with oxygen therapy, analgesics, and reassurance. Occasionally, surgery may be necessary to repair painfully persistent fractures of the ribs and sternum. Pleural infection can arise from a retained hemothorax or foreign body and can result in empyema, pleurisy, and fibrothorax.[34] Thoracotomy, pleural drainage, antibiotics, and pleural decortication are frequently used to correct poorly responding pleural infections and to avert the formation of a fibrothorax.

Penetrating and blunt chest injuries can lead to pulmonary artery-to-vein fistula, aortic aneurysm, cardiac valvular insufficiency, constrictive pericarditis, diaphragmatic herniation, and esophageal stricture or fistula.[36] Retained foreign bodies have been found to migrate or erode into other areas many years after the initial injury. Foreign-body migration can result in embolic events. Erosion of a sharp body can result in hemoptysis, pneumonia, and lung abscess. These long-term complications often require acute and rehabilitative care coupled with surgical repairs.

Clinical Features and Laboratory Findings

Gathering a proper history about the events of the trauma is vital to understanding the extent of injuries. Information about the nature of the motor vehicle accident (e.g., whether seat restraints were used, whether the victim was ejected, the size of vehicle), the caliber or type of gun used, and how long the victim went untreated or was in shock are examples of useful information. It is important to gather any information regarding preexisting heart, lung, vascular, and renal disease, as well as a history of substance abuse, because they often complicate the response to trauma.

A rapid and careful physical examination should include evaluation of the patient's airway, breathing rate and effort, heart rate, blood pressure, signs of flail chest, presence of subcutaneous emphysema, and symmetry and quality of breath sounds. A rapid and systematic method of initial evaluation of the nervous, circulatory, and respiratory systems is found in the trauma score.[37] This scoring system is a simple method for evaluating trauma patients and determining the severity of their injuries (Table 14–3). The findings dictate which additional tests should be performed and what type of care should be provided.

A variety of studies and laboratory procedures are frequently used to obtain a bet-

TABLE 14-3   **Trauma Score**

Glasgow Coma Scale	Systolic Blood Pressure	Respiratory Rate	Points
13–15	>89	10–29	4
9–12	76–89	>29	3
6–8	50–75	6–9	2
4–5	1–49	1–5	1
3	0	0	0

EXAMPLE

	POINTS
Glasgow coma scale* = 14	4
Blood pressure = 80	3
Respiratory rate = 35	3
Trauma score:	10

*Glasgow coma scale is a simple neurologic examination system that awards points according to the patient's best eye movement, verbal response, and motor response to various stimuli (see Chapter 12 for a more detailed explanation of the Glasgow coma scale).
SOURCE: Adapted from Champion, HR, et al: A revision of the trauma score. J Trauma 29:623, 1989.

ter concept of the nature and extent of chest injuries. The portable anteroposterior chest radiograph is necessary in virtually all cases for further evaluation of the patient and for helping guide emergent care. Complete blood count (CBC), electrolytes, arterial blood gases (ABGs), and ECG are taken on admission and then serially. More specialized studies, such as bronchoscopy, CT scanning, magnetic resonance imaging, and angiography, are done to gain a more precise determination of the extent of injuries.

Treatment

Approximately 80 percent of all trauma-related deaths occur in the first few hours after injury (Fig. 14-5).[38] Victim survival improves with rapid access to advanced life support and trauma center care. Acute care for chest trauma includes maintenance of a patent airway; supplementary oxygen therapy with 100 percent FIO_2 via non-rebreathing mask; resuscitation bag with reservoir or high-flow oxygen delivery system; mechanical ventilation; placement of arterial and intravenous (IV) catheters for monitoring blood pressure and for fluid or blood administration; chest tube placement; and possibly direct admission to the operating room for emergency thoracotomy. Placement of a pulmonary artery catheter is useful when managing a patient who is either hemodynamically unstable or requires large amounts of fluids to maintain fluid balance and blood pressure, or both. Pain management is also important. Use of patient-controlled analgesia devices for the infusion of pain medication (e.g., systemic infusion or thoracic epidural analgesia) improves the patient's pain toleration, cooperation in deep breathing, and pulmonary function and avoids ventilatory support.[39,40]

Airway Management

Airway obstruction after trauma is believed to be the leading cause of preventable death.[38] Airway obstruction is most commonly caused by the tongue's slipping back

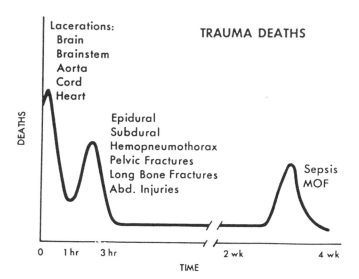

FIGURE 14-5 The trimodal distribution and principal causes of death following trauma. The initial 50 percent die almost immediately, another 30 percent within hours of admission to the hospital, and the remaining 20 percent later from complications (multiple organ failure [MOF]). (From Trunkey, DD: Organization of trauma care. In Burke, JF, Boyd, RJ, and McCabe, CJ (eds): Trauma Management. Year Book Medical, Chicago, 1988, with permission.)

into the oropharynx. Aspiration of vomitus, blood, excessive saliva, dentures, and oral or laryngeal injuries with swelling are also causes of airway obstruction. Manual reposition of the victim's head and placement of an oropharyngeal airway facilitates a patent airway and bag-mask ventilation with 100 percent oxygen prior to intubation.

A properly sized cuffed oral endotracheal tube is the airway of choice for most cases involving emergency airway maintenance. It permits positive pressure ventilation, facilitates endotracheal suctioning, and helps protect the lungs from gastric contents. If the patient has a suspected cervical fracture, bronchoscopically assisted placement of a nasotracheal tube is recommended because this method does not require extension of the head for placement. Inadequate preoxygenation, mainstem intubation, esophageal intubation, respiratory alkalosis secondary to excessive ventilation, vasovagal reflex bradycardia, or a combination of these, may result in cardiac arrest during attempted endotracheal tube placement.

Careful examination of the endotracheal tube placement should be done to ensure bilateral ventilation. Right mainstem bronchial intubation occurs in approximately 30 percent of victims that require resuscitation.[41] A chest radiograph and fiberoptic bronchoscopy are indicated to evaluate excessive blood being suctioned from the airway. Diagnostic and therapeutic fiberoptic bronchoscopy is often very useful in patients with persistent or reoccurring atelectasis. A double-lumen endotracheal tube may be required in cases of severe asymmetric lung contusion or tracheobronchial rupture necessitating independent lung ventilation. In situations where endotracheal intubation and tracheostomy tube placement are difficult or impossible, cricothyrotomy can be performed until it is possible to place a tracheostomy tube. In situations where no other airway access is available, the insertion of one or several 12-gauge cricothyroid needles can provide short-term percutaneous transtracheal oxygenation and ventilation until a tracheostomy tube can be placed.[42]

Ventilatory Support

Patients who present with apnea, frank respiratory failure (PaO_2 less than 60 mm Hg, $PaCO_2$ greater than 50 mm Hg, and pH less than 7.20), or who have impending respiratory failure (respiratory rate greater than 35/minute and very shallow breathing) will require ventilatory support. Initial ventilator settings for a patient with an unknown degree of chest injury should be directed toward complete support with volume-controlled ventilation at a tidal volume (V_T) setting of 7 to 10 mL/kg, set rate of 15/minute, flow setting to provide an inspiratory:expiratory (I:E) ratio of 1:3, and an FIO_2 of 1.0. Adjustments can then be made after further clinical examination and ABG results are reviewed. A PEEP of 5 to 15 cm H_2O is frequently necessary to improve lung volume and oxygenation. Caution is always necessary, however, when using positive pressure ventilation and PEEP in chest trauma victims because of their higher risk of hypotension and barotrauma. When they can effectively breathe spontaneously, synchronized intermittent mandatory ventilation (SIMV) combined with pressure support is useful for matching the ventilator with the patient's breathing pattern. Weaning from ventilatory support is frequently done by decelerating SIMV to pressure or volume support alone. Next, the RCP reduces the amount of support during each breath to a point where the patient can effectively maintain a V_T of 4 to 5 mL/kg while breathing comfortably at a respiratory rate of less than 20 to 25/minute.

A variety of more complex modes of ventilation are available for management of more complicated cases. In severe cases of ARDS the use of pressure-controlled inverse-ratio ventilation may improve oxygenation and ventilation and reduce high peak airway pressure.[43-46] Patients who present with severe asymmetric lung injury, and who show signs of poor oxygenation despite the application of 100 percent oxygen and PEEP during conventional mechanical ventilation, may improve with independent lung ventilation through a double-lumen endotracheal tube.[47-50] High-frequency jet ventilation or independent lung ventilation may support the ventilatory needs of patients with bronchopleural fistula.[51,52] Extracorporeal membrane oxygenation (ECMO) is beneficial for stabilizing and improving gas exchange and improving neurologic outcomes in some victims of trauma.[19,53] Initial experience with ECMO in the treatment of ARDS, however, demonstrated no major survival benefit compared to standard treatment.[54]

Other Techniques of Respiratory Care

The patient with chest trauma often requires additional forms of respiratory care. Therapy using heated or cooled humidity, or both, is frequently used for the management of secretions. Airway clearance is very important for those who have prosthetic airways and secretion retention. Chest physical therapy is often effective in mobilizing retained airway secretions and may help reexpand atelectatic areas. Aerosolized bronchodilator therapy is frequently employed to reduce airway resistance, facilitate lung expansion, and reduce the work of breathing. These "low-tech" forms of respiratory care are important in the acute as well as long-term phases of treatment for chest trauma patients.

CASE STUDY

History

Ms. M, a 20-year-old woman, was in good health but not wearing her seat belt when she accidentally drove off the roadway at high speed and struck a tree head-on. She was conscious when discovered a short while later, resuscitated in the field, and had a reported trauma score of 10. She was initially taken to a community hospital, where she was assessed and trauma life support begun.

QUESTIONS

1. What signs and symptoms will need to be evaluated immediately upon her arrival?

2. What diagnostic techniques can be used to help determine the severity of her injuries?

3. What therapeutic support should be available upon her arrival?

ANSWERS

1. Signs of a patent airway, spontaneous breathing, quality of breath sounds and their symmetry, pulse rate, blood pressure, and level of consciousness should be evaluated.

2. The nature and severity of her injuries can be better understood by determining the nature of the motor vehicle accident. A careful and rapid physical evaluation followed by radiographs of her spine, chest, abdomen, and extremities will be needed as indicated. Other important features include the degree and duration of shock, signs of gastric aspiration, signs of hypothermia, and any underlying medical conditions or history of substance abuse that may complicate her injuries.

3. Oxygen therapy (cannula or non-rebreathing mask), intubation equipment, manual resuscitation bag with proper mask, oxygen reservoir and a PEEP capability, venous and arterial line placement equipment, fluids for vascular support, resuscitation drugs, chest tube placement equipment, and medications for pain and agitation should be available. Patients in shock as a result of internal bleeding must have direct access to the operating room upon arrival to the hospital.

Physical Examination

General: A tall woman with an approximate weight of 55 kg; awake with a cervical collar on, combative, and moving all extremities while breathing air; Glasgow coma scale of 13

Vital Signs: Temperature 35.5°C (96.0°F); respiratory rate 32/minute; blood pressure 91/61 mm Hg; heart rate 138/minute; nail bed refill 5 seconds

HEENT: Pupils equal and reactive to light; no obvious nasal flaring, no signs of blood or vomit in mouth

Neck: Trachea somewhat shifted to the left of midline; no signs of inspiratory stridor or contusion to the larynx; carotid pulses ++ bilaterally without bruit; no signs of lymphadenopathy or thyroidomegaly; some jugular vein distention noted with the patient elevated; some tensing of sternocleidomastoid and scalene muscles noted during inspiration

Chest: Abrasions over the right chest; obvious flail motion of the right lateral and anterior chest with 1 to 2 cm depression on inspiration; subcutaneous air felt over the anterior and lateral right chest; breath sounds diminished in the right lung compared to the left lung; some thoracoabdominal paradoxical motion noted

Heart: Regular rhythm at a rate of 135 to 145/minute; distant S_1 and S_2 sounds without murmurs, gallops, or rubs

Abdomen: Abrasions over the right upper quadrant; somewhat distended and tender; bowel sounds hypoactive

Extremities: Moving all extremities; no signs of fracture or dislocation; no clubbing and no obvious cyanosis

QUESTIONS

4. What signs and symptoms indicate chest injuries?

5. How will the chest injuries influence respiratory function?

6. What are the possible causes of her respiratory distress?

7. In addition to the physical examination, how should the patient's cardiorespiratory status be further evaluated?

8. What other laboratory tests would be helpful?

ANSWERS

4. Chest injuries are indicated by the presence of chest wall abrasions, flail motion, tachypnea, accessory muscle tensing, tracheal deviation, subcutaneous emphysema, diminished breath sounds in the right lung, and thoracoabdominal wall paradoxical motion.

5. Flail chest will result in increased work of breathing and decreased efficiency of gas exchange. ABGs are almost always abnormal as a result of this type of injury.

6. Her respiratory distress is probably due in part to the flail chest and pain from broken ribs. Other possible causes include pneumothorax or hemopneumothorax, lung contusion, tracheobronchial rupture, cardiac contusion, great vessel fracture, diaphragmatic herniation, and intra-abdominal injuries. These changes may be inducing increased airway resistance, decreased pulmonary compliance, $\dot{V}/\dot{Q}$ mismatching, hypoxemia, and ventilatory failure.

7. To evaluate her cardiorespiratory distress further, ABGs, ECG monitoring, and a chest radiograph are needed. Placement of peripheral venous, central venous, and arterial lines will be needed to guide and maintain hemodynamic stability.

8. Laboratory assessment of CBC, electrolytes, and standard blood chemistry and screening for alcohol and illegal drugs are indicated. Her hypothermia secondary to exposure after the accident may be contributing to her hypotension and altered mental status and will require care and continued monitoring. Abdominal injuries should be evaluated by peritoneal lavage for the presence of blood. Blood in the peritoneum signifies ruptured abdominal organs and requires explorative and corrective surgery.

Bedside and Laboratory Evaluations

ECG: Sinus tachycardia of 137/minute without any other abnormalities

Chest Radiograph:

Subcutaneous air over the right hemothorax

Ribs 3 through 8 fractured on the right

Hemopneumothorax in the right pleural space

Mediastinal shift to the left, indicating tension pneumothorax

Signs of hazy infiltrate in the right, which is consistent with pulmonary contusion

Normal mediastinal width and no sign of pneumomediastinum

No foreign bodies visible

ABGs: pH 7.07, $PaCO_2$ 61 mm Hg, PaO_2 31 mm Hg, HCO_3^- 18 mEq/liter while breathing room air

Hematology: Hematocrit (Hct) 21 percent, hemoglobin (Hb) = 7 g/dL, red blood cells (RBCs) $2.3 \times 10^6/mm^3$, white blood cells (WBCs) 9.2×10^3, platelets = 210×10^3

Chemistry and Toxicology: Results pending

QUESTIONS

9. How would you interpret the ECG and blood pressure?

10. What does the chest radiograph indicate, and what should be done based on these findings?

11. How would you interpret the ABG data?

12. What do the hematologic data indicate?

13. What respiratory care is indicated at this time, and how should it be evaluated?

14. What hemodynamic support is indicated at this time, and how should it be evaluated?

15. What complications may occur in the next 24 to 48 hours?

ANSWERS

9. The ECG findings indicate a compensatory tachycardia in response to blood loss, hypotension, and stress.

10. The chest radiographic findings reveal the magnitude of injuries after a severe blunt-impact injury to the right chest. The tension hemopneumothorax indicates the need for emergent chest tube placement to drain both blood and air.

11. The ABG shows severe respiratory and metabolic acidosis, hypoventilation, and hypoxemia. After severe blunt chest injuries, these findings are consistent with one or more of the following: shock, $\dot{V}/\dot{Q}$ abnormality, diffusion defect, and venous-arterial intrapulmonary shunting.

12. The hematologic data indicate anemia secondary to severe blood loss and requires immediate fluid replacement and transfusion. Peritoneal lavage revealed substantial blood in the peritoneal cavity and the need for emergent exploratory laparotomy.

13. The patient will need to be fully supported. After intubation, visual inspection of chest motion and breath sounds will be needed for initial determination of proper tube placement. To help correct the hypoxemia and acidosis, her initial ventilator support could include the following parameters:

volume control mode, set V_T at 800 mL, set rate at 16/minute, provide adequate inspiratory flow to maintain an I:E ratio of 1:3, set PEEP at 0 cm H_2O, and set FIO_2 at 100 percent. Place chest tubes in the right hemithorax. A repeat physical examination, vital signs, ABG, and chest radiograph should be done to determine the patient's initial response to therapy.

14. Fluid resuscitation with crystalloid IV infusion should be started. Blood should be given as soon as available. Evaluation of central venous pressure, systemic blood pressure, and renal output should be monitored to avoid hypotension or fluid overload. If hemodynamic instability persists, placement of a pulmonary artery balloon catheter for monitoring preload pressures, cardiac output, and afterload may be needed.

15. The severity of her blunt-impact injuries and shock provide multiple risk factors for the development of ARDS and multiple organ failure. She will require intensive care for continued ventilatory support, IV fluid administration, and monitoring of neurologic, cardiovascular, pulmonary, and renal function.

CASE STUDY—continued

In the operating room, Ms. M was anesthetized, orally intubated with a 7.5-mm cuffed tube, and placed on mechanical ventilation with 100 percent O_2. Peripheral venous and arterial lines were placed, and fluid resuscitation was begun. Two 36-French chest tubes were placed in the right pleural space, and 25 cm H_2O of suction was applied by underwater seal drainage systems. Air and 600 mL of blood were immediately removed. Exploratory laparotomy resulted in discovery and removal of a large amount of free blood, a ruptured spleen, and a lacerated right lobe of the liver. The peritoneal cavity was then lavaged with warm saline and povidone-iodine (Betadine). During surgery and over the next 12 hours, she received 35 units of packed RBCs and 3.5 L of Ringer's lactate. A CT scan of her head was done after admission to the intensive care unit, and no signs of closed head injury were found despite persistent reduction in her level of consciousness. After 24 hours of care and stabilization at the community hospital, she was transferred to the regional trauma center.

On admission to the trauma center her problem list included the following:

1. Status after shock and respiratory failure from blunt trauma to the chest and abdomen

2. Multiple rib fractures, flail chest, lung contusion, and subcutaneous emphysema on the right side with chest tubes

3. Midline abdominal incision after repair of multiple abdominal injuries

4. Possible closed head injury or hypoxic brain injury

5. Rule out spinal injuries and pelvic fractures

6. Status after hypothermia

7. Positive disseminated intravascular coagulation screen

The goals of her initial treatment at the trauma center concentrated on improving cardiovascular stability and respiratory function. A central venous catheter was placed, and the administration of fluids, fresh frozen plasma, and blood continued along with full ventilatory support.

Shortly after her arrival at the trauma center, her bedside findings, vital signs, chest radiograph, ventilator settings, and laboratory data were as follows:

Ms. M is lying in a semi-Fowler's position and is orally intubated, with two chest tubes exiting her right thorax. Bandages cover a distended abdomen that has a bandaged midline incision. A small amount of blood (less than 20 mL/hour) is continuously draining from the chest tubes, and no air leaks are crossing the water seal. She is moving all four extremities and periodically becomes combative, requiring reassurance and analgesics for sedation. She is spontaneously initiating approximately every other breath from the Siemens Servo 900C ventilator through an endotracheal tube (7.5-mm internal diameter). The endotracheal tube has 25 cm H_2O pressure in the cuff, and no gas leakage is heard over the cuff site. The airway is secured to the upper lip with waterproof tape and is showing the 23-cm mark at the lip. The right hemithorax is noted to have a flail motion when she becomes agitated and makes spontaneous efforts to breathe. Her breath sounds are generally diminished over the right lung, with better aeration noted in the left lung with occasional expiratory rhonchi heard. On suctioning her airway, small amounts of mucoid sputum are removed. In-line ventilator circuit delivery of 2.5 mg albuterol diluted in 3 mL of saline is being given every 4 hours and as needed (prn).

Bedside Findings

Vital Signs, Hemodynamics, and Urine Output:

Rectal temperature 37.2°C (99.0°F)

Respiratory rate 20/minute

Heart rate 100/minute

Systemic arterial blood pressure 123/78 mm Hg

Central venous pressure 6 mm Hg

Urine output ranged from 65 to 80 mL/hour since admission

Chest Radiograph: See Figure 14–6.

Ventilator Settings and Findings:

SIMV + pressure support (PS) mode

Rate set 17/minute

PS 10 cm H_2O

SIMV V_T set 0.75 liter

SIMV V_T exh 0.78 liter

PS V_T 0.435 liter

FIO_2 1.0

Inspiratory flow 51 liters/minute

Gas temperature 35°C (95°F)

Total respiratory rate 22/minute

$\dot{V}_E$ 14.3 liters/minute

Peak pressure 38 cm H_2O

Plateau pressure 30 cm H_2O

set PEEP 10 cm H_2O

auto-PEEP 11 cm H_2O

Static compliance 41 mL/cm H_2O

Effective airway resistance 9 cm H_2O/liter per second

Laboratory Evaluation

ABGs: pH 7.35, $PaCO_2$ 44 mm Hg, PaO_2 350 mm Hg, HCO_3^- 23 mEq/liter, $P(A - a)O_2$ 308 mm Hg, PaO_2/FIO_2 350, SaO_2 100 percent (calculated), SpO_2 = 99 percent (pulse oximeter)

Hematology: Hct 38 percent, Hb 12.7 g/dL, RBCs $4.1 \times 10^6/mm^3$, WBC = $10.4 \times 10^3/mm^3$, platelets $135 \times 10^3/mm^3$

Electrolytes and Chemistry: Na^+ 144 mEq, K^+ 4.1 mEq, Cl^- 100 mEq, glucose 116 mg/dL, blood urea nitrogen 18 mg/dL, creatinine = 0.9 mg/dL

Toxicology: No alcohol or other drugs found

Microbiology: Blood, sputum, and wound smear and cultures pending

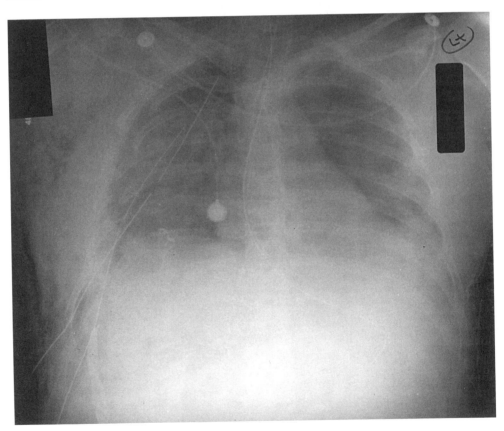

FIGURE 14-6   Portable chest radiograph shortly after admission to the trauma center.

QUESTIONS

16. What do her airway care and breath sounds indicate? What would be recommended at this time?

17. How would you describe her hemodynamics?

18. How would you describe the radiographic findings?

19. How would you describe the ventilator settings, breathing pattern, pulmonary mechanics, and ABG findings? Are the ventilator settings appropriate for the patient's condition? What should be recommended at this time?

20. What do her other laboratory findings indicate?

ANSWERS

16. The airway is appropriate, and its position appears acceptable. Cuff pressure is effectively sealing the trachea at a safe pressure and high enough to help avoid silent aspiration of saliva around the cuff. Placement of a tracheostomy tube is not indicated at this time. Breath sounds indicate reduced ventilation of the right lung and retained secretions. The in-line aerosolization of albuterol is appropriate; however, its dosage may need to be increased, or use of an in-line metered dose inhaler with 4 to 10 puffs may be more efficacious. The sputum removed from the airway does not suggest pulmonary hemorrhage or infection at this time. Special attention to the airway, its maintenance, and sterile technique are necessary to help avoid complications.

17. The hemodynamics are acceptable after massive transfusion and fluid replacement. The right heart filling pressure (central venous pressure) indicates that she has an adequate blood volume at this time.

18. The portable anteroposterior chest radiograph taken shortly after admission to the trauma center (Fig. 14–6) shows subcutaneous emphysema in the lateral right hemothorax with generalized loss of lung volume. Ribs 3 through 8 are fractured along the right posterior and lateral margin with bilateral pleural effusions, right lung pulmonary contusion with air bronchograms, bilateral atelectasis, and abdominal compression of the thorax. Two chest tubes are seen in the right thorax, the endotracheal tube is 3 cm above carina, a central venous line ends in the right atrium, and a nasogastric tube terminates in the stomach. There is no evidence of a pneumothorax.

19. The ventilator settings indicate that she is receiving substantial ventilatory support while in a state of mild tachypnea with a potentially toxic FIO_2. The V_T setting of 0.75 liter (14 mL/kg) is at the upper limit of acceptable for her frame size. She is triggering the ventilator at a rate beyond the set SIMV rate of five pressure-supported breaths. The pressure-supported V_Ts should be increased (e.g., 0.6 liter) to improve their gas-exchange effectiveness and to reduce her respiratory rate. A better approach would be to return her to an assist-control mode of ventilation with sedation for better stabilization of her chest and reduction of her work of breathing. The peak and plateau pressures during volume-limited breaths are elevated as a result of the moderately reduced compliance and increased airway resistance. The PEEP is necessary to improve $\dot{V}/\dot{Q}$ matching, prevent further development of atelectasis, and allow FIO_2 reduction. Her respiratory pattern is not resulting in any additional auto-PEEP, although she may start gas trapping if her rate increases.

Her PaO$_2$ is excessive, and her FIO$_2$ should be tapered with continuous pulse oximetry to maintain a targeted SpO$_2$ of greater than 90 percent. The P(A − a)O$_2$ is significantly increased and indicates a diffusion defect, shunting, V̇/Q̇ mismatching, or a combination of these. Her oxygen content is acceptable at 18 mL/dL. The PaCO$_2$ is normal, but is requiring an elevated minute ventilation as a result of an increased metabolic rate, dead space ventilation, or both. The acid-base balance is acceptable.

20. The hematologic data indicate an acceptable RBC count and hemoglobin concentration after massive transfusion. A mildly elevated WBC count is not uncommon after this degree of trauma and the stress response to it. The reduced platelet count is consistent with the disseminated intravascular coagulation. The electrolytes and renal function are normal, considering the amount of blood and fluid that she has received. The slight hyperglycemia may be a result of glucocorticoid and catecholamine release secondary to the trauma or the IV fluids being given, or both.

CASE STUDY—continued

After assessment of Ms. M's condition, her FIO$_2$ was gradually reduced to 50 percent over the next 2 hours, and a third chest tube was placed in the left chest to drain the pleural effusion. Sputum cultures and sensitivity showed a heavy growth of *Streptococcus pneumoniae*, and she was started on appropriate antibiotics. Aerosolized bronchodilation continued with a trial of postural drainage via a modified Trendelenburg's position. Postural drainage was discontinued after first attempt when she became extremely short of breath and her pulse oximeter saturations dropped from 94 to 88 percent.

For the next week her ventilatory requirements continued at the same level, and she could not tolerate an SIMV rate reduction of less than 15/minute and a pressure support of less than 10 cm H$_2$O without becoming excessively tachypneic, desaturated (pulse oximetry), tachycardic, and hypertensive. Cyclic fever spikes and episodic atelectasis with infiltrates occurred during this period. These pulmonary changes required rigorous pulmonary hygiene and therapeutic bronchoscopy for removal of mucus plugs. One of the right chest tubes was eventually removed without recurrence of pneumothorax. Her abdominal wound required reexploration and lavage because of a small abscess, and the abdomen remained excessively swollen. Her nutritional status was maintained through regular central line alimentation until nasogastric tube feedings were tolerated.

Eleven days after her accident her temperature spiked up 39.3°C (102.7°F) accompanied by tachycardia, tachypnea with obvious flail motion on the right side, and increasing FIO$_2$ requirements from 40 to 60 percent to maintain an SpO$_2$ of greater than 92 percent. Breath sounds became progressively more course sounding, with bilateral inspiratory and expiratory rhonchi and wheezes, and were diminished on the right. Sputum suctioned from her became purulent and somewhat foul smelling. A chest radiograph taken at this time (Fig. 14–7) showed increasing bilateral infiltrates with a loss of lung volume and no signs of pneumothorax. The endotracheal tube, chest tube, central venous catheter, and nasogastric tube all appeared to be in their proper positions. Sputum smears showed 3+ gram-positive cocci and 1+ gram-positive bacilli. Her antibiotics were adjusted, and airway care and aerosolized bronchodilators were intensified to help clear the retained secretions. She was still unable to tolerate chest physiotherapy. Over the next 48 hours her breath sounds, sputum production, and chest radiograph improved. Ventilatory support was gradually reduced to an SIMV of 6/minute with a PS of 12 cm H_2O and 40 percent FIO_2. Over the next week, this pattern of fever spike, breath-sound changes, purulent sputum with heavy bacterial counts, chest radiographic findings consistent with pneumonia, increasing ventilatory support requirements, antibiotic treatment, and intensive airway care was repeated two more times. In each case, her ventilatory support was increased and then reduced back to the same level. During this period, her chest tubes were successfully removed. It was believed that she was ready to be removed from ventilatory support on the 16th day after admission to the trauma center, and she was extubated. Shortly after extubation, her respiratory rate climbed to 45 to 50/minute with obvious flail motion of the right hemithorax, heart rate increased to 140 to 150/minute, and oxyhemoglobin saturation declined to 88 percent despite the use of 60 percent FIO_2 via high-flow oxygen therapy. She was reintubated and returned to an SIMV of 12/minute and a PS of 14 cm H_2O with 60 percent FIO_2. She stabilized rapidly and was able to tolerate reduction of her ventilatory support to PS ventilation alone with an FIO_2 of 30 percent over the next 2 days.

Twenty-three days after her initial injury she was again evaluated for extubation. Her bedside findings, vital signs, chest radiograph, ventilator settings, and laboratory data were as follows:

Ms. M is sitting up in bed, orally intubated, alert, and communicative through a writing tablet. She is spontaneously initiating every breath from the Siemens Servo 900C ventilator through an endotracheal tube (7.5-mm internal diameter). The airway has 25 cm H_2O pressure in the cuff, no gas leakage is heard over the cuff site, and it is secured to the upper lip with waterproof tape and showing the 22 cm mark at the lip. The right hemithorax is still noted to have some flail motion when she makes vigorous efforts to breathe. Her breath sounds are generally diminished over the right lung with better aeration noted in the left lung; inspiratory and expiratory rhonchi are heard bilaterally. Moderate amounts of mucoid sputum are periodically removed during airway care. In-line ventilator circuit delivery of 2.5 mg of albuterol diluted in 3 mL of saline continues every 4 hours and prn.

Bedside Findings

Vital Signs, Hemodynamics, and Urine Output:

Temperature 38.3° C (100.9°F)

Respiratory rate 23/minute (total rate observed while on ventilator)

Heart rate 102/minute

Systemic arterial blood pressure 128/81 mm Hg

Urine output continuing at about 70 mL/hour

Chest Radiograph:

Multiple rib fractures on the right

A few patchy infiltrates bilaterally, which are in the process of clearing

No signs of pneumothorax

Endotracheal tube, central venous catheter, and nasogastric tube apparently in their proper positions

Ventilator Settings and Findings:

PS + PEEP mode

PS = 10 cm H_2O

PS exhaled VT 0.425 to 0.635 liter

FIO_2 30 percent

set PEEP 5 cm H_2O

Gas temperature 34°C (93.2°F)

Total respiratory rate = 23/minute

$\dot{V}E$ 12.7 liters/minute

Peak pressure 15 cm H_2O

Laboratory Evaluation

ABGs: pH 7.42, $PaCO_2$ 38 mm Hg, PaO_2 96 mm Hg, HCO_3^- 24 mEq/liter, $P(A - a)O_2$ 68 mm Hg, PaO_2/FIO_2 = 320, Hb 14 g/dL, SaO_2 98 percent (calculated), SpO_2 =97 percent (pulse oximeter), CaO_2 = 18.6 mL/dL

Spontaneous Ventilation Study: (After 5 minutes of breathing 40 percent FIO_2 via non-rebreathing valve): respiratory rate 36/minute, $\dot{V}E$, 11.2 liters/minute, VT = 0.31 liter, rate/VT = 116, forced vital capacity 0.68 liter, maximum inspiratory pressure (MIP) −20 cm H_2O, SpO_2 = 92 percent, heart rate 129/minute, blood pressure 133/88 mm Hg.

CASE STUDY—continued

Ms. M became somewhat anxious toward the end of the trial and began to exhibit some flail motion of the right chest and increasing tachypnea (45/minute).

QUESTIONS

21. How would you interpret her vital signs?
22. What do the current ventilator settings and breathing pattern indicate about her ventilator support?
23. What do the ABGs indicate?
24. How would you assess the spontaneous ventilation data?
25. What course of action would you recommend at this time? Why?

ANSWERS

21. Her vital signs indicate a mild stress response with the presence of mild tachypnea and tachycardia. Urine output and temperature are within normal limits.
22. She is currently in a spontaneous mode of pressure support ventilation with a low level of PEEP. Her respiratory pattern shows mild tachypnea, acceptable tidal ventilation (7 to 11 mL/kg), and moderately elevated minute ventilation. Approximately 75 percent or more of her pressure support is overcoming the airway resistance imposed by the endotracheal tube. The FIO_2 is modestly elevated, but well below a toxic level.
23. Her most recent ABG data indicate acceptable oxygenation with slight elevation of the $P(A - a)O_2$ consistent with persistent but improving $\dot{V}/Q$ mismatching. The $PaCO_2$ indicates normal alveolar ventilation despite the elevated minute

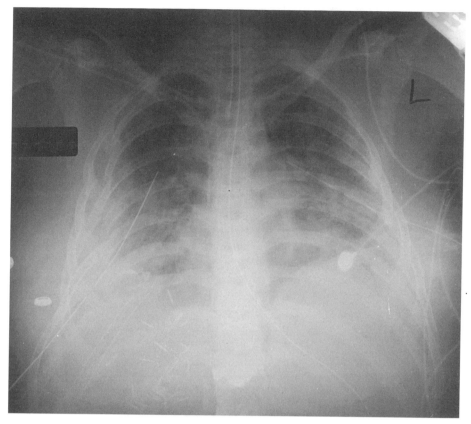

FIGURE 14-7   Portable chest radiograph 11 days after admission to the trauma center.

ventilation. The relatively high minute ventilation may be due to elevated metabolism or dead space, or both. The acid-base data indicate a normal balance.

24. The spontaneous ventilation data after a 5-minute trial with a non-rebreathing valve supplied with an FIO_2 of 40 percent show marked tachypnea, elevated minute ventilation, and relatively shallow tidal ventilation. The ratio of rate/VT is markedly elevated and greater than 100, indicating a rapid and shallow respiratory pattern that is not predictive of successful spontaneous ventilation.[54] The best vital capacity was twice the VT, indicating that she may not have an effective cough. The MIP is barely acceptable and consistent with a weakened ventilatory muscle capability. When viewed together with her anxiety, desaturation of hemoglobin to 92 percent, increasing heart and respiratory rate, and the presence of a flail motion at the end of the trial, these measurements all indicate that she is not yet ready for spontaneous unsupported ventilation and extubation.

25. She should be returned to PS ventilation to stabilize her respiratory, cardiovascular, and psychological status. It is clear that a more gradual approach to her weaning from ventilatory support will be necessary. The placement of a tracheostomy tube should facilitate her weaning and secretion management and should prevent further laryngeal injury from the endotracheal tube.

   A number of weaning strategies can be used. Short trials of low-level PS (e.g., 5 cm H_2O) for 5 to 30 minutes three to four times per day could be tried. These trials can then be lengthened as she develops more respiratory muscle endurance and less dyspnea. Her flail chest motion continues to retard her progress; however, this should gradually improve. Continued assessment of her abdominal wound; respiratory tract secretions; pain; and nutritional, psychological, and fluid and electrolyte status should be made.

CASE STUDY—continued

She was returned to PS ventilation, and it was decided to attempt T-tube trials with adequate oxygen three times per day for 30 minutes, as tolerated. A cuffed tracheostomy tube (7.5-mm internal diameter) was placed. T-tube trials continued over the next week until she was able to remain off the ventilator throughout the day and most of the night without excessive dyspnea and flail motion. During this period, she began to first stand at the bedside for a few minutes and then take short walks in and outside her room while having ventilation assisted with manual bag ventilation. Thirty-two days after her accident, she tolerated removal from the ventilator. She did well on 30 percent oxygen via cool aerosol to a tracheostomy collar (Fig. 14–8). Over the next 6 days, she increased her ability to walk and her tracheostomy tube was intermittently plugged and the cuff deflated until she was decannulated. Forty days after the initial injury she was discharged to her home.

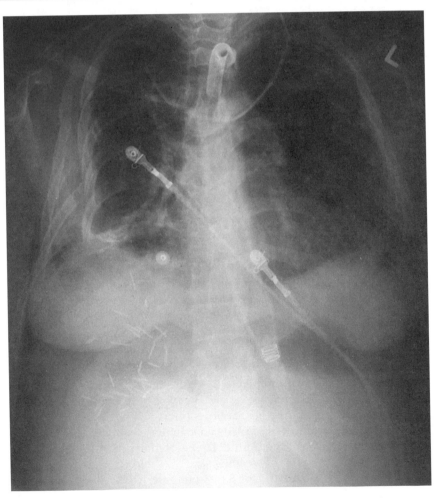

FIGURE 14–8   Portable chest radiograph 2 days after successful weaning from ventilatory support.

REFERENCES

1. Statistical Abstracts of the United States, National Data Book, ed 114. US Department of Commerce, 1994.
2. Glinz, W: Evaluation of thoracic injuries. In Border, JR (ed): Blunt Multiple Trauma. Marcel Dekker, New York, 1990.
3. Wilson, RF: Trauma. In Shoemaker, WC, et al (eds): Textbook of Critical Care, 2nd ed. WB Saunders, Philadelphia, 1989.
4. LoCicero, J, and Mattox, KL: Epidemiology of chest trauma. Surg Clin North Am 69:15-19, 1989.
5. Kirsh, MM: Acute thoracic injuries. In Siegel, JH (ed): Trauma: Emergency Surgery and Critical Care. Churchill Livingstone, New York, 1987.
6. Gaillard, M, et al: Mortality prognostic factors in chest injury. J Trauma 30:93-96, 1990.
7. Wilson, RF, et al: Shock and acute respiratory failure after chest trauma. J Trauma 17:697-705, 1977.
8. Marcus, NA, et al: Low-velocity gunshot wounds to extremities. J Trauma 20:1061-1064, 1980.
9. Grimes, WR, et al: A clinical review of shotgun wounds to the chest and abdomen. Surg Gynecol Obstet 160:148-156, 1985.
10. Wilson, RF, et al: Nonpenetrating thoracic injuries. Surg Clin North Am 57:17-36, 1977.
11. Baldino, WA, and Cernaianu, AC: Tracheal and bronchial disruptions. Trauma Q 6:19-26, 1990.
12. Meredith, JW: Chest wall injury. In Trunkey, DD, and Lewis, FR (eds): Current Therapy of Trauma. BC Decker, Philadelphia, 1991.
13. Besson, A, and Saegesser, F: Color Atlas of Chest Trauma and Associated Injuries, Vol 1. Medical Economics Company, Oradell, NJ, 1983.
14. Pate, JW: Chest wall injuries. Surg Clin North Am 69:59-70, 1989.
15. Rodriquez, A: Injuries of the chest wall, the lungs, and the pleura. In Turney, SZ, et al (eds): Management of Cardiothoracic Trauma. Williams & Wilkins, Baltimore, 1990.
16. Ashbaugh, DB, et al: Chest trauma: Analysis of 685 patients. Arch Surg 95:546-555, 1967.
17. Christensson, P, et al: Early and later results of controlled ventilation in flail chest. Chest 75:456-460, 1979.
18. Wilkins, EW: Noncardiovascular thoracic injuries: Chest wall, bronchus, lung, esophagus, and diaphragm. In Burke, JF, et al (eds): Trauma Management. Year Book, Chicago, 1988.
19. Van Way, CW: Advanced techniques in thoracic trauma. Surg Clin North Am 69:143-155, 1989.
20. Regel, G, et al: Occlusion of bronchopleural fistula after lung injury and treatment by bronchoscopy. J Trauma 29:223-226, 1989.
21. Hudson, LD, et al: Clinical risks for development of the acute respiratory distress syndrome. Am J Respir Crit Care Med 151:293-301, 1995.
22. Fuhrman, GM, et al: Blunt laryngeal trauma: Classification and management protocol. J Trauma 30:87-92, 1990.
23. Pate, JW: Tracheobronchial and esophageal injuries. Surg Clin North Am 69:111-123, 1989.
24. Ecker, RR, et al: Injuries of the trachea and bronchi. Ann Thorac Surg 11:289-298, 1971.
25. Fulda, G, et al: Blunt traumatic rupture of the heart and pericardium: A ten-year experience (1979-1989). J Trauma 31:167-172, 1991.
26. Ivantry, RR, and Rohman, M: The injured heart. Surg Clin North Am 69:93-110, 1989.
27. Carasquilla, C, et al: Gunshot wounds of the heart. Ann Thorac Surg 13:208-213, 1972.
28. Doty, DB, et al: Cardiac trauma: Clinical and experimental correlations of myocardial contusion. Ann Surg 180:452-458, 1974.
29. Hilgenberg, AD: Trauma to the heart and great vessels. In Burke, JF, et al (eds): Trauma Management. Year Book, Chicago, 1988.
30. Gewertz, B, O'Brien, C, Kirsh, MM: Use of the intra-aortic balloon support for refractory low cardiac output in myocardial contusion. J Trauma 17:325-327, 1977.
31. Rodriquez, A, and Turney, SZ: Blunt injuries of the heart and pericardium. In Turney, SZ, et al (eds): Management of Cardiothoracic Trauma. Williams & Wilkins, Baltimore, 1990.
32. Parmley, LF, et al: Non-penetrating traumatic injury to the heart. Circulation 18:371-386, 1958.
33. Van Vugt, AB, and Schoots, FJ: Acute diaphragmatic rupture due to blunt trauma: A retrospective analysis. J Trauma 29:683-686, 1989.
34. Symbas, PN, and Gott, JP: Delayed sequela of thoracic trauma. Surg Clin North Am 69:135-142, 1989.
35. Kishikawa, M, et al: Pulmonary contusion causes long-term respiratory dysfunction with decreased functional residual capacity. J Trauma 31:1203-1208, 1991.
36. Hix, WR, and Aaron, BL (eds): Residua of Thoracic Trauma. Futura, Mount Kisco, 1987.
37. Champion, HR, et al: A revision of the trauma score. J Trauma 29:623-629, 1989.
38. Trunkey, DD: Organization of trauma care. In Burke, JF, et al (eds): Trauma Management. Year Book, Chicago, 1988.
39. Worthley, LIG: Thoracic epidural in the management of chest trauma: A study of 161 cases. Intensive Care Med 11:312-315, 1985.
40. Cicala, RS, et al: Epidural analgesia in thoracic trauma: Effects of lumbar morphine and thoracic bupivacaine on pulmonary function. Crit Care Med 18:229-231, 1990.
41. Dronen, S, et al: Endotracheal tip position in the arrested patient. Ann Emerg Med 11:116-120, 1982.
42. Jorden, RC, et al: A comparison of PTV and endotracheal intubation in an acute trauma model. J Trauma 25:978-983, 1985.
43. Gurevitch, MJ: Selection of the inspiratory:expiratory ratio. In Kacmarek, RM, and Stoller, JK (eds): Current Respiratory Care. BC Decker, Philadelphia, 1988.
44. Tharatt, RS, et al: Pressure controlled inverse ratio ventilation in severe adult respiratory failure. Chest 94:755-762, 1988.
45. Abraham, E, and Yoshihara, G: Cardiorespira-

tory effects of pressure controlled inverse ratio ventilation in severe respiratory failure. Chest 96:1356–1359, 1989.

46. Enderson, BL, et al: Inverse ratio ventilation can improve oxygenation in respiratory distress syndrome (abstract). Crit Care Med 17:S152, 1989.

47. Kanarek, DJ, and Shannon, DC: Adverse effect of positive end expiratory pressure on pulmonary perfusion and arterial oxygenation. Am Rev Respir Dis 112:457–459, 1976.

48. Glass, DD, et al: Therapy of unilateral pulmonary insufficiency with double lumen endotracheal tube. Crit Care Med 4:323–326, 1976.

49. Branson, RD, et al: Synchronous independent lung ventilation in the treatment of unilateral pulmonary contusion: A report of two cases. Respir Care 29:361–367, 1984.

50. Ray, C: Independent lung ventilation. In Kacmarek, RM, and Stoller, JK (eds): Current Respiratory Care. BC Decker, Philadelphia, 1988.

51. Turnbull, AD, et al: High frequency jet ventilation in major airway or pulmonary disruption. Ann Thorac Surg 32:468–474, 1981.

52. Kopec, IC, et al: High frequency jet ventilation. In Kacmarek, RM, and Stoller JK (eds): Current Respiratory Care. BC Decker, Philadelphia, 1988.

53. Higgins, RS, et al: Mechanical circulatory support decreases neurologic complications in the treatment of traumatic injuries of the thoracic aorta. Arch Surg 127:516–521, 1992.

54. Zapol, WM, et al: Extracorporeal membrane oxygenation in severe acute respiratory failure: A randomized prospective study. JAMA 242: 2193–2196, 1979.

CHAPTER **15**

Postoperative Atelectasis

Thomas P. Malinowski, BS, RRT

Key Terms

air bronchograms
atelectasis
bronchial breath
  sounds

chest physiotherapy
  (CPT)
continuous positive airway
  pressure (CPAP)

late-inspiratory crackles
surfactant

Introduction

Atelectasis is a clinical condition characterized by regions of the lung that are collapsed or airless. Atelectasis is commonly seen after major surgery; it can lead to pneumonia and respiratory failure and is a common cause of increased hospital stays. Obesity, old age, smoking history, general anesthesia, and history of heart or lung disease increase a patient's risk for postoperative atelectasis.[1] The most significant risk factor, however, is a history of chronic obstructive pulmonary disease (COPD) (e.g., chronic bronchitis, emphysema). For this reason, all surgical patients must be screened for chronic lung disease, especially if the surgery involves the upper abdomen or chest.

Adults are not the only patients susceptible to postoperative atelectasis. Atelectasis has been reported to occur in about 10 to 30 percent of postoperative surgical cases involving infants and children.[2]

Etiology

Three factors may combine or independently contribute to the development of atelectasis: inadequate lung distending force, obstruction of the airways, and insufficient surfactant levels.[3] All three of these factors may occur in the surgical patient, especially during the postoperative period.

Inadequate Lung Distention

Lung expansion depends on (1) the ability of the respiratory muscles to generate negative intrapleural pressures and (2) an intact chest cage. Factors that weaken the respiratory muscles or reduce the effect of normal negative inspiratory pressures will reduce lung inflation and encourage atelectasis.

For example, elderly patients who are malnourished may be unable to generate the inspiratory force necessary for deep breathing and coughing. Patients with chest wall abnormalities (e.g., kyphosis, scoliosis) have limited lung expansion because of their thoracic cage malformation (Table 15-1). Diaphragmatic movement may be limited in obese patients or those with neuromuscular disease (see Chapter 17). Pulmonary fibrosis causes the lung to expand poorly in response to normal negative intrapleural pressures (Table 15-2).

Numerous intraoperative factors may also affect lung distention. The diaphragm relaxes and displaces upward when patients are given anesthetics and paralytics.[4] In addition, prolonged use of paralytic agents have been associated with diaphragmatic muscle atrophy, resulting in a reduction in diaphragmatic strength. Use of steroidal preparations in combination with paralytic agents has been clearly shown in many patients to result in a neuromyopathy and weaning failure.[5] The type, location, and duration of the surgical procedure also affect lung distention.[1,6-8] Upper abdominal procedures present the greatest risk for atelectasis, followed by thoracic, lower abdominal, and peripheral procedures. Diaphragmatic function may be compromised by fluid accumulation in the abdominal space (ascites, peritoneal fluid) and pleural space (pleural effusion). Postoperative pain is often associated with decreased respiratory effort and a reduction in pleural and intra-abdominal pressures, resulting in atelectasis after upper abdominal surgery.[1] Patients who have thoracic surgery are also at risk for postoperative atelectasis. Topical cooling of the left phrenic nerve, which commonly occurs during cardiac surgery, can cause inadequate diaphragmatic movement postoperatively and can contribute to left lower lobe atelectasis.[9] In the postoperative period, the inadequate lung distention may persist for 7 to 14 days, especially in the presence of complications such as excessive pain or pleural effusion.[10]

Newborns and infants are particularly susceptible to atelectasis in the postoperative period. Lung expansion is limited by poor ventilatory reserve (i.e., less diaphragmatic muscle mass and strength) and a less effective cough secondary to muscle weakness. In addition, diaphragmatic innervation may be immature or insufficient to respond to an increased ventilatory need.

Obstruction of the Airways

The development of postoperative atelectasis can also occur as a result of retained secretions in the bronchi.[3,11] Secretion retention occurs when mucociliary transport is diminished, cough is weak or absent, secretion volume is excessive, or hydration is

TABLE 15-1   **Factors That Decrease Ability to Generate Negative Pressures**

Anesthesia
Pain
Reduction in lung volume
Diaphragmatic apraxia: phrenic neuropathy, myopathy
Chest wall disorders
Ascites
Malnutrition

TABLE 15-2   **Factors That Reduce the Effect of Normal Inspiratory Pressures**

Reclining position
Pleural effusion
Pneumothorax
Pleural mass
Pulmonary fibrosis

inadequate. Anesthetic agents impair mucociliary activity and depress tidal volume and cough. Humidity is rarely added during anesthesia, and the anesthesiologist will frequently administer pharmacological agents that, as a side effect, dry respiratory secretions.[4] Pathologic conditions associated with excessive secretions and impaired mucus transport (i.e., smoking history, chronic bronchitis, asthma) will increase the risk of secretion retention.[8] Mucus plugs lead to atelectasis with absorption of gases distal to the obstruction. This condition is enhanced during breathing of anesthetic gases or high fraction of inspired oxygen (FIO_2) concentrations because these gases are more readily absorbed into the pulmonary blood flow.[12,13] Intubated infants and children are particularly susceptible to secretion retention and partial obstruction of the airways. Limited collateral ventilation (pores of Kohn) and reduced airway diameter make neonatal and pediatric patients susceptible to lobar atelectasis due to secretion retention.

Surfactant Depletion

An adequate quantity and quality of **surfactant** is necessary to maintain alveolar stability and prevent collapse. The quantity and quality of surfactant can be reduced with pulmonary edema, smoke inhalation, inhaled anesthetics, lung contusion, pulmonary embolus, adult respiratory distress syndrome (ARDS), high FIO_2 concentrations, and prolonged breathing at low tidal volumes.[3] Cardiopulmonary bypass may cause an inadequate perfusion of the lung and alveolar epithelium, leading to insufficient release of surfactant.[14]

Pathophysiology

Atelectasis results in a decrease in functional residual capacity and lung compliance. This results in alterations in the distribution of the inhaled gas without corresponding changes in perfusion. As a result, ventilation-perfusion ($\dot{V}/\dot{Q}$) mismatching occurs, which leads to hypoxemia. General anesthesia also inhibits hypoxic pulmonary vasoconstriction reflexes in the lung, which further contributes to $\dot{V}/\dot{Q}$ mismatching and hypoxemia.[14]

Surface tension holds collapsed alveoli shut, requiring higher distending pressures to reinflate the affected regions of the lung. Unaffected lung regions are more compliant and easier to inflate. The more compliant regions receive more of the tidal volume than the atelectatic areas and may be easily overinflated when large tidal volumes are used with mechanical ventilation.

Patients with moderate to severe atelectasis exhibit significant increases in work of breathing. Increased work of breathing adds a significant work load to the muscles of breathing and contributes to the onset of respiratory failure, especially in those with preexisting lung disease.

Clinical Features

Signs and symptoms of atelectasis vary with the amount of lung involved, the patient's previous health status, and the duration of the problem. Dyspnea is the most common symptom associated with atelectasis, but this may not be present if the patient has minimal lung involvement and has been previously healthy. When the atelectasis involves larger portions of the lung or when the patient has a chronic lung disease, the dyspnea can become severe. Atelectasis is the likely diagnosis in patients with a recent history of abdominal or thoracic surgery.

Tachypnea is commonly associated with atelectasis. Respiratory rates usually increase in proportion to the amount of lung involved. Decreased lung compliance results in the patient's breathing smaller tidal volumes with minimal variations in the depth of the breath.[11,15] To maintain adequate gas exchange, the patient must breathe with a more rapid rate to compensate for the smaller tidal volume. Tachycardia and fever may indicate infection associated with retention of secretions.

Auscultation of breath sounds is often helpful in detecting the onset of atelectasis. **Late-inspiratory crackles** are heard on deep inspiratory efforts and represent the sudden opening of atelectatic regions. These inspiratory crackles are usually heard initially in the dependent regions of the lung and may clear after the patient takes several deep breaths. **Bronchial breath sounds** and bronchophony over the affected region indicate airway patency in the atelectatic area. Diminished or absent breath sounds indicate that the airways are plugged or collapsed in the affected region, which results in little or no ventilation into the affected area. Accessory muscle usage indicates a significant increase in the work of breathing, which is typically the result of a decreased lung compliance.

Abnormal or adventitious breath sounds may be of little value in diagnosing atelectasis in the intubated infant. An alternate technique is observation of chest expansion. Chest expansion in the mechanically ventilated infant is often unequal or reduced with severe atelectasis.

The chest radiograph is a helpful tool in the diagnosis of chest atelectasis.[3,11] Chest radiographs may reveal a reduction in lung volume and opacification that is not clinically apparent. Obliteration of typical radiographic shadows may indicate the location of involvement. For example, the right heart border is often obscured with right middle lobe atelectasis but is present with right lower lobe atelectasis. Other signs of lung volume loss include elevation of the hemidiaphragm and mediastinal shifts toward the affected side. **Air bronchograms,** frequently observed on chest radiograph with atelectasis, are caused by collapse of the lung tissue around inflated airways. When present, air bronchograms indicate that the atelectasis is not due to mucus obstruction of the airways. Arterial blood gases (ABGs) often reveal hypoxemia in the postoperative patient with atelectasis. The severity of hypoxemia does not necessarily correlate with the extent of atelectasis on the chest radiograph. Profound hypoxemia may exist as a result of microatelectasis that is not apparent radiographically. Hypoxemia frequently causes mild respiratory alkalosis.

Because patients with pulmonary disease are at greater risk for postoperative complications, bedside spirometry is useful to identify high-risk patients before surgery. Spirometry is especially useful to assess patients with a significant smoking history or those scheduled for upper abdominal or thoracic surgery.[16] After surgery, bedside spirometry is also useful to detect the severity of the decrease in lung volumes (vital capacity [VC] and inspiratory capacity) associated with atelectasis. Severe decreases in VC indicate that the simple techniques to correct atelectasis may not be sufficient (see later discussion).

Treatment

The preoperative evaluation by the respiratory care practitioner (RCP) should identify factors that might contribute to the onset of postoperative complications. Patients with a long history of smoking or pulmonary symptoms should be evaluated with spirometry to identify whether obstructive or restrictive lung disease is present. Patients with moderate to severe COPD have a greater risk for postoperative respiratory complications. Preoperative bronchial hygiene techniques and smoking cessation may be useful.

Once the diagnosis of postoperative atelectasis has been made, the severity of respiratory compromise will determine the therapy. If there is no significant respiratory distress and the patient is ambulating, treatment may not be needed. Patients with atelectasis who are distressed or unable to ambulate need postoperative respiratory care.

Lung Inflation Techniques

Deep breathing and coughing are often as effective as any other of the more costly techniques for the treatment and prevention of atelectasis in the cooperative patient.[17] Incentive spirometry may benefit patients who require additional coaching, and it can serve as an indicator of improvement in pulmonary function.

Intermittent application of 10 to 15 cm H_2O **continuous positive airway pressure** (CPAP) or positive expiratory pressure (PEP) is often effective in the treatment of atelectasis.[18-20] Concise guidelines for the application of CPAP and PEP can be found in the AARC clinical practice guidelines on positive airway pressure adjuncts to bronchial hygiene therapy.[21] In adults, most complications associated with CPAP are observed in the greater than 20 to 25 cm H_2O range. In infants and children, complications may develop at lower pressures. Periodic application of CPAP (every 1 to 3 hours) is also frequently effective in clearing atelectasis and may be beneficial to those patients who are not able to cooperate or who have recurrent or persistent forms of atelectasis. PEP has been effective in improving postoperative pulmonary function when applied on an hourly basis.[19]

Intermittent positive-pressure breathing (IPPB) may be indicated in patients who are unable to perform more simple maneuvers for lung inflation and whose VC is less than 10 to 15 mL/kg. Volume-oriented IPPB can be instrumental in improving lung volumes and can help promote a more effective cough.[22]

Even though the complication rate is low, patients treated with positive-pressure ventilation (e.g., CPAP, IPPB) should be closely monitored for the adverse effects of raised intrathoracic pressure (i.e., hyperinflation, reduced perfusion, barotrauma, and gastric inflation). The application of positive pressure must be used in conjunction with bronchial hygiene techniques when secretion retention is the cause of the atelectasis.

Secretion Removal

When the cause of the lobar atelectasis is retained mucus, treatment should be aimed at removal of airway secretions in addition to lung inflation. Encouraging the patient to generate an effective cough is often all that is necessary. If this therapy is not effective and radiographic evidence suggests the characteristic lobar atelectasis pattern (i.e., radiographic density, absent air bronchograms, fissure displacement, mediastinal shift, diaphragmatic elevation, compensatory hyperinflation), then **chest physiotherapy (CPT)** may be indicated. The use of CPT in postoperative atelectasis should be limited to patients with large amounts of secretions.

Lobar atelectasis often responds to a short, vigorous course of CPT, usually within 6 hours, and is frequently as effective as bronchoscopy at removing retained secretions.[23,24] If this program is inadequate, removal of central secretions by the use of endotracheal suctioning or bronchoscopy is indicated.[25] Postoperative management of patients with COPD should also include bronchodilators to facilitate a better cough and secretion expectoration. CPT has not been shown to be effective in preventing postoperative atelectasis in infants and newborns, and on the contrary, may be associated with an increased risk of atelectasis.[26]

The simulated cough maneuver has recently been advocated as a treatment regimen in children with various degrees of lung collapse unresponsive to conventional CPT.[27] The therapy consists of endotracheal instillation of saline, followed by manual lung inflation with a momentary inflation hold, release of the hold, and simultaneous forced exhalation and vibration to simulate cough. The procedure is completed by endotracheal suctioning. The maneuver is usually repeated three to five times. The maneuver has been most successful in infants with airway occlusion secondary to mucus (without air bronchograms on x-ray).

Intrapulmonary percussive ventilation (IPV) is a positive-pressure maneuver that delivers a high-velocity gas into the airways at rates of 100 to 300 cycles/minute. The IPV device (Percussionaire, Sand Point, Idaho) is a pneumatic high-frequency positive-pressure ventilator. Treatments are administered on an intermittent basis (e.g., every 2 hours, every 4 hours) for a duration of 15 to 20 minutes. Peak airway pressures from the device may vary from 5 to 25 cm H_2O. Theoretically, IPV loosens secretions and maintains positive airway pressures, allowing secretions to migrate to larger airways for clearance. Published case reports have identified IPV as a safe and effective therapy in enhancing secretion removal and reversing lung consolidation in children and adults unresponsive to conventional therapy.[28]

Mechanical Ventilation

Mechanical ventilation will be needed in some patients after major surgery, especially if underlying pulmonary disease is present. In cardiac surgery patients, mechanical ventilation is useful in the postoperative period until all hemodynamic parameters are stable.[12] In some cardiac surgery patients, extubation can occur within a few hours after surgery; however, those with arrhythmias, mediastinal bleeding, or decreased cardiac output will need mechanical ventilation for a longer period.[12]

CASE STUDY

History

Mrs. M is a 67-year-old white woman who was admitted to the emergency room for complaints of dyspnea, chest pain, and diaphoresis. Further workup on this admission revealed a diagnosis of duodenal ulcer. On admission day she was taken to the operating room, where a perforated prepyloric ulcer was repaired and purulent fluid removed from the peritoneal space. After surgery she returned to the surgical intensive care unit and was maintained on continuous mechanical ventilation for 1 day. She was extubated on day 2 and placed on a 40 percent high-flow oxygen aerosol mask. Two days after extubation, she began complaining of "not being able to catch her breath."

Her past medical history includes systemic hypertension, which is adequately managed with medication; and a four-vessel coronary artery bypass graft procedure performed 2 years earlier. She denies any history of smoking, alcohol abuse, or drug abuse.

QUESTIONS

1. What clinical conditions could cause the patient's acute dyspnea?

2. What is the significance of the anatomic location of the surgical procedure?

3. What physical examination procedures would you suggest be done at this point?

ANSWERS

1. Dyspnea may be due to an increased work of breathing associated with decreased lung compliance from pulmonary edema, atelectasis, or diaphragmatic compression from the abdomen. Other potential causes of dyspnea in this case would include pulmonary embolus and pneumonia.

2. There is a direct relationship between postoperative complications and the proximity of the surgical incision to the diaphragm. Upper abdominal surgery is much more likely to be associated with atelectasis than peripheral surgery.

3. Assessment of the respiratory rate, pulse rate, body temperature, breathing pattern, and breath sounds would help evaluate Mrs. M's pulmonary status. Cardiac examination for a third or fourth heart sound, jugular venous distention, and hepatojugular reflex would help rule out pulmonary edema. Abdominal evaluation for a pleural friction rub and palpation of the calf muscles for tenderness would help rule out pulmonary embolism.

Physical Examination

General: Patient fatigued and in moderate respiratory distress; mildly diaphoretic, lying in a semi-Fowler's position in bed

Vital Signs: Temperature 38.5°C (101.3°F), respiratory rate 38/minute, blood pressure 148/57 mm Hg, pulse 124/minute

HEENT: Pupils equal, round, and reactive to light and accommodation (PERRLA); tympanic membranes clear; no nasopharyngeal lesions, masses, or exudates; nasal flaring with inspiration

Neck: Trachea midline and mobile to palpation; no stridor; no carotid bruits, lymphadenopathy, thyromegaly, or jugular venous distention; tension of sternocleidomastoid muscles noted during inspiration

Chest: Symmetrical chest expansion with rapid, shallow breathing pattern; decreased resonance to percussion of lower lung fields

Heart: Regular rhythm with a rate of 124/minute; no murmurs, gallops, or rubs

Lungs: Late-inspiratory crackles heard in the bases, with diminished breath sounds in mid and upper lung fields

Abdomen: Distended, tender; no bowel sounds

Extremities: No clubbing, cyanosis, or edema; capillary refill less than 3 seconds; pulses and reflexes +1 and symmetrical

QUESTIONS

4. What pathophysiology is suggested by the rapid, shallow breathing pattern?
5. What is the cause of the late-inspiratory crackles in the bases? What characteristic of these crackles should the RCP identify?
6. What could be causing the patient's tachycardia?
7. Why is the patient using her accessory muscles to breathe?
8. What laboratory tests would you recommend at this point?

ANSWERS

4. Rapid, shallow breathing suggests that the patient is experiencing a significant drop in her lung compliance. This leads to breathing with smaller tidal volumes and a more rapid rate. Common causes of decreased lung compliance include pulmonary edema, atelectasis, and pneumonia.

5. Late-inspiratory crackles are caused by the sudden opening of many collapsed peripheral airways. This occurs when the patient with atelectasis inhales deeply enough to reexpand atelectatic regions. The RCP should determine whether the crackles diminish as the patient repeatedly inhales deeply. This would suggest that the crackles are due to atelectasis.

6. Tachycardia could be due to a number of causes: hypoxemia, inadequate pain management, fever, and anxiety. The patient has had cardiac disease in the past and may have an abnormal cardiac rhythm because of the heart disease.

7. The diaphragm, the primary inspiratory muscle, is much less effective for several weeks or months after abdominal surgery. Lungs are also less compliant and more difficult to expand after major surgery. Atelectasis may worsen the problem, and assistance may be needed from the accessory breathing muscles to maintain ventilation. This increases the patient's total work of breathing.

8. Laboratory tests that would be helpful are aimed at narrowing the list of problems that could cause the patient's current distress. Such tests include a chest radiograph, ABG analysis, bedside spirometry, complete blood count (CBC) and electrolyte evaluation, and an electrocardiogram (ECG).

Laboratory Evaluation

Chest Radiograph: See Figure 15–1

ABGs: pH 7.46, $PaCO_2$ 33 mm Hg, PaO_2 54 mm Hg on FIO_2 0.40, HCO_3^- 24 mEq/liter

Spirometry: Slow inspiratory capacity 1.0 liter; patient unable to perform a VC maneuver

CBC:

White blood cells (WBCs) 16,500/mm³, with 65 percent segmented neutrophils and 11 percent bands

Red blood cells (RBCs) 3.9 million/mm³

Hemoglobin (Hb) 9.9 g/dL

Hematocrit (Hct) 37 percent

Platelets 155,000/mm³

Chemistry: Na^+ 139 mEq/liter, K^+ 3.2 mEq/liter, Cl^- 102 mEq/liter, blood urea nitrogen 17 mg/dL, total proteins 6.7 g/dL (albumin 3.2 g/dL), glucose 78 mg/dL

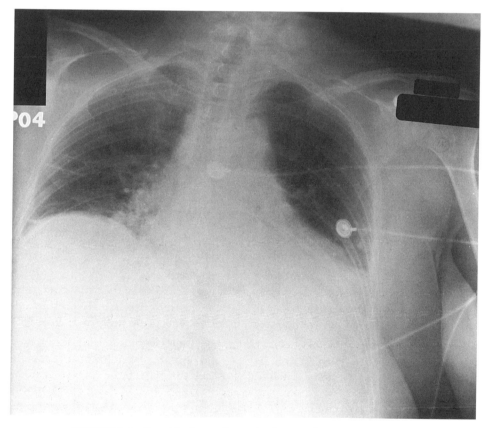

FIGURE 15-1   Portable chest radiograph of Mrs. M 48 hours after surgery.

QUESTIONS

9. How would you interpret the ABG and spirometry results?

10. How would you interpret the chest radiograph?

11. How would you interpret the CBC and electrolyte values?

12. What are your therapeutic objectives for respiratory care?

13. What would be your treatment plan?

14. How would you evaluate the patient's response to therapy?

ANSWERS

9. The ABGs reflect moderate hypoxemia with mild uncompensated respiratory alkalosis, suggesting that the patient is hyperventilating. The Pao_2 of 54 mm Hg on 0.40 Fio_2 suggests the hypoxemia is somewhat refractory to oxygen therapy. The spirometry results are consistent with a poor effort or a severely restrictive condition. The patient's inability to perform a VC maneuver indicates significant fatigue.

10. The chest radiograph suggests poor inspiratory effort or reduced lung volumes. Obliteration of the right heart border is consistent with right middle lobe atelectasis. Presence of air bronchograms suggests a lack of mucus plugs in the affected regions.

11. The WBCs are elevated, consistent with infection. The increase in bands indicates that young WBCs have been recruited to fight an acute infection. Hb, Hct, and RBCs are reduced, indicating hemodilution or blood loss. This reduces oxygen-carrying capacity, requiring an increased cardiac output to maintain adequate oxygen delivery. The potassium is slightly reduced and should be replenished, especially if heart rhythm abnormalities develop. Circulating total proteins and albumin are reduced, which is a common finding after major surgery. This slightly reduces oncotic pressure, making the patient susceptible to fluid accumulation in the lungs.

12. The therapeutic goals are to reexpand collapsed areas of the lung via lung inflation techniques and to treat the hypoxemia.

13. Initial recommendations for treatment should focus on simple lung inflation techniques and correction of hypoxemia:

    a. Incentive spirometry (IS) with multiple, maximal inspiratory capacity maneuvers should be performed hourly.

    b. Lung volume improvement should be monitored.

    c. Poor response to IS would warrant PEP mask therapy or intermittent CPAP, usually with initial pressures of 8 to 10 cm H_2O. Pressures may need to be increased if the initial settings do not prove effective.

    d. Supplemental oxygen therapy should continue, using a high-flow oxygen system at a specific Fio_2. A high-flow system helps ensure that Fio_2 concentrations will not vary with changes in the tidal volume, pattern, or rate. Because the patient's ventilation ($Paco_2$) is adequate, monitoring improvement in oxygenation can be done with intermittent pulse oximetry. A repeat ABG analysis is indicated if the clinical condition fails to improve or deteriorates.

    e. Hb and Hct should be monitored; transfusion may be indicated if values continue to drop.

    Patient compliance and proper coaching is extremely important for successful lung inflation therapy. Excessive secretions do not appear to be the cause of this patient's atelectasis, so CPT or bronchoscopy are not indicated.

14. The RCP should evaluate the patient's response to oxygen therapy by monitoring heart rate, respiratory rate, perceived dyspnea, pulse oximetry, and ABGs.

CASE STUDY—continued

Initial treatment included IS along with encouraging deep breathing and coughing. Six hours after IS was initiated by the RCP, the patient remained alert and oriented but continued to complain of dyspnea. Her inspiratory capacity was 1.3 liters, respiratory rate 26/minute, and pulse 116/minute. She remained febrile, continued to use her accessory muscles for breathing, and continued to have diminished breath sounds in the bases along with some inspiratory crackles. Pulse oximetry revealed an oxygen saturation of 92 percent on an F_{IO_2} of 45. Results of a repeat chest radiograph are pending.

QUESTIONS

15. Are the therapeutic objectives being met?
16. What is your assessment of the patient's condition after IS therapy for 6 hours?
17. Would you suggest any changes in the treatment plan?
18. What is this patient at risk for with regard to her pulmonary status?

ANSWERS

15. The therapeutic objectives were to improve oxygenation and lung expansion. It appears that oxygenation has improved, although it remains less than optimal. Lung expansion has not improved significantly.

16. Assessment of the patient after 6 hours of IS reveals persistent atelectasis. This assessment is based on the continued tachypnea, diminished breath sounds and crackles, and reduced inspiratory capacity.

17. Treatment at this point should include the application of intermittent CPAP or PEP. This is needed because of the slow resolution of the atelectasis with IS.

18. The patient is at high risk for respiratory failure. Respiratory failure could occur when the excessive work of breathing tires the respiratory muscles and results in fatigue. This would be recognized by deterioration of the ABGs, vital signs, and sensorium.

CASE STUDY—continued

PEP-mask therapy was started every hour for 15 breaths at 8 cm H_2O and increased to 12 cm H_2O. Four hours after initiating PEP, dyspnea improved, respiratory rate was 18/minute, and pulse oximetry was 97 percent on an F_{IO_2} of 40. A repeat of the chest radiograph demonstrated improvement (Fig. 15–2). PEP frequency was reduced to every 3 hours, and IS was maintained every hour while awake. The patient was switched to nasal cannula at 4 liters/minute, and 24 hours later transferred to a step-down unit. IS and oxygen orders continued for 2 days after her transfer.

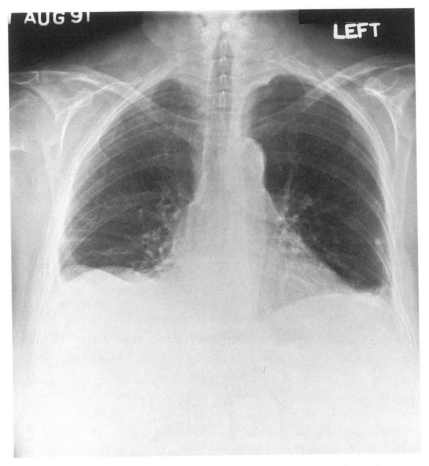

FIGURE 15-2 Portable chest radiograph demonstrating improvement with better lung expansion.

REFERENCES

1. Luce, JM: Clinical risk factors for postoperative pulmonary complications. Respir Care 29:484, 1984.
2. Rivera, R, and Tibballis, J: Complications of endotracheal intubation and mechanical ventilation in infants and children. Crit Care Med 20:193–199, 1992.
3. Johnson, NT, and Pierson, DJ: The spectrum of pulmonary atelectasis: Pathophysiology, diagnosis, and therapy. Respir Care 31:1107, 1986.
4. Didier, EP: Some effects of anesthetics and the anesthetized state on the respiratory system. Respir Care 29:463, 1984.
5. Fluegel, W, et al: Risk factors for acute myopathy in patients with severe asthma who require mechanical ventilation (abstract). Am J Respir Crit Care Med 149:A342, 1994.
6. Stein, M, and Cassara, EL: Preoperative pulmonary evaluation and therapy for surgery patients. JAMA 211:787, 1970.
7. Wightman, JAK: A prospective survey of the incidence of postoperative pulmonary complications. Br J Surg 55:85, 1968.
8. Hodgkin, JE: Preoperative assessment of respiratory function. Respir Care 29:496, 1984.
9. Benjamin, JJ, et al: Left lower lobe atelectasis and consolidation following cardiac surgery: The effect of topical cooling on the phrenic nerve. Radiology 142:11, 1982.
10. Craig, DG: Postoperative recovery of pulmonary function. Anesth Analg 60:46, 1981.
11. Marini, JJ: Postoperative atelectasis: Pathophysiology, clinical importance, and principles of management. Respir Care 29:516, 1984.
12. Dale, WA, and Rahn, H: Rate of gas absorption during atelectasis. Am J Physiol 170:606, 1952.
13. Webb, SJS, and Nunn, JF: A comparison between the effect of nitrous oxide and nitrogen on arterial PO_2. Anaesthesia 22:69, 1967.
14. Matthay, MA, and Wiener-Kronish, JP: Respiratory management after surgery. Chest 95:424, 1989.
15. Askanazi, J, et al: Patterns of ventilation in postoperative and acutely ill patients. Crit Care Med 7:41, 1979.

16. Stroller, JK: Pulmonary function testing as a screening technique. Respir Care 34:611, 1989.

17. Celli, BR, et al: A controlled trial of intermittent positive pressure breathing, incentive spirometry, and deep breathing exercises in preventing pulmonary complications after surgery. Am Rev Respir Dis 130:12, 1984.

18. Branson, RD: PEEP without endotracheal intubation. Respir Care 33:598, 1988.

19. Ricksten, SE, et al: Effects of periodic positive pressure breathing by mask on postoperative pulmonary function. Chest 89:774, 1986.

20. Ford, TG, and Guenter, CA: Toward prevention of postoperative complications. Am Rev Respir Dis 130:4, 1984.

21. American Association for Respiratory Care: AARC clinical practice guideline: Use of positive airway pressure adjuncts to bronchial hygiene therapy. Respir Care 38:516–521, 1993

22. O'Donohue, WJ Jr: Maximum volume IPPB for the management of pulmonary atelectasis. Chest 76:683, 1979.

23: Marini, JJ, et al: Acute lobar atelectasis: A prospective comparison of fiberoptic bronchoscopy and respiratory therapy. Am Rev Respir Dis 119:971, 1979.

24. Stiller, KB, et al: Acute lobar atelectasis: A comparison of two chest physiotherapy regimens. Chest 98:1336, 1990.

25. Mahajan, VK, et al: The value of fiberoptic bronchoscopy in the management of pulmonary collapse. Chest 73:817, 1978.

26. Al-Alaiyan, S, et al: Chest physiotherapy and post-extubation atelectasis in infants. Pediatr Pulmonol 21:227–230, 1996.

27. Galvis, A, et al: Bedside management of lung collapse in children on mechanical ventilation. Pediatr Pulmonol 17:326–30, 1994.

28. Birnkrant, D, et al: Persistent pulmonary consolidation treated with intrapulmonary percussive ventilation: A preliminary report. Pediatr Pulmonol 21:246–249, 1996.

CHAPTER 16

Interstitial Lung Disease

N. Lennard Specht, MD

Key Terms

asbestosis
drug-induced interstitial
  lung disease
honeycomb lung

hypersensitivity
  pneumonitis
pneumoconiosis
pulmonary fibrosis

sarcoidosis
silicosis

Introduction

Interstitial lung disease comprises a group of diseases that cause inflammation and fibrosis of the lower respiratory tract. The term **pulmonary fibrosis** is also applied to these diseases because fibrosis of the lung is the ultimate result of interstitial lung disease. As many as 81 of every 100,000 Americans have some form of interstitial lung disease.[1] Many conditions lead to interstitial lung disease, including diseases that have no known etiology, such as **sarcoidosis,** rheumatoid arthritis, and idiopathic pulmonary fibrosis. Causes of interstitial lung disease in which the etiology is known include diseases of inhalation, such as asbestosis, **silicosis,** and **hypersensitivity pneumonitis.** Cancer chemotherapy, high-concentration oxygen therapy, and radiation therapy may also cause pulmonary fibrosis.

The earliest descriptions of interstitial lung disease involved workers exposed to inorganic dusts. Hypocrites told stories of miners who had difficulty breathing. Dutch pathologists noted a sandy texture to the lungs in patients who had worked in mines. Nineteenth-century English medical literature contains many good descriptions of dust-related lung disease (**pneumoconiosis**).[2,3] Coalminer's pneumoconiosis generated a tremendous amount of publicity in the early 20th century. Worker safety concerns generated intense political debate and resulted in the "Black Lung Laws." These laws allow employees with coalminer's pneumoconiosis to be compensated financially for their lung disease.

Cutaneous sarcoidosis was first described in 1869 by two dermatologists. Sarcoid

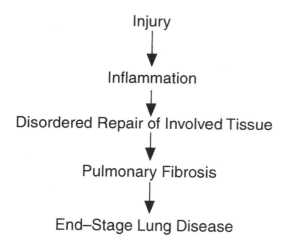

Injury

↓

Inflammation

↓

Disordered Repair of Involved Tissue

↓

Pulmonary Fibrosis

↓

End–Stage Lung Disease

FIGURE 16-1   Cascade of events thought to represent the steps leading from the initiation of interstitial lung disease and culminating with pulmonary fibrosis and end-stage lung disease. Each of these stages may be present simultaneously in a given patient.

lung involvement was noted several decades later.[4] Idiopathic pulmonary fibrosis was first described in 1944—a recent discovery in comparison to other forms of interstitial lung disease.[5]

All forms of interstitial lung disease follow a common chain of events (Fig. 16-1). In this scheme, the disease is initiated by an injury. The injury promotes a vigorous immune reaction and inflammation. Inflammation leads to destruction of lung tissue and is followed by a disorganized repair process. The disordered repair leads to pulmonary fibrosis and eventually to end-stage lung disease.

Etiology

An extremely large number of diseases can induce interstitial lung disease. These diseases are usually classified according to the type of agent that causes the lung injury (Table 16-1). About one third of patients with interstitial lung disease have an identifiable agent responsible for inducing lung injury. Typical inorganic dusts that may induce interstitial lung disease include asbestos, silica (sand), coal, and talc. These agents injure the epithelium or endothelium of the lung directly via a toxic effect,[6] or indirectly by leading to the production of toxic metabolites or activating immune responses.[7] Perhaps the most infamous disease caused by the inhalation of inorganic dusts is coalminer's pneumoconiosis, which occurs in about 0.4 percent of people who regularly work with coal dust.[8]

TABLE 16-1   Classification of Interstitial Lung Disease

Known Etiology	Unknown Etiology
Inorganic dusts	Sarcoidosis
Hypersensitivity pneumonitis	Collagen vascular disease
Drugs	Idiopathic pulmonary fibrosis
Toxins	Other
Oxygen	
Radiation	
Infection	

Inhalation of organic dusts may create a form of interstitial lung disease known as hypersensitivity pneumonitis. Hypersensitivity pneumonitis is associated with repeated exposure to organic antigens. In susceptible patients, repeated exposure to the antigen leads to an abnormal allergic response that is destructive to the lung. Many different antigens can cause hypersensitivity pneumonitis. One of the more notorious antigens is from a group of bacteria called thermophilic *Actinomyces,* which thrive at temperatures between 45°C (113°F) and 60°C (140°F) (temperatures present during vegetation decompositions). Repeated exposure to dusts from decomposing vegetation containing thermophilic *Actinomyces* will precipitate the disease in susceptible individuals. A number of forms of hypersensitivity pneumonitis are named for organic materials that contain thermophilic *Actinomyces* as they decompose. These forms include humidifier lung (air conditioning or humidifier ducts), bagassosis (sugar cane), mushroom worker's lung (mushroom compost), farmer's lung (hay), and grain handler's lung (grain). Thermophilic *Antinomyces* is only one group in a wide array of organisms that provide antigens that cause hypersensitivity pneumonitis. These organisms include various fungi, actinomycetes, bacteria, parasites, insects, and mammals.

Drug-induced interstitial lung disease is an important medical problem because the disease is frequently the result of therapy. Early recognition of drug-induced injury will allow discontinuation of the offending drug, will usually stop further injury, and may reverse the disease process. A large number of drugs are known to induce lung injury (Table 16–2).

The majority of drugs that are well known for causing interstitial lung disease are used in the treatment of cancer. Drug-induced lung disease is a major cause of morbidity and mortality in patients undergoing cancer chemotherapy.[9] Of patients undergoing chemotherapy who are found to have diffuse infiltrative changes in their lungs, up to 20 percent are diagnosed with interstitial lung disease.[10] Many patients die as a result of chemotherapy-induced interstitial lung disease.[11] Most chemotherapy agents induce a pulmonary reaction within weeks of exposure, but some may result in lung disease many months after the last dose.

Amiodarone is a potent antiarrhythmic drug used for patients with serious cardiac arrhythmias that do not improve with other treatments. The development of amiodarone lung disease is related to the dose the patient receives.[12] Patients receiv-

TABLE 16–2   **Partial List of Drugs Associated with Development of Interstitial Lung Disease**

Amiodarone
Antibiotics
Anti-inflammatory agents
Aspirin
Bleomycin
Busulfan
Cancer chemotherapy
Cardiovascular drugs
Cyclophosphamide
Cytosine arabinoside
Gold
Illicit drugs (e.g., heroin)
Methotrexate
Nitrofurantoin
Propoxyphene

ing high doses of amiodarone have a greater incidence of toxicity than those who receive a lower dose.[12] The incidence of pulmonary complications due to amiodarone is between 1 and 18 percent. Because of the risk of toxicity, it is used only after most other antiarrhythmic agents have proved ineffective. If lung disease develops, it becomes a difficult decision whether to reduce or stop amiodarone and thereby risk sudden cardiac death or to continue the drug and risk worsening of the fibrosis.

Nitrofurantoin is a particularly effective antibiotic for treating urinary tract infections, but on rare occasions, its use gives rise to interstitial lung disease.[13] The pulmonary toxicity from nitrofurantoin is either an acute reaction that begins hours to a few days following the first dose, or a chronic reaction that develops after months to years of drug use.

Illicit drugs, particularly narcotics such as heroin, may produce an acute form of noncardiogenic pulmonary edema. Talc is occasionally mixed into illicit drugs either because it was used to dilute ("cut") the drug or because the drug was prepared for injection from talc-containing tablets. The intravenous (IV) injection of talc creates a granulomatous reaction in small blood vessels and the interstitium of the lung.

Oxygen at high concentrations over several hours or days may induce acute lung injury. Pathologic pulmonary changes develop in animals after 12 hours of exposure to 100 percent oxygen. Pulmonary edema develops after 48 hours of exposure to 100 percent oxygen. Adult respiratory distress syndrome (ARDS) follows the development of pulmonary edema.

Pathology and Pathophysiology

The architecture of the lung can be viewed as a very delicate collection of small bubbles (alveoli). The bubbles connect to the trachea through a complex network of airways. The walls of the alveoli consist of an extremely thin layer of tissue and blood vessels and provide little resistance to the diffusion of gas between the capillary and alveolar air. The epithelial cells responsible for most of the alveolar lining are type I alveolar cells (pneumocytes). These cells are very flat with a large surface area that conforms to the shape of the underlying capillary bed. Scattered among the type I cells are a few type II cells that are much rounder and thicker; these are responsible for the secretion of surfactant. This fragile structure becomes the principal focus of the events associated with interstitial lung disease (Fig. 16-1).

The pathologic appearance of the lungs in patients with early interstitial lung disease is characterized by inflammation. Some forms of interstitial lung disease develop characteristic patterns of inflammation on microscopic examination. The pattern of inflammation is used to assist in determining the underlying disease responsible for lung injury; however, most forms of pulmonary fibrosis are virtually indistinguishable by the time they reach the end stage.

The initial event leading to interstitial lung disease is lung injury. In most cases of interstitial lung disease, no injuring agent is visible on microscopic evaluation; however, certain inorganic agents such as asbestos and talc are typically visible on microscopic inspection.

In patients with interstitial lung disease, pulmonary inflammation develops after lung injury. The alveoli are the most frequent sites of inflammation, but the vasculature and smaller airways may be involved as well. The inflammatory response is characterized by migration into the alveolus and alveolar wall of one or more of the following: neutrophils, eosinophils, lymphocytes, macrophages, and plasma cells. The influx of immune cells is accompanied by fluid accumulation in the alevolar walls and alveolar airspace. This immune reaction damages the alveoli. The flat type I pneumocytes are destroyed and replaced with the secretory type II cells. The alveolar walls become thickened and distorted by the inflammation. The alveoli are eventually destroyed as the disease progresses and are eventually replaced with fibrotic connective tissue and cystic airspaces. The cystic airspaces that result from this process are lined with cuboidal or columnar epithelium and do not participate in gas exchange.[14]

Clinical Features

Medical History

The symptoms of lung involvement are similar regardless of the underlying cause. In addition, the symptoms of lung involvement are nonspecific and could suggest many other causes, including obstructive lung disease, heart disease, or pulmonary vascular disease. The first symptom of pulmonary fibrosis is usually progressive dyspnea on exertion or a nonproductive cough. Patients initially notice dyspnea only during heavy exertion. Lower levels of exertion induce breathlessness as the process advances. In very advanced stages of the disease, dyspnea occurs at rest.

Interstitial lung disease may lead to pulmonary hypertension and then right heart failure (cor pulmonale). Cor pulmonale causes edema to accumulate primarily in the lower extremities and causes patients to complain of swollen ankles.

A careful history must include an employment record and a review of the patient's environment. A thorough review of the patient's past medical history, and along with current and previous medications, is also important. The goal of these questions is to determine whether the patient was exposed to agents known to cause interstitial lung disease. Evaluation and treatment may be greatly altered if the patient was exposed to any of these agents.

Physical Examination

Results of the physical examination in patients with interstitial lung disease are often very nonspecific. There may be no abnormal findings early in the course of the disease. As the process progresses, tachypnea and fine, inspiratory crackles are present. A prominent pulmonic component of the second heart sound (loud P_2) will occur if pulmonary hypertension is present. Distention of the jugular veins and edema of the lower extremities are signs of cor pulmonale and suggest more severe disease. Clubbing of the digits is a frequent finding, particularly with asbestosis and idiopathic pulmonary fibrosis.

If the cause of pulmonary fibrosis is a systemic disease, then additional abnormalities specific to the disease can often be found on examination. For example, rheumatoid lung is almost always accompanied by arthritis. Patients with sarcoidosis may have a rash, swollen lymph nodes, or cardiac rhythm irregularities. A complete physical examination is vital because it may guide the clinician to the etiology of pulmonary fibrosis and it provides an indication of the severity of the disease.

Laboratory Data

Arterial blood gas (ABG) levels are normal early in the disease. As the process develops, the alveolar-arterial difference in partial pressure of oxygen ($P[A-a]O_2$) increases.[15,16] Hypoxemia during exercise is a frequent finding that may progress to hypoxemia at rest in advanced disease. Hypercapnia may occur during the terminal stages of pulmonary fibrosis.

Lung volumes and flow rates are initially normal, but both decrease throughout the course of the disease.[17] Pulmonary function testing usually shows a purely restrictive defect in most patients with interstitial lung disease. This is characterized by a decrease in forced vital capacity (FVC) and forced expiratory volume in 1 second (FEV_1). The loss of FEV_1 is proportional to FVC loss, so that the ratio of FEV_1 to FVC remains normal. Other measurements of lung volume, such as total lung capacity (TLC) and residual volume (RV), are also usually reduced.

The compliance of the lungs decreases as lung involvement progresses. This is due in part to fibrosis of the pulmonary parenchyma and the formation of cystic airspace.[18] Diffusion capacity of the lung (D_{LCO}) is a good reflection of alveolar capillary surface area. Destruction of lung parenchyma results in a reduction in D_{LCO} as interstitial lung disease progresses. An abnormal D_{LCO} may be the earliest evidence of interstitial lung disease found on standard pulmonary function tests.[16,19]

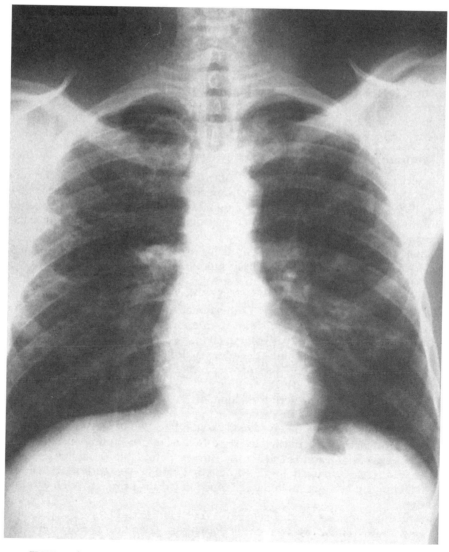

FIGURE 16-2   A diffuse reticular nodular pattern is visible throughout both lungs.

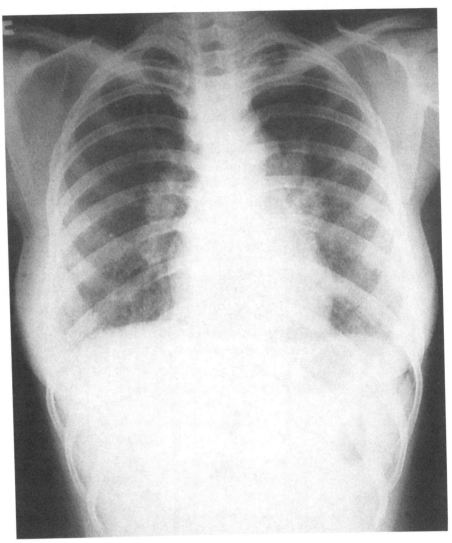

FIGURE 16-3   This chest radiograph shows a reticular pattern throughout both lungs. In addition, lymphadenopathy is visible in both hilar regions.

Oxygen desaturation during exercise is a frequent finding in patients with interstitial lung disease and is usually the earliest detectable pulmonary abnormality.[15,16] Exercise desaturation is caused by an alveolar capillary diffusion limitation and a worsening of ventilation-perfusion $(\dot{V}/\dot{Q})$ matching.[20]

The chest radiograph is normal early in the course of interstitial lung disease. The initial abnormality on the chest radiograph is referred to as a ground-glass appearance of the lungs. Later in the course of the disease, both lungs are seen to be diffusely affected on the typical chest radiograph.

Another radiographic presentation of this disease is diffuse pulmonary opacification (infiltrate). These opacities have three characteristic patterns: small nodules (nodular), lines (reticular), or both (reticulonodular; see Fig. 16-2). Some chest radiographs contain specific findings that are suggestive of a particular disease process. For example, sarcoidosis is often associated with swelling of the lymph nodes in the hilum of the lung (hilar lymphadenopathy [Fig. 16–3]). Wegener's granulomatosis is associated with lower lobe cavities and nodules. Asbestosis is often associated with calcified pleural plaques (Fig. 16–4).

Most interstitial lung diseases cause a progressive increase in the opacities on the radiograph and culminate with the development of **honeycomb lung.** The honeycomb-like appearance is created by the cysts that characterize the pathology of end-stage interstitial lung disease (Fig. 16–5).

Interstitial lung disease causes characteristic changes to the lung parenchyma that can be seen using computed tomography (CT). A normal CT scan examines a 10-mm-thick slice of tissue for each image. The densities in the 10-mm slice of lung are then averaged to create each image. The lung parenchyma is so delicate that its structure is

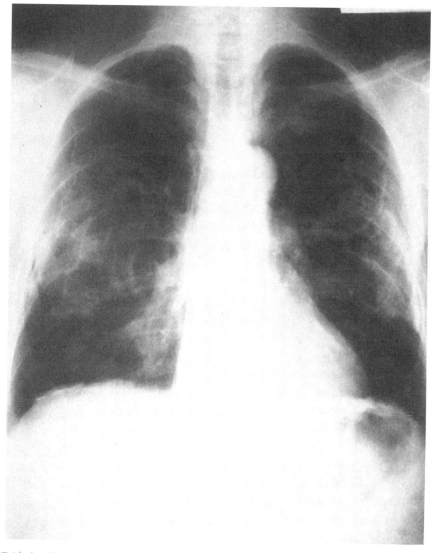

FIGURE 16–4   This chest radiograph discloses asbestos-related calcified pleural plaques. The plaques are easiest to see on the diaphragmatic surface as dense raised areas on both hemidiaphragms. Pleural plaques are also visible, superimposed over the middle of both lungs. The plaques overlying the lung are more difficult to see than the diaphragmatic plaques because visualization is through the flat surface rather than the end of the plaque.

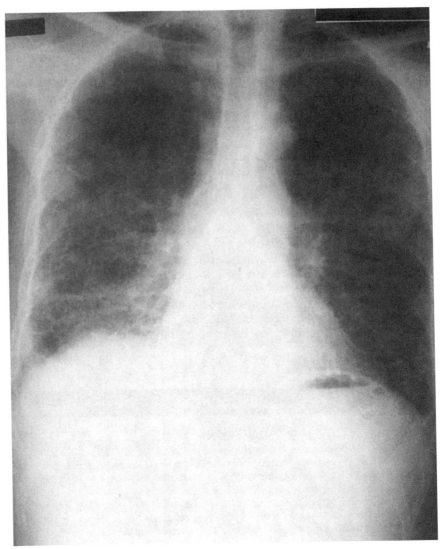

FIGURE 16-5   Dense reticular changes and cystic air spaces can be seen on this film—a pattern often called "honeycomb lung." This film is typical of end-stage pulmonary fibrosis.

lost by averaging such a thick slice of tissue for each image (Fig. 16–6). The best way of viewing the lung parenchyma is to use a high-resolution CT scan, which examines only 1 mm of lung at each level, thus revealing some of the lung parenchyma's delicate architecture (Fig. 16–7).

A high-resolution CT scan provides a wealth of information on the structural changes of the lung caused by the disease processes.[21,22] This information can be used to assist in the diagnosis of interstitial lung disease and evaluate the severity of the disease (Fig. 16–8). The negative aspect of high-resolution CT scans is that they expose patients to as much as 2.8 times the radiation of a normal CT scan.[21]

Radioactive gallium-67 is absorbed in areas of inflammation. Gallium scans of the lungs frequently show uptake of the isotope in patients with interstitial lung disease. The presence of inflammation may correlate with the presence of gallium-67 uptake in the lungs. Gallium scanning has been used to follow the effectiveness of therapy.[18,23]

Confirmation of interstitial lung disease frequently requires a lung biopsy in ad-

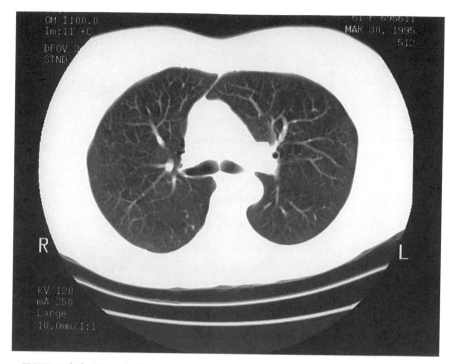

FIGURE 16–6   Normal CT scan of the chest with 10-mm thick slice, averaged for image.

dition to a meticulous history and physical examination, as well as laboratory and radiographic evaluations. Pulmonary fibrosis typically involves all lobes of both lungs. When the lung is examined microscopically, however, the stage of involvement is extremely variable from one area of the specimen to another. Portions of lung that re-

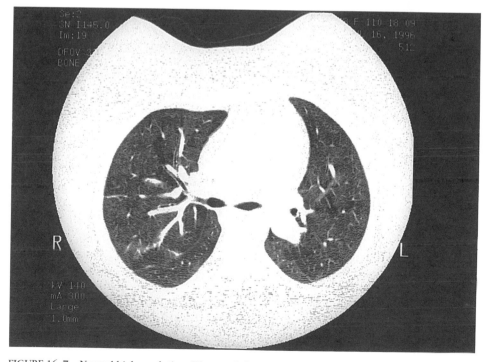

FIGURE 16–7   Normal high-resolution CT scan of chest, using a 1-mm thick slice, averaged for image.

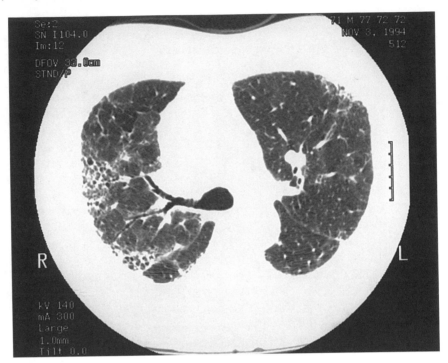

FIGURE 16-8   High-resolution CT scan of a patient with interstitial lung disease. Notice the large number of cystic air spaces typical of honeycomb lung.

veal characteristic pathologic findings are often scattered among areas of normal lung and areas of end-stage fibrosis. To be certain that areas with characteristic changes are sampled, an open lung or thoracoscopic[24,25] biopsy is often required. Sarcoidosis is one disease that has such diffuse and characteristic pathologic changes that only very small pieces of lung are required to establish the diagnosis. These smaller specimens can be obtained with a bronchoscope using a technique called *transbronchial biopsy.* To perform transbronchial biopsy, the bronchoscope is positioned in a smaller airway and a forceps is passed beyond the view of the operator into the periphery of the lung. The forceps can then be used to take small biopsies of lung tissue.

Bronchoalveolar lavage is another diagnostic technique performed by passing a bronchoscope into a segmental or smaller bronchus. The area beyond the bronchoscope is washed with saline. The saline that is then aspirated back through the bronchoscope contains a small number of cells. The cells that are recovered include many from the alveoli and are representative of the cells associated with the inflammatory process. The pathologic evaluation of these cells may provide data on the cause of the interstitial lung disease and may also be useful to follow the inflammatory activity of the lung during therapy.

Treatment

The events that cause interstitial lung disease begin with lung injury (Fig. 16-1), which leads to lung inflammation, which in turn results in irreversible pulmonary fibrosis and end-stage lung disease. The goal of therapy is to prevent further irreversible damage to the lung. This is achieved by prevention of further injury and suppression of the inflammatory response. The most obvious treatment for lung injury induced by a known agent is preventing the patient from being further exposed to the injurious substance. Although such avoidance of exposure is often adequate treatment and arrests the disease, an offending agent is identified in only about one third of patients with interstitial lung disease. If the source of injury cannot be removed, or if removal of the source of injury is insufficient to avoid disease progression, treatment is aimed at suppressing inflammation. The drug most commonly used to suppress inflammation initially is prednisone. In addition to prednisone, other immunosuppressive drugs such as cyclophosphamide[26] and azathioprine[27] are also used.

Exertional dyspnea associated with exercise hypoxemia is frequently improved by the addition of supplemental oxygen.[28] Oxygen at rest is required in the latter stages of the disease when resting hypoxemia develops.

Patients with progressive interstitial lung disease that continues to progress despite immunosuppressive therapy may require lung transplantation. Transplanting only one of the patient's diseased lungs is usually adequate.[29] Lung transplantation is appropriate for interstitial lung disease only when the patients are in the end stages of the disease. Although this therapy is successful at improving lung function and quality of life, as many as 40% of patients who undergo lung transplantation die within the first 2 years following the surgery.[30]

Prognosis

The prognosis for patients with interstitial lung disease is extremely variable. Early therapy can be helpful but does not alter the prognosis for a large number of interstitial lung diseases. The most common of these diseases include sarcoidosis, silicosis, hypersensitivity pneumonitis, and amiodarone toxicity. Some diseases are progressive and difficult to control even with aggressive therapy. These diseases include idiopathic pulmonary fibrosis, many forms of drug-induced lung disease, and some of the lung diseases associated with collagen vascular disease.

CASE STUDY

History

RJ is a 28-year-old black man currently employed as a savings-and-loan computer analyst. He noticed increasing fatigue over the last several months, which progressed to the point where he stopped jogging and he felt listless and tired most of the time. This began as a flulike illness and left him with a nonproductive cough. He denied having fever, chills, sore throat, coryza, headaches, or wheezing. He noted no sputum production, hemoptysis, or abnormalities in his hands or feet. After further questioning he agreed that the fatigue he experienced was probably dyspnea. He could walk indefinitely on level ground, but if he were to climb more than one flight of stairs, he would have to stop to catch his breath. He did not awaken with breathlessness, nor did he notice having dyspnea at rest.

As a child he had had chickenpox, but not measles or mumps. He has had no surgeries but had broken his leg in a skiing accident at age 22. RJ never smoked and drank alcoholic beverages only socially. The only prescription medication he took was ampicillin once or twice for upper respiratory infections. He took aspirin for minor pain control, usually once a month. His mother has hypertension, but his father is healthy; his maternal grandfather has lung carcinoma, but his maternal grandmother is well. Both of his paternal grandparents died in an automobile accident. He has two children, and both are well. Two healthy birds are kept as pets in the house.

RJ works as a manager of a small group of computer technicians. He has not been exposed to any dusts or fumes while performing his duties. He has worked as a computer manager since graduating from college. While in college he worked in a gas station pumping gas; in high school he worked at a local drive-through restaurant

He is an avid sports fan and spends his leisure time watching professional sports. None of his hobbies places him at risk for lung disease.

QUESTIONS

1. What is RJ's principal problem? Is there anything in the history that would help you characterize the problem?

2. What possible diagnosis could explain this man's dyspnea on exertion?

3. Do the jobs this man has performed place him at risk for lung disease? What jobs are typically related to exposure to inhaled inorganic dusts?

4. Although this patient denies using illicit drugs, what form of lung disease do these drugs cause?

5. What are your goals for the physical examination.

ANSWERS

1. RJ's principal complaint is dyspnea. The dyspnea is present only on exertion and has been progressive.

2. The four major types of illness that can cause exertional dyspnea include (1) obstructive lung diseases, such as asthma, emphysema, or chronic bronchitis; (2) interstitial lung disease; (3) pulmonary vascular disease, such as primary pulmonary hypertension or chronic thrombotic obstruction of the pulmonary artery; and (4) heart diseases, such as ischemic or valvular heart disease. This patient lacks the typical symptoms of obstructive lung disease, such as wheezing and experiencing episodic dyspnea that occurs at rest or awakens him from sleep. He also lacks a history of previous cardiac problems that are typical of many patients with exertional dyspnea due to heart problems. There is no history of previous deep vein thrombosis to suggest chronic thrombotic obstruction of the pulmonary artery.

   Despite a careful history, none of these diagnoses can be excluded from consideration. The history does, however, clarify the problem we are dealing with and allows one to formulate a preliminary differential diagnosis.

3. RJ is young and has worked primarily as a manager. None of the jobs he describes are likely to have caused lung disease. A careful exposure history should also include a history of exposure to pets and hobbies. The birds that are kept in his home as pets are a possible source of hypersensitivity pneumonitis or infection.

   The most common forms of inorganic pneumoconiosis are coalminer's pneumoconiosis, asbestosis, and silicosis. Coalminer's pneumoconiosis is caused by repeated exposure to coal dust. This occurs in miners and people who load coal for shipment. Asbestosis occurs in workers who are exposed to dust from asbestos. These people have usually worked directly with asbestos as it is machined or installed. Asbestos is hazardous only when it is in the form of a dust that can be inhaled. Asbestos-containing products that do not shed dust are not dangerous. Silicosis occurs in miners, sand blasters, foundry workers, or anyone who deals with sand dust on a regular basis.

4. Illicit drugs can cause lung disease in two ways: (1) by inducing noncardiogenic pulmonary edema or (2) by vasculitis induced by the IV injection of talc. Talc is sometimes used to dilute (cut) the active drug or may have contaminated the drug as it was extracted from talc-containing tablets.

5. The major goal of the physical examination is to help clarify the cause of RJ's dyspnea. Obstructive lung disease may be associated with an increase in the anteroposterior (AP) diameter of the chest and wheezes over the lung. Interstitial lung disease is usually associated with pulmonary crackles. Pulmonary vascular disease is characterized by the signs of pulmonary hypertension. The physical examination findings in pulmonary hypertension are a loud pulmonic component to the second heart sound (P_2) and possibly right ventricular heave or lift. Patients with chronic heart disease may have an abnormal heart rhythm. Abnormal extra heart sounds, such as a cardiac murmur and an S_3 or S_4, suggest valvular heart disease and heart failure, respectively.

Physical Examination

Vital Signs: Temperature 36.3°C (97.3°F), pulse 62/minute, respiratory rate 14/minute, blood pressure 155/97 mm Hg

General: An athletic-appearing black man in no respiratory distress

HEENT: Head normal; nose patent without discharge; pupils equal, round, and reactive to light; mucous membranes moist without cyanosis

Neck: Carotid arteries normal in contour and intensity; jugular neck veins not distended; trachea in midline of neck; swelling of submandibular salivary glands and several 1- to 2-cm lymph nodes in anterior cervical region

Chest: Configuration and expansion of the chest normal; diffuse, fine, inspiratory crackles throughout both lungs without wheezing found upon auscultation; normal resonance noted over all portions of the chest with percussion

Heart: Regular rate with no murmur or gallop; S_1 and S_2 have normal intensity and splitting; cardiac impulse in the fourth interspace 1 cm medial to the midclavicular line

Abdomen: Soft, nontender; bowel sounds active; no masses or organ enlargement noted; abdominal wall rising with each inspiration

Extremities: No edema noted; no clubbing or cyanosis seen; extremities warm with good capillary refill

---

QUESTIONS

6. What is your interpretation of the vital signs?

7. How would you interpret the pulmonary findings? How might they affect your assessment of this patient?

8. How would you interpret the cardiac findings? How might they affect your assessment?

9. Does this patient have evidence of cor pulmonale?

10. What is the significance of the swelling of multiple structures in the neck?

11. Describe the normal relationship between the respiratory cycle and movement of the abdominal wall.

12. What pathology typically accounts for the fine, inspiratory crackles heard in this patient? Are crackles commonly heard in patients with restrictive lung disease or obstructive lung disease?

13. Does the lack of cyanosis indicate that hypoxemia is not present?

14. What laboratory work would be most useful to determine the etiology of this person's dyspnea?

ANSWERS

6. With the exception of the blood pressure, the vital signs are normal. The elevation of blood pressure may be due to hypertension, or it may be a response to stress in a healthy person. Treatment of hypertension of this magnitude is not necessary unless multiple measurements have shown chronic elevation of blood pressure.

7. It was noted that RJ had diffuse, fine, inspiratory crackles over both lungs, which is consistent with the diagnosis of interstitial lung disease or pulmonary edema due to heart failure. Wheezing and increased AP diameter of the chest, signs of obstructive lung disease, are absent.

   The lung examination indicates that heart failure and interstitial lung disease are the most likely explanations for RJ's exertional breathlessness. It is still possible, though much less likely, that this represents an atypical presentation of obstructive lung disease or pulmonary vascular disease.

8. Results of the heart examination were normal. There were no extra heart sounds and no increase in P_2. The location of the cardiac impulse was normal. The lack of abnormal findings on cardiac examination makes it less likely, but not impossible, that RJ's dyspnea is related to pulmonary hypertension or heart failure.

9. Cor pulmonale is right heart failure that is the result of lung disease. Right heart failure causes systemic venous congestion, which is characterized by distention of the jugular veins, pedal edema, and hepatojugular reflux. In addition to systemic congestion, the heart examination is also abnormal when cor pulmonale is present. Right ventricular strain causes an abnormal pulsation (heave) over the lower left sternal border and an S_3 or S_4 that can be heard over this same area. RJ has none of these findings and therefore does not have cor pulmonale.

10. Swelling of lymph nodes (lymphadenopathy) can result from an infection or inflammatory process occurring either in the area drained by the lymph node or in the lymph node itself. Sarcoidosis is associated with cervical lymphadenopathy and enlargement of salivary glands.

11. The diaphragm is the major muscle of respiration. Contraction of the

diaphragm causes it to descend, drawing air into the lungs. Diaphragmatic descent also causes the abdominal wall to rise during inspiration, as is seen in this patient. If a patient has a very high inspiratory muscle load or diaphragmatic fatigue, the diaphragm rises on inspiration. This paradoxical movement of the diaphragm causes the abdominal wall to fall on inspiration. This would be a sign of respiratory failure.

12. Inspiratory crackles are caused by sudden opening of peripheral lung units with inspiration. This finding is typical of patients with interstitial lung disease, atelectasis, or pulmonary edema.

13. A lack of cyanosis does not indicate that hypoxemia is not present.

14. The disease process that is causing RJ to experience dyspnea is probably an interstitial lung disease, but this has not been proved. Pulmonary function testing including spirometry and DLCO would help to determine whether restrictive or obstructive lung disease is present and would also determine the severity of the disease. A chest radiograph should be ordered to help classify the pulmonary disease. An ABG analysis should be ordered to determine RJ's ability to ventilate and oxygenate.

Laboratory Evaluation

Chest Radiograph: (Fig. 16–9)

ABG (on Room Air):

pH	7.45
Pao_2	65 mm Hg
$Paco_2$	32 mm Hg
HCO_3^-	21 mEq/liter
$P(A-a)O_2$	44 mm Hg
O_2 content	17.5 mL/dL

Complete Blood Count:

	Observed	Normal
White blood cells/mm³	9100	4000–11,000
Red blood cells (million/mm³)	4.3	4.1–5.5
Hemoglobin (g/dL)	14.2	14–16.5
Hematocrit (%)	41	40–54
Differential		
Segmented neutrophils (%)	69	40–75
Band neutrophils (%)	9	0–6
Lymphocytes (%)	17	20–45
Monocytes (%)	3	2–10
Eosinophils (%)	1	0–6
Basophils (%)	1	0–1

Chemistry:

Na$^+$ (mEq/liter)	142	137–147
K$^+$ (mEq/liter)	4.1	3.5–4.8
Cl$^-$ (mmol/dL)	108	98–105
HCO$_3^-$ (mEq/liter)	22	22–29
Blood urea nitrogen (mg/dL)	19	7–20
Creatinine (mg/dL)	1.1	0.7–1.3
Calcium (mmol/liter)	2.5	2.1–2.55
Phosphate (mg/dL)	2.9	2.7–4.5
Uric acid (mg/dL)	6.9	4.5–8.2
Albumen (g/dL)	4.8	3.5–5.0
Protein (g/dL)	8.2	6.4–8.3

Pulmonary Function Testing:

	Value	*(%) of Predicted*
Spirometry		
FVC (liters)	2.79	63
SVC (liters)	2.61	59
FEV$_1$ (liters)	2.12	67
FEV$_1$/FVC (%)	76	
FEF$_{25-75\%}$ (liters/minute)	4.11	98
Body plethysmography		
RV (liters)	1.20	118
TLC (liters)	3.99	74
D$_{LCO}$ (mL/minute per mm Hg)	11.35	38%

FEF = forced expiratory flow; SVC = slow vital capacity

QUESTIONS

15. How do you interpret the chest radiograph?

16. How would you evaluate and interpret this patient's ABG values?

17. Interpret the results of the pulmonary function test. How do these tests affect possible diagnosis of interstitial lung disease or obstructive lung disease?

18. What testing may be helpful in determining whether the patient will be helped by supplemental oxygen?

19. What additional testing will be needed to determine the cause of this patient's disease?

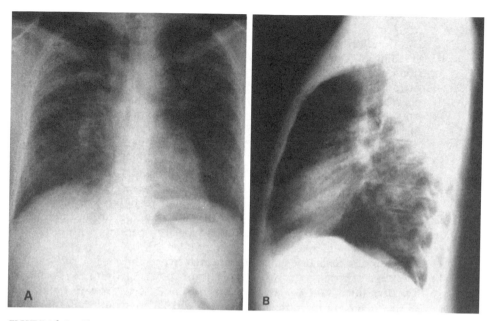

FIGURE 16-9   Chest radiograph of RJ at presentation. (*A*) Posteroanterior (PA) view; (*B*) lateral view.

ANSWERS

15. The chest radiograph shows diffuse reticulonodular opacification of both lungs. There is bilateral hilar enlargement as well. The heart is of normal size and configuration. This chest radiograph is consistent with interstitial lung disease. The presence of hilar lymphadenopathy suggests the diagnosis of sarcoidosis.

16. Chronic respiratory alkalosis is demonstrated in these ABG values. The patient has mild hypoxemia with an increase in the $P(A-a)O_2$.

17. The reduction of lung volumes on spirometry suggests restrictive lung disease. The loss of FEV_1 is proportional to the loss of vital capacity (FEV_1/FVC is normal), suggesting restrictive lung disease. Measurements obtained from body plethysmography suggest restrictive lung disease. TLC is decreased. The normal RV indicates that some obstructive lung disease may also be present. The abnormal DLCO indicates a loss of alevolar capillary surface area and strongly suggests that lung destruction is occurring. These findings are consistent with interstitial lung disease.

18. The initial ABG analysis does not indicate that supplemental oxygen is required. Patients with interstitial lung disease become desaturated upon exercise and may benefit from supplemental oxygen during exercise. Treadmill exercise testing with ABG samples and exhaled gas collection would determine whether RJ requires oxygen with exertion.

19. At this point there is strong evidence that RJ has a form of interstitial lung disease. It is important to determine the type of interstitial lung disease in order to devise an appropriate therapeutic plan. Lung biopsy is the most effective way to determine with accuracy what disease is responsible for RJ's symptoms. There are several reasons to suspect that RJ has sarcoidosis. Because sarcoidosis is the most likely diagnosis, transbronchial biopsy is the diagnostic test of choice.

Additional Diagnostic Data

The patient underwent pulmonary stress testing. He exercised for 8 minutes and 32 seconds using a modified Bruce protocol exercise test. He stopped because of extreme dyspnea. No cardiac abnormalities were noted on the electrocardiogram.

	Value	% of Predicted
$\dot{V}O_2$ max (mL/min)	1201	37
$\dot{V}CO_2$ max (mL/min)	1528	
RQ	1.27	
Lowest O_2 saturation (%)	81	

RQ = respiratory quotient; $\dot{V}CO_2$max = maximum CO_2 consumption; $\dot{V}O_2$max = maximum O_2 consumption

ABGs (on room air at rest and during peak exercise):

ABG at Rest	Value
pH	7.43
PaO_2	65 mm Hg
$PaCO_2$	33 mm Hg
HCO_3^-	22 mEq/liter
$P(A-a)O_2$	44 mm Hg
O_2 content	17.5 mL/dL

Peak Exercise	Value
pH	7.31
PaO_2	47 mm Hg
$PaCO_2$	28 mm Hg
HCO_3^-	14 mEq/liter
$P(A-a)O_2$	67 mm Hg
O_2 content	15.6 mL/dL

A bronchoscopy with transbronchial biopsy and a bronchoalveolar lavage were performed. The airways appeared normal on examination. A modest amount of bleeding was encountered following transbronchial biopsy. The transbronchial biopsy contained numerous noncaseating granulomas without infectious organisms. The pathologic diagnosis was sarcoidosis. The bronchoalveolar lavage showed numerous lymphocytes with alveolar macrophages and occasional neutrophils.

QUESTIONS

20. What is a plausible explanation of RJ's dyspnea on exertion?
21. Interpret the ABG analysis taken at peak exercise. What physiologic changes are responsible for each of the changes you see?
22. What is a respiratory quotient? What does RJ's RQ indicate?

23. How is a transbronchial biopsy obtained? What type of tissue will it provide for examination?

24. How is bronchoalveolar lavage obtained? What types of samples will it provide for examination?

25. Will oxygen therapy help relieve RJ's breathlessness? If oxygen is given to this patient, how should he use it?

26. What therapy should RJ receive for his sarcoidosis? What is the goal of that therapy?

ANSWERS

20. There are many reasons for persons with interstitial lung disease to experience dyspnea. In RJ, hypoxemia develops with exercise. This exertional desaturation may in part explain the breathlessness he develops when jogging.

21. There is profound hypoxemia with exercise. There is also a mixed acid-base disorder with a respiratory alkalosis and a metabolic acidosis. The hypoxemia in this case is caused by worsening of $\dot{V}/\dot{Q}$ matching and reduction in the red blood cell transit time through the alveolar capillaries. The drop in $Paco_2$ may be driven by hypoxia and acidosis. The drop in HCO_3^- is caused by lactic acidosis due to anaerobic metabolism of exercising muscle.

22. The RQ is the ratio of carbon dioxide produced to oxygen consumed. At rest, the RQ of a healthy person is about 0.8. With anaerobic metabolism, such as occurs during vigorous exercise, the amount of carbon dioxide produced exceeds the amount of oxygen consumed. When an individual makes a transition from aerobic to anaerobic metabolism, he or she is said to have crossed the "anaerobic threshold." RJ had an EQ of 1.27, which indicates that he crossed his anaerobic threshold.

23. Transbronchial biopsy is a technique for sampling alveoli and small airways without performing major surgery. A bronchoscope is used to locate the airway that leads to the portion of the lung that is to be sampled. Biopsy forceps are then passed several inches beyond the bronchoscope, and the biopsy is taken from the small airways. The samples of tissue that are obtained are very small and therefore inadequate for diagnosing many forms of interstitial lung disease. This technique is popular, however, because it can easily diagnose diseases such as sarcoidosis, tumors, and infections and does not require a general anesthetic or skin incision.

24. Like transbronchial biopsy, bronchoalveolar lavage is a bronchoscopic technique. The purpose of the lavage is to wash a small number of cells from the alveoli for pathologic examination. The bronchoscope is passed into the smallest airway it can enter. Saline (50 to 200 mL) is injected into the bronchial lumen. The saline washes out to the small airways and is then aspirated back out through the bronchoscope. Unlike biopsy, bronchoalevolar lavage obtains cells with no surrounding structure. This technique is useful for diagnosing and staging interstitial lung disease; diagnosing certain lung infections (particularly *Pneumocystis carinii* pneumonia); and diagnosing some forms of lung cancer.

25. Yes, RJ has a marked tendency toward desaturation with moderate exercise levels. The use of supplemental oxygen with exertion may help his exertional dyspnea. There is no need at this time to have him use oxygen 24 hours a day.

26. Sarcoidosis is one of the forms of interstitial lung disease that has no known cause. As a consequence, therapy cannot be directed at preventing further exposure to an injuring agent. Instead, therapy is aimed at suppressing inflammation, which is usually accomplished with corticosteroids, cyclophosphamide, or azathioprine, or a combination of these drugs. In sarcoidosis, therapy with corticosteroids such as prednisone is usually very effective at stopping progression of the disease.

CASE STUDY—continued

Follow-up

One year after the initial diagnosis of sarcoidosis, RJ felt much better. He had taken prednisone for 1 year, after which his chest radiograph showed improvement. He had less dyspnea on exertion and no longer required oxygen therapy. He continued to have a restrictive defect on spirometry and a reduction in his DLCO, but both of these parameters improved.

QUESTION

28. If the sarcoidosis had progressed to its end stage, what would RJ's lungs have been like radiographically and pathologically?

29. If pulmonary fibrosis were to progress to its end stage despite anti-inflammatory medication, what treatment options would be available?

ANSWER

28. End-stage interstitial lung disease is characterized by replacement of normal lung tissue by cystic airspaces and fibrotic tissue. On radiograph, the cystic airspaces can be seen surrounded by fibrous connective tissue in a pattern called honeycomb lung (Fig. 16–5).

29. End-stage pulmonary fibrosis may require single lung transplantation to control the symptoms of interstitial lung disease. Single lung transplantation improves a patient's symptoms, exercise tolerance, and quality of life if they survive the surgery.

REFERENCES

1. Coultas, DB, et al: The epidemiology of interstitial lung diseases. Am J Respir Crit Care Med 150:967, 1994.
2. Morgan, WKC, and Seaton, A: Occupational Lung Diseases, ed 2. WB Saunders, Philadelphia, 1984.
3. Becklake, MR: Pneumoconiosis. In Murray, JF, and Nadel, JA (eds): Textbook of Respiratory Medicine. WB Saunders, Philadelphia, 1988, pp 1556–1592.
4. Johns, CJ: Sarcoidosis. In Fishman, AP (ed): Pulmonary Disease and Disorders. McGraw-Hill, New York, 1988, pp 619–641.
5. Hammon, L, and Rich, AR: Acute interstitial fibrosis of the lung. Bull Johns Hopkins 74:177, 1944.
6. Stachura, I, et al: Mechanisms of tissue injury in desquamative interstitial pneumonitis. Am J Med 68:733, 1980.
7. Fox, RB, et al: Pulmonary inflammation due to

oxygen toxicity: Involvement of chemotactic factors and polymorphonuclear leukocytes. Am Rev Respir Dis 123:521, 1981.

8. Guidotti, TL: Coal workers' pneumoconiosis and medical aspects of coal mining. South Med J 72:456, 1979.

9. Batist, G, and Andrews, JL: Pulmonary toxicity of antineoplastic drugs. JAMA 246:1449, 1981.

10. Cockerill, FJ, et al: Open lung biopsy in immunocompromised patients. Arch Intern Med 145:1398, 1985.

11. Rosenow, EC, and Martin, WJ: Drug induced interstitial lung disease. In Schwarz, MI, and King, TE (eds): Interstitial Lung Disease, BC Decker, Toronto, 1988, pp 123–137.

12. Kndenchyk, PJ, et al: Prospective evaluation of amiodarone pulmonary toxicity. Chest 86:541, 1984.

13. Suntres, ZE, and Shek, PN: Nitrofurantoin-induced pulmonary toxicity: In vivo evidence for oxidative stress-mediated mechanisms. Biochem Pharmacol 43:1127, 1992.

14. Flint, A: Pathologic features of interstitial lung disease. In Schwarz, MI, and King, TE (eds): Interstitial Lung Disease. BC Decker, Toronto, 1988, pp 45–62.

15. Crystal, RG, et al: Idiopathic pulmonary fibrosis: Clinical, histologic, radiographic, physiologic, scintigraphic, cytologic and biochemical aspects. Ann Intern Med 85:769, 1976.

16. Fulmer, JD: The interstitial lung diseases. Chest 82:172, 1982.

17. Carrington, CB, et al: Natural history and treated course of usual and desquamative interstitial pneumonia. N Engl J Med 298:801, 1978.

18. Fulmer, JD: An introduction to the interstitial lung diseases. Clin Chest Med 3:457, 1982.

19. Crystal, RG, et al: Interstitial lung disease: Current concepts of pathogenesis staging and therapy. Am J Med 70:542, 1981.

20. Wagner, PD: Ventilation-perfusion matching during exercise. Chest 101:192S, 1992.

21. Engeler, CE, et al: Volumetric high resolution CT scan in the diagnosis of interstitial lung disease and bronchiectasis: Diagnostic accuracy and radiation dose. AJR 163:31, 1994.

22. Nishimura, K, et al: The diagnostic accuracy of computed tomography in diffuse infiltrative lung diseases. Chest 104:1149, 1993.

23. Line, BR, et al: Gallium-67 scanning to stage the alveolitis of sarcoidosis: Correlation with clinical studies, pulmonary function studies and bronchoalveolar lavage. Am Rev Respir Dis 123:440, 1981.

24. Nasim, A, et al: Video-thoracoscopic lung biopsy in diagnosis of interstitial lung disease. J R Coll Surg Edin 40:22, 1995.

25. Krasna, MJ, et al: The role of thoracoscopy in the diagnosis of interstitial lung disease. Ann Thorac Surg 59:348, 1995.

26. Johnson, MA, et al: Randomized controlled trial comparing prednisolone alone with cyclophosphamide and low dose prednisolone in combination in cryptogenic fibrosing alveolitis. Thorax 44:280, 1989.

27. Raghu, G, et al: Azathioprine combined with prednisone in the treatment of idiopathic pulmonary fibrosis: A prospective double-blind randomized placebo-controlled clinical trial. Ann Rev Respir Dis 144:291, 1991.

28. Harris-Eze, AO, et al: Oxygen improves maximal exercise performance in interstitial lung disease. Am J Respir Crit Care Med 150:1616, 1994.

29. Egan, TM, et al: Isolated lung transplantation for end-stage lung disease: A viable therapy. Ann Thorac Surg 53:590, 1992.

30. Cooper, JD, et al: Current status of lung transplantation: Report of the St. Louis International Lung Transplant Registry. Clin Transpl 77:81, 1992.

CHAPTER **17**

Neuromuscular Diseases

N. Lennard Specht, MD
Robert L. Wilkins, PhD, RRT

Key Terms

acute postinfectious
  polyneuropathy
  (Guillain-Barré
  syndrome [GBS])
amyotrophic lateral
  sclerosis (ALS) (Lou
  Gehrig's disease)

diplopia
fasciculations
myasthenia gravis
myopathy
paresthesia

primary alveolar
  hypoventilation
ptosis
Tensilon test

Introduction

Neuromuscular disorders can threaten every activity from walking to breathing. They may occur suddenly, as with a spinal cord fracture, or more slowly, as with amyotrophic lateral sclerosis. They may be temporary and completely resolve, or they may be permanent, resulting in paralysis or even death. Regardless of the specific type of neuromuscular disorder present, the patient needs to be accurately diagnosed so that the best treatment can be given and the most optimal outcome obtained.

    Respiratory care practitioners (RCPs) often play a key role in the evaluation and care of the patient with neuromuscular disease, especially when the disorder threatens use of the muscles of breathing or the reflexes that protect the lungs from aspiration. Dyspnea is a frequent problem associated with neuromuscular disease, but it is often inappropriately attributed to other problems, such as asthma or chronic obstructive pulmonary disease (COPD). RCPs are often in the best position to recognize impending respiratory failure and unusual response to therapy for common lung diseases. For this reason, it is vital that RCPs be familiar with this type of medical problem. A review of the anatomy and physiology associated with the neuromuscular system controlling breathing is helpful as an introduction to the subject of specific neuromuscular diseases.

Normal Neuromuscular Function in Breathing

Normal breathing during rest, exercise, and sleep requires a healthy respiratory pump for effective movement of air in and out of the chest. The respiratory pump consists of four major components: the *respiratory center* in the brain to control breathing, *chemoreceptors* to respond to blood levels of oxygen and carbon dioxide, the *nerves* to conduct impulses from the brain to the respiratory muscles, and the *respiratory muscles* to provide ventilation.

Respiratory Centers

The respiratory centers are located diffusely within the medulla and pons in the brain stem. Three major components form the respiratory centers: The *medullary center* is responsible for maintaining a regular rhythmic respiratory pattern. The *apneustic center* and the *pneumotaxic center* work together to regulate respiratory frequency and volume.[1]

The respiratory centers receive input from oxygen sensors in the carotid bodies, hydrogen ion sensors in the brain stem, mechanoreceptors in the lung, and the cerebral cortex. The respiratory centers interpret this information and produce a signal that is sent through peripheral nerves to the respiratory muscles. As the impulse leaves the brain stem, it travels down the spinal cord, exits to the peripheral nerves, and travels to the neuromuscular junction. Here the impulse connects to the respiratory muscles, which respond to the stimulus by contraction.

Chemoreceptors

There are two types of chemoreceptors: one type senses the concentration of oxygen in the surrounding fluid; the other senses the concentration of carbon dioxide. Both create neural impulses based on the concentration of oxygen or carbon dioxide and transmit these impulses to the respiratory centers.

The *oxygen chemoreceptors* are located in the carotid bodies and the aortic bodies. The carotid bodies are located in the back of the bifurcation of the common carotid arteries, and the aortic bodies are located in the arch of the aorta. The output of these receptors increases as the PaO_2 drops.

The *carbon dioxide (central) chemoreceptors* are located in the ventral surface of the medulla. These receptors are responsive to the concentration of hydrogen ions in the surrounding cerebrospinal fluid (CSF). The extracellular fluid is largely controlled by the blood-brain barrier. This barrier strictly regulates the flow of ions and water into the brain. Three ions are the major determinants of CSF: bicarbonate (HCO_3^-), hydrogen ($H^+[pH]$), and carbon dioxide (CO_2). HCO_3^- and H^+ movement is carefully regulated by the blood-brain barrier, whereas CO_2 can freely cross it. The enhanced mobility of CO_2 makes the central chemoreceptors much more responsive to changes in blood CO_2 than to changes in blood pH.

Nerve Transmission

The three nerve groups that are most important to respiration are the phrenic, the intercostal, and the abdominal wall muscle nerves (Fig. 17–1). The *phrenic nerves* arise from the cervical spinal cord at the C3 to C5 level. These nerves leave the spinal canal,

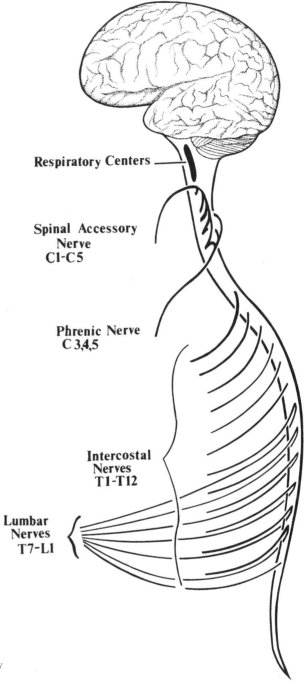

FIGURE 17-1   The neural pathways necessary
for the respiratory pump.

travel through the neck and into the mediastinum and then over the pericardium, and
insert into the diaphragm on either side of the heart. The *intercostal nerves* arise from
the thoracic spinal cord at levels T1 to T12. These nerves each course under a rib and
supply the intercostal muscles. The *abdominal muscle nerves* arise from the thoracic
and lumbar spine (T7 to L1).

Neuromuscular Junction

Each nerve ending is connected to a muscle fiber by a neuromuscular junction. An impulse transmitted along a nerve reaches a nerve ending at the neuromuscular junction. The nerve ending releases acetylcholine when stimulated by a nerve impulse. The presence of acetylcholine at the neuromuscular junction causes the muscle to contract. Acetylcholine is rapidly degraded by acetylcholinesterase to prevent excessive muscle stimulation.

Respiratory Muscles

There are several muscles of respiration (Fig. 17–2). The diaphragm is the largest and most important *inspiratory muscle.* Contraction of the diaphragm pushes down on the abdominal contents, which are held in place by the abdominal wall, and uses them as a fulcrum to raise the ribs. Raising the ribs causes a negative intrapleural pressure, which causes the lungs to inflate. Other inspiratory muscles include the external intercostal, scalene, and sternocleidomastoid muscles. They become active during heavy exercise in healthy persons or at rest in patients with a dysfunctional diaphragm.

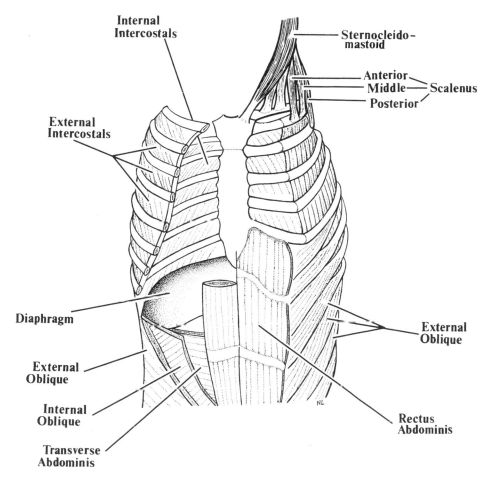

FIGURE 17–2   The major respiratory muscles.

The *expiratory muscles* are the internal intercostal and abdominal wall muscles, including the rectus abdominus, internal and external oblique, and transverse abdominus muscles. They are called on only during forceful exhalation, as with a cough. They are not needed during passive exhalation to the point of functional residual capacity in healthy persons.

Pathology and Pathophysiology

The respiratory pump is an efficient servomechanism in healthy people that evaluates respiratory requirements and translates these requirements into ventilation. However, the respiratory pump is vulnerable to injury; damage to even the smallest portion of the pump can lead to respiratory failure.

Respiratory Centers

Because the respiratory centers are located in diverse parts of the body, they are relatively invulnerable to direct injury. In fact, the respiratory centers are frequently one of only a few neurologic functions still operating in patients with severe cerebral injury. A number of disease processes and agents affect the respiratory centers; conversely, several diseases are thought to result from abnormalities of the respiratory centers.

Sedative drugs, particularly narcotics, can suppress respiration by depressing the respiratory centers. An overdose of narcotics or barbiturates can lead to hypoventilation or even apnea in severe cases.

Central sleep apnea is an example of a disease caused by an abnormality in the respiratory center. It is characterized by lapses of breathing effort during sleep. This disorder most often affects adults with cerebrovascular disease, but it may also play a role in sudden infant death syndrome (SIDS).

Primary alveolar hypoventilation is another example of a disease caused by insufficient respiratory drive in the absence of an obvious defect of the respiratory pump or lungs. These patients hypoventilate while awake and during sleep and can voluntarily lower their $PaCO_2$ to normal levels.

Nerve Interruption

If signals from the respiratory centers to the respiratory muscles are interrupted, the respiratory pump will be unable to provide ventilation. There are many sites along the pathway where nerve damage can result in compromise of the respiratory system.

Trauma is the most frequent cause of nerve damage that affects the respiratory pump. Spinal cord injury blocks transmission of nerve impulses below the level of injury. Nerves that arise from the spinal cord below the level of injury, as well as muscles supplied by those nerves, are therefore nonfunctional. Injuries to the cervical spinal cord create much more difficulty than injuries to the thoracic and lumbar spine (Table 17–1). Damage to the midthoracic spine leads to loss of function of the abdominal and some of the intercostal muscles. Cervical spine injuries in the C6 to C7 area lead to loss of function of all intercostal and abdominal muscles. A cervical spinal cord transection to the C1 to C3 area will lead to apnea because all respiratory muscles are affected.

TABLE 17-1   **Respiratory Muscle Innervation**

Spinal Cord Level	Peripheral Nerve(s)/Muscle(s)
C1–2	Spinal accessory/sternocleidomastoid
C3–5	Phrenic/diaphragm
C4–8	Cervical/scalene
T1–12	Intercostal/intercostal
T7–L1	Abdominal/abdominal wall

The phrenic nerve, which arises from C3 to C5, is the most peripheral nerve that may be injured. Temporary interruption of a phrenic nerve may occur during coronary artery bypass surgery. Cooling measures used to protect the heart from ischemia while the bypass grafts are being completed may cool the phrenic nerves excessively. Excessive cooling of the phrenic nerve causes interruption of the nerve and resultant diaphragmatic paralysis. This paralysis is frequently temporary but may take months to resolve.

Nerves can also be interrupted by nontraumatic processes. Polio is a viral illness that destroys the motor neurons in the anterior horn of the spinal cord. The destruction of motor neurons may involve nerves that innervate respiratory muscles. Paralysis of the respiratory muscles from polio may become so pronounced that respiratory failure and apnea develop. Respiratory failure from polio was a common occurrence until the development of the polio vaccine in the 1950s.

Amyotrophic lateral sclerosis (ALS) is a progressive fatal neurological disease also known as **Lou Gehrig's disease**. Despite extensive research, no etiology for ALS has been discovered. As in polio, patients with ALS lose muscle function because of loss of motor neurons in the anterior horn of the spinal cord. Respiratory failure invariably develops in ALS patients (Table 17–2).

Patients with **Guillain-Barré syndrome** (GBS) have a progressive, ascending paralysis caused by an inflammatory destruction of the myelin sheath around peripheral nerves. GBS, also known as **acute postinfectious polyneuropathy,** is frequently preceded by a viral-type illness. The viral syndrome is followed by inflammation of spinal roots and peripheral nerves. The inflammation of the spinal roots causes destruction of the myelin sheaths. The loss of myelin sheaths causes the associated

TABLE 17-2   **Neuromuscular Disorders**

Location of Defect	Disorder
Central nervous system	Ondine's curse
	Central sleep apnea
	Primary alveolar hypoventilation
	Sedative hypnotic overdose
Neuronal pathway	Spinal cord injury
	Multiple sclerosis
	Amyotrophic lateral sclerosis
Neuromuscular junction	Myasthenia gravis
	Botulism poisoning
	Organophosphate poisoning
Muscular function	Muscular dystrophy
	Myotonic dystrophy

nerve to malfunction. Most often, the inflammation resolves and the myelin sheaths regenerate.

Neuromuscular Junction. The nervous impulse can be interrupted at the synapse of the neuromuscular junction. This interruption can be caused by failure of a nerve to release acetylcholine, as in botulism poisoning. Destruction of acetylcholine receptors on the muscle, as in myasthenia gravis, will also lead to muscle weakness and potentially respiratory pump failure (Table 17–2). Some toxins, such as organophosphate insecticides and chemical-warfare nerve gases, block the breakdown of acetylcholine in the neuromuscular junction. Blocking the breakdown of acetylcholine causes muscle spasms, tetany, and respiratory failure. **Myasthenia gravis** is a classic example of a neuromuscular disease that affects the neuromuscular junction. It is probably a immunologic disease resulting from circulating antibodies directed against acetylcholine receptors in the junction. As a result, nerve impulses do not result in forceful muscle contraction when stimulated.

Muscle Diseases. A **myopathy** is a disorder of the muscle. Several congenital abnormalities lead to progressive muscular weakness. Muscular dystrophies are one of the most common examples of this type of disease. Muscular dystrophy leads to progressive muscle weakness and loss of function. Loss of muscle function eventually becomes so profound that a poor cough develops, lung volumes become reduced, and eventually respiratory failure develops. Patients with muscular dystrophy frequently die of respiratory failure or pneumonia.

Clinical Features

The patient with neuromuscular disease may not initially develop respiratory complications. Signs and symptoms of respiratory failure will occur, however, as the muscular weakness progresses to the point where the muscles of breathing are compromised. As the inspiratory muscles weaken, the patient's lung volumes decrease, and a rapid and shallow breathing pattern develops. The patient often complains of dyspnea, especially on exertion. Weakness of expiratory muscles leads to a poor cough and inability to clear excessive secretions from the airways. Retention of sputum in the lung may lead to mucus plugging, atelectasis, and pneumonia, which are common complications of neuromuscular disease.[2]

Initial arterial blood gas (ABG) findings may be normal in the patient with mild neuromuscular disease; however, with severe weakness of the respiratory muscles, the ABG values demonstrate hypoxemia, an increased $Paco_2$, and decreased pH. Hypoxemia is common because of ventilation-perfusion ($\dot{V}/\dot{Q}$) mismatching and the increase in alveolar Pco_2 ($Paco_2$), but it typically responds to supplemental oxygen therapy. If the patient also has a complicating pneumonia, more severe hypoxemia may be present. In general, ABG abnormalities are a late sign of acute respiratory failure in patients with neuromuscular disease and should not be relied on to determine the severity of the disease or when to intubate the patient.

Bedside assessment of pulmonary function will reveal a reduced vital capacity (VC). Severe disease is marked by a reduction in the VC below 1.0 to 1.5 liters in the adult. The maximum inspiratory pressure (MIP) decreases as the inspiratory muscles weaken. MIP is a useful tool for quantifying the degree of muscle weakness and identifying trends in the course of the disease. An MIP measurement of less than −20 to

−30 cm H_2O usually indicates severe weakness of the inspiratory muscles. Bedside clinicians should measure MIP against a closed mouthpiece after the patient has exhaled to residual volume. Exhaling to residual volume provides the inspiratory muscles with the best mechanical advantage for performing the MIP maneuver.[3]

GBS may occur at any age and has no discernible geographic or seasonal distribution. A preceding viral infection is commonly seen in patients diagnosed with GBS.[4] Initial symptoms often include weakness of the lower extremities and **paresthesia** (sensations of numbness or tingling) in the fingers and toes. The lower extremity weakness is usually symmetrical, and the weakness progresses to the muscles of the abdomen, diaphragm, arms, and face. The patient with GBS may experience difficulty swallowing and a poor gag reflex as the muscles of the throat become involved. This may lead to aspiration if the airway is not protected. Hypertension or cardiac dysrhythmias develop in some GBS patients owing to involvement of the autonomic nervous system. Cardiac dysrhythmias may be serious enough to cause death if appropriate treatment is not implemented. Measurement of CSF protein level may be useful in making the diagnosis of GBS. CSF protein levels above 100 mg/100 mL are consistent with GBS.[5]

Myasthenia gravis can occur at any age, but the incidence increases in early adulthood and in the elderly. In young adults, women outnumber men 2 to 1 in the incidence of the disease.[6] The patient with myasthenia gravis usually presents with weakness of certain muscles when used repeatedly. The extraocular muscles are often affected initially and cause the patient to experience blurred vision (**diplopia**) and droopy eyelids (**ptosis**). The symptoms increase with repeated use of the involved muscles and may improve with rest. In fact, they may disappear after a good night of sleep. Some patients with myasthenia gravis experience gradual progression of the disease to other muscle groups, including the pharyngeal, laryngeal, arm, trunk, and leg muscles. Respiratory symptoms usually do not develop in individuals with milder cases of myasthenia gravis; however, respiratory failure is likely to occur when the diaphragm is affected by the disease. A number of factors (e.g., infection, surgery, menstruation, immunizations, certain drugs, emotional distress) can precipitate a myasthenia gravis crisis in a patient with a previously stable case.

The **Tensilon test** helps to establish the diagnosis of myasthenia gravis. This test involves intravenous (IV) injection of 10 mg of Tensilon (edrophonium) while the areas of major muscle weakness are carefully observed. Muscle weakness will resolve within 20 to 30 seconds and remains nearly normal for a few minutes if myasthenia gravis is the cause of the patient's weakness.

Patients with ALS most often initially experience progressive weakness of distal muscle groups, such as the hands. Occasionally, the initial symptom is difficulty with swallowing. The disease may cause asymmetric weakness, atrophy, and tremors. A characteristic feature of ALS is the development of muscle fiber twitching called **fasciculations.** ALS advances over a period of 2 to 7 years and eventually causes weakness of all four extremities as well as the breathing muscles. Dyspnea occurs at rest, and the patient begins having difficulty coughing, swallowing, and talking as the disease progresses. Respiratory failure and death most often occur 3 to 4 years after the onset of symptoms.[7]

Respiratory symptoms of the patient with a spinal cord injury will vary with the location of the lesion. High cervical injuries above the C3 level produce nearly complete respiratory muscle paralysis. In these cases the patient is unable to breathe effectively, talk, or cough. The lack of effective breathing causes the rapid onset of respiratory acidosis and hypoxemia. Breath sounds are very diminished or absent. The diaphragm is elevated and immobile. Bedside VC is at best 20 percent of predicted.[8]

The patient with a spinal lesion at the level of C4 to C8 is quadriplegic but usually retains some use of the respiratory muscles. VC is markedly reduced immediately after the injury but improves somewhat over the initial 12 months. Pneumonia or atelectasis commonly complicate the care of patients with spinal cord injury because of their inability to breath deeply and cough effectively. ABG results usually demonstrate mild hypoxemia and a normal $PaCO_2$ during the daytime.[8]

Disruption of the spinal cord below C8 does not usually cause a significant reduction in lung volumes. A mid to low spinal-cord lesion often attenuates expiratory muscle function to the point where the patient's cough may be weak and ineffective. As a result, secretion retention and atelectasis is a potential complication.

Treatment

Neuromuscular disease may weaken the respiratory muscles and cause the patient to have difficulty clearing airway secretions. Bronchial hygiene techniques, including postural drainage, cough assistance, and aerosol therapy, are often beneficial. Intermittent positive-pressure breathing may be useful to prevent or treat atelectasis and dyspnea. Intubation may be needed when aspiration is likely to occur as a result of loss of the gag reflex.

Careful monitoring of the vital signs, breathing pattern, ability to cough, VC, and MIP is essential to identify the need for ventilatory assistance. A decline in the ABG measurements is often a late clinical manifestation and should not be relied on to determine the need for mechanical ventilation. Intubation and mechanical ventilation is warranted if the patient demonstrates a respiratory rate greater than 30/minute at rest, a VC less than 15 mL/kg of ideal body weight, the inability to clear airway secretions, progressive dyspnea, or an increasing $PaCO_2$. Once the patient is intubated, the RCP should keep the airway clear with postural drainage and suctioning. Tracheostomy is useful when long-term mechanical ventilation is needed, as in the case of a high cervical spine fracture. Tracheostomy is usually not used during the first 2 weeks of mechanical ventilation for reversible conditions such as GBS or myasthenia gravis. After 10 to 14 days of intubation, however, if the patient has not shown any signs of improvement, tracheostomy should be considered.

Clinicians caring for the patient with neuromuscular disease should anticipate complications such as pneumonia and pulmonary emboli. Antibiotics should be given if fever and pulmonary infiltrates develop. Prophylactic use of heparin is useful in reducing the incidence of deep venous thrombosis and pulmonary embolism.

Weaning from mechanical ventilation is reasonable when the patient is free of infection, is hemodynamically stable, and has significantly improved respiratory muscle function. Signs of improvement include a VC greater than 1.5 liter, an MIP greater than -30 cm H_2O, and a spontaneous tidal volume (VT) greater than 300 mL. Improvement in lung mechanics is not likely to occur in patients with high neck fractures or ALS.

Treatment of the GBS patient is primarily supportive. Plasmapheresis has been used with some success and is reserved for severe cases. It involves removal of a portion of the circulating blood, which is then centrifuged to separate the red blood cells (RBCs) from the plasma. The plasma is discarded, and the RBCs are mixed with fresh plasma and re-infused into the patient. This process is continued until a major portion of the plasma is replaced, causing dilution of the offending antibody. Corticosteroids are controversial and are not commonly used to treat the GBS patient. Careful monitoring of the patient is crucial because respiratory failure represents the most immediate threat of life.[9] Mechanical ventilation is needed in about 25 percent of cases.[10] After a period of stability the patient will usually begin to recover, but it often takes several weeks or months for complete recovery. The prognosis is usually very good unless serious complications occur.

Specific treatment of myasthenia gravis include anticholinesterase medications such as neostigmine. The patient with myasthenia gravis should be admitted to the hospital any time he or she has difficulty breathing or swallowing. Careful monitoring of respiratory function is essential, as previously mentioned. Plasmapheresis and thymectomy (surgical removal of the thymus gland) have been used with some success to treat severe cases.[11,12] Because patients with myasthenia gravis may have thymus gland enlargement, they may improve after thymectomy.

Treatment for the patient with ALS is nonspecific and supportive. Careful monitoring of respiratory function is important, as respiratory failure can occur with little warning. Intermittent mechanical ventilatory support using a negative-pressure body respirator may prove useful for the patient with a severe case of chronic neuromuscular disease, as occurs with ALS. Nocturnal ventilation with a body respirator has a distinct advantage in that an artificial airway does not need to be placed in order to achieve ventilation. This type of mechanical ventilation may allow the fatigued diaphragm to rest at night and subsequently results in better gas exchange and sleep during the night.[13,14] Nocturnal nasal-mask intermittent positive-pressure ventilation (NIPPV) is an alternative to negative-pressure ventilation for patients with severe, chronic neuromuscular disease.[15] NIPPV appears to be safe and effective and is less cumbersome to implement compared to negative-pressure ventilation.[16]

Care of patients with spinal cord injury must be tailored according to the location of the lesion. Those with a high neck fracture (above the level of C3) require intubation and mechanical ventilation to survive. Once stabilized, tracheostomy is needed for long-term ventilatory assistance. Patients with fractures below C3 require careful assessment to determine the extent of respiratory muscle paralysis. Most patients with neck fracture below the C3 level do not need continuous mechanical ventilation but may need nocturnal ventilatory support and assistance with secretion removal. In general, the lower the site of the neck fracture, the less respiratory care the patient will need.

CASE STUDY NO. 1

History

Ms. M is a 25-year-old white woman who came to the emergency room complaining of extremity weakness and difficulty swallowing. The patient stated that 10 days earlier she had an episode of fever, headache, and general malaise. Her physician diagnosed her condition as influenza. She was given acetaminophen for the headache and told to drink plenty of fluids and rest until the symptoms resolved. The next day she noticed dizziness, extremity weakness, and numbness. The extremity weakness had progressed to the point where she could not stand without assistance. During the past 24 hours, she had difficulty swallowing and frequently choked. She stated that she became short of breath during moderate exertion. She denied having dyspnea at rest, chest pain, cough, sputum, fever, or nausea.

QUESTIONS

1. What conditions are suggested by this medical history?

2. What is the significance of the patient's having difficulty swallowing?

3. What is the significance of the recent history of flu symptoms?

4. Should the patient be admitted? If so, why?

ANSWERS

1. The symptoms suggest either a neuromuscular disease (e.g., myasthenia gravis, GBS, ALS), or flu with dehydration.

2. The difficulty with swallowing is significant because it suggests that neuromuscular control of the gag reflex may be in jeopardy, which could result in aspiration.

3. A recent history of flu symptoms is common in patients with GBS. Approximately 65 percent of patients diagnosed with GBS have had a recent episode of respiratory or gastrointestinal flu within the previous 8 weeks.

4. This patient should be admitted because of her difficulty swallowing and because the respiratory muscles may weaken, resulting in a rapid onset of respiratory failure.

Physical Examination

General: The patient is alert, well oriented, and in no apparent distress. She is moderately obese for her height (height 5 feet 4 inches, weight 155 lb)

Vital Signs: Temperature 36.6°C (97.9°F), heart rate 88/minute, respiratory rate 20/minute, blood pressure 150/110 mm Hg

HEENT: Normocephalic with no signs of trauma; pupils equal, round, and reactive to light and accommodation (PERRLA); tympanic membranes intact; carotid pulses ++ bilaterally; trachea midline and without stridor; no ptosis noted, even upon repeated blinking

Lungs: Clear breath sounds bilaterally; normal chest configuration; no evidence of trauma

Heart: Irregular rate and rhythm without murmurs; normal first and second heart sounds (S_1 and S_2), with no third or fourth heart sounds (S_3 or S_4); point of maximal intensity not palpable

Abdomen: Obese, soft, nontender; positive bowel sounds; no hepatomegaly

Extremities: Deep tendon reflexes of the extremities absent; noticeable weakness of legs and feet; grip weak in both hands; no evidence of cyanosis, edema, or clubbing; extremities warm to touch

---

QUESTIONS

5. What are the key findings of the physical examination, and what problems do they suggest?

6. What may explain the hypertension and irregular heartbeat?

7. Why did the examining physician ask the patient to blink her eyelids repeatedly?

8. What neuromuscular disease usually causes an ascending paralysis, as seen in this case?

9. What laboratory and bedside tests would be useful in this case to identify the cause of the problem?

10. Should the attending physician administer the Tensilon test? What is the purpose of this test?

ANSWERS

5. The key findings on the physical examination are the muscular weakness and loss of deep tendon reflexes of the extremities, and the irregular heartbeat and hypertension. The extremity weakness and loss of reflexes suggests that the neuromuscular system is not functioning properly.

6. The hypertension and irregular heartbeat may indicate that the neuromuscular disease is involving the autonomic nervous system. It is also possible, however, that the irregular heartbeat is the result of an unrelated heart condition.

7. Asking the patient to blink repeatedly is useful to check for myasthenia gravis. The eyelids will rapidly tire and begin to droop if myasthenia gravis is present. In Ms. M's case, myasthenia gravis is not the likely diagnosis, as the eyelids remained functional.

8. GBS typically causes an ascending paralysis, as is seen in this case.

9. Laboratory tests that would be useful include a CSF protein count, a bedside analysis of VC and MIP, a complete blood count (CBC), and an electrolyte measurement. A chest radiograph may be useful to assess the condition of the lungs. An ABG assessment is not needed at this point, as there is no evidence of respiratory complications.

10. The Tensilon test is useful to confirm the diagnosis of myasthenia gravis. Because the evidence suggests that myasthenia gravis is not the cause of Ms. M's weakness, the Tensilon test would not be useful.

Laboratory Evaluation

CBC:

White blood cells (WBCs)	9.5 thousand/mm^3
Segmented neutrophils	71 percent
Bands	6 percent
Lymphocytes	14 percent
Monocytes	8 percent
Basophils	1 percent
Red blood cells (RBCs)	4.2 million/mm^3
Hemoglobin (Hb)	13 g/100 mL
Hematocrit (Hct)	38 percent

Electrolytes: Normal, except for reduced total CO_2 (21 mEq/liter)

MIP: −35 cm H_2O

Bedside VC: 2.4 liters (predicted normal 3.6 liters)

Chest Radiograph: Low lung volumes bilaterally with no evidence of infiltrates

---

QUESTIONS

11. How would you interpret the CBC results?

12. What could explain the reduced CO_2 on the electrolyte panel?

13. How would you interpret the bedside MIP and VC?

14. Is the chest radiograph consistent with the tentative diagnosis of neuromuscular disease? If so, why?

ANSWERS

11. The CBC is normal.

12. The reduced total CO_2 on the electrolyte panel represents reduced plasma HCO_3^-. This is commonly seen in patients who have been hyperventilating long enough for the kidneys to compensate for the resultant respiratory alkalosis by excreting plasma HCO_3^-. A reduced plasma HCO_3^- concentration also indicates metabolic acidosis.

13. The MIP and VC are reduced, which suggests that the respiratory muscles are probably affected by the disease and that the patient needs careful monitoring.

14. The chest radiograph finding of reduced lung volume is consistent with neuromuscular disease. As the inspiratory muscles weaken, the lung recoil is less opposed and the lung volumes tend to diminish.

CASE STUDY—continued

The diagnosis at this point was neuromuscular disease, probably due to GBS. Ms. M was admitted to the intensive care unit (ICU) for careful monitoring. A spinal tap was done to measure the CSF protein level, which was found to be elevated. This provided more evidence to support the diagnosis of GBS. Plasmapheresis was started. Four hours after admission, the patient began complaining of shortness of breath after minimal exertion. Bedside assessment revealed a VC of 1.6 liters and a MIP of -20 cm H_2O. The patient's respiratory rate had increased to 36/minute, and her heart rate was 128/minute. Her blood pressure remained moderately elevated. ABG results at this point were as follows: pH 7.45, $Paco_2$ 30 mm Hg, Pao_2 89 mm Hg, arterial oxygen saturation (Sao_2) 95.9 percent; HCO_3^- 19 mEq/liter on room air.

QUESTIONS

15. What is plasmapheresis, and why is it used to treat GBS?

16. How would you interpret the changes in the VC and MIP measurements?

17. How would you interpret the ABG results?

18. What therapy is indicated at this point?

ANSWERS

15. Plasmapheresis is the process of removing a portion of the patient's blood and centrifuging it to separate the blood cells from the plasma. The plasma is discarded, and the remaining blood cells are mixed with fresh plasma and reinfused into the patient. The purpose of plasmapheresis is to dilute the offending antibody present in the plasma.

16. The VC and MIP are reduced significantly from the previous measurement. This suggests that the respiratory muscles are weaker and that the patient is at high risk for respiratory failure.

17. The ABG results demonstrate compensated respiratory alkalosis with adequate oxygenation on room air. The ABG results reflect adequate lung function. Respiratory failure, however, may occur in the very near future despite the relatively normal ABG results.

18. Based on the downward trend of decreasing respiratory muscle strength, increasing respiratory rate, and increasing dyspnea, intubation and mechanical ventilation are indicated. It is usually better to perform the intubation while the patient with neuromuscular disease remains somewhat stable. Once respiratory failure is present, attempts to intubate are often rushed and the patient is at greater risk for complications.

CASE STUDY—continued

After being given an explanation regarding the procedure, Ms. M was intubated nasally and placed on mechanical ventilation. Initial settings were assist-control mode with a backup rate of 12/minute and a tidal volume (V_T) of 800 mL, a fraction of inspired oxygen (F_{IO_2}) of 0.35, and no positive end-expiratory pressure (PEEP). A chest film confirmed appropriate placement of the endotracheal tube. The ABG results 20 minutes after the initiation of mechanical ventilation with a mechanical rate of 16/minute were as follows: pH 7.45, Pa_{CO_2} 32 mm Hg, Pa_{O_2} 105 mm Hg, HCO_3^- 20 mEq/liter, and Sa_{O_2} 98 percent. The patient continued to complain of weakness and extremity numbness.

QUESTIONS

19. What changes in the ventilator settings would you suggest based on the ABG findings.

20. What complications should be anticipated in this case?

21. What should the patient be told about her prognosis?

22. Should a tracheostomy be performed to avoid permanent damage to the larynx by the endotracheal tube?

ANSWERS

19. Because the oxygenation is more than adequate, a slight reduction in the F_{IO_2} from 0.35 to 0.30 is reasonable. A reduction in the mechanical $\dot{V}_E$ would help increase the Pa_{CO_2} to normal range. This could be accomplished by reducing the V_T; however, a smaller V_T may promote atelectasis. Lowering the backup rate may decrease the minute volume, but only if the patient does not trigger the ventilator. Sedation may help reduce the patient's anxiety and reduce the hyperventilation. An alternative would be to switch the ventilator to the intermittent mandatory ventilation (IMV) mode (see Chapter 3). This would allow the patient to take spontaneous breaths between the mechanical breaths and should lower the overall minute volume. The IMV rate should be set high enough, however, to maintain adequate ventilation and allow the muscles to rest (e.g., 10 to 12/minute).

20. Complications in this case could include pulmonary embolus, atelectasis, pneumonia, cardiovascular compromise from the mechanical ventilation, and pneumothorax.

21. The patient should be told that a full recovery is expected. A majority of GBS patients recover fully within a few weeks or months.

22. At this point, a tracheostomy is not needed. It is possible that the patient will recover enough to breathe on her own within 1 to 2 weeks. A tracheostomy should be considered if after 7 to 10 days the patient has not made any progress toward recovery.

CASE STUDY—continued

During the next week, Ms. M was maintained on mechanical ventilation with an IMV rate of 10/minute and a mechanical V_T of 800 mL. Plasmapheresis was repeated daily. The patient's spontaneous V_T varied but usually was in the range of 200 to 300 mL. On day 7 her MIP was −25 cm H_2O, and she stated that she felt stronger. The bilateral extremity numbness was greatly reduced, and her grip was noticeably stronger. Her vital signs remained stable except for an elevation in body temperature to 38.3°C (100.9°F). Secretions suctioned from the endotracheal tube were white. The chest radiograph demonstrated bibasilar atelectasis. The ABG findings on day 7 were as follows: pH 7.43, $Paco_2$ 36 mm Hg, Pao_2 84 mm Hg, and Fio_2 0.30.

QUESTIONS

23. What treatment should be given for the bibasilar atelectasis?

24. Should weaning from mechanical ventilation be started? Why or why not?

ANSWERS

23. The bibasilar atelectasis should be treated with chest physical therapy and postural drainage. Frequent changes in position and occasional deep breaths with the volume ventilator may also be helpful. The sputum sample should be sent to the laboratory for a Gram stain and culture. If the sputum demonstrates numerous pus cells and bacterial growth, antibiotics should be started.

24. It appears that the patient is improving, but weaning from mechanical ventilation should not begin until the fever and atelectasis have cleared.

CASE STUDY—continued

On day 14 the patient had a normal body temperature, and the chest radiograph demonstrated significant clearing of the infiltrates. The weaning parameters at this point were VC 2.1 liters, MIP −35 cm H_2O, and spontaneous V_T 350 mL. The patient tolerated an IMV rate of 4/minute, which yielded normal ABG results. On the evening of day 14 the patient was extubated, and she tolerated the procedure well. She stated that she still felt weak but much improved. Her cough was weak but improved daily. Her breath sounds remained clear and vital signs stable. Neurologic examination revealed improved deep tendon reflexes and nearly normal responses to stimuli. The patient was transferred from the ICU to the rehabilitation unit on day 18 and was sent home on day 21 without further complications.

CAST STUDY NO. 2

History

BR is a 62-year-old man with a 6-month history of ALS. Approximately 8 months earlier, he noticed weakness in his hands and legs. His initial problem involved gripping objects such as a cup or doorknob. He then had difficulty getting out of a chair. The disease had progressed rapidly over the last 6 months until he was unable to walk, grip anything, or lift anything more 1 to 2 lb with his arms. Speaking had become more difficult, but his mind was clear and he still communicated well with his family. His neurologist had referred him for an evaluation of his respiratory status.

BR was experiencing mild dyspnea, most notably when he talked or assisted in transferring himself to a wheelchair. His family noted that he could not complete a sentence without stopping to catch his breath. When he was at rest and not talking, he appeared in no distress. One month before his visit, he acquired pneumonia of the right lower lobe, which was treated with ampicillin and resolved.

No other significant problems in BR's past history were identified. He was a dentist who had been in practice until 8 months ago, when the ALS was first discovered.

BR understood that this disease would lead to respiratory failure and was terminal. He felt that his quality of life was good enough at present and that he would like to have ventilatory support, if needed, to prolong his life. In addition, BR expressed that if his ALS progressed to the point where his quality of life did not warrant continued ventilatory support, he would like to have mechanical ventilation discontinued at that time.

QUESTIONS

1. What part of the nervous system does ALS affect, and what is the etiology of the disease?

2. The initial sign of BR's muscle weakness was a weak grip. Is this pattern of weakness typical of proximal or distal muscle weakness?

3. Is it reasonable to provide mechanical ventilation for BR considering that his disease is progressive and terminal?

4. If you were to initiate mechanical ventilation for BR and he later decided he wanted to stop ventilatory support and die, should you assist his death by discontinuing mechanical ventilation?

5. What characteristic muscle movements would you expect to see during your examination of the patient?

ANSWERS

1. ALS is a degenerative disease of motor neurons that has no known cause. The disease specifically destroys the Betz neurons in the cerebral cortex and the motor neurons in the anterior horns of the spinal cord.

2. Weakness of the hands and feet are signs of distal muscle weakness. The fact that distal muscle weakness was the initial symptom suggests that the disease is a neuromuscular disorder such as ALS or GBS. Proximal muscle weakness is characteristically seen in the arm and thigh, most notably when a patient gets up from a chair. Proximal muscle weakness is characteristic of muscle diseases such as muscular dystrophy.

3. Patients do have the right to decide which therapies they are willing to undergo (see Chapter 2). Because BR is approaching respiratory failure, mechanical ventilation is a treatment option. Ideally, one of the roles of health care providers is to educate patients regarding the benefits and costs of such therapy. It is important that BR's caregivers inform him of the discomfort associated with such therapy, as well as the intrusion into his life associated with mechanical ventilation. In addition, he needs to understand the nature and prognosis of the disease process that led to the requirement for this therapy. Only after patients (or close family members) have been fully educated in all aspects of their disease and the proposed therapy can they make an educated decision.

4. As discussed in the previous answer, the patient has the right to decide whether to initiate therapy and when to terminate therapy. If BR were to decide to discontinue life support, it would probably be wise to make certain that he arrived at his decision after careful consideration, and that the family understands and respects the decision before discontinuing mechanical support.

5. Muscle fasciculations, which are characterized by a visible twitching of muscle fibers from the affected muscles, develop in ALS patients.

Physical Examination

General: Patient sitting in wheelchair and in no respiratory distress; vital signs stable; respiratory rate 24/minute

Head and Neck: No significant abnormalities

Heart: Regular, with a normal rate; both S_1 and S_2 normal; no murmurs

Lungs: A few fine, inspiratory crackles heard over the bases of both lungs; weak cough

Abdomen: Soft, nontender; normal, active bowel sounds; no masses palpated

Extremities: Equal pulses in all extremities; no peripheral edema noted

Neurological: Alert, articulate; short sentences spoken, with pauses to take a breath every three to five words; cranial nerve function normal except for weakness of sternocleidomastoid, trapezius, and facial muscles; sensory examination normal; extreme weakness of extremities revealed upon motor examination; legs move and gestures weak; fasciculations noted over forearm and thigh muscles

---

QUESTIONS

6. In this setting, what is the most likely reason for BR's pulmonary crackles? Why do the crackles remain after coughing?

7. What tests are most important in determining when mechanical ventilation should be instituted?

8. Should the patient be admitted to the hospital at this time?

ANSWERS

6. The principal pulmonary problem that patients with neuromuscular disease have is weakness of the respiratory pump. Weakness of respiratory muscles predisposes patients to difficulty expanding lung units, resulting in atelec-

tasis. In addition, these patients may have difficulty clearing secretions; thus atelectasis may develop as a result of mucus plugging. In patients with neuromuscular disease the airway may not be protected, which is why aspiration and subsequent pneumonia can develop.

The profound respiratory muscle weakness that is common among patients with neuromuscular disease makes it difficult for these patients to breath deeply and cough well enough to reverse atelectasis completely.

7. The test that is most commonly used to determine whether patients with neuromuscular disease require mechanical ventilation is the measurement of VC. If the VC is less than 1 liter, then mechanical ventilation is usually indicated.

8. If mechanical ventilation becomes necessary, the patient will then be admitted, and both the patient and family will be trained in the use of the ventilator. The physician may need to perform a tracheostomy if long-term mechanical ventilation is required.

Laboratory Evaluation

CBC:

	Observed	*Normal*
WBCs/mm^3	5100	4000–11,000
RBCs (million/mm^3)	4.2	4.1–5.5
Hb (g/dL)	14	14–16.5
Hct (%)	41	37–50
Differential		
Segmented neutrophils (%)	61	38–79
Bands (%)	4	0–7
Lymphocytes (%)	29	12–51
Monocytes (%)	5	0–10
Eosinophils (%)	1	0–8
Basophils(%)	0	0–2

CHEMISTRY:

	Observed	*Normal*
Na$^+$ (mEq/liter)	141	136–146
K$^+$ (mEq/liter)	4.2	3.5–5.1
Cl$^-$ (mEq/liter)	93	98–106
HCO$_3^-$ (mEq/liter)	37	22–29
Blood urea nitrogen (mg/dL)	8	7–18
Creatinine (mg/dL)	0.5	0.5–1.1
Calcium (mmol/liter)	2.2	2.1–2.55
Phosphate (mg/dL)	2.9	2.7–4.5
Uric acid (mg/dL)	2.1	4.5–8.2
Albumin (g/dL)	3.9	3.5–5.0
Protein (g/dL)	7.2	6.4–8.3

Chest Radiograph: See Figure 17–3

ABG (on room air):

pH	7.38
PaO_2	67 mm Hg
$PaCO_2$	58 mm Hg
HCO_3^-	33 mEq/liter
Alveolar-arterial oxygen gradient ($P[A-a]O_2$)	10 mm Hg
O_2 content	16.8 mL/dL

Spirometry:

Forced vital capacity (FVC)	0.92 liters
Negative inspiratory pressure	-12 cm H_2O

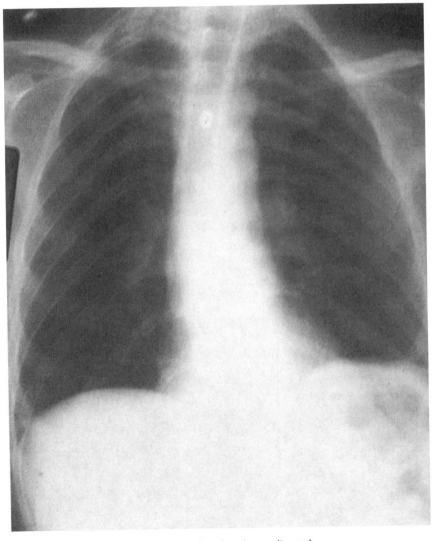

FIGURE 17–3   Portable chest radiograph.

QUESTIONS

9. How would you interpret the chest radiograph?

10. How would you interpret the results of the ABG?

11. How would you interpret the spirometry results?

12. What treatment options would you recommend to the physician at this point?

ANSWERS

9. The lungs are hyperinflated as a result of preexisting COPD. A slight degree of scoliosis is visible.

10. The ABG indicates chronic respiratory acidosis, indicating that the hypoxemia is primarily due to the hypoventilation. The $P(A-a)O_2$ is normal.

11. The spirometry is consistent with profound respiratory muscle weakness.

12. Having chronic respiratory acidosis and profound respiratory muscle weakness, this patient is at risk for acute respiratory failure due to ALS. This patient wanted to begin mechanical ventilation when necessary, and this is an appropriate time to do so. The patient should be admitted and educated, along with the family members, regarding the procedure.

    There are two different mechanical-ventilation options for patients in neuromuscular respiratory failure. One option is to perform a tracheostomy and initiate volume-cycled mechanical ventilation; the other option is to begin mechanical ventilation with nasal mask intermittent positive-pressure ventilation (NIPPV). The advantage of the second option is that no tracheostomy is required. At home, NIPPV or a negative-pressure body respirator may prove useful.

CASE STUDY—continued

BR was admitted to the hospital. NIPPV was instituted for nocturnal use. The patient and family were instructed in the use of the ventilator, and after a few days of stabilization on the new regimen, the patient was discharged home.

For several weeks after the institution of NIPPV, the patient felt more energetic and found breathing and talking easier. His ABGs improved, showing a normal $PaCO_2$ during NIPPV use and during the daytime.

Over the next several months his functioning deteriorated as the ALS progressed. His ventilatory requirements increased, and his breathlessness worsened. He found that he required NIPPV 24 hours a day and could not easily talk or communicate with his family. He was now unable to perform even the simplest task without assistance. At this point BR decided that the cost of the NIPPV was greater than the benefits he was deriving. He did not want tracheostomy or other, more invasive forms of mechanical ventilation. He decided he would stop using the NIPPV. He and his family fully understood the consequences of this step. After talking with his family and caregivers, he stopped the ventilator on his own. He died a few minutes later.

REFERENCES

1. West, JB: Control of ventilation. In West, JB (ed): Respiratory Physiology. Williams & Wilkins, Baltimore, 1985, p 113.
2. Rochester, OF, and Findley, LJ: The lungs and neuromuscular and chest wall diseases. In Murray, JF, and Nadel, JA (eds): Textbook of Respiratory Medicine. WB Saunders, Philadelphia, 1988.
3. Marini, JJ: Monitoring during mechanical ventilation. Clin Chest Med 9:73, 1988.
4. Derdak, S: Guillain-Barré. In Civetta, JM, et al (eds): Critical Care. JB Lippincott, Philadelphia, 1988, p 1251.
5. Andreoloi, TE, et al (eds): Cecil's Essentials of Medicine. WB Saunders, Philadelphia, 1986, p 721.
6. Derdak, S: Myasthenia gravis. In Civetta, JM, et al (eds): Critical Care. JB Lippincott, Philadelphia, 1988, p 1257.
7. Fallat, RJ, et al: Spirometry in amyotrophic lateral sclerosis. Arch Neurol 36:74, 1979.
8. Ledsome, RJ, and Sharp, JM: Pulmonary function in acute cervical cord injury. Am Rev Respir Dis 124:41, 1981.
9. Luce, JM: Neuromuscular diseases leading to respiratory failure. In Hall, JB, et al (eds): Principles of Critical Care. McGraw-Hill, New York, 1992, pp 1783–1792.
10. Ropper, AH: Severe acute Guillian-Barré syndrome. Neurology 36:429, 1986.
11. Gracey, DR, et al: Plasmapheresis in the treatment of ventilator-dependent myasthenia gravis patients. Chest 85:739, 1984.
12. Dau, PC: Respiratory failure in myasthenia gravis. Chest 85:721, 1985.
13. Holtackers, TR, et al: The use of the chest cuirass in respiratory failure of neurologic origin. Respir Care 27:271, 1982.
14. Curran, FJ: Night ventilation by body respirators for patients in chronic respiratory failure due to late stage Duchenne muscular dystrophy. Arch Phys Med Rehabil 62:270, 1981.
15. Hess, DR, and Kacmarek, RM: Essentials of Mechanical Ventilation. McGraw-Hill, New York, 1996, p 115.
16. Leger, P, et al: Home positive pressure ventilation via nasal mask for patients with neuromuscular weakness or restrictive lung or chest-wall disease. Respir Care 34:73, 1989.

CHAPTER 18

Bacterial Pneumonia

Robert L. Wilkins, PhD, RRT
James R. Dexter, MD, FCCP

Key Terms

bronchopneumonia
community-acquired
   pneumonia
lobar pneumonia

necrotizing pneumonia
nosocomial pneumonia
Pneumocystis carinii
   pneumonia

pneumonia
viral pneumonia

Introduction

The term **pneumonia** refers to inflammation of the lung parenchyma and is most often used to describe inflammation caused by infection. Pneumonia is caused by a variety of infectious agents, including bacteria, viruses, and fungi; however, this chapter focuses on bacterial pneumonia. This type of pneumonia continues to be a common medical problem despite the advent of antibiotics, and it is now is returning as a serious public health problem because of the emergence of antibiotic-resistant organisms.

Each year approximately four million persons contract pneumonia in the United States, about one fifth of whom need to be hospitalized.[1] Most cases of pneumonia are contracted outside the hospital and are referred to as **community-acquired pneumonia.** This type of pneumonia is often easily treated on an outpatient basis. Pneumonia that occurs in the hospitalized patient is referred to as **nosocomial pneumonia.** Although other types of nosocomial infections (e.g., urinary tract infection) occur more often in hospitalized patients, pneumonia is the most common fatal nosocomial infection. Pneumonia represents a more serious medical problem among hospitalized and elderly patients whose immune systems are often inadequate.

Etiology

The distal airways are usually sterile because of the wide variety of mechanical and chemical systems that protect the lungs from infectious agents (Table 18–1). These

TABLE 18-1   **Summary of the Protective Mechanisms of the Respiratory System**

Mechanical
    Filtration by nares
    Sneezing
    Gag reflex
    Cough
    Ciliary movement
Immunological
    Phagocytosis by macrophages and leukocytes
    Immunoglobulins, such as IgA, in secretions
    Cell-mediated immunity
    Opsonization by complement

protective systems may be sabotaged by factors such as cigarette smoking, alcohol abuse, chronic lung disease, neuromuscular disease, or acute viral upper respiratory tract infection. Pneumonia is increasingly common in the elderly and those with co-existing illness.[1] Neuromuscular disorders are particularly troublesome because they may reduce the effectiveness of the patient's cough and interfere with the protective reflexes of the upper airway that prevent aspiration.

The distal airways can become contaminated with pathogenic organisms once the protective upper airway mechanisms are damaged. Infection is much more likely if the defense mechanisms of the lower airways are also compromised or if the organism is particularly virulent. Systemic disorders such as diabetes, cirrhosis, renal failure, malnutrition, acquired immune deficiency syndrome (AIDS), or cancer may render the patient's immune system compromised and contribute to the onset of pneumonia (Table 18-2). AIDS patients frequently acquire *Pneumocystis carinii* **pneumonia.** The use of steroids can suppress a patient's immune system and may contribute to the onset of pneumonia. For example, steroids used to treat obstructive lung disease may contribute to the onset of atypical infections in the lung, such as fungal pneumonia.[2]

In addition to aspiration, potentially pathogenic organisms can enter the lung by inhalation and through the blood stream. Inhalation of small pathogen-carrying droplets is not common when the upper airway is healthy and capable of filtering the inspired gas. If the upper airway is diseased or bypassed, as with tracheotomy or intubation, organisms are more likely to be deposited in the lower airways. Systemic infections may result in the offending organism's traveling to the lung via blood flow. Once the organism reaches the lung from the blood stream or airways and begins to grow, pneumonia is likely to result.

Pathology and Pathophysiology

Infections of the lung parenchyma incite a reaction that causes an outpouring of fluid, inflammatory proteins, and white blood cells (WBCs). Interstitial and alveolar spaces become flooded with edema and exudative material. The inflammatory exudate makes the distal lung spaces dense and consolidated. Some cases of bacterial pneumonia are limited to small areas of lung parenchyma, but others quickly spread to surrounding tissue and to the pleura and pericardium.

Some bacterial organisms such as *Staphylococcus* and *Pseudomonas* can become severe enough to permanently damage lung tissue. Pneumonia causing permanent damage to the lung tissue is called **necrotizing pneumonia.**

TABLE 18-2   **Factors That Predispose Patients to Pneumonia**

PULMONARY FACTORS
Airway disease
    Chronic bronchitis
    Asthma
    Bronchiectasis
    Obstructed bronchus due to tumor
    Positive smoking history
Poor cough
    Neuromuscular disease
    Emphysema
    Abdominal pain
    Drug overdose
Reduced gag reflex and aspiration
    Drug overdose
    Alcohol abuse
    Stroke
    Neuromuscular disease

SYSTEMIC FACTORS
Immunosuppression
    Leukemia
    Chemotherapy
    AIDS
    Transplantation
Chronic systemic disease
    Diabetes
    Cirrhosis
    Renal failure
    Heart failure

IATROGENIC PROCEDURES
Intubation
Mechanical ventilation
Use of humidifiers and aerosol generators
Lack of hand washing
Lack of sterile technique

Acute inflammation and consolidation of the lung leads to a reduction in ventilation and gas exchange in the affected region. Perfusion of the affected lung segments in areas that have poor ventilation results in severe ventilation-perfusion ($\dot{V}/\dot{Q}$) mismatching, or shunt.

Lung consolidation associated with pneumonia reduces lung compliance in the affected region. This increases the patient's work of breathing and causes a sensation of breathlessness. Lung volumes are typically reduced during the acute stages of pneumonia, but will usually return to normal once the infection resolves.

Clinical Features

The patient with bacterial pneumonia usually complains of fever, cough, and sputum production and may complain of shortness of breath and chest pain. Dyspnea is more common when the pneumonia involves multiple regions of the lung or when it is superimposed on chronic pulmonary disease. When chest pain is present, it is usually pleuritic. Symptoms such as headache, skin rash, and diarrhea may be present with some types of pneumonia. The past medical history is often positive for a chronic systemic or pulmonary disorder in the patient with acute pneumonia. The patient with a past history of chronic obstructive pulmonary disease (COPD) is prone to pneumonia.

The patient often appears acutely ill at the onset of common bacterial pneumonia. Assessment of the vital signs often reveals a rapid heart and respiratory rate. Rapid breathing occurs with the drop in lung compliance and when fever or hypoxemia is present. Fever increases the patient's metabolic rate, which increases demand on the heart and lungs to provide additional oxygen to the tissues.

In the presence of severe pneumonia, inspection may reveal cyanosis and use of accessory muscles to breathe. A unilateral reduction in chest expansion may be seen with lobar pneumonia. This finding results from the poor expansion of the involved lobe caused by consolidation. Increased tactile fremitus and bronchial breath sounds are commonly found over the consolidated lung if the lobar bronchus associated with the affected region is patent. Sound travels more readily through consolidated lung tissue, so the turbulent flow sounds of the larger airways are more easily heard over areas of consolidation. The breath sounds will be markedly diminished or absent if the bronchus is obstructed. Reduced resonance to percussion is present over areas of consolidated lung. Inspiratory crackles are often present. Coarse crackles imply excessive airway mucus

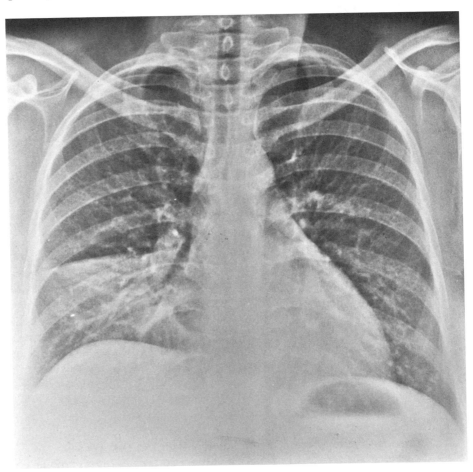

FIGURE 18–1   Lobar pneumonia as seen on posteroanterior (PA) chest radiograph. In this case the pneumonia is located in the right middle lobe.

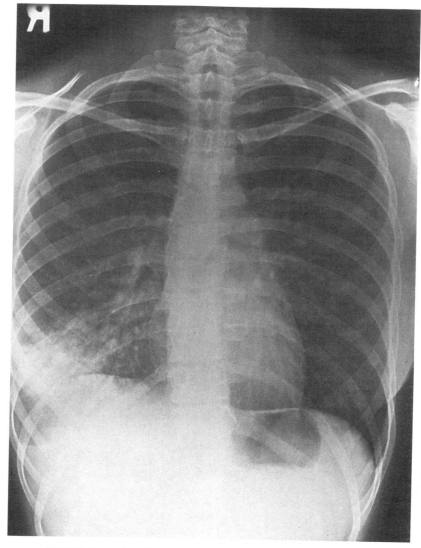

FIGURE 18-2   Bronchopneumonia as seen on PA chest radiograph.

and are a common finding late in the course of bacterial pneumonia. A pleural friction rub may be present when pleural inflammation is complicating the pneumonia.

Examination of the peripheral blood sample will reveal leukocytosis in most cases of bacterial pneumonia. Acute bacterial infection stimulates the bone marrow to increase the neutrophils in the circulating blood. As the infection worsens, the number of immature WBCs (bands) also increases. Leukopenia is seen in cases of severe bacterial pneumonia that overwhelm the immune system. A normal WBC count is commonly encountered with *Mycoplasma* or nonbacterial pneumonias.

The chest radiograph is almost always abnormal when pneumonia is present. It also provides information about the extent of lung involvement and the onset of complications such as pleural effusion. Radiographic changes associated with pneumonia include areas of increased density with air bronchograms. In some cases, the pneumonia may involve an entire lobe (**lobar pneumonia**), whereas in other cases the infiltrates occur along the airways and have a patchy segmental distribution (**bronchopneumonia**) (Figs. 18-1 and 18-2). Necrotizing pneumonia produces areas of radiolucency (caused by lung destruction) seen in the areas of increased density. **Viral pneumonia** most often causes interstitial infiltrates throughout both lungs (Fig. 18-3). The chest film may take as long as 3 months to clear completely after bacterial pneumonia. There is no need to document complete resolution of the infiltrate if the patient improves clinically unless he or she is at risk for bronchogenic carcinoma (e.g., a cigarette smoker more than 40 years of age).

Arterial blood gases (ABGs) often reveal hypoxemia and respiratory alkalosis. Respiratory acidosis is uncommon unless the patient also has COPD or neuromuscular disease.

Microbiological evaluation of sputum is done in an effort to identify the pathogen responsible for the respiratory infection and is best performed before antibiotics are administered. In many cases, a representative sample of lung pathogens is difficult to obtain because most sputum specimens are contaminated with oral secretions as they pass through the mouth. Screening of the sputum sample is useful to identify significant contamination with oral secretions. Sputum samples should be discarded when 10 or more squamous epithelial cells per low-power field (lpf) are present because this signifies that the sample is heavily contaminated by oral secretions. A good sample is recognized by identifying many (greater than 25/lpf) polymorphonuclear WBCs in the presence of few epithelial cells. A Gram stain and culture are more likely to be helpful when a good specimen has been obtained. The Gram stain does not take long, and often (40 to 60 percent of the time) identifies the general category of bacteria causing the infection. If positive, the Gram stain allows the physician to start more specific antibiotic therapy before culture results are available. Cultures may identify the specific pathogen responsible for a pneumonia, and the sensitivity testing identifies effective antibiotics for the organism.

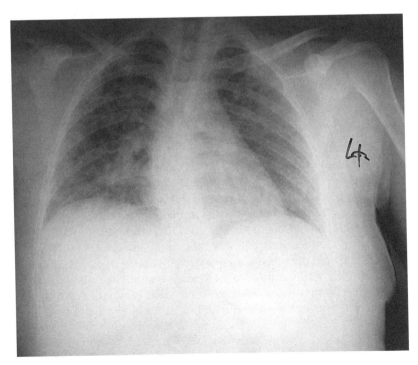

FIGURE 18-3   Viral pneumonia as seen on PA chest radiograph.

Many severely ill patients with pneumonia have trouble expectorating a sputum sample. In these cases, invasive procedures such as transtracheal and transthoracic aspiration, bronchoscopy, and open lung biopsy are needed to obtain a representative sputum sample.

Treatment

Some patients may be treated for pneumonia as outpatients, but severe cases should be managed in the hospital. Severe pneumonia is more common in the elderly and those with a coexisting illness. The criteria for severe pneumonia are listed in Table 18-3. Severe cases generally require supportive care, including fluid and nutritional therapy. Oxygen therapy is important in the presence of hypoxemia; 3 to 5 liters/minute by nasal cannula is adequate unless the pneumonia is widespread. Aerosol or humidity therapy can be useful when thick secretions are difficult to expectorate. Chest physical therapy is not useful in treating the typical case of bacterial pneumonia unless it is complicated by bronchiectasis.[3] Respiratory failure requiring mechanical ventilation is uncommon unless the pneumonia is unusually severe or is superimposed on a chronic lung disease.

The attending physician can predict the offending organism causing the pneumonia in most cases simply by careful bedside examination or radiographic analysis. Therefore, the choice and dosage of initial antibiotic therapy is necessarily determined *empirically* (i.e., on the basis of experience) in most cases. The initial empirical antibiotic therapy is based on the severity of the pneumonia and the presence of either coexisting illness or advanced age (more than 65 years).[1] Patients with severe pneumonia, coexisting illness, or advanced age often have different pathogens causing the infection compared to other patient groups, and therefore they need a different antibiotic therapy.

An appropriate antibiotic should be started as soon as possible, although several days of the drug are needed to reach full effectiveness. In the patient who is not severely ill, a short delay in the onset of antibiotic therapy is reasonable while appropriate sputum and blood samples are obtained. The preliminary diagnostic results, such as the Gram stain and chest x-ray, may provide important clues regarding the offending organism. If gram-positive, elongated diplococci typical of pneumococci are seen, penicillin is the drug of choice. The presence of gram-negative coccobacilli on the sputum sample suggests that ampicillin or a second-generation cephalosporin would be preferred. Once the culture results are available, the most specific agent that is effective against the offending organism should be given. In many cases, however, the responsible pathogen is not identified, even with extensive testing.[4]

The decision to admit the patient with pneumonia is based not only on the severity of the infection, but also on the presence of certain risk factors.[5] Patients with ad-

TABLE 18-3   **Criteria for Diagnosis of Severe Pneumonia***

Respiratory rate > 30/minute at rest
$PaO_2 < 60$ mm Hg on $FIO_2 > 0.30$
Chest radiograph showing multiple lobe involvement
Evidence of shock (systolic BP < 90 mm Hg or diastolic BP < 60 mm Hg)
Low urine output (<20 mL/hour)

*Severe pneumonia is diagnosed when a patient presents with one or more of these clinical signs.

vanced age, coexisting illness, high fever, or leukopenia are at greater risk for severe, life-threatening pneumonia and should be more strongly considered for admission.

The patient admitted for pneumonia is at risk for acquiring a nosocomial infection (*superinfection*), especially if the patient requires ventilator therapy.[6,7] Careful hand washing between visits with each patient and use of sterile technique during airway care is crucial for preventing the spread of organisms from one patient to the next in the intensive care unit (ICU). This point is emphasized by the fact that many nosocomial pneumonias are caused by gram-negative organisms, which are spread most commonly by fluid and contact with another person's hands. Gram-negative organisms are often relatively resistant to therapy, which makes treatment difficult and increases the risk of infection-related death.

CASE STUDY

History

MC is a 60-year-old black man who lives in his 1958 Nash Rambler. He earns money by collecting aluminum cans along the roadside and from trash dumpsters. He states that he has been coughing up about ¼ cup of white sputum each morning for the past 20 years. About 1 week ago, he noticed a sudden onset of shaking, chills, fever, sweating, malaise, chest pain, and shortness of breath at rest. He also began coughing up rust-colored sputum that was thicker than his normal sputum production. MC admits to current consumption of two packs per day of cigarettes (i.e., a 70 pack-year smoking history). He admits to occasional alcohol use but denies having orthopnea, ankle edema, nausea, vomiting, diarrhea, weight loss, dysuria, wheezing, or hemoptysis.

QUESTIONS

1. What are the key symptoms in this case, and what disease do they suggest?
2. What is the significance of the place of residence and source of income?
3. What is the significance of the smoking history?
4. What is the significance of the patient's chronic sputum production?
5. What physical examination techniques are useful in this case, and what purpose do they serve?

ANSWERS

1. The key symptoms in this case are fever, sputum production, shortness of breath, and chest pain. These symptoms strongly suggest pneumonia.
2. The fact that MC lives in his car and earns money from collecting aluminum cans suggests that he may not have adequate nutritional intake. This decreases immune response and makes him more prone to pneumonia. It also makes him more likely to develop a severe or overwhelming pneumonia.
3. MC's smoking history is very significant and suggests that he is a candidate for lung cancer, COPD, and heart disease. COPD would increase his susceptibility to infections. His current use of cigarettes adds to his susceptibility to pneumonia, since they reduce the defensive mechanisms of the lung.
4. Chronic sputum production is typical of patients with chronic bronchitis.

Poor clearance of secretions in the lung makes infection, including pneumonia, more common.

5. The physical examination should begin with a general assessment and evaluation of the patient's vital signs. This will help assess the severity of MC's illness and provides a baseline for later comparison. The chest should be inspected for chest wall configuration and breathing pattern, percussed for resonance, palpated for tactile fremitus, and auscultated for the presence of bronchial breath sounds, adventitious lung sounds, and pleural friction rubs. This will help identify the presence of lung consolidation and help determine whether the pleura is involved. The heart should be auscultated for evidence of failure (gallops) and murmurs. The extremities are examined for the presence of cyanosis, edema, or clubbing. The examiner should look for evidence of COPD.

Physical Examination

General: Chronically ill–appearing elderly male in mild to moderate respiratory distress at rest; alert, oriented to person and place, and of nearly normal intellect, with long-term memory better than short-term

Vital Signs: Temperature 39°C (102.2°F), heart rate 122/minute, respiratory rate 32/minute, blood pressure 110/60 mm Hg, height 150 cm, weight 65 kg

HEENT: Cyanosis of the lips and mouth

Neck: Supple with full active range of motion; trachea midline and mobile and without stridor or wheezing; carotid pulsation ++ and symmetrical with no bruits; mild supraclavicular and cervical lymphadenopathy bilaterally; no jugular venous distention

Chest: Anteroposterior diameter abnormally large, with diminished excursion noted on right side with each inspiratory effort; diminished resonance to percussion and increased tactile fremitus noted over right lower lobe posteriorly

Lungs: Bronchial breath sounds over right lower lobe posteriorly; clear but diminished breath sounds over entire left lung and right middle and upper lobes; pleural friction rub heard over right lateral chest wall

Heart: Regular rate and rhythm; no murmurs, gallops, or rubs noted; point of maximal impulse felt in epigastric area

Abdomen: Normal in appearance, without tenderness to palpation; bowel sounds present; no masses, and no organomegaly

Extremities: Cool, moist, and slightly dusky; cyanosis noted in fingertips; no clubbing or edema; pulses slightly diminished and symmetrical

QUESTIONS

6. What is the significance of the patient's poor short-term memory?
7. How would you interpret the vital signs?
8. What is the significance of an increase in anteroposterior diameter?
9. What explains the unilateral chest expansion?
10. What explains the decrease in resonance and increase in tactile fremitus?
11. What is the cause and significance of the bronchial breath sounds?

12. What is the significance of the pleural friction rub?

13. Why are the extremities cool, moist, and dusky?

14. What laboratory tests are useful in this case?

ANSWERS

6. Poor memory is an indication of reduced mental acuity and may be related to a number of adverse events, including hypoxia, alcohol abuse, sepsis, and chronic disease. Short-term memory is usually affected more severely by any cerebral insult compared to long-term memory.

7. The vital signs demonstrate fever, tachycardia, and tachypnea. The blood pressure is within normal limits, though on the low end of normal. These findings are consistent with a more severe case of acute pneumonia.

8. The increase in anteroposterior diameter is consistent with COPD. Since COPD is a common predisposing factor for pneumonia, and since it may influence treatment, clinicians should be careful to note such findings.

9. A unilateral reduction in chest expansion is commonly seen in lobar pneumonia. The affected lobe does not expand as well as the unaffected side with inspiration and lags behind the normal contralateral side.

10. The decrease in resonance with percussion suggests that the tissue underlying the chest wall in the affected region is dense, which is common with pneumonia. Other conditions, such as pleural effusion and lung tumors, may cause the same finding. An increase in tactile fremitus is also consistent with lung consolidation. The vibrations generated at the larynx travel much better through dense lung tissue compared to air-filled tissue.

11. The bronchial breath sounds are consistent with lung consolidation. The turbulent flow sounds of the larger airways travel through consolidated lung more directly as compared to normal air-filled lung. The bronchus leading into the affected lung region must be patent to hear bronchial breath sounds over the affected region.

12. The pleural friction rub suggests that pleural inflammation is present. This finding indicates that the pneumonia is adjacent to the pleura.

13. The extremities are cool, moist, and cyanotic because of the release of catecholamines in response to stress. The catecholamines cause sweating and peripheral vasoconstriction, which reduces blood flow to the extremities. As a result, the hands and feet become sweaty, cool, and cyanotic.

14. Useful laboratory tests in this case would include a complete blood count (CBC), blood culture, chemistry profile, sputum Gram stain with culture and sensitivity, ABG, and chest x-ray.

Laboratory Evaluation

CBC: WBCs 4000/mm^3, segmented neutrophils 60 percent, bands 30 percent, lymphocytes 10 percent, hemoglobin 10.4 g

ABG on room air: pH 7.47, Paco$_2$ 32 mm Hg, Pao$_2$ 44 mm Hg, HCO$_3^-$ 23 mEq/liter

Chest X-Ray: Right middle lobe consolidation; right heart border not visible (Fig. 18–4)

Sputum: Numerous gram-positive cocci with many WBCs and no epithelial cells

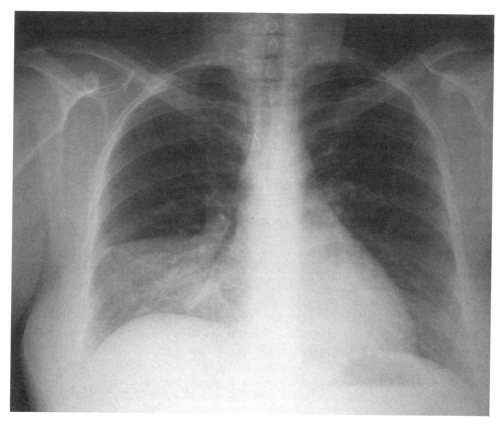

FIGURE 18-4   Right middle lobe pneumonia as seen on PA chest radiograph.

QUESTIONS

15. How would you interpret the CBC?

16. How would you interpret the ABG results? Why are the $Paco_2$ and Pao_2 reduced?

17. What is the significance of the lack of visibility of the right heart border on the chest x-ray?

18. What is the significance of gram-positive cocci found on the sputum Gram stain? What is the significance of the numerous WBCs and no epithelial cells?

19. Should this patient be treated as an outpatient, on the ward, or in the ICU?

20. What treatment should be provided?

ANSWERS

15. The reduced WBC count in the presence of infection is consistent with an overwhelming infection. The WBC differential shows a large number of immature neutrophils (bands) that are not usually called into action unless the infection is severe. The hemoglobin is consistent with mild anemia.

16. The ABG measurements are consistent with acute respiratory alkalosis and moderate hypoxemia. The Pao_2 would be lower if the patient were not hyperventilating. The patient may be hyperventilating in response to both hypoxemia and sepsis. The Pao_2 is reduced because of $\dot{V}/\dot{Q}$ mismatching in the lung.

17. The inability to see the right heart border is evidence that the pneumonia is located in the right middle lobe. If the density were located in the right lower lobe, the right heart border would probably be visible.

18. The gram-positive cocci found on the Gram stain indicate that antibiotics such as penicillin derivatives and first-generation cephalosporins should be effective. The numerous leukocytes and lack of epithelial cells indicate a valid sputum sample representative of lower airway secretions.

19. The patient should be admitted to the ICU, where he can be closely monitored. This is needed because he is at risk for respiratory failure and there is evidence (via the low WBC count) that the pneumonia is overwhelming the patient's immune system.

20. The patient should be started on intravenous (IV) antibiotics, either a first-generation cephalosporin or a penicillin derivative. Respiratory care should start the patient on oxygen with an FIO_2 of 0.40 to 0.50 and titrate his FIO_2 to an arterial oxygen saturation (SaO_2) of approximately 90 percent. After his SaO_2 is stable, a follow-up ABG would confirm his ventilatory, acid-base, and oxygenation status. IV fluids are needed to maintain hydration, as sepsis often decreases vascular tone and causes a relative hypovolemia. Sepsis-related vascular relaxation can result in profound hypotension requiring large amounts of fluid. Central venous pressure monitoring would be important if hypotension were to develop.

CASE STUDY—continued

MC was admitted to the ICU, where IV fluids and penicillin were started. Oxygen was given by mask at an FIO_2 of 0.40 with a heated aerosol. A cardiac monitor was attached to his chest to allow continuous assessment of heart rate and rhythm. Repeat ABGs 30 minutes after the start of oxygen therapy revealed the following: pH 7.47, $PaCO_2$ 33 mm Hg, and PaO_2 = 53 mm Hg. Vital signs at this time were as follows: pulse 134/minute, respiratory rate 36/minute, body temperature 38.2°C (100.8°F), and blood pressure 105/65 mm Hg. MC complained of increased dyspnea and cough. No change was noted in his right pleuritic chest pain. A blood sample was sent to the laboratory for culture.

QUESTIONS

21. How would you interpret the repeat ABG results?

22. What probably explains why the PaO_2 did not increase very much with the increase in FIO_2 to 0.40?

23. Why is the $PaCO_2$ not lower in response to the severity of the hypoxemia?

24. What is your assessment of the patient's condition in the ICU as compared to previously?

25. What treatment is indicated based on your updated assessment? Should the caregivers be concerned about oxygen-induced hypoventilation?

ANSWERS

21. The acid-base status of the repeat ABG has not changed significantly from the initial ABG. Respiratory alkalosis with moderate hypoxemia continues.

22. Simple $\dot{V}/\dot{Q}$ mismatching causes hypoxemia that usually improves with supplemental oxygen therapy. Shunt is the likely explanation when the Pao_2 increases little or not at all in response to an increase in Fio_2. Pneumonia can lead to lung consolidation, which prevents air from entering the alveoli and coming in contact with blood in the pulmonary capillaries. An increase in Fio_2 will not increase the Pao_2 significantly unless the affected region is participating in gas exchange.

23. The $Paco_2$ is not lower in this case because of the presence of COPD. A high work of breathing and a large physiologic dead space associated with COPD make it difficult for the patient to increase ventilation enough to reduce his $Paco_2$ more than the ABG now shows.

24. The patient's condition appears to be deteriorating. The fever will increase his metabolic rate, which will require increased ventilation and blood flow, putting additional stress on his heart and lungs. Most patients do not tolerate respiratory rates greater than 30/minute for a prolonged time, and an increasing respiratory rate is evidence of respiratory distress. The patient is experiencing increased dyspnea, which also suggests that he may be tiring and on the brink of respiratory failure.

25. The Fio_2 should be increased in an effort to obtain a Pao_2 of 60 to 80 mm Hg. Given this patient's poor response to initial increases in the Fio_2 and the deteriorating vital signs, he will probably need intubation and mechanical ventilation to ensure adequate gas exchange. Oxygen-induced hypoventilation is not a concern in this case because the patient's previous ABGs reveal a reduced $Paco_2$. Adequate oxygenation should never be sacrificed to avoid an increase in $Paco_2$, even when $Paco_2$ is already elevated.

CASE STUDY—continued

MC's dyspnea and vital signs deteriorated further during the next hour. The cardiac monitor demonstrated frequent premature ventricular contractions and tachycardia with a rate of 144/minute. An endotracheal tube was placed, and mechanical positive pressure ventilation was started when MC became confused and disoriented.

QUESTIONS

26. What is the significance of the patient's sudden confusion and frequent premature ventricular contractions seen on the ECG monitor?

27. What mode of ventilation, tidal volume (V_T), respiratory rate, and Fio_2 would you recommend?

28. How should the intubation and mechanical ventilation be assessed?

ANSWERS

26. The sudden confusion and premature ventricular contractions suggest that the patient has become more hypoxic or septic, or both, and that he has inadequate cerebral perfusion. This is a sign that the patient's cardiopulmonary system is failing.

27. The patient can be ventilated with assist/control or intermittent mandatory

ventilation. A mechanical respiratory rate of 10 to 14/minute with a VT of 650 to 900 mL (10 to 15 mL $\times$ 65 kg = 650 to 900 mL). An FIO_2 of 1.0 should be used initially, since the patient is demonstrating signs of hypoxia.

28. Placement of the endotracheal tube can be assessed by the following:

    a. Listening for airflow at the tube orifice as the patient makes respiratory efforts

    b. Auscultating for bilateral breath sounds on the lateral chest wall

    c. Listening for air entering the stomach with ventilator (or bag-valve-mask) driven breaths

    d. Examining a chest x-ray

    The mechanical ventilation can be assessed by ABG, breathing pattern, and vital signs.

CASE STUDY—continued

MC was placed on a volume ventilator in the assist/control mode with a backup rate of 12/minute, a VT of 800 mL, and an FIO_2 of 1.0. Initial auscultation revealed bilateral breath sounds with bronchial breath sounds over the right lower lobe. ABGs 20 minutes later revealed the following: pH 7.46, PaO_2 125 mm Hg, $PaCO_2$ 35 mm Hg, and HCO_3^- 27 mEq/liter. MC had the following initial vital signs while on the ventilator: heart rate 128/minute, respiratory rate 16/minute, blood pressure 110/68 mm Hg, and temperature 38.5°C (101.3°F). A repeat chest x-ray revealed appropriate placement of the endotracheal tube and no change in the right lower lobe infiltrate. A Foley catheter was placed, and initial urine output was 25 mL for the first hour.

QUESTIONS

29. What changes in the ventilatory settings would you recommend based on the most recent assessment data?

30. What is the significance of the urine output of 25 mL for the first hour?

31. Is this patient at risk for nosocomial infection? If so, why? How can bedside clinicians reduce the risk?

ANSWERS

29. The initial ABG shows a relatively high PaO_2 on an FIO_2 of 1.0. The oxyhemoglobin dissociation curve demonstrates that nearly as much O_2 is carried by blood with a PaO_2 of 60 mm Hg as by blood with a PaO_2 greater than 100 mm Hg. An FIO_2 of 1.0 puts the patient at risk for oxygen toxicity and it should be titrated down to achieve an SaO_2 of approximately 90 percent (PaO_2 of about 60 to 65 mm Hg). Since the $PaCO_2$ is within normal range, no change in the VT or rate is needed.

30. The initial urine output of 25 mL/hour suggests that the patient has poor renal perfusion, which may be caused by low relative blood volume. A normal urine output is approximately 60 mL/hour. IV fluid therapy is usually provided as initial therapy for patients with low urine output or low blood pressure associated with sepsis. Evidence that fluids might not be

appropriate would include elevated jugular venous pressure, gallops in heart rhythm (third or fourth heart sound), hepatojugular reflex, and peripheral edema.

31. MC is at high risk for nosocomial infection because of his compromised immune system, intubation, and mechanical ventilation. Careful hand washing by all bedside clinicians before caring for each ICU patient is very important to prevent spread of bacteria from one patient to the next. The use of sterile technique for suctioning the airway is also important.

CASE STUDY—continued

Over the next 24 hours, MC improved steadily. His temperature dropped to 37.5°C (99.5°F), and his heart rate dropped to 95/minute. A repeat CBC revealed a WBC of 6000/mm^3 with 65 percent segmented neutrophils and 20 percent bands. IV penicillin and fluids were continued. ABGs at this time were as follows: pH 7.44, PaCO$_2$ 39 mm Hg, PaO$_2$ 72 mm Hg, and FiO$_2$ 0.50.

On day 3, the patient's weaning parameters were good, and he was weaned from mechanical ventilation without difficulty. His vital signs were normal except for a respiratory rate of 28/minute. The endotracheal tube was removed, and he tolerated spontaneous breathing well. He was given heated aerosol by mask with an FiO$_2$ of 0.50 after extubation. A repeat chest x-ray on day 3 demonstrated that the right middle lobe infiltrate was less dense. The patient was switched to a nasal cannula at 3 liters/minute, which he tolerated well. After the patient's temperature was normal for 24 hours, the IV antibiotics were discontinued and oral antibiotics were started. The patient was sent home on day 5 on oral penicillin. A follow-up visit with his physician was scheduled for 1 week later.

QUESTIONS

32. What risk factors placed MC at risk for pneumonia?

33. How long might it take for the infiltrate to completely clear on the chest film? Should this patient have follow-up chest films to document complete resolution of the pneumonia? If so, why?

ANSWERS

32. MC's risk factors included a positive smoking history, COPD, possible alcohol abuse, and malnutrition.

33. The infiltrate of bacterial pneumonia seen on the chest film generally clears in 2 weeks in young, healthy patients but may take as long as 3 months to clear in older patients with lung disease.

    Yes, this patient should have follow-up chest films taken to document complete resolution of the pneumonia. He is also at high risk for bronchogenic carcinoma (see Chapter 21). The chest radiograph is needed because the infiltrate may be caused by airway obstruction from bronchogenic carcinoma; in such cases, the infiltrate will not clear completely with antibiotics. A nonresolving pneumonia requires further evaluation, most likely with bronchoscopy.

REFERENCES

1. Guidelines for the initial management of adults with community-acquired pneumonia: Diagnosis, assessment of severity, and initial antimicrobial therapy. Am Rev Respir Dis 148:1418–1426, 1993.
2. Rodrigues, J, et al: Nonresolving pneumonia in steroid-treated patients with obstructive lung disease. Am J Med 93:29–34, 1992.
3. Eid, N, et al: Chest physiotherapy in review. Respir Care 36:270, 1991.
4. Bates, JH, et al: Microbial etiology of acute pneumonia in hospitalized patients. Chest 101:1005–1012, 1992.
5. Fine, MJ, et al: Hospitalization decision in patients with community-acquired pneumonia: A prospective cohort study. Am J Med 89:713–721, 1990.
6. Craven, DE, and Steger, KA: Pathogenesis and prevention of nosocomial pneumonia in the mechanically ventilated patient. Respir Care 34:85, 1989.
7. Celis, R, et al: Nosocomial pneumonia: A multivariate analysis of risk and prognosis. Chest 93:318, 1988.

CHAPTER **19**

Pneumonia in the Immunocompromised Patient

N. Lennard Specht MD, FACP

Key Terms

acquired
  immunodeficiency
  syndrome (AIDS)
antigens
Aspergillus

autoimmune diseases
delayed hypersensitivity
helper T lymphocytes
lymphadenopathy
opportunistic infections

oral thrush
phagocytosis
Pneumocystis carinii
pneumocystis pneumonia

Introduction

The respiratory system has an extremely large surface area that is exposed to inhaled gases. At times, inhaled gases contain microorganisms that predispose the lungs to the development of serious infections. In healthy individuals, the immune system is one of several factors that resist the development of pulmonary infections. Highly infectious microorganisms such as *Streptococcus pneumoniae,* however, can cause pulmonary infections despite a strong immune system. Less infectious organisms that are easily controlled and eradicated by a normal immune system can cause serious pulmonary infections if the immune system is damaged. Infections caused by organisms that do not usually affect people with a healthy immune system are called **opportunistic infections.**

Defects in the immune system can be mild, causing only a slight increase in the frequency of infections, or severe, causing life-threatening infections. The source of the defect can be congenital (primary) or acquired (secondary). One example of a primary immunodeficiency is selective IgA deficiency; drugs, infections, radiation, and malnutrition are factors that can cause acquired immunodeficiencies.

Respiratory care practitioners are treating patients with immunodeficiencies with increasing frequency. The emergence of **acquired immunodeficiency syn-**

drome (AIDS), the increasing use of transplantation, and aggressive chemotherapy regimens have all contributed to this trend.

Etiology

Basic Function of the Immune System

The immune system is a complex group of defense mechanisms that are responsible for eliminating foreign organisms. Immunity has three principal characteristics that govern its behavior: ability to differentiate self from nonself, specificity, and memory. The vast majority of immune attacks are directed at invading microorganisms, not the host. This selectivity is critical to avoid indiscriminate immune responses damaging the host. In diseases such as rheumatoid arthritis, systemic lupus erythematosis, or scleroderma, the immune system attacks the host. These diseases are called **autoimmune diseases.**

The immune response detects molecules with specific shapes unique to the organism it is attacking. These uniquely shaped molecules are called **antigens**. The use of specific antigens to recognize and attack invading organisms assists the immune system in recognizing invaders and differentiating host from nonhost. The immune system remembers when it has been invaded by an organism and provides a more rapid, larger response when it is invaded by the same organism a second time. This principle, called *immune memory,* is the basis of vaccinations. A vaccination consists of a collection of antigens that resemble an organism, which when given to a patient, provides protection against that organism.

Anatomy of the Immune System

The immune system is not confined to one area of the body. There are collections of immune cells scattered throughout the body that mobilize and circulate to specific areas as they are needed. Polymorphonuclear cells, such as neutrophils, basophils, and eosinophils, originate in the bone marrow. Lymphocytes congregate in the spleen, thymus, and lymph nodes.

The immune system is made up of many different types of cells (Fig. 19–1). Lymphocytes and monocytes make up the majority of the immune cells. The populations of lymphocytes are broadly divided into T and B lymphocytes. B lymphocytes can develop into antibody-secreting cells called *plasma cells.* Antibodies, also called *immunoglobulins (Ig),* are molecules that identify and bind to specific foreign antigens to assist the immune system in recognizing and destroying foreign invaders.

There are five classes of immunoglobulins: IgG, IgM, IgE, IgA, and IgD. IgM antibodies are usually the first antibody produced at the onset of an infection. The level of IgM quickly rises to a peak and then declines as IgM is replaced by IgG as the primary antibody fighting the infection. IgA antibodies are produced in tissue adjacent to mucous membranes. These antibodies are then secreted onto the surface of the mucosa. On the mucosal surface, IgA inhibits binding of organisms to the membrane's surface and forms the initial barrier to entry of organisms across the mucosa. IgE antibodies mediate allergic reactions.

T lymphocytes mature into three different types of lymphcoytes that serve distinct functions. One subpopulation, called natural killer cells, have a direct cytotoxic effect on targeted cells. Another subgroup, called **helper T lymphocytes,** promote

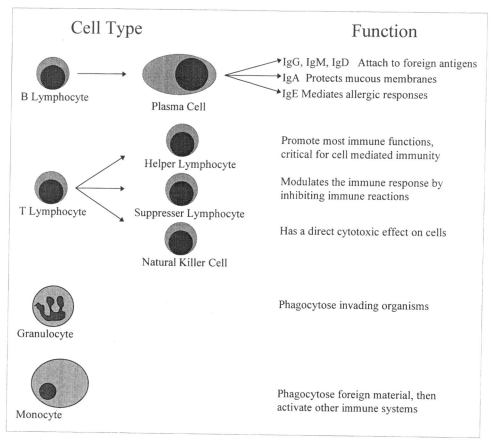

FIGURE 19-1   The major cells of the immune system and their function.

the development of antibodies by B lymphocytes and assist in the development of natural killer cells. Helper T lymphocytes have the CD4+ antigen on their surface. The CD4+ antigen is used to recognize helper T cells in the clinical laboratory. Suppressor T cells inhibit the immune responses. This effect is important for inhibiting attacks on the host and regulating immune response following antigen exposure. Suppressor T cells have the CD8+ antigen on their surface.

Helper T lymphocytes are a significant factor in cell-mediated immunity. They are responsible for defense against specific types of organisms, including *Mycobacterium tuberculosis*. The reaction of the cell-mediated immunity to an antigen is called **delayed hypersensitivity**. The strength of the delayed hypersensitivity reaction can be assessed with a skin test.

Monocytes and macrophages are larger than lymphocytes. These mononuclear cells play a critical role in the immune response. *Monocytes* circulate in the blood and may migrate into tissue to become macrophages. *Macrophages* engulf foreign material and degrade it (**phagocytosis**). Important antigens in the degraded foreign material are then used by macrophages to activate the immune response by other cells, such as helper T lymphocytes.

Because of their phagocytic function, granulocytes provide another important defense against infection. *Granulocytes* are formed in the bone marrow and circulate in the blood as neutrophils, eosinophils, or basophils. As granulocytes develop, their nucleus becomes segmented with multiple lobules, giving these cells the appearance of multiple nuclei. For that reason they are often called polymorphonuclear cells. Neutrophils are the most common granulocyte. They are responsible for detecting invading microorganisms, phagocytosing them, killing them, and degrading their remains. Neutrophils often die in the process of destroying invading organisms. Neutrophils—both living and dead—are the major constituent of pus, which is found in infected tissue (e.g., boils).

Pathology and Pathophysiology

Immunosuppression and Disease

There are numerous causes of depressed immunity. Each form of immunosuppression leads to decreased function of a distinct portion of the immune system (Table 19-1). When a portion of a patient's immune system is not functioning properly, the patient is prone to infection. Infections are frequently caused by organisms that are normally best controlled by the portion of the immune system that is damaged. To understand an opportunistic infection, you must also understand the immune system of the patient who has acquired the infection. An understanding of a particular patient's immune defect allows one to predict the most likely organisms that may be causing an infection. Some of the more commonly encountered forms of immune diseases are discussed here to illustrate the interaction among immune disease, the resulting infection, and optimal therapy.

Antibody Deficiency

An inadequate level of antibodies increases a patient's susceptibility to infection. In patients with this form of immunosuppression, infections are usually caused by organisms that can also affect individuals with normal immunity. In patients with an antibody deficiency, however, these infections are more frequent and severe than they would be if their immune systems were normal. Infections in these patients are therefore not typically classified as opportunistic because they can also occur in patients with normal immunity.

A complete or partial absence of antibodies leads to repeated infections with bacteria such as *S. pneumoniae* or *Haemophilus influenzae* and other encapsulated bacteria. The respiratory tract is the usual target for these infections, but meningitis or septicemia can also develop. The most severe form of antibody deficiency is X-

TABLE 19-1   **Types of Immune System Deficiencies**

Type of Immunity	*Cause of Deficiency*	*Example*
Antibodies	Congenital	IgA deficiency
Cell-mediated immunity	Infection	AIDS
	Congenital	MHC class II deficiency
	Medications	Transplantation immunosuppression
Phagocytic immunity	Chemotherapy	Neutropenia
	Congenital	Chronic granulomatous disease

MHC = major histocompatibility complex

linked agammaglobulinemia. Starting 6 to 9 months after birth, infants affected with this disorder begin to acquire successive infections if they are not treated. Without treatment, patients with this disorder will die at a very young age. Immunoglobulin replacement therapy is effective, but these patients may still be susceptible to respiratory infections because transfused IgA is not secreted onto the surface of mucous membranes.

Selective IgA deficiency is the most common form of immunoglobulin deficiency. IgA deficiency can lead to chronic, recurrent pulmonary infections. Not every patient with IgA deficiency acquires an unusual number of infections. Many of these patients are asymptomatic throughout life. Patients with IgA deficiency do not benefit from IgA transfusions and must rely on treatment of infections as they develop.

Defects in Cellular Immunity

Cell-mediated immunity is the portion of the immune system provided by T lymphocytes. A good example of this immunity is the body's defense against intracellular pathogens, such as *M. tuberculosis*. Cell-mediated immunity is regulated by helper T lymphocytes and suppressor T lymphocytes. Helper T lymphocytes have an important part in determining which antigens will be reacted to. Helper T cells also determine which immune cells are most effective for a given situation. They then mobilize that immune cell type into the area of infection.

Another cell-mediated response is cytotoxicity. Cytotoxic cells, like natural killer lymphocytes, bind to target cells and lyse them. Cytotoxic reactions are triggered when the host's natural killer lymphocytes recognize antigens or antibodies bound to the cell surface. A good example of antigens that are recognized and attacked as foreign are the major histocompatibility complex (MHC) antigens. The MHC antigens are expressed on the surface of the host's cells in a pattern unique to each individual. Cytotoxic cells recognize the unique MHC pattern as self and will attack any cells that do not express that pattern. The MHC antigens are an important factor in transplantation. Ideally the MHC pattern of a donor graft should be as close as possible to the recipient's pattern.

Deficiencies of cell-mediated immunity include rare, inherited forms and the more common acquired deficiencies (Table 19–2). AIDS is by far the most common defect of cell-mediated immunity.

Defects in Phagocyte Function

Phagocytic cells are important in fighting infections caused by pyogenic bacteria. A significant decrease in the number of circulating phagocytes, or their ability to func-

TABLE 19–2   **Types of Cell-Mediated Immunodeficiencies**

Inherited
  MHC class II deficiency
  DiGeorge's syndrome
  Hereditary ataxia-telangiectasia
  Wiskott-Aldrich syndrome
Acquired
  Acquired immunodeficiency syndrome

MHC = mayor histocompatibility complex

tion, may result in overwhelming bacterial infections. Most of the circulating phagocytes are neutrophils.

Neutropenia (an abnormally low number of circulating neutrophils, usually less than 500/dL) can be congenital or acquired. Hereditary defects in phagocyte function include chronic granulomatous disease and leukocyte adhesion deficiency. Acquired neutropenia is frequently caused by cancer chemotherapy. Chemotherapy drugs can reduce the number of circulating granulocytes for several days. If an infection develops during the period of granulocytopenia, the infection can rapidly become overwhelming. Because infections in patients with neutropenia are so serious, patients are treated with intravenous antibiotics at the first sign of fever.

Clinical Features

General

History and Physical Examination. Opportunistic pulmonary infections occur when the effectiveness of the immune system has been reduced. Frequently, the cause of immunocompromise is clear when a patient presents for care. On occasion, however, immunosuppression may not be obvious on initial evaluation. A careful history and review of the laboratory data will usually uncover evidence suggesting that immunosuppression is present. Opportunistic pneumonia should be considered in any patient with recurrent bouts of pneumonia or a case of pneumonia that does not resolve with treatment. The interview should document whether the patient has a history of an acquired or inherited immunodeficiency or is at risk of an acquired immunodeficiency (Table 19-3).

In most cases, opportunistic pneumonias have signs and symptoms similar to more common pneumonias. The symptoms of cough, dyspnea, and fever are common but not universal. Fever, when a patient is neutropenic following chemotherapy, usually represents a serious infection. Patients with pyogenic pneumonias may also experience pleuritic chest pain, the production of purulent sputum, occasional hemoptysis, malaise, and recent weight loss.

The physical examination of an immunocompromised patient with pneumonia will usually reveal features of both the acute pulmonary infection and the immunosuppression. Localized crackles over the chest usually indicate localized pneumonia, whereas diffuse crackles indicate widespread infection. In an immunocompetent patient, an opportunistic pneumonia is more likely to be widespread than a bacterial pneumonia.

TABLE 19-3   **Risk Factors for Acquired Immunodeficiency Syndromes**

AIDS
   Multiple sexual partners
   Intravenous drug abuse
Neutropenia
   Leukemia
   Lymphoma
   Recent chemotherapy
Miscellaneous
   Immunosuppression for prevention of a transplant rejection
   Corticosteroid use

Laboratory Evaluation. Several laboratory tests may indicate immunosuppression. An abnormally low number of lymphocytes, particularly CD4+ cells, indicates a defect in cell-mediated immunity (e.g., AIDS). Neutropenia is characterized by a neutrophil count less than 500/μL on a blood count. Patients with pneumonia, either diffuse or localized, will have some deterioration in gas exchange. This may be seen either as hypoxemia in severe cases or as an increase in the alveolar-arterial difference in partial pressure of oxygen ($P[A-a]O_2$) in milder cases.

The chest radiograph of a patient with a healthy immune system who acquires pyogenic pneumonia usually reveals a localized area of increased density (frequently called an infiltrate) in the infected portion of the lung. In patients with an immunodeficiency, pneumonia is diffuse, often affecting all portions of the lung. The chest radiograph of an immunocompromised patient with **pneumocystis pneumonia** usually reveals a diffusely increased density that ordinarily occurs in all portions of the lung.[1] The diffuse chest radiograph markings from pneumocystis pneumonia are occasionally subtle, having a ground-glass appearance; however, as the disease progresses the markings become obvious, diffuse, interstitial infiltrates. If symptoms are suggestive of pneumocystis pneumonia but the chest radiograph is normal, a gallium scan or an evaluation of lung diffusion capacity (DLCO) may be useful[2,3] for determining whether such an infection is present. Chest radiographs of patients with mild immunocompromise and tuberculosis reveal unilateral or bilateral upper lobe cavitating densities. These findings are similar to those of patients with tuberculosis but without evidence of immune compromise.[4] Chest radiographs of patients with severe immunocompromise may show diffuse pulmonary infiltrates and lymph node enlargement without cavitation.[5]

Microbiological Diagnosis. A wide variety of organisms can infect the immunocompromised patient, including bacteria, fungi, parasites, and viruses. Empiric treatment for all of these possibilities may be necessary, but it is very toxic and expensive. For this reason it is important to identify the organism causing pneumonia in an immunocompromised patient as rapidly as possible. Unfortunately it is not always possible to identify the infecting organism, even with invasive testing procedures. These procedures should be used as soon as possible after opportunistic pneumonia is suspected. Empiric treatment is started until the results of diagnostic testing are available. The type of immunosuppression will dictate which empiric treatment is best.

Culture and microscopic examination of the sputum are the least invasive and most readily available techniques for identifying infectious agents. Initially, a Gram stain and acid-fast stain are used to stain the sputum. Cultures are performed for bacteria, acid-fast bacilli, and fungi. A stain should also be performed for ***Pneumocystis carinii*** if the patient has a defect in cell-mediated immunity. To obtain optimal sputum samples, many centers are meticulous in their sputum collection. Specimens are collected in the early morning, just after the patient has awakened. The patient brushes his or her teeth and oral cavity extensively and then gargles with water. Next a 3% saline solution is nebulized to induce the specimen. Using these techniques patients with pneumocystis pneumonia can be identified without an invasive test in as many as 75% of cases.[6] Specimens to be cultured are collected in a sterile container and sent immediately to the microbiology laboratory. For *P. carinii* evaluation, specimens are sent to a cytopathology laboratory for staining and review for the organism. A number of stains are used to identify the *Pneumocystis* organisms, including monoclonal antibodies, Papanicolaou, Giemsa, and Grocott.[7]

If an induced sputum fails to determine which organism is responsible for the infection, a bronchoscopy with bronchoalveolar lavage[8,9] or transbronchial biopsy[10] may help establish the diagnosis. An open lung biopsy may be required to establish the etiology if bronchoscopy fails to reveal the infectious organism and the patient is not improving.[11]

Specific Immune Syndromes

Some diseases that cause immunodeficiency are very uncommon. A few immunodeficiencies have become progressively more frequent. It is useful to focus our discussion on the more common immunodeficiency syndromes that respiratory care practitioners may encounter in their practice.

Acquired Immunodeficiency Syndrome. An infection by the human immunodeficiency virus (HIV) causes AIDS. HIV infection usually causes an unrelenting, slowly progressive loss of cell-mediated immunity. A patient infected with HIV is said to have developed AIDS when the immunocompromise becomes so severe that it causes an opportunistic infection or another complication, such as a tumor. HIV preferentially infects cells that have the CD4+ antigen. As the infection progresses, the helper T lymphocytes that express the CD4+ antigen are destroyed. The immune system becomes compromised when the number of helper T cells decreases from a normal concentration of 800 to 1200/μL to less than 600/μL. The risk of both opportunistic and nonopportunistic infections progressively increases as the CD4+ count drops. The number of circulating CD4+ cells is a rough indication of AIDS severity and the infections that are most likely to occur (Table 19-4).

The most common opportunistic pulmonary infections include *P. carinii, Mycobacterium avium* (a bacteria closely related to *M. tuberculosis*) complex, and *Candida albicans.* The defect in cellular immunity also predisposes AIDS patients to nonopportunistic infections, such as bacterial infections, tuberculosis, coccidioidomycosis, and histoplasmosis (Table 19-5).[12] In addition to being prone to infections, patients with AIDS are at increased risk of some forms of cancer, such as Kaposi's sarcoma[13] and lymphoma.[14] Interstitial pulmonary diseases, such as lymphoid interstitial pneumonitis or interstitial pneumonitis not associated with any identifiable infection, may also develop in AIDS patients.

AIDS patients may have constitutional symptoms, such as fever, chills, malaise, and weight loss due to the HIV infection alone. **Lymphadenopathy** develops in the early stages of the disease. The lymph nodes enlarge throughout the body and are usu-

TABLE 19-4　**Frequent Infections in Patients with Acquired Immunodeficiency Syndrome**

Number of Circulating CD4+ Cells	Likely Infections
CD4 + >200/μL	*Mycobacterium tuberculosis*
	Candida albicans
CD4 + 150–200/μL	Cryptosporidiosis
	Kaposi's sarcoma
	Lymphoma
CD4 + 75–125/μL	*Pneumocystis carinii*
	Mycobacterium avium complex
	Herpes simplex virus
	Toxoplasma gondii
	Cryptococcus neoformans
	Mucocutaneous candidiasis
CD4 + <50/μL	Cytomegalovirus retinitis

TABLE 19-5   **Organisms That Frequently Cause Pneumonia in Patients with Defects of Cell-Mediated Immunity**

Opportunistic Infections	*Nonopportunistic Infections*
Pneumocystis carinii	Pyogenic bacteria
Mycobacterium avium complex and other nontuberculous mycobacteria	
Cryptococcus neoformans	
Cytomegalovirus	*Mycobacterium tuberculosis*
Herpes simplex virus	*Coccidioides immitis*
Toxoplasma gondii	*Histoplasma capsulatum*

ally not tender when palpated. Most patients in the latter stage of the disease experience severe weight loss. Many patients will also experience dyspnea on exertion if a pulmonary infection develops. These patients often have symptoms of a cough, frequently productive, and occasionally have pleuritic chest pain. Fever may be absent in patients with pneumocystis pneumonia. Symptoms of pneumocystis pneumonia may be very subtle, including simply a chronic cough and dyspnea on exertion. Uncommonly, a pneumothorax or large pleural effusion develops in patients with pulmonary infections associated with AIDS. Examination of the respiratory tract may reveal whitish plaques adherent to the tongue and mouth. These plaques are characteristic of mucocutaneous infection with *C. albicans* (**oral thrush**) and indicate that a form of immunocompromise is probably present. In patients with immunosuppression, the *Candida* plaques may extend from the mouth to the throat and may involve the trachea and esophagus. Patients with HIV infection may have diffuse lymphadenopathy either due to the HIV infection itself or to an AIDS-related malignancy.

Patients with pneumocystis pneumonia often completely recover. The mortality for all cases of pneumocystis pneumonia in AIDS patients is approximately 10 percent.[15] However, patients who go into respiratory failure as a result of AIDS-associated pneumocystis pneumonia have a mortality of 80 to 90 percent.[15,16] Treatment of AIDS-associated pneumocystis infections is complicated by the inability of many AIDS patients to tolerate the commonly prescribed antibiotics. Adverse reactions to these medications may lead to a skin rash or more serious problems, such as neutropenia. When a severe reaction develops, the antibiotics must be changed. Unfortunately, the alternate drugs are often more toxic and no more effective than the initial medications.

Transplantation. Transplantation is an increasingly popular treatment for patients with end-stage organ failure. Transplanting the organ of one person into a patient who is not genetically identical provides a stimulus for the recipient's immune system to attack the transplanted organ. The host's immune system recognizes the different pattern of MHC antigens on the surface of the transplanted organ and attacks it. This attack is called *transplant rejection.* A patient who has received a transplant takes immunosuppressive medications such as cyclosporin and corticosteroids to control transplant rejection. Although these immunosuppressive medications control transplant rejection, they also increase a patient's risk of pulmonary infection. The most common pulmonary infections seen in patients using immunosuppressive medications are listed in Table 19-6. The risk of pulmonary infection increases if the patient has received a bone marrow transplant or if high doses of immunosuppressive medications are required.

Symptoms of post-transplantation infection include a nonproductive cough,

TABLE 19-6   **Pulmonary Infections Associated with Transplantation**

Post-Transplantation Stage	Organism
Early (up to 30 days)	Pyogenic bacteria
	Fungi, particularly *Aspergillus* and *Candida*
	Viruses
Mid (30–100 days)	Cytomegalovirus
	Aspergillus
	P. carinii
	Pyogenic bacteria
Late (>days)	Pyogenic bacteria
	Fungi
	Viruses
	P. carinii
	Mycobacteria

dyspnea, and fever. The fever may not be severe if the immunosuppression is significant. The chest examination findings may be localized (e.g., in pyogenic bacterial infections) or diffuse (e.g., in infections due to cytomegalovirus or *P. carinii*).

Neutropenia. Cancer chemotherapy is designed to kill cells that are multiplying rapidly. Most cancers are made up of rapidly dividing cells. A large percentage of cancer cells are killed each time chemotherapy is used. Unfortunately, chemotherapy kills not only cancer cells, but also some normal cells. Cells that generate hair and white blood cells are very sensitive to chemotherapy. For this reason, chemotherapy often causes hair loss and a low white blood cell (WBC) count (neutropenia). The number of circulating granulocytes may drop to very low levels when some forms of chemotherapy are given. Neutropenia occurs when the granulocyte count is less than 500/μL. Neutropenia may begin 7 days after chemotherapy is initiated and may continue for 2 to 3 weeks. During the period of neutropenia, a patient is prone to infection because of the small numbers of circulating phagocytic cells. These infections are generally caused by pyogenic bacteria of fungal organisms such as *Aspergillus.* An infection in a neutropenic patient advances quickly if the cause of the infection is not promptly treated. Fever is a very important sign of infection in a neutropenic patient. The first sign of a fever is often the initial clue of a serious infection. The patient will experience dyspnea and a cough if the lungs are the site of infection. Examination of the chest of a patient with neutropenia-associated pneumonia may disclose localized crackles.

Immunosuppressive Drugs. Many drugs used to treat inflammatory diseases such as rheumatoid arthritis, systemic lupus erythematosis, scleroderma, or asthma can suppress the immune system. Drugs such as corticosteroids, cyclophosphamide, and azathioprine increase the patient's risk of both opportunistic and nonopportunistic pneumonia.

Treatment

Empiric Therapy

In immunocompromised patients, pneumonia can progress very rapidly. The rapid progression often forces clinicians to begin therapy without waiting for the results of diagnostic tests that determine the microorganism causing the infection (*empiric therapy*). A patient's particular type of immune defect helps predict which organisms are most likely to be responsible for the infection. Empiric therapy is selected on this basis. A patient with neutropenia is usually treated with antibiotics against pyogenic bacteria such as *Pseudomonas aeruginosa* or fungi such as *Aspergillus* organisms. Patients with AIDS are usually empirically treated with a combination of trimethoprim and sulfamethoxazole because they are likely to have pneumonia due to *P. carinii*.

Specific Therapy

Empiric therapy is replaced by treatment directed at the specific organism if diagnostic testing discloses which organism has caused the pneumonia. Patients with pyogenic bacterial infections are treated with at least one and frequently two antibacterial agents. The microbiology laboratory uses sensitivity testing to determine the best antibiotics to use for a given infection.

Pneumonia due to *P. carinii* is diagnosed by identifying these small organisms with a high-powered microscope in specially strained lung secretions. These infections are usually treated with a combination of sulfa antibiotics. Patients who cannot tolerate sulfa antibiotics may be given pentamidine intravenously or by aerosol. Other treatment regimens have been developed, including dapsone, primaquine, atovaquone, and trimetrexate.[17] These drugs are usually reserved for patients who cannot tolerate either of the more common therapies. Patients who have moderate to severe pneumonia due to *P. carinii* benefit from high-dose corticosteroid treatments with methylprednisolone.[18,19]

Fungal pneumonia due to *Aspergillus* organisms or other fungal infections is treated with antifungal antibiotics. Treatment is begun with amphotericin B for most immunocompromised patients with a fungal pneumonia. Oral antifungal agents classified as imidazoles are available. These drugs (e.g., itraconazole,[20] ketoconazole, fluconazole) are reserved for patients with mild infections or those who have responded well to amphotericin B but for whom further oral therapy is desired.

AIDS patients in whom tuberculosis develops require intensive therapy with multiple drugs. The first 2 months should include the following four drugs: isoniazid, rifampin, pyrazinamide, and ethambutol. Isoniazid and rifampin are continued for the remaining 7 months.[21]

Prophylactic Therapy

Patients with immunodeficiencies such as AIDS are at risk for several forms of opportunistic pneumonia. As a preventive measure, it is often wise to institute prophylactic antibiotic therapy.[22] In AIDS cases, prophylactic therapy is started either to follow an acute infection in order to prevent a recurrence or when the number of circulating CD4+ lymphocytes becomes so low that infection is likely. Antibiotics should be started to prevent pneumocystis pneumonia when the number of CD4+ lymphocytes is less than 200/µL. The first choice for prophylactic treatment is a daily tablet of trimethoprim-sulfamethoxazole. Aerosolized pentamidine or dapsone tablets may be used if a patient cannot tolerate sulfa antibiotics (e.g., trimethoprim-sulfamethoxazole). Rifampin and clarithromycin are recommended for prevention of *M. avium* complex if the CD4+ count is less than 100/µL.

CASE STUDY

History

KW is a 35-year-old man. Three years ago he was found to be infected with the HIV virus. Since the discovery of his infection, he has been well. Despite regular use of azidothymidine (AZT) he has lost 20 pounds over the last 2 months and experienced a progressive decrease in the number of circulating CD4+ lymphocytes. The most recent count revealed a CD4+ level of 97/μL. Two weeks prior to the office visit, he noticed mild dyspnea on exertion and a nagging, nonproductive cough. He did not experience fever or myalgias. A chest radiograph was normal, and his initial evaluation was unremarkable. Following that clinic visit, a DLCO was ordered, and KW was instructed to return for a follow-up visit in 2 weeks. During the next 2 weeks, KW found that his cough persisted and his exercise tolerance progressively deteriorated. The DLCO was 42% of predicted.

QUESTIONS

1. In what manner does HIV affect the immune system?

2. List several organisms that cause opportunistic pneumonia in patients infected with HIV.

3. How do you interpret the number of circulating CD4+ lymphocytes in KW, and what is the significance?

4. KW has a nonproductive cough and dyspnea on exertion. What opportunistic infections can cause these symptoms?

5. What is the significance of the reduced DLCO?

ANSWERS

1. The human immunodeficiency virus attacks several cell types in the body. It most severely affects helper T lymphocytes, which are critical for the proper function of cellular immunity. As the helper T lymphocytes are destroyed, cellular immunity is destroyed along with them.

2. Infections that would not normally occur in a person with a healthy immune system are called opportunistic infections. Table 19–4 lists several organisms that cause opportunistic pneumonia in patients with deficient cellular immunity; the most common is *P. carinii*. Other organisms include *M. avium* complex, *Cryptococcus neoformans*, *Toxoplasma gondii*, cytomegalovirus, herpes simplex virus, and nontuberculous mycobacterial organisms.

3. KW's CD4+ cell count is very low (normal levels are 800–1200/μL). This reduction in the number of circulating helper T cells indicates that KW is at risk for several forms of opportunistic infections (Table 19–3).

4. Any pneumonia could cause dyspnea on exertion. Most pneumonias increase the mucus production of the pulmonary mucosa and therefore cause a productive cough. The cough may be nonproductive if there is little immune reaction to the infection or if the patient has an insufficient cough to expectorate the secretions.

5. The reduction of DLCO indicates a functional decrease in the alveolar capillary surface area. A reduction in DLCO suggests that pulmonary disease is present, but it cannot specify which disease has caused KW's pulmonary symptoms.

Physical Examination

General: A chronically thin, ill-appearing man who is in no acute distress; no respiratory distress exhibited at rest

Vital Signs: Temperature 37.2°C (99.0°F), pulse 77/minute, respiratory rate 21/minute, blood pressure 125/76 mm Hg

HEENT: Whitish plaques seen on tongue and palate; plaques firmly adhere to the mucosa and bleed when scraped.

Neck: Diffuse, nontender lymphadenopathy in the neck; no jugular venous distention

Chest: Normal configuration and resonance to percussion; normal expansion with respiration

Heart: Regular, without murmurs or gallops

Lungs: Air movement good, with harsh breath sounds over the entire chest; fine inspiratory crackles heard over both lungs diffusely, primarily in the bases

Abdomen: Normal appearance; bowel sounds active, and abdomen nontender; no masses or organomegaly noted

Extremities: warm, well perfused, and without edema; pulses strong and symmetric

QUESTIONS

6. Why does KW have diffuse lymphadenopathy?

7. What does the distribution of inspiratory crackles over KW's lungs indicate?

8. What is the most likely source of the whitish plaques on the oral mucosal surface?

9. What is the most likely diagnosis for KW's symptoms?

10. How can the suspected diagnosis be confirmed?

ANSWERS

6. HIV infections cause a diffuse lymphadenopathy in most patients. This adenopathy is usually nontender and can be found in most lymph node–bearing regions. Another less likely possibility is that KW has developed an HIV-associated lymphoma. HIV-associated lymphomas usually occur in extranodal sites[23] and can be of either the Hodgkin's or the non-Hodgkin's variety.

7. The distribution of crackles scattered diffusely over both lungs, primarily the bases, suggest that a diffuse process is affecting the lungs. Many pulmonary diseases associated with AIDS are diffuse. Possible diseases include lymphoid interstitial pneumonitis, idiopathic interstitial pneumonitis, and pneumonia due to *P. carinii,* cytomegalovirus, and many other organisms.

8. The appearance of the oral mucosa is indicative of mucocutaneous candidiasis, caused by *C. albicans.* This is a frequent infection in patients who use corticosteroids (particularly inhaled) or who have depressed cellular immunity. Patients with severely depressed cellular immunity may have the *Candida* infection in the esophagus, trachea, bronchi, or lungs in addition to the mouth. The presence of mucocutaneous candidiasis suggests that KW has a significant deficiency in cell-mediated immunity.

9. KW probably has pneumonia. By far the most common cause of diffuse lung

disease in AIDS patients is an infection. The most common pulmonary infection in patients with AIDS is pneumocystis pneumonia.

10. To confirm the diagnosis of pneumonia, a current chest radiograph should be reviewed. A stained sputum sample is useful to help establish the organism responsible for the pneumonia. If the patient cannot produce sputum, bronchoscopy can provide specimens for a definitive diagnosis.

Laboratory Evaluation

Complete Blood Count (CBC) (See Appendix for normal values): WBC 3800/µL, granulocytes 3150/µL, monocytes 370/µL, lymphocytes 280/µL, hemoglobin 8.2 g/dL

Electrolytes: Na^+ 139 mEq/liter, K^+ 4.3 mEq/liter, Cl^- 104 mEq/liter, CO_2 23 mEq/liter, blood urea nitrogen 27 mg/dL, creatinine 1.4 mg/dL

Arterial Blood Gases (ABGs): pH 7.45, $Paco_2$ 32 mm Hg, PaO_2 71 mm Hg, HCO_3^- 22 mEq/liter on room air

Chest Radiograph: See Figure 19–2

Sputum Gram Stain: Numerous squamous epithelial cells with occasional gram-positive rods, gram-positive cocci, and rare gram-negative rods; numerous yeasts and pseudohyphae seen.

QUESTIONS

11. How would you interpret the CBC results?

12. How would you interpret the ABG results? Are these ABGs normal for a man of this age?

13. How would you interpret the results of the chest radiograph?

14. What do the findings of the sputum Gram stain represent? Does the absence of *P. carinii* organisms on the Gram stain indicate that infection with *P. carinii* is unlikely?

15. Should KW be admitted to the hospital, or could further evaluation and treatment be delivered to him as an outpatient?

16. What are the best steps to take at this time to determine the source of KW's pulmonary disease?

17. If a repeat sputum sample is induced, what steps should be taken to ensure that the patient is properly prepared so that an optimal specimen can be obtained?

ANSWERS

11. The WBC count is low, primarily because of a reduction in the number of circulating lymphocytes (lymphopenia). It is not uncommon for patients with AIDS to have a lymphopenia. Anemia is also present.

12. The ABGs indicate a chronic respiratory alkalosis. In addition, the $P(A-a)O_2$ is 39 mm Hg, which is far wider than one would predict for a 35-year-old man.

13. The findings indicate a diffuse process. The possibilities for such a process include infections due to *P. carinii,* cytomegalovirus, or many other organisms; or a form of interstitial lung disease. Tumors such as lymphoma and Kaposi's sarcoma rarely create lung disease as diffuse as KW has developed.

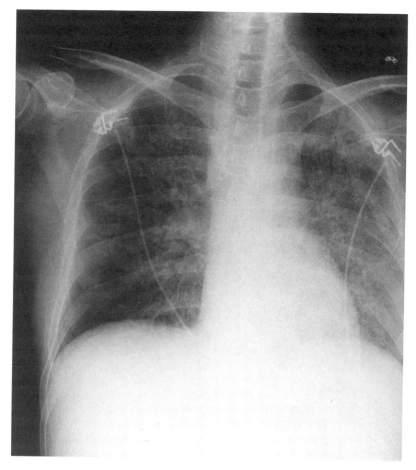

FIGURE 19-2   Chest radiograph from KW.

14. The initial sputum Gram stain shows extensive contamination of the specimen with oral secretions. The large number of squamous epithelial cells come from the oral pharynx; thus, the sample is not representative of bronchial secretions. The bacterial organisms seen are probably from the mouth. The presence of yeast and pseudohyphae suggests that KW has yeast organisms infecting or colonizing his mouth, and this correlates well with the physical examination findings. Pneumocystis organisms cannot be seen on a Gram stain, but require specialized stains.

15. Initial assessment and ABG data suggest that KW is quite ill. Initial diagnostic studies and treatment could be done on an outpatient basis, but the rapid deterioration in his condition would make hospital admission reasonable. Once he is clearly stable and the medication he needs can be administered at home, he could be discharged and cared for as an outpatient.

16. The diffuse lung disease that KW has developed could be caused by an infection. The most common diffuse pneumonia in AIDS patients is due to *P. carnii.* An induced sputum specimen is likely to diagnose this and most other forms of pneumonia in AIDS patients. If, after a careful examination of an induced sputum specimen, no cause of the pulmonary disease is established, a bronchoscopy with bronchoalveolar lavage and possibly a

transbronchial biopsy is often performed. If the diagnosis is still lacking after bronchoscopy, an open lung biopsy may be helpful.

17. Specimens should be collected in the early morning, just after the patient has awakened. The patient should brush his teeth and oral cavity extensively and then gargle and rinse his mouth with water. Then a 3% saline solution is nebulized to induce the specimen. A high percentage of patients with AIDS-associated pneumonias can be diagnosed on the basis of such a specimen. By careful attention to proper patients preparation, the physician can avoid ordering invasive tests such as bronchoscopy.

CASE STUDY—continued

KW was admitted to the hospital and placed in respiratory isolation. Sputum inductions were performed, and KW began treatment with trimethoprim-sulfamethoxazole. The day after admission, KW experienced increasing respiratory distress. He appeared diaphoretic, dusky in color, and was in moderate respiratory distress. He had inspiratory crackles scattered over his entire chest. His ABGs were pH 7.49, $PaCO_2$ 27 mm Hg, PaO_2 46 mm Hg, HCO_3^- 20 mEq/liter on room air. He was transferred to the intensive care unit (ICU), started on oxygen by a 50% Venturi mask, and intravenous methylprednisolone. His respiratory distress improved and his ABGs on an FIO_2 of 0.50 were pH 7.39, $PaCO_2$ 36 mm Hg, PaO_2 97 mm Hg, and HCO_3^- 21 mEq/liter.

QUESTIONS

18. In the absence of blood or body fluid contamination of a health care worker, KW's HIV infection cannot be spread by casual contact, such as caring for a patient in the hospital. What is the value of placing this patient in respiratory isolation?

19. What is the purpose of administering trimethoprim-sulfamethoxazole?

20. Interpret the results of both ABGs. What do the changes in KW's ABG while in the ICU indicate in relation to the ABG findings on admission?

21. Does the PaO_2 of 97 mm Hg on 0.50 FIO_2 indicate correction of the patient's hypoxemia? Is it an indication that the patient has stabilized or even improved?

ANSWERS

18. Respiratory isolation is of no benefit in protecting a health care worker or family member from contracting an HIV infection. Many of the infections that patients with HIV disease get are opportunistic infections and cannot be spread to an immunocompetent health care worker. The one pulmonary infection that can be spread to persons with a normal immunity is tuberculosis. If there is a question whether a patient could be infected with *M. tuberculosis,* respiratory isolation should be instituted until the infection has either been partially treated or ruled out.

19. The most likely pulmonary infection in an HIV-infected patient with a CD4+ lymphocyte count less than 100/μL is *P. carinii.* Trimethoprim and sulfamethoxazole are the drugs most often used for treatment of *P. carinii.* When KW was first admitted, there were a number of signs that suggested that he was very ill with pneumonia. These signs included weight loss, the widened $P(A-a)O_2$ gradient, and the diffuse nature of the densities observed on the chest radiograph.

20. The initial ABG was measured on room air. There is an acute respiratory alkalosis with hypoxemia. The second ABG discloses a normal acid-base balance with no hypoxemia and a very wide $P(A-a)O_2$ gradient. These ABGs indicate that KW's lung disease has progressed significantly.

21. KW has a much better PaO_2 and is no longer hypoxemic on an FIO_2 of 0.50. Despite the improvement in his PaO_2, his gas exchange is still much worse than it was on admission and indicates that his acute lung disease has not stabilized, but has progressed.

CASE STUDY—continued

The sputum specimen that was induced on the first hospital day revealed organisms consistent with *P. carinii.* No acid-fast bacilli or fungal organisms were identified. Sputum culture had *C. albicans* and a mixture of organisms that normally colonize the upper respiratory tract. The chest radiograph taken the day KW moved into the ICU showed a marked increase in the diffuse pulmonary opacification not unlike the pattern of acute respiratory distress syndrome (ARDS). Respiratory isolation was discontinued after three induced sputum specimens stained for acid-fast bacilli disclosed no tuberculosis-like organisms. After receiving a 1-week course of sulfa antibiotics, oxygen therapy, oral antifungal therapy, and AZT, KW improved. He never required mechanical ventilation.

QUESTIONS

22. What organisms are usually identified by an acid-fast stain?

23. The chest radiograph from the day KW was admitted to the ICU indicated a diffuse pulmonary process. This process could be due to a diffuse pneumonia, ARDS or pulmonary edema. How would a pulmonary artery catheter help you decide which of these problems is the most likely cause of KW's pulmonary disease?

ANSWERS

22. Acid-fast stains are most useful in identifying mycobacterial species such as *M. tuberculosis.* In addition, the acid-fast process will stain a few other organisms, such as *Actinomyces* and *Nocardia.*

23. A pulmonary artery catheter provides many important hemodynamic measurements. One of these measurements is the pulmonary capillary wedge pressure (PCWP), which if elevated usually indicates left ventricular failure. Left ventricular failure is the most common cause of pulmonary edema. If a chest radiograph shows diffuse infiltrates but the PCWP is normal or low, pulmonary edema due to heart failure is unlikely; rather, ARDS or diffuse pneumonia is a more likely diagnosis (see Chapter 8).

CASE STUDY—continued

After 23 days of hospitalization, KW improved enough to go home. He no longer had dyspnea on exertion when he did not require oxygen. His lung examination improved, with only occasional inspiratory crackles. His chest radiograph cleared. His room-air ABGs were pH 7.42, $PaCO_2$ 38 mm Hg, PaO_2 52 mm Hg, and HCO_3^- 24 mEq/liter. During the last days of treatment with trimethoprim-sulfamethoxazole, leukopenia developed. He was discharged home with instructions to receive a monthly treatment of aerosolized pentamidine.

QUESTIONS

24. Should KW receive supplemental oxygen at home?

25. What is the purpose of the aerosolized pentamidine?

ANSWERS

24. Yes: Although he has improved markedly, he is still hypoxemic on room air.

25. Patients with AIDS frequently experience another pneumocystis pneumonia episode after their first infection. KW could either receive trimethoprim-sulfamethoxazole or monthly aerosolized pentamidine. Pentamidine is the drug of choice for KW because of the leukopenia he developed while receiving trimethoprim-sulfamethoxazole.

REFERENCES _____

1. Suster, B, et al: Pulmonary manifestations in AIDS: Review of 106 episodes. Radiology 161: 87-93, 1986.

2. Mitchell, DM, et al: Pulmonary function in human immunodeficiency virus infection: A prospective 18 month study of serial lung function in 474 patients. Am Rev Respir Dis 146:745-751, 1992.

3. Vanarthos, WJ, et al: Diagnostic uses of nuclear medicine in AIDS. Radiographics 12:731-749, 1992.

4. Chaisson, R, et al: Tuberculosis in patients with AIDS: A population based study. Am Rev Respir Dis 136:570-574, 1987.

5. Small, PM, et al: Treatment of tuberculosis in patients with advanced human immunodeficiency virus infection. N Engl J Med 324:289-294, 1991.

6. Ng, VL, et al: The use of mucolysed induced sputum for the identification of pulmonary pathogens associated with human immunodeficiency virus infection. Arch Pathol Lab Med 113:488-493, 1989.

7. Wazir, JF, et al: EB9, a new antibody for the detection of trophozoites of *Pneumocystis carinii* in bronchoalveolar lavage specimens in AIDS. J Clin Pathol 47:1108-1111, 1994.

8. Murry, T, et al: Is transbronchial biopsy necessary for diagnosis of pulmonary infections with AIDS? Am Rev Respir Dis 133:A182, 1986.

9. Golden, JA, et al: Bronchoalveolar lavage as the exclusive diagnostic modality for *Pneumocystis carinii* pneumonia. Chest 90:18-22, 1986.

10. Milligan, SA, et al: Transbronchial biopsy without fluoroscopy in patients with diffuse roentgenographic infiltrates and the acquired immunodeficiency syndrome. Am Rev Respir Dis 137:486-488, 1988.

11. Fitzgerald, W, et al: The role of open-lung biopsy in patients with the acquired immunodeficiency syndrome. Chest 91:659-661, 1987.

12. Wallace, JM, et al: Respiratory illness in persons with human immunodeficiency virus infection. Am Rev Respir Dis 148:1523-1529, 1993.

13. Northfelt, DW: In Cohen, PT, et al (eds): The AIDS Knowledge Base. Little, Brown & Co, Boston, 1994.

14. Kaplan, LD, et al: AIDS associated non-Hodgkin's lymphoma in San Francisco. JAMA 261:719-724, 1981.

15. Hawley, PH, et al: Decreasing frequency but worsening mortality of acute respiratory failure secondary to AIDS-related Pneumocystis carinii pneumonia. Chest 106:1456-1459, 1994.

16. De Palo, VA, et al: Outcome of intensive care in patients with HIV infection. Chest 107:506-510, 1995.

17. Lane, HC, et al: NIH conference: Recent advances in the management of AIDS-related opportunistic infections. Ann Intern Med 120:945-955, 1994.

18. Bozzette, SA, et al: A controlled trial of early adjunctive treatment with corticosteroids for Pneumocystis carinii pneumonia in the acquired immunodeficiency syndrome: California Cooperative Treatment Group. N Engl J Med 323:1451-1457, 1990.

19. McLaughlin, GE, et al: Effect of corticosteroids on survival of children with acquired immunodeficiency syndrome and Pneumocystis carinii-related respiratory failure. J Pediatr 126:821-824, 1995.

20. Denning, D, et al: Treatment of invasive aspergillosis with itraconazole. Am J Med 86:791-800, 1989.

21. Centers for Disease Control, Advisory Committee for the Elimination of Tuberculosis: Recommendation for the elimination of tuberculosis. MMWR 38:236-250, 1989.

22. Simonds, RJ, et al: Prophylaxis against Pneumocystis carinii pneumonia among children with perinatally acquired human immunodeficiency virus infection in the United States. Pneumocystis carinii Pneumonia Prophylaxis Evaluation Working Group. N Engl J Med 332:786-790, 1995.

23. Knowles, DM, et al: Lymphoid neoplasia associated with the acquired immunodeficiency syndrome (AIDS): The New York University Center experience with 105 patients (1981-1986). Ann Intern Med 108:744-753, 1988.

CHAPTER **20**

Tuberculosis

David Lopez, MA, RRT
Arthur B. Marshak, BS, RRT

Key Terms

anorexia
Ghon complex
granuloma

miliary tuberculosis
Mycobacterium tuberculosis
night sweats

purified protein derivative
  (PPD)
tuberculosis (TB)

Introduction

According to the World Health Organization, **tuberculosis** (TB) has become the number-one cause of infectious disease–related death in the world. Globally, 1.9 billion persons were reported to have TB in a 1996 report.[1] As a result of increases in world travel, the burgeoning number of immunocompromised patients, and decreasing expenditures on public health programs, TB is showing a remarkable resurgence in the United States. Long thought to be "under control" in the U.S., TB is now producing increased morbidity and mortality rates among U.S. citizens.[2-4]

The following facts about TB have been documented:

- TB kills more individuals than all other infectious diseases combined.
- TB is the leading killer of HIV-positive individuals, causing more than 30 percent of AIDS-related deaths.
- One new person acquires TB every second.
- One third of the world's population is infected with TB.[5]

Asian immigrants from Vietnam, Cambodia, Laos, China, and the Philippines are routinely screened for TB on entrance to the U.S. This has greatly facilitated treatment of persons at risk and has reduced potential spread of the disease. However, immigrants from Mexico, Central America, Haiti, and other countries frequently enter the U.S. without undergoing any systematic screening.[6] A community-based survey of 1871 Latinos in San Francisco found a 53 percent prevalence of positive tuberculin tests in the foreign-born population compared to 7 percent for those born in the U.S. Infection rates among U.S.-born Latino children were higher than reported for whites and African Americans from other large cities. In 1990, 91 percent of Asians/Pacific Islanders and 51 percent of Latinos with TB were born outside of the U.S.[6] In California, 40 percent of TB cases were reported among foreign-born persons.[7-10] Figure 20–1 demonstrates the increase in TB cases among foreign-born persons in the U.S.

Although the reported incidence of TB increased significantly in the early 1990s, recent data from the Centers for Disease Control (CDC) has found a decline in the number of reported TB cases (Fig. 20–2).[11] The U.S. government has increased its efforts to combat TB and has been successful in controlling the spread of infection; however, the problems of immigration and multidrug-resistant TB continue to be major concerns.

The incidence of TB in the U.S. is affected not only by changes in population demographics, but also by the number of individuals who are highly susceptible to it as a result of a poor immune system, malnutrition, and institutional housing (e.g., nursing homes, prisons, homeless shelters).[12-18] TB is sometimes difficult to diagnose, and many individuals are misdiagnosed. Other individuals with TB do not seek medical care because of the gradual onset of the disease, or because they belong to a segment of society that does not have ready access to medical care.[19] Many who are diagnosed and treated do not follow through with the medication regimen, which requires patient compliance for months on end. Failure to treat TB adequately has also produced drug-resistant strains.[20-22] For these reasons, in the U.S. TB has become a disease of the elderly, of foreign-born persons from high-prevalence countries, of nonwhite minorities, and of persons with immunodeficiency.[23-25]

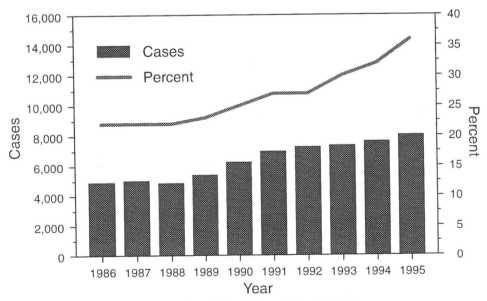

*Comprises the 50 states, the District of Columbia, and New York City.

FIGURE 20–1   Number and percentage of tuberculosis cases in foreign-born persons in the United States, 1986–1995. (From the Centers for Disease Control, with permission.)

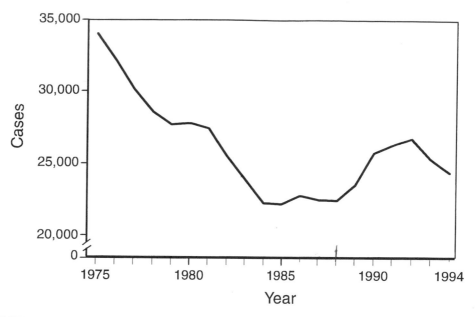

FIGURE 20-2   Number of tuberculosis cases by year in the United States, 1975-1994. (From the Centers for Disease Control, with permission.)

Etiology and Transmission

The agent that causes TB, **Mycobacterium tuberculosis,** is a nonmotile, non-sporulating, rod-shaped, acid-fast bacillus (AFB) with a dimension of approximately 0.2×5.0 μm. It is a slow-growing aerobe, multiplying faster in the presence of an abundant supply of oxygen. Therefore, it grows best in areas of the body where Po_2 is highest (lung apices) and immunity lowest (spinal discs).

    M. tuberculosis is almost exclusively transmitted by very small, aerosolized droplets usually less than 8 to 10 μm in diameter.[26] These minuscule particles are aerosolized into the environment by infected individuals through coughing, sneezing, or talking. The particles remain suspended in the air by brownian motion. Once in-haled by a susceptible person, they will cause infection if they get deep into the lung, past the mucociliary transport system.

    Other reported means of contracting the disease include ingestion of unpas-teurized milk from cattle infected with the pathogen (usually *M. bovis*); direct inoc-ulation through the skin, as occurs in laboratory accidents and during postmortem ex-aminations; and inhalation of aerosolized fluid from contaminated materials (e g , urine, sinus drainage, feces, sputum) that are improperly handled.[27] TB is not, how-ever, contracted through contact with *fomites*—objects or material on which the bac-teria are present, such as clothing, eating utensils, writing objects, and paper.

Pathology and Pathogenesis

Primary Infection

Inhaled *Mycobacterium* particles initially settle in the distal parenchyma of the lung with the greatest amount of ventilation (i.e., the lung bases). The bacilli multiply despite the body's defense mechanisms and slowly migrate throughout the body by way of the lymph and circulatory systems. Approximately 6 to 8 weeks after this initial infection, the host's immune system causes localized inflammation and containment of the infection by forming **granulomas.**

A granuloma develops in the infected lung tissue and results in a fibrin mass; necrosis and parenchymal breakdown of this mass produces a cheesy material at the center, known as *caseation.* The regional lymph nodes also become infected and enlarged. The infection is often walled off by fibrosis. The initial lung lesion is called a Ghon nodule, and the combination of the initial lung lesion and the affected lymph node is known as the **Ghon complex.** Although difficult to detect on a chest radiograph at this stage, the lesions may be seen as small, sharply defined opacities. This initial stage of TB usually heals completely in the majority of infected individuals, leaving only small scars that may later become calcified.

The body's cell-mediated immune response is usually effective in controlling the infection at this point, but it may not kill all the bacteria. Pockets of bacteria may lie dormant in either the primary or the metastatic sites, sometimes for many years, until some event precipitates reactivation and reinfection. Between the primary and reinfection phases is a dormant or "healthy" period known as *tuberculosis infection without disease.* Clinically there is no evidence of disease, except for a positive skin test and possibly residual scarring on the chest radiograph. This positive reaction indicates the presence of live tuberculin bacilli in the body.

Postprimary or Reactivation Infection

Some time after the initial infection has occurred, reinfection may take place in up to 10 percent of infected individuals. Reinfection is most common within the first 2 years after initial infection, but may occur up to several decades later.[28] The exact cause of reinfection is poorly understood, but the following are among the known predisposing factors: aging, malnutrition, alcoholism, diabetes, immunocompromising diseases, silicosis, postpartum period, gastrectomy, chronic hemodialysis, and other chronic debilitating disorders. Because the bacilli grow best in an aerobic environment, they usually present as an infiltrate in the apical and posterior segments of the upper lobes, where the relative oxygen concentration is highest in the lung. Reactivation may also occur at extrapulmonary sites with a good oxygen supply or poor immune potential, to which the original infection had metastasized.

The majority of TB patients seen at medical clinics present with reactivated TB, rather than the primary disease. Extrapulmonary disease accounts for about 15 percent of active disease. Granulomas (or tubercules) with central caseation are typical pathological changes associated with reactivated TB. Fibrosis and cavity formation take place as the body continues its fight against the organism. Eventually fibrosis encases the granulomatous lesions, resulting in loss of lung volume. The affected lobe retracts, and calcification may become evident. These retractions and morphological changes may cause the bronchi to become distorted and dilated.[29]

In some cases a disseminated form of the disease may develop, known as **miliary tuberculosis.** This is usually an acute, generalized TB spread throughout the region or organ system characterized by the radiographic appearance of many small nodules. Miliary TB usually occurs in immunocompromised patients and predominantly involves newborns and older men. About half of the adult cases are associated with an underlying disease state such as chronic alcoholism, immunosuppression therapy (e.g., for organ transplantation), immunodeficiency diseases (e.g., AIDS), or neoplasia.[30]

Pathophysiology

The continuous destruction of infected lung parenchyma leads to scarring and loss of lung volume along with the destruction of blood vessels, which is why ventilation-perfusion ($\dot{V}/\dot{Q}$) mismatching is usually not seen. Hypoxemia and hypercapnia are unusual findings unless the patient has concurrent lung disease, such as chronic obstructive pulmonary disease (COPD). Pulmonary function is initially not greatly affected, but as the disease progresses, the lung volumes and flows decrease.

Clinical Features

Medical History

The medical history is important in the patient suspected of having TB. The interview is done to determine whether (1) the patient has been exposed to TB, (2) the patient has risk factors for TB reactivation, and (3) symptoms are consistent with TB.

A careful history of the patient suspected of having TB must include recent travel outside the U.S. and travel of close family or friends who might be infected with TB. Other factors to identify are nutritional status, immunosuppression, institutionalized care, and previous or current treatment for TB. Exposure of the patient to a person with active TB is extremely helpful to document, especially if this contact has been significantly close.[31]

TB is a chronic disease with an insidious onset. It may not be recognized as a serious illness by either the patient or the physician. The attending physician must document clues in the patient's medical history that are suggestive of TB, such as pleurisy with pleural effusion or a past diagnosis of prolonged pneumonia. History of associated illnesses should also be documented, such as uncontrolled diabetes, alcoholism, malnutrition due to a variety of causes, or occupational exposure to quartz dust or silica. It is important to note recent nursing home admission, incarceration, or institutional care.[32,33]

TB patients commonly have the following complaints:

- Fatigue, low-grade fever, **night sweats,** and chills
- Chronic cough, sputum production, and hemoptysis
- Pleuritic chest pain
- Weight loss

TB symptoms may progress so slowly over a period of weeks that they are recognized only in retrospect. Some patients may never have obvious symptoms, despite having extensive bilateral cavitation. Nonspecific systemic symptoms include progressive onset of fatigue; mild digestive disturbances; malaise; slow onset of weight loss; **anorexia;** irregular menses; night sweats; and low-grade fevers lasting for weeks to months. Fevers occur more often in the afternoon or evening and dissipate at night. Less common is an acute onset of spiking temperatures, chills, myalgia, sweating, and weakness in association with parenchymal infiltrates on the chest radiograph; this is usually attributed to a secondary pneumonia or viral illness.[34-36]

Physical Examination

Physical examination findings in the patient with TB are not specific enough to make the diagnosis. Physical examination can, however, help determine the extent of the progression of the disease, and whether other areas of the body outside the chest are involved.

Vital signs are not initially suggestive of TB unless the infection is severe enough to produce changes in heart rate, respiratory rate, blood pressure, or body temperature. The pulmonary lesions associated with TB usually give rise to varying degrees of impaired resonance to percussion, bronchial breath sounds, and coarse crackles. Endobronchial disease or bronchial compression by lymph nodes (more common in children) may produce localized wheezing, which can be accentuated by forced expiration while the patient assumes different positions. The trachea may be deviated if the upper lobes have undergone loss in volume.[37]

Evidence of extrapulmonary TB in other areas of the body (e.g., spine tenderness; swollen lymph nodes; joint tenderness; enlarged abdominal organs, including the liver and spleen) should also be documented. Changes in skin color or blood pressure due to adrenocortical involvement may be present. Digital clubbing and hypertrophic osteoarthropathy are rare findings of TB.[38]

A pleural effusion, whether or not it is associated with TB, is characterized by dullness to percussion and absence of breath sounds over the affected region as well as diminished transmission of spoken or whispered sounds. The size of the effusion determines the degree of underlying lung compression and subsequent lung dysfunction.[39]

Laboratory Data

The microbiology laboratory provides the basis for TB diagnosis, but routine laboratory data are minimally helpful in the absence of any other underlying infections.[40] The white blood cell (WBC) count is usually normal in primary pulmonary TB. A WBC count greater than 15 to $20 \times 10^3/\mu L$ is generally suggestive of another type of infection except in cases of miliary TB (TB dissemination into the blood), which can result in significant leukocytosis.[41] A mild anemia may be seen in chronic TB. The following laboratory data may be increased with TB, yet are considered nonspecific because other problems can also make them abnormal:

- Increase of immature WBCs (left shift) as the TB spreads
- Elevated erythrocyte sedimentation rate
- Increase in α_2-globulins and γ-globulin
- Elevated transaminases and alkaline phosphatase

Arterial blood gas assessment is rarely helpful in evaluating the initial presentation of TB. In a mild infection, the patient will compensate for mild $\dot{V}/\dot{Q}$ mismatching and hypoxemia by hyperventilation, which results in respiratory alkalosis. Respiratory acidosis and hypoxemia are seen only in end-stage TB patients in respiratory failure.

Posteroanterior and lateral chest films show the extent of pulmonary involvement and location of the disease. Together with bacteriologic examinations of sputum and a positive skin test, the chest radiograph provides a valuable tool in the diagnosis of TB (Fig. 20–3). The chest radiograph may also show involvement of the hilar and paratracheal lymph nodes. Atelectasis, pleural effusions, and empyema may be seen on the chest film.[42,43]

Bacteriologic Diagnosis. Numerous nontuberculous strains of *Mycobacteria* can show up on AFB smears. Therefore, a culture of *M. tuberculosis* is a necessary test to confirm TB[44,45]; unfortunately, these cultures take up to 6 weeks to complete. New in-

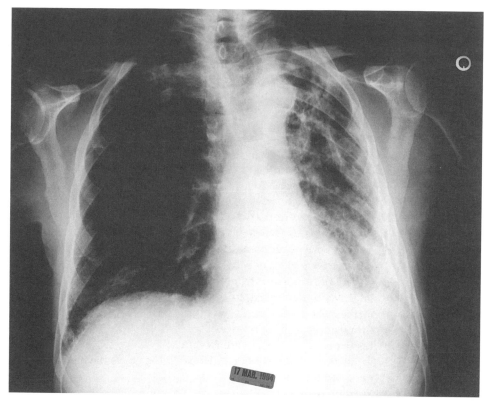

FIGURE 20-3   Typical chest radiograph for tuberculosis. Note the cavity lesion in the right upper lobe.

novations to circumvent this problem include DNA probe, polymerase chain reaction assay (from sputum), or mycolic acid pattern on high-pressure chromatography.[46-49]

An early morning collection of expectorated sputum is best for laboratory evaluation by stain and culture.[50,51] The least invasive method of collecting sputum is to have the patient produce the sample by coughing. If the patient is unable to produce a sputum sample, a sputum induction can be done to collect the specimen. The health care worker must be protected from exposure to TB during sputum collection and subsequent treatment of the patient. Whenever TB is suspected, universal precautions should be instituted to protect against potentially contaminated, aerosolized fluid.[52] In sputum induction, aerosolized hypertonic saline is administered for 15 to 20 minutes to stimulate the patient to cough and produce sputum. Saline helps the patient produce sputum by providing moisture and stimulation of expectoration.

TB patients often swallow their sputum during sleep; thus, in some cases where the patient is unable to expectorate sputum, a gastric aspirate culture is helpful. A sample of stomach contents is aspirated in the early morning before the patient arises. The use of a gastric aspirate smear has limited value, however, because of the presence of nontuberculous AFB in the gastric contents.

Bronchoscopy may also be used to collect a sputum sample if other, less invasive techniques are not effective. Use of local anesthetics during bronchoscopy, such as xylocaine, can decrease the viability of the *M. tuberculosis* organism. RCPs that assist physicians in the bronchoscopy procedure need to be aware of this fact and minimize the use of xylocaine in this setting.

Skin Testing. An estimated 10 to 15 million persons in the U.S. have dormant *M. tuberculosis* infection. The Mantoux skin test for TB is an intracutaneous injection of a standardized dose of **purified protein derivative (PPD).** A positive reaction is indicated by a visible or palpable induration (i.e., raised, hardened area) caused by prior sensitization to the TB organism. The CDC classifies the positive skin test reactions for specific groups as follows:

- **5 mm or more**
  - Persons who have recently had close contact with an individual with infectious TB
  - Persons whose chest radiographs showing fibrotic lesions are likely to represent old, healed TB
  - Persons with known or suspected HIV infection
- **10 mm or more in those who do not meet the above criteria, but have other risk factors**
  - Persons with other medical risk factors known to pose a substantially increased risk of TB once infection has occurred
  - Foreign-born persons from high-prevalence countries
  - Medically underserved, low-income populations, including high-risk minorities
  - Intravenous drug users
  - Residents of long-term care facilities
  - Populations that have been identified locally as having an increased prevalence of TB.
- **15 mm or more**
  - All other persons

Older patients should have a repeat skin test in 2 to 4 weeks if the first skin test is negative. A positive second skin test indicates that the first test was a false-negative and that the patient has been infected with TB. Approximately 5 to 8 percent of the overall population are considered anergic (i.e., nonreactive to the PPD). In addition to the above populations, skin-test screening for TB infection is also recommended in high-risk populations, including the following:

- Persons with signs or symptoms, or both, that are suggestive of TB
- Individuals in close contact with persons known to have pulmonary TB
- Persons with medical conditions that increase the risk of TB (see later discussion)
- Alcoholics
- Health care workers

It is important to remember that the absence of a reaction to the tuberculin test does not exclude the diagnosis of TB.[53]

Treatment

After the diagnosis of active TB has been established by culture and the extent of the lung disease defined by chest radiograph, treatment can be started. The decision as to which treatment regiment should be used is based on the extent of the TB infection, the skin test reaction, and the sensitivity of the *M. tuberculosis* organism to the drug. The following are the basic principles of TB therapy:

- An effective multidrug regimen must be included in each program.
- Organisms must be susceptible to at least two of the drugs used.
- Bacteriologic response should occur within the expected time.
- A single drug should never be added to a program that is failing.
- Drug treatment must continue for a sufficient period of time.
- Patient compliance must be monitored.

The first-line drugs are relatively effective and pose a relatively low risk of toxic side effects. In addition to the above basic principles, the CDC has recommended the following treatment criteria:

- **6-month regimen**
  - 2-month period of daily isoniazid, rifampin, pyrazinamide, and either ethambutol or streptomycin, followed by isoniazid and rifampin given daily or twice weekly for 4 months
- **9-month regimen**
  - 1 to 2 months of daily isoniazid and rifampin followed by twice-weekly isoniazid and rifampin for a duration of 9 months
- **Regimens of less than 6 months**
  - Not recommended[54]

Treatment Considerations

The most common side effect of rifampin, isoniazid, and pyrazinamide is hepatitis. It can usually be avoided by stopping treatment when liver enzymes reach three to five times the upper limits of normal. Rifampin also has the further potential side effects of gastrointestinal upset, skin eruptions, flulike symptoms, and red-orange discoloration of urine and other body fluids (permanent discoloration of soft contact lenses may occur). Side effects of ethambutol are ocular toxicity (optic nerve); however, at the doses currently recommended, this condition is rare. During pregnancy, treatment should continue for a minimum of 9 months, and breastfeeding should not be discouraged.[54]

Directly Observed Treatment

One of the most cost-effective methods of combating TB is called directly observed treatment (DOT). DOT calls for health care workers to ensure appropriate treatment by watching that their TB patients take each dose of the medications.[55-57] New treatment regimens that require only 2 or 3 days of medication each week have made DOT a more practical approach.

Prophylactic Therapy

Patients without active disease but with a positive skin test can decrease their risk for the development of active disease by taking a 6- to 9-month course of isoniazid. Unfortunately, isoniazid-associated hepatitis increases in frequency in older patients; hepatitis will develop in nearly 2.5 percent of isoniazid-treated patients over the age of 65. The risk-benefit ratio thus mandates prophylactic therapy for 9 months for any patient with a positive TB skin test who is less than 35 years of age and for any patient older than 35 who has had a recent TB skin test conversion.

CASE STUDY

History

ST is a 52-year-old mechanical engineer from Thailand who was referred to the pulmonary department by the public health service after his skin test was found to be positive. His brother, who lives with him, recently started a three-drug therapeutic course for a confirmed case of active TB. The patient denies having cough, sputum, fever, chills, night sweats, weight loss, change in exercise tolerance, or dyspnea. He reports, however, that in the early morning he has been producing one to two small globs of yellow sputum.

QUESTIONS

1. What kind of reaction was responsible for the positive TB skin test?
2. Does the positive TB skin test prove that the patient has active TB?
3. How would you determine whether the patient was merely infected with TB or had active disease?
4. What further tests should be done to clarify the situation?
5. Is this patient likely to be contagious, and should he be isolated from his family, friends, and coworkers?

ANSWERS

1. Cellular immunity is responsible for the positive skin test.
2. No, the positive skin test does not prove that active TB is present. It indicates only that TB infection is present, which could be either dormant or active.
3. Results of a sputum AFB smear and culture would determine whether active disease were present.
4. A positive skin test alone could occur with dormant disease; a positive skin test and a positive sputum TB culture indicates active TB.
5. The patient's contagiousness depends on the number of TB organisms in the lung, the amount of sputum production, and the severity of his cough. ST does not need to be isolated, but until the sputum smear results are obtained, he should limit his exposure only to those family members with whom he has already had recent contact. A negative sputum smear but positive culture usually means that relatively few organisms are present in the sputum and that the risk of transmission is low. Those who are susceptible to catching TB are the very young (especially infants) and the immunocompromised. If the smear and culture are negative, the patient may resume social activities.

Physical Examination

General: A thin, vigorous Asian man in no respiratory distress at rest

Vital Signs: Temperature 37°C (98.6°F), heart rate 80/minute, respiratory rate 14/minute, blood pressure 120/72 mm Hg

HEENT: Noncontributory to the current problem; neck supple with full, active range of motion; trachea midline and mobile with palpation; no stridor or wheezes; thyroid normal; carotid pulsations +2 and symmetrical with no bruits; no jugular venous distention; no cervicular or supraclavicular lymphadenopathy

Chest: Anteroposterior diameter of chest normal; normal expansion of chest with respiration; chest nontender to palpation; normal resonance of chest with percussion; axillae without lymphadenopathy

Heart: Regular rhythm; rate approximately 80/minute without murmurs, gallops, or rubs

Lungs: Clear on auscultation

Abdomen: Soft, nondistended, and nontender to palpation; no masses noted; no organomegaly; bowel sounds present

Genitourinary: Rectal examination is deferred at the patient's request

Extremities: No cyanosis, clubbing, or edema; pulses and reflexes +2 and symmetrical; Homans' sign bilaterally negative

QUESTIONS

6. Did the physical examination add any significant information to the history?

7. Has your impression changed about ST's risk of simple dormant infection versus active disease?

8. Should treatment be instituted at this time? If so, what sort of treatment?

9. Should the patient be isolated at this time? If so, for how long?

10. What tests should be done now, and how soon can results be expected?

ANSWERS

6. Yes, the physical examination suggests that if active disease is present, it is probably mild. There is no evidence of pleural effusion, lung collapse, or extensive tubercular pneumonia.

7. The physical examination does not reveal any evidence of active disease, since the breath sounds are clear and the vital signs are normal. So far, the only evidence of any disease is the history of recent TB exposure and morning sputum production. The recent exposure could result in either dormant or active disease. The sputum production suggests active TB or an unrelated problem, such as chronic bronchitis.

8. No, treatment should not be started yet. Further evaluation is warranted. We must know whether the patient has had exposure without infection, exposure with dormant infection, or active infection before deciding on treatment.

9. No, the patient should not be isolated yet. There is not enough evidence suggesting active disease. He should, however, be warned against visiting young, sick, or elderly persons. He should also be instructed to cover his mouth and nose with a tissue when he coughs.

10. Skin testing should be performed for TB and, in California, for cocci. Results should be available in 2 days. A chest radiograph is needed, and results should be available the same day. It is necessary to obtain a sputum AFB smear (results within about 3 days) and sputum AFB culture (final results in 6 weeks).

Laboratory Evaluation

Complete Blood Count (CBC): See Appendix for normal values

WBC 8000/μL:

Hemoglobin 14.2

Electrolytes normal

Creatinine normal

Normal liver profile (enzymes AST, ALT, and LDH normal)

Chest Radiograph: See Figure 20–4

AFB Stain (early morning sample): Few AFB organisms

Gram Stain: 2+ WBCs, 1+ gram-positive cocci

Sputum Culture: Normal flora

QUESTIONS

11. Would you expect the WBC to become abnormal during a TB infection? Why or why not?

12. The electrolytes, liver profile, and creatinine are normal. Is this more important for evaluating the tuberculous disease or for determining the dose of therapy?

13. The liver enzymes are normal. Would this finding affect your choice of therapy? Why or why not?

14. What are the typical chest radiograph abnormalities associated with TB infection?

15. Does ST's chest radiograph show typical evidence of active TB infection?

16. Does the presence of AFB organisms in the sputum smear prove that ST has TB infection?

17. Is the sputum Gram stain and culture helpful at this time?

18. What medications should be started at this time?

ANSWERS

11. No, the WBC count is not expected to increase with TB infection. Generally, WBCs do not play a role in the body's fight against AFB.

12. The normal chemistry, liver profile, and creatinine are useful in determining the dose and risk of therapy. The liver and kidneys both play a role in breaking down the TB medications. If these organs are damaged, the dose must be reduced to prevent toxicity.

13. Normal liver enzymes suggest that the patient should tolerate multiple drugs.

14. The typical chest radiograph in the patient with primary TB shows pneumonia or a small peripheral nodule. In post–primary TB infection with active disease, upper lobe cavity is common.

15. Yes, the patient's chest film shows typical evidence of active disease: A small upper lobe cavity is present.

16. The presence of AFB organisms does not prove that TB is present. Other nontuberculous mycobacteria can be present in the sputum (especially in HIV patients, elderly patients, and those with chronic lung disease). These

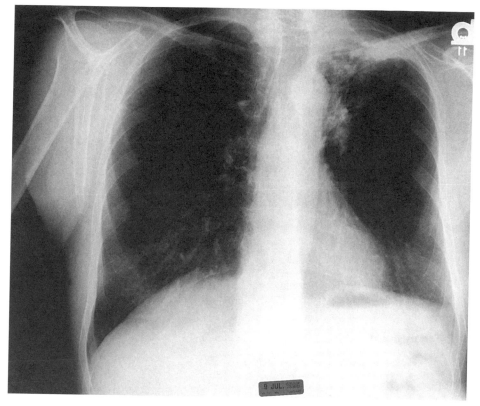

FIGURE 20–4   Posteroanterior chest film for patient ST.

bacteria are called atypical organisms, and culture is required to distinguish them from *M. tuberculosis.*

17. Yes, the sputum Gram stain and culture are helpful at this time because they help rule out concurrent pneumonia.

18. The physician should prescribe a combination of three of the four first-line drugs: isoniazid, rifampin, ethambutol, and pyrazinamide. Since ST is Asian and foreign-born, he is at higher risk of having disease resistant to one or more of the first-line medications. The initial use of three drugs to start is reasonable until culture and sensitivity results are back. The patient has no risk factors for drug complications.

CASE STUDY—continued

Follow-up

Two months later, ST continues to feel well. Sputum AFB cultures are positive for TB, and the organism is sensitive to all drugs. No further sputum is produced. His liver profile reveals elevation of liver enzymes to approximately two times normal, and his chest radiograph is minimally changed from the initial film.

QUESTIONS

19. Should the treatment be discontinued? If so, what new form of treatment should be instituted? If not, how should the patient be monitored?

20. Can any of the medications be stopped at this time?

21. How long should therapy be continued?

ANSWERS

19. No, treatment should not be discontinued.

20. Yes, the isoniazid and rifampin would be adequate for the treatment protocol.

21. A classic treatment regimen calls for continuation of isoniazid and rifampin for 6 more months.

CASE STUDY—continued

One Month Later

Weekly follow-up liver profiles have slowly returned toward normal levels, and ST continues to feel well. His chest radiograph is not significantly changed, but he is not coughing and no longer produces sputum.

REFERENCES

1. World Health Organization: Groups at Risk: WHO Report on the Tuberculosis Epidemic 1996. Arata Kochi, Executive Summary, Geneva, Switzerland, 1996.
2. Wenzel, RP: Airline travel and infectious tuberculosis. N Engl J Med 334(15):981–982, 1996.
3. Keyon, TA, et al: Transmission of multidrug resistant Mycobacterium tuberculosis during a long airplane flight. N Engl J Med 334(15): 933–938, 1996.
4. Riley, DK, et al: Tuberculosis: Yesterday, today, tomorrow. Ann Intern Med 124(4):455–456, 1996.
5. World Health Organization: WHO Report on the Tuberculosis Epidemic 1995. Hiroshi Nakajima, Executive Summary, Geneva, Switzerland, 1995.
6. Centers for Disease Control: Tuberculosis among foreign-born persons entering the United States: Recommendations of the Advisory Council for the Elimination of Tuberculosis. MMWR 39(RR-18):1–21, 1990.
7. Centers for Disease Control: Prevention and control of tuberculosis in U.S. communities with at risk minority populations. MMWR 41(RR5):1–11, 1992.
8. Stead, WW, et al: Racial differences in susceptibility to infection by Mycobacterium tuberculosis. N Engl J Med 322(7):422–427, 1990.
9. Chretien, J: Tuberculosis today. Eur Respir J Suppl 20:617S–619S, 1995.
10. Rubel, AJ, and Garro, LC: Social and cultural factors in the successful control of tuberculosis. Public Health Rep 107(6):626–636, 1992.
11. Centers for Disease Control: Tuberculosis morbidity: United States 1995. MMWR 45(18): 1–5, 1996.
12. Braun, MM, et al: Trends in death with tuberculosis during the AIDS era. JAMA 269:2865–2868, 1993.
13. Centers for Disease Control: Screening for tuberculosis and tuberculosis infection in high-risk populations; and the use of preventive therapy for tuberculosis infection in the United States: Recommendations of the Advisory Committee for elimination of tuberculosis. MMWR 39(RR-8):1–12, 1990.
14. Nazar-Stewart, V, and Nolan, CM: Results of a directly observed intermittent isoniazid preventive therapy program in a shelter for homeless men. Am Rev Respir Dis 146:57–60, 1992.
15. Centers for Disease Control: Prevention and control of tuberculosis in migrant farm workers: Recommendations of the Advisory Council for the Elimination of Tuberculosis. MMWR 41(RR-17):1–14, 1992.
16. Centers for Disease Control: Tuberculosis prevention in drug-treatment centers and correctional facilities: Selected U.S. sites, 1990–1991. MMWR 42(RR-11):210–213, 1993.
17. Perlman, DC, et al: Tuberculosis in drug users. Clin Infect Dis 21(5):1253–1264, 1995.
18. Rosenberg, T, et al: Two-step tuberculin testing in staff and residents of a nursing home. Am Rev Respir Dis 148:1537–1540, 1993.
19. Nardell, EA: Beyond four drugs: Public health policy and the treatment of the individual patient with tuberculosis. Am Rev Respir Dis 148:2–5, 1993.
20. Mahmoudi, A, and Iseman, MD: Pitfalls in the care of patients with tuberculosis: Common errors and their association with the acquisition of drug resistance. JAMA 270(1)65–68, 1993.
21. Frieden, TR, et al: The emergence of drug-resistant tuberculosis in New York City. N Engl J Med 328(8):521–526, 1993.

22. Sumartojo, E: When tuberculosis treatment fails: A social behavioral account of patient adherence. Am Rev Respir Dis 147:1311-1320, 1993.
23. Rieder, HL, et al: Tuberculosis in the United States. JAMA 262:385-389, 1989.
24. Glassroth, J, et al: Why tuberculosis is not prevented. Am Rev Respir Dis 141:1236-1240, 1990.
25. American Thoracic Society/Centers for Disease Control: Treatment of tuberculosis and tuberculosis infection in adults and children. Am Rev Respir Dis 149:1359-1374, 1994.
26. Fishman, AP (ed): Pulmonary Diseases and Disorders, ed 2, Vol 3. McGraw-Hill, New York, 1988, p 1802.
27. Baum, GL, and Wolinsky, E: Textbook of Pulmonary Diseases, ed 5, Vol 1. Little, Brown & Co, Boston, 1994, p 523.
28. Fishman, AP (ed): Pulmonary Diseases and Disorders, ed 2. Companion Handbook, McGraw-Hill, New York, 1994, p 355.
29. Farzan, S: A Concise Handbook of Respiratory Diseases, ed 3. Appleton & Lange, Norwalk, CT, 1992, p 81.
30. Fishman, AP (ed): Pulmonary Diseases and Disorders, Vol 3, ed 2, McGraw-Hill, New York, 1988, p 1827.
31. Fischl, MA, et al: Clinical presentation and outcome of patients with HIV infection and tuberculosis caused by multiple-drug-resistant bacilli. Ann Intern Med 117:184-190, 1992.
32. Fischl, MA: Clinical presentation and outcome of patients with HIV infection and tuberculosis caused by multiple drug resistant bacilli. Ann Intern Med 117:184, 1992.
33. Stead, WW, et al: The clinical spectrum of primary tuberculosis in adults: Confusion with reinfection in the pathogenesis of chronic tuberculosis. Ann Intern Med 68:731, 1968.
34. van der Ende, J, and Gompel, AV: Clinical problem solving: If at first you don't succeed. N Engl J Med 334(14):191-120, 1996.
35. Chaulk, CP, et al: Eleven years of community-based directly observed therapy of tuberculosis. JAMA 274:945-951, 1995.
36. Pitchenik, AE, and Fertel, D: Tuberculosis and nontuberculous mycobacterial disease. Med Clin North Am 76(1):121-171, 1992.
37. Fishman, AP: Clinical Forms of Mycobacterial Disease: Pulmonary Disease and Disorders, ed 2. McGraw-Hill, New York, pp 1843-1861, 1988.
38. Hernandez-Pando, R, et al: Adrenal changes in murine pulmonary tuberculosis: A clue to pathogenesis. FEMS Immunol Med Microbiol 12(1):63-72, 1995.
39. McColloster, P, and Neff, NE: Outpatient management of tuberculosis. Am Fam Phys 53(5):1511-1512, 1996.
40. Rolfs, A, et al: Amplification of Mycobacterium

41. Proudfoot, AT, et al: Miliary tuberculosis in adults. Br Med J 2:273-276, 1969.
42. Cohen, R, et al: The validity of classic symptoms and chest radiographic configuration in predicting pulmonary tuberculosis. Chest 109(2):420-423, 1996.
43. Bobrowitz, ID: Active tuberculosis undiagnosed until autopsy. Am J Med 22:650-658, 1982.
44. Daniel, TM: The rapid diagnosis of tuberculosis: A selective review. J Lab Clin Med 116(3):277-282, 1990.
45. Eisenach, KD, et al: Detection of Mycobacterium tuberculosis in sputum samples using a polymerase chain reaction. Am Rev Respir Dis 144:1160-1163, 1991.
46. Brisson-Noel, A, et al: Diagnosis of tuberculosis by DNA amplification in clinical practice evaluation. Lancet 338:364-366, 1991.
47. Choi, YJ, et al: Clinical significance of a polymerase chain reaction assay for the detection of Mycobacterium tuberculosis. Am J Clin Pathol 105(2):200-204, 1996.
48. Wilson, SM, et al: Progress toward a simplified polymerase chain reaction and its application to diagnosis of tuberculosis. J Clin Microbiol 31(4):776-782, 1993.
49. Condos, R, et al: Peripheral blood based PCR assay to identify patients with active pulmonary tuberculosis. Lancet 347(9008):1082-1085, 1996.
50. Harries, AD, et al: Sputum smears for diagnosis of smear positive pulmonary tuberculosis. Lancet 347(9004):834-835, 1996.
51. Richeldi, L, et al: Molecular diagnosis of tuberculosis. Eur Respir J Suppl 20:689S-700S, 1995.
52. Chaisson, RE, and McAvinue, S: Control of tuberculosis during aerosol therapy administration. Respir Care 36(9):1017-1025, 1991.
53. Centers for Disease Control: Diagnosis of TB infection and TB Disease. Doc. #250102. March 21, 1996.
54. Centers for Disease Control: Treatment of Tuberculosis Disease. Doc. #250111. March 21, 1996.
55. Combs, DL, et al: The USPHS tuberculosis short-course chemotherapy trial 21: Effectiveness, toxicity and acceptability: The report of final results. Ann Intern Med 112:397-406, 1990.
56. Iseman, MD, et al: Directly observed treatment of tuberculosis: We can't afford not to try it (editorial). N Engl J Med 328(8):576-578, 1993.
57. Weis, SE, et al: The effect of directly observed therapy on the rates of drug resistance and relapse in tuberculosis. N Engl J Med 330:1179-1184, 1994.

tuberculosis from peripheral blood. J Clin Microbiol 33(12):3312-3314, 1995.

CHAPTER 21

Lung Cancer

Gregory A.B. Cheek, MD, MSPH

Key Terms

bronchoscopy
carcinogens
chemotherapy
cytology

hemoptysis
Horner's syndrome
metastatic malignancy
primary lung cancer

ptosis
radiation therapy

Introduction

Lung cancer, also called *bronchogenic carcinoma,* is now the most common fatal cancer in both men and women in the United States. The American Cancer Society estimated that there would be 177,000 new cases of lung cancer diagnosed in 1996.[1] Currently, about 32 percent of cancer deaths in men and 25 percent of cancer deaths in women are due to lung cancer.[1] Despite advances in methods of cancer diagnosis and therapy, overall survival for lung cancer has changed little over the past 30 years. About 1 in 10 patients lives beyond 5 years from the time of diagnosis.[2] Earlier diagnosis and more effective therapy become ever more important as the worldwide incidence of lung cancer rises.

This chapter discusses cancer that arises within the lung itself (**primary lung cancer**). Cancer that arrives in the lung from other tissues (**metastatic malignancy**) is not discussed.

Etiology

Most scientists, except perhaps those employed by the tobacco industry, agree that cigarette smoking causes lung cancer. There is a strong association between smoking exposure and the incidence of bronchogenic carcinoma. Ten percent of all smokers eventually get lung cancer, and about 83 percent of all lung cancer patients smoke or have smoked.[3] The risk of lung cancer is related to the number of cigarettes smoked, the duration (in years) of smoking, the age at initiation of smoking, the depth of in-

TABLE 21-1 **Relative Risk of Lung Cancer**

Patient History	Risk Ratio*
Never smoked; no significant industrial contact	1
Cigarette smoker	
$<\frac{1}{2}$ pack/day	15
$\frac{1}{2}$–1 pack/day	17
1–2 packs/day	42
>2 packs/day	64
Cigar smoker	3
Pipe smoker	8
Ex-smoker	2–10
Nonsmoking spouse exposed to spouse's smoke	1.4–1.9
Asbestos worker	
Nonsmoker	5
Cigarette smoker	92
Uranium miner	
Nonsmoker	7
Cigarette smoker	38
Relatives of lung cancer patients	
Nonsmokers	4
Smokers	14

SOURCE: Adapted from Murray, JF, and Nadel, JA: Textbook of Respiratory Medicine. WB Saunders, Philadelphia, 1988, p 1177, with permission.
*The risk ratio is the relative risk of developing lung cancer compared to the risk of comparable individuals without the listed exposure.

halation, and the tar and nicotine content in cigarettes smoked. There is a 10- to 25-fold greater risk of lung cancer among smokers than among nonsmokers.[4] A person's lung cancer risk gradually declines for about 13 years after smoking cessation, but it never quite reaches a nonsmoker's risk level.[5]

A nonsmoker in the vicinity of a smoker inhales "sidestream" smoke that contains higher concentrations of **carcinogens** than the smoke inhaled by the smoker. There is about a twofold increased risk of lung cancer in individuals exposed to passive smoke.[6,7] Exposure to certain irritant fibers, ionizing radiation, and fumes from various chemicals has also been linked to an increased incidence of lung cancer. These agents include asbestos, chromium, nickel, uranium, vinyl chloride, bis(chloromethyl)ether, and decay products of radon gas.[8] Many of these materials potentiate the effect of cigarette smoke in the induction of bronchogenic carcinoma. Asbestos exposure in nonsmokers has been associated with a fivefold increase in the incidence of lung cancer. Asbestos exposure in cigarette smokers is associated with a 92-fold increase in the incidence of lung cancer (Table 21-1).[9,10]

A familial predisposition to lung cancer increases individual susceptibility to the disease. Compared to the general population, lung cancer is three times more likely to develop in persons who have close relatives with the disease.[11]

Pathology

The four major histological types of lung cancer are squamous cell (epidermoid) carcinoma (25 percent), adenocarcinoma (30 percent), large cell carcinoma (15 percent), and small cell carcinoma (25 percent).[12] The clinical effect of small cell carcinoma is much different from that of the other three forms of lung cancer, which is why lung cancers are usually classified in terms of small cell and non–small cell carcinomas (NSCLCs).

Squamous cell carcinoma is named for the appearance of cells that resemble those of the skin (epidermis). These cells usually contain the skin protein called *keratin*. Squamous cell carcinomas arise most often from the bronchial lining and may grow to obstruct air passages.

Adenocarcinoma resembles poorly formed glandular tissue. It may be difficult to determine whether an adenocarcinoma is a primary lung cancer or a metastatic tumor from elsewhere in the body. Many organs in the body can develop adenocarcinoma that may metastasize to the lungs.

Large cell carcinomas are characterized by a collection of poorly formed large cells that have abundant cytoplasm. These tumors may exhibit a glandlike structure and produce some mucin.

Small cell carcinomas are characterized by very "small" cells with scant cytoplasm. Small cell carcinoma is a very rapidly growing tumor that usually metastasizes to distant tissue (e.g., brain, liver, bone) while the tumor is quite small.

Lung cancer can affect lung function in a variety of ways, depending on the size and location of the tumor. Small, peripheral lung tumors may not impair lung function in a noticeable way. Larger tumors may invade the lung parenchyma and reduce lung volume in an amount proportional to the size of the growth. Cancerous growths may obstruct a major airway and result in pooling of secretions and little or no gas exchange distal to the obstruction. The affected lung region will typically become atelectatic and susceptible to pneumonia.

Clinical Features

It is essential to obtain a complete medical history and physical examination when evaluating a patient for lung cancer. Emphasis must be placed on identifying (1) symptoms that are commonly associated with cancer (Table 21–2) and (2) symptoms that describe the extent of the tumor spread and define surgical resectability.

Approximately 15 percent of patients are asymptomatic at the time of diagnosis (i.e., incidental nodule seen on chest radiographs).[3] Symptoms due either to local intrathoracic or to distant metastatic effects of tumor are present in about 70 percent of all lung cancer patients on presentation.[13]

Pulmonary symptoms associated with lung cancer may include a change in cough or sputum production, hemoptysis, wheezing, dyspnea, stridor, chest pain, or fever. These findings may provide the first clue that lung cancer is present and often are the result of the cancer's obstructing airways and lymphatics.

Cough and sputum production are not specific symptoms, as the majority of lung cancer patients suffer from chronic bronchitis and emphysema due to cigarette smoking. However, a change in the character of the cough, a change in the quality and quantity of sputum, or unresponsiveness to previously effective therapy (e.g., bronchodilators, antibiotics, steroids) should raise the suspicion that a tumor is present.

Shortness of breath may be associated with lung cancer when the tumor obstructs a large airway. Large pleural effusions or paralysis of a hemidiaphragm resulting from phrenic nerve involvement may also cause dyspnea.

TABLE 21-2   **Clinical Manifestations of Bronchogenic Carcinoma**

Cough	74%
Weight loss	68%
Dyspnea	58%
Chest pain	49%
Sputum production	45%
Hemoptysis	29%
Malaise	26%
Bone pain	25%
Lymphadenopathy	23%
Hepatomegaly	21%
Fever	21%
Clubbing	20%
Neuromyopathy	10%
Superior vena cava syndrome	4%
Dizziness	4%
Hoarseness	3%
Asymptomatic	12%

SOURCE: Adapted from Doyle, LA and Aisner, J: Clinical presentation of lung cancer. In Roth, JA, Ruckdeschel, JC, and Weisenburger, TH (eds): Thoracic Oncology. WB Saunders, Philadelphia, 1989, p 53.

Hemoptysis associated with lung cancer is caused by ulceration of the bronchial mucosa. The quantity of blood is usually small, but it can become massive and life-threatening. Hemoptysis usually prompts the patient to seek medical attention and is suggestive of endobronchial tumor.

Chest pain in lung cancer may indicate local invasion of the pleura, ribs, and nerves. It may be dull, constant, and debilitating or intermittent and sharp, varying with the respiratory cycle. It may localize to the chest wall, or it may radiate to the midback, scapula, shoulder, or arm on the side of the tumor.

In the lung cancer patient with a small tumor, physical examination findings may be relatively normal. Auscultation may reveal wheezing if an airway is partially obstructed. The wheezing is usually monophonic and localized, and does not disappear after a cough. Wheezing may be heard on both inhalation and exhalation. Percussion reveals diminished resonance over lung tissue affected by a large tumor, pleural effusion, or pneumonia (consolidation). Careful examination may reveal distant metastasis to skin or regional lymph nodes. Clubbing of the fingers or toes, or both, may indicate hypertrophic pulmonary osteoarthropathy (paraneoplastic syndrome) associated with lung cancer.

Physical examination evidence for surgical nonresectability includes hoarseness, facial edema, arm pain, bone pain, or changes in mental or emotional status. Hoarseness suggests left vocal cord paralysis caused by recurrent laryngeal nerve compression by tumor. Facial edema suggests compression of the superior vena cava by tumor. Tumor compression of the cervical sympathetic nerve plexus causes **Horner's syndrome,** which consists of **ptosis** (drooping eyelid), myosis (pinpoint pupil), and anhydrosis (lack of sweating of the cheek). Arm and shoulder pain suggests invasion of the brachial nerve plexus by a superior sulcus tumor (Pancoast's syndrome combined with Horner's syndrome).[14] Bone pain suggests metastasis to the bone. Change in mental status, emotional status, or coordination suggests brain metastasis.

Diagnosis

The 5-year survival rate for all patients with carcinoma of the lung is only about 10 percent.[2] This dismal statistic reflects the fact that the disease is usually advanced when first detected. Routine, frequent cytological and radiographic screening for lung cancer unfortunately has not proved to alter the mortality rate and is not cost-effective.[15] There are no official recommendations for screening patients for lung cancer, except for a high clinical suspicion based on risk factors discussed earlier.[16]

The aim of diagnostic procedures is twofold: (1) to confirm the clinical diagnosis by sputum cytology or histology; and (2) to establish the extent of dissemination (stage) of the disease in order to determine the most suitable treatment (i.e., surgery, irradiation, chemotherapy, a combination of procedures, or hospice care).

Radiographic Data

The chest radiograph may demonstrate asymptomatic lung cancer and is almost always abnormal when the patient is symptomatic. A tumor nodule must be at least 2 to 3 mm before it is visible on a chest radiograph and greater than 1 to 2 cm before fluoroscopically guided transthoracic needle aspiration biopsy (TNAB) has a reasonable chance of making the diagnosis.[17]

A common dilemma associated with small pulmonary nodules is whether the

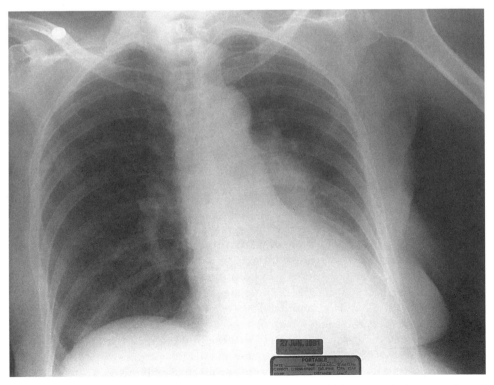

FIGURE 21-1   Chest radiograph demonstrating tumor obstruction of left lower lobe bronchus ("cutoff sign") leading to atelectasis distal to obstruction and mediastinal shift toward the lung volume loss.

nodule is a small bronchogenic cancer or a benign granuloma. Clues as to the probability of malignancy include growth rate, margin configuration, and presence of calcification. Malignant tumors grow at a rate such that the number of cells in the tumor doubles at least every 120 days, but not more often than every 30 days.[18] Careful measurement is important because a tumor or granuloma is a three-dimensional sphere: A doubling of its volume changes its diameter only by a factor of 1.27. Tumor margins are most often irregular and indistinct because tumors invade neighboring tissue, whereas granulomas often develop around a central area of inflammation and therefore have very smooth, distinct borders. Tumors may rarely develop asymmetric calcification, whereas granulomas develop central, well-defined calcification. A rare benign tumor called a *hamartoma* is noted for developing a pattern of calcification with a "popcorn ball" configuration.[19]

The heart and other thoracic structures obscure large portions of the lung tissue, and it is important to evaluate both a frontal and side view before calling a chest radiograph "normal." The four most common types of bronchogenic carcinoma (squa-

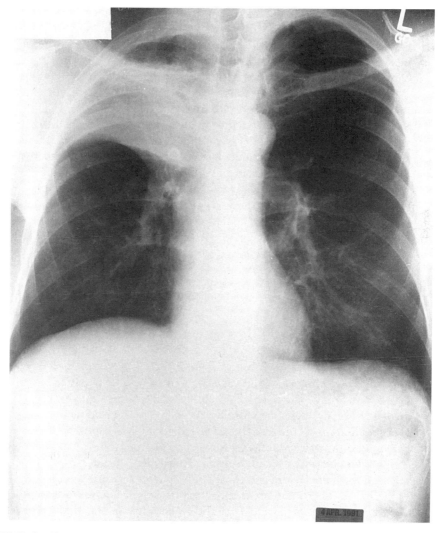

FIGURE 21–2   Chest radiograph demonstrating right upper lobe pneumonia and atelectasis from tumor obstruction of a major airway.

mous cell, adenocarcinoma, small cell, and large cell) usually present with slightly different chest radiographic patterns, but there is so much overlap that only biopsy and histological examination provide reliable evidence about the cell type.

Obstruction of a main or segmental bronchus may be associated with atelectasis. *Atelectasis* is collapse of lung alveoli distal to an obstructing lesion causing volume loss in a portion of lung. If the loss is large, a shift of the mediastinum toward the lesion is best seen on a maximal inspiratory chest radiograph (Fig. 21–1). Airway obstruction can also cause refractory pneumonia (Fig. 21–2).

Laboratory Studies

Other diagnostic tests that may reflect local, metastatic, or paraneoplastic effects of lung cancer include serum chemistry, complete blood count (CBC), liver function, arterial blood gas (ABG), the 12-lead electrocardiogram (ECG), and pulmonary function tests. Hyponatremia occurs in the presence of ectopic antidiuretic hormone (ADH), most often from small cell carcinoma. Hypercalcemia in lung cancer occurs either due to metastatic tumor spread to bone or from a parathyroid hormone–like substance most often associated with squamous cell carcinoma. Alkaline phosphatase may be elevated in the presence of bone or liver metastases. Liver dysfunction may occur due to intrahepatic spread or extrahepatic obstruction, or both, from metastatic disease. *Anemia* (low hemoglobin), *thrombocytopenia* (low platelet count), *leukoerythroblastic peripheral blood pattern* (immature blood cell forms resembling leukemia), and even *pancytopenia* (low count of all blood cell types) may occur from metastatic spread of tumor to bone marrow. ABGs may show hypoxemia resulting from ventilation-perfusion abnormalities or shunting.

The ECG may show low voltage or pulsus alternans (i.e., amplitude of QRS waveform varies with respiration) due to pericardial effusion or a conduction block from metastatic disease. A murmur may indicate *marantic endocarditis* (noninfectious vegetations on heart valves) or spread of tumor via the pulmonary vein to form an intracardiac mass. Pulmonary function tests may indicate restrictive disease owing to lymphatic spread.

Diagnostic Procedures

Methods available for diagnosing bronchogenic carcinoma include sputum cytology, fiberoptic bronchoscopy with transbronchial needle or forceps biopsy, percutaneous TNAB (also termed fine-needle aspiration), thoracentesis, pleural biopsy, thoracoscopy, mediastinoscopy, and thoracotomy (wedge resection/lobectomy/pneumonectomy). Each method has its inherent benefits, risks, and limitations.

Sputum **cytology** is useful for diagnosing central squamous cell carcinomas. It is much less helpful in diagnosing peripheral lesions because relatively few cells are released from the lesion, and those that are released rarely get to the central airways.

Flexible fiberoptic **bronchoscopy** is an invaluable tool for diagnosing bronchogenic carcinoma. The extent and operability of the tumor are assessed by observing the site of the tumor and extent of airway involvement. When lesions are visible endobronchially, bronchial washings have a diagnostic yield of approximately 80 percent; bronchial brushings and bronchial mucosal forceps biopsy samples provide diagnosis of tissue in nearly 98 percent of visualized tumors.[15] False-negative results may occur in deeper, submucosal lesions because they cannot be grasped and sampled adequately. Under fluoroscopic control, transbronchial forceps biopsies, brushings, and washings can diagnose peripheral, parenchymal lesions up to 60 percent of the time. Blind transbronchial fine-needle aspiration biopsies are commonly directed toward submucosal lesions or known areas of adenopathy evident on computed tomography (CT) of the chest.[17]

The use of TNAB is most suitable for peripheral pulmonary nodules (i.e., tumors located away from mediastinal vascular structures and emphysematous bullae). Fluoroscopic guidance is adequate for nodules that are 2 cm or greater in diameter and visible on both frontal and lateral chest radiographs. For lesions as small as 2 cm, the diagnostic accuracy is about 95 percent for malignant lesions.[3] Nodules smaller than 2 cm in diameter are usually aspirated under CT guidance. The incidence of pneumothorax is 15 to 35 percent and is more common in emphysematous patients. Only 5 to 10 percent of patients with TNAB require any kind of thoracostomy tube placement for lung reexpansion after biopsy.[20] Bronchoscopy carries less risk of pneumothorax (less than 5 percent with transbronchial biopsy).[21]

A positive pleural fluid cytology proves the spread of malignancy to the pleural space. Definitive diagnosis may be obtained from a cell block of centrifuged pleural fluid or positive histology from pleural biopsy. Thoracentesis and pleural biopsy combined provide up to a 90 percent diagnostic yield in patients with malignancy.[3] Most malignant pleural effusions are exudative in nature. Exudative effusion has a pleural protein level of greater than 3.5 g/dL and a lactate dehydrogenase (LDH) level of greater than 200; pleural/serum protein ratios are greater than 0.5, and pleural/serum LDH ratios are greater than 0.6.

Thoracoscopy improves the diagnostic yield of exudative pleural effusions. Biopsy specimens are taken under direct vision with a diagnostic yield of 93 to 96 percent for malignant pleural effusions.[22]

Mediastinal lymph nodes are involved at initial presentation in about half of lung cancer patients.[23] Patients with evidence of mediastinal lymphadenopathy (lymph nodes greater than or equal to 1 cm) and with central or large (greater than 6 cm) peripheral lesions should have a diagnostic mediastinoscopy before having a thoracotomy. Anterior cervical mediastinoscopy allows direct visualization and biopsy of mediastinal nodes with less risk than an exploratory thoracotomy. Its use has decreased the percentage of unnecessary exploratory thoracotomies.[24]

Staging

Staging the extent of lung cancer is essential in selecting appropriate therapy and avoiding unnecessary surgery. The modified staging classification system developed by the American Joint Committee and the Union Contre le Cancer in 1986 provides a nomenclature that is widely accepted: the *TNM system* (T = primary *tumor*; N = regional lymph *nodes*; M = distant *metastasis* [spread of cancer to distant site identified on biopsy]). T describes the size of the tumor (Table 21–3). N describes the lymph nodes involved (Table 21–4). M is either present (M1) or absent (M0) metastasis (Table 21–5).

TNM classification is used as a basis upon which to formulate five stages of severity of lung cancer (Table 21-6). This system is primarily used in the management of NSCLC. In stages I and II, the cancer is considered surgically resectable. Stage IIIA cancer may be surgically curable, but the perioperative risk is high and the survivor benefit marginal. Cancers in stages IIIB and IV are not surgically resectable.

TABLE 21-3 **Definition of Primary Tumor (T) Characteristics in Lung Cancer According to TNM System**

Descriptor	*Definition*
TX	Tumor proved by the presence of malignant cells in bronchopulmonary secretions but not visualized on chest radiograph or by bronchoscope, or any tumor that cannot be assessed as in a retreatment staging
T0	No evidence of primary tumor
TIS	Carcinoma in situ
T1	A tumor that is 3.0 cm or less in greatest dimension, surrounded by lung or visceral pleura, and without evidence of invasion proximal to a lobar bronchus at bronchoscopy
T2	A tumor >3.0 cm in greatest dimension, or a tumor of any size that either invades the visceral pleural or has associated atelectasis or obstructive pneumonitis extending to the hilar region; at bronchoscopy, the proximal extent of demonstrable tumor must be within a lobar bronchus or at least 2 cm distal to carina
T3	A tumor of any size with direct extension into the chest wall, diaphragm, or mediastinal pleura or pericardium without involving the heart, great vessels, trachea, esophagus, or vertebral body, or a tumor in the main bronchus within 2 cm of the carina without involving the carina
T4	A tumor of any size with invasion of mediastinum or involving heart, great vessels, trachea, esophagus, vertebral body, or carina, or presence of malignant pleural effusion

TABLE 21-4 **Definition of Nodal Involvement (N) in Lung Cancer by TNM Classification**

Descriptor	*Definition*
N0	No demonstrable metastasis to regional lymph nodes
N1	Metastasis to lymph nodes in the peribronchial or ipsilateral hilar region, or both, including direct extension
N2	Metastasis to ipsilateral mediastinal lymph nodes and subcarinal lymph nodes
N3	Metastasis to contralateral mediastinal lymph nodes, contralateral hilar lymph nodes, ipsilateral or contralateral scalene or supraclavicular lymph nodes

TABLE 21-5 **Definition of Distant Metastasis (M) in Lung Cancer by TNM Classification**

Descriptor	*Definition*
M0	No (known) distant metastasis
M1	Distant metastasis present; specify sites

TABLE 21-6   **TNM Stage Grouping for Lung Cancer**

Stage	T	N	M
	TNM Subsets		
Occult cancer	TX	N0	M0
0	TIS	Carcinoma in situ	
I	T1	N0	M0
	T2	N0	M0
II	T1	N1	M0
	T2	N1	M0
IIIA	T3	N0	M0
	T3	N1	M0
	T1-3	N2	M0
IIIB	Any T	N3	M0
	T4	Any N	M0
IV	Any T	Any N	M1

Treatment and Prognosis

The majority of lung cancer patients present with extensive disease and have a poor prognosis. The choice of therapy and the survival rate are related to the histological cell type of the tumor and the stage of the disease at the time of diagnosis.

One of the most important indices of long-term survival is the patient's performance status at the time the lung cancer is diagnosed. The performance status is an objective assessment of the effect that the cancer has on the patient's ability to carry on with daily activities and work. Two scales are widely used in the United States: the Karnofsky Performance Scale and the Eastern Cooperative Oncology Group (ECOG) or Zubrod Performance Scale.[24] A poor performance status with a low-stage lung cancer indicates that the cancer may actually be more widespread than believed or that the patient's physiological status is such that he or she will not tolerate therapy well. There is a very strong relationship between performance index and length of survival.

Surgery

Surgical resection provides a cure in 60 to 80 percent of patients with stage I NSCLC.[12] A segmented wedge resection may provide the best risk-benefit ratio in patients with small tumors (stage I) and poor pulmonary reserve. Patients with stage I NSCLC and inadequate pulmonary reserve or severe concurrent medical problems are candidates for radiation therapy with or without chemotherapy and have an anticipated cure rate of about 20 to 30 percent.[12] Radiation therapy does not improve cure rate after surgical resection of stage I NSCLC.[12]

Surgery is the only curative modality for stage II and IIIA NSCLC. The treatment of choice is lobectomy or pneumonectomy with resection of regional and mediastinal lymph nodes, depending on the tumor size and location. Although 15 to 25 percent of patients who undergo surgical resection for stage II or IIIA NSCLC have local tumor recurrence, radiation therapy is not used because of the toxicity and lack of proven benefit on survival.

Stage IIIB (unresectable) cancer is treated with radiation therapy, especially when symptoms of pain, hemoptysis, or airway obstruction are present. Chemotherapy has provided relatively brief partial remissions in some patients.

Radiation Therapy

Radiation therapy can be beneficial for palliation of hemoptysis, bronchial obstruction, and bone pain from metastatic disease, but it is not a comparable alternative to curative surgical therapy. Candidates include patients who have inoperable NSCLC because of advanced stage or other medical problems. These patients should have a good performance scale status and be able to tolerate postirradiation pulmonary fibrosis. Complications include radiation pneumonitis and fibrosis, esophagitis, pericarditis, and damage to the spinal cord. Preoperative radiation is recommended only for superior sulcus (Pancoast's) tumor.

Chemotherapy

Chemotherapy is not used as a primary form of treatment for NSCLC, but it is recommended for small cell lung cancer.[25] Chemotherapy for lung cancer requires relatively toxic agents and is not generally easy for the patient to tolerate. Adverse side effects of chemotherapy depend on the specific drug regimen chosen. The most common side effects include bone marrow suppression, nausea, vomiting, renal and liver toxicity, and neuropathy. Some agents cause severe tissue necrosis if leaked into the skin around the IV catheter site. Inoperable NSCLC may be treated with radiation therapy or chemotherapy, or both. Chemotherapy can extend a patient's life for several months if he or she is responsive to it.

Small Cell Disease

Limited Disease

Chemotherapy is much more effective for small cell carcinoma than for NSCLC. The overall response rate (measured by remission of tumor growth or shrinkage of primary tumor mass, or both) with limited small cell disease ranges from 70 to 90 percent, with a long-term remission rate of 40 to 50 percent.[12] Concurrent radiation therapy of the thorax may decrease incidence of local recurrence. Prophylactic cranial radiation is used because metastasis to the brain is common and chemotherapy does not cross the blood-brain barrier.

Extensive Disease

Systemic chemotherapy results in an overall response rate of 60 to 80 percent.[12] Unfortunately, response rates are temporary and chemotherapy is palliative. The median survival rate ranges from 9 to 12 months.[12] Prophylactic cranial and early chest irradiation have no value in patients with extensive disease. Radiotherapy is important for palliation of brain and bone metastases.

Preoperative Evaluation

Among patients undergoing thoracotomy for diagnosis or cure, several parameters must be measured to estimate the patient's risk of perioperative pulmonary complications. One of the most important is *pulmonary function*. Postoperative survival depends on adequate preoperative pulmonary reserve. The desired postoperative forced expiratory volume in 1 second (FEV_1) is greater than 0.8 liter. In patients with borderline or poor lung function, a differential lung perfusion study helps to predict postoperative effective FEV_1. The percent of flow to the "good" lung that is to remain is multiplied by the preoperative FEV_1 to estimate postoperative FEV_1. This estimate is most helpful when large portions of lung are to be removed. Exercise testing is performed in some patients considered at high risk for surgery (i.e., preoperative FEV_1 less than 40 percent predicted and $Paco_2$ greater than 45 mm Hg) to measure oxygen consumption at peak exercise. In several studies, a peak oxygen consumption value of greater than 15 mL/kg per minute carried a significantly lower risk for perioperative cardiopulmonary complications and death compared to a lower value.[26,27]

CASE STUDY

History

CS is a 65-year-old man who presents with fever, chills, progressive dyspnea, and cough, which has produced one-quarter cup of yellow-green sputum each day for 2 weeks, and the sputum has been blood-tinged for 2 days. His exercise tolerance has been decreasing over the past 6 months, but he has not sought medical attention until now. He has also noticed a 30-lb weight loss over the past 6 months. He had smoked two packs of cigarettes per day for 40 years, but quit four months ago because "they didn't taste good anymore." He stated that he has had difficulty swallowing solids for 4 months and hoarseness for 3 months. He had been seen in the emergency room 2 days earlier for a diagnosis of "pneumonia" and given a course of oral antibiotics.

Surgical History: Transurethral resection of the prostate (TURP) 2 years earlier; basal cell carcinoma of the lip removed 1 year earlier

Medications: Amoxicillin 500 mg three times per day; metaproterenol inhaler two puffs every 4 hours as needed

Occupational Exposure: Worked in the boiler room on a ship in the Navy for 3 years during the Korean War, then as a sandblaster in a shipyard for 2 years; denies symptoms of tuberculosis (TB) or fungal disease, as well as exposure to these diseases

Current Occupation: Car mechanic and garage manager

QUESTIONS

1. What risk factors for bronchogenic carcinoma in this man's history can you identify? How many pack-years has he smoked?
2. What symptoms in the history suggest lung cancer?
3. Would old granulomatous disease increase the risk of lung cancer?
4. What would the following symptoms suggest in a patient suspected of having cancer?

a. Chest pain

b. Bone pain

c. Hoarseness

d. Dysphagia (difficulty swallowing)

e. Weakness of extremities or change in mental status

ANSWERS

1. Age is a significant risk factor for lung cancer,[28] but tobacco smoking is the most significant. The number of pack-years is calculated by multiplying the packs smoked per day times the number of years smoked. Ten percent of long-term smokers get lung cancer and about 80 percent of all lung cancer patients smoke or have smoked.[1] This patient has a 80–pack-year smoking history.

   Asbestos exposure (working in a boiler room without protective respiratory apparatus) is a risk factor for lung cancer; concurrent smoking and asbestos exposure vastly increases the risk (up to approximately 90-fold).[8,9] Exposure to silicates (sandblasting) also increases the risk of lung cancer in smokers.

2. Change in cough and sputum production may be a sign of lung cancer. Hemoptysis has many causes, including acute bronchitis, tuberculosis, pulmonary embolus, trauma, or tumor, but tumor is a likely cause of the bleeding in this case.

   Progressive dyspnea may be due to large airway obstruction from a tumor or worsening of the preexisting emphysema. Other possible causes for the dyspnea include pleural effusion, diaphragmatic paralysis, pulmonary embolus, or pericardial effusion.

   Unexplained weight loss should prompt a search for hidden malignancy.

3. Old granulomatous disease is associated with a slightly higher risk of lung cancer, especially if extensive scarring is present.

4. In the patient suspected of having cancer, specific symptoms may be suggestive of specific cancers:

   a. Lung tissue does not have pain receptors; therefore, chest pain indicates spread of the lung cancer to parietal pleura, ribs, or other chest wall structures.

   b. Bone pain may indicate bone metastasis or osteoarthropathy.

   c. The recurrent laryngeal nerve travels from the neck around the aorta and back to the vocal cord. Compression of the recurrent laryngeal nerve by tumor or enlarged para-aortic lymph nodes may cause hoarseness. Hoarseness indicates that the tumor has involved vital structures and is unresectable.

   d. Dysphagia (difficulty swallowing) may indicate esophageal compression from mediastinal adenopathy or invasion by lung tumor.

   e. Arm or leg weakness or change in mental status suggests metastasis to the brain. A metastatic brain tumor may be manifested initially by relatively subtle signs, but these signs gradually progress to overt mental, emotional, or physical dysfunction.

Physical Examination

General: Height, 5 feet 8 inches; weight, 120 lb; lethargic, thin, chronically ill–appearing white man who appears older than stated age, with mild respiratory distress; patient alert but mildly confused (disoriented to place and time) and unable to provide coherent history

Vital Signs: Temperature 37.6°C (99.7°F), pulse 102/minute, respiratory rate 22/minute, blood pressure 110/50 mm Hg

HEENT: Pupils equally round and responsive to light and accommodation (PERRLA); no ptosis, funduscopically normal; tympanic membranes clear bilaterally, edentulous; no jugular venous distention, facial edema, or adenopathy

Chest:

Chest Wall: Nontender

Heart: Regular rhythm, no murmur, gallop, or rub; point of maximum impulse below xiphoid process

Lungs: Markedly decreased breath sounds over lower right lung with inspiratory coarse crackles; localized, monophonic expiratory wheeze in right midlung; no pleural rub; right lower lobe dull to percussion

Abdomen: Soft, nondistended, with bowel sounds active; slightly enlarged liver at 4 cm below right costal margin

Extremities: Abnormally small muscle mass; no edema or cyanosis; mild enlargement (clubbing) of distal fingertips

QUESTIONS

5. What do the vital signs and general appearance indicate?
6. What does the decreased resonance to percussion over the right lower lobe indicate?
7. What does the monophonic wheeze indicate?
8. What would be the significance of facial edema?
9. What would be the significance of ptosis (drooping of the eyelid)?

ANSWERS

5. Low-grade fever is consistent with pneumonia. Respiratory rate is elevated slightly, indicating compromised respiratory mechanics, compromised gas exchange, psychogenic stress (anxiety) or a combination of these. There is no evidence of accessory respiratory muscle use or paradoxical breathing to indicate diaphragmatic fatigue (i.e., impending respiratory failure). Weight loss in conjunction with tumor is a poor prognostic sign. Confusion and lethargy suggest one or more of the following: cerebral metastasis, hypoxia, or hypercapnia.
6. Dullness to percussion indicates lung consolidation.
7. The localized right monophonic wheeze indicates partial airway obstruction of a single, large conducting airway in the right lung.
8. Tumor-related facial edema is most often caused by compression of the superior vena cava by enlarging tumor.

9. Eye ptosis is a sign of Horner's syndrome, which is caused by tumor compression of the sympathetic nerves (from lower cervical and upper thoracic spinal nerves).

Diagnostic Data

Chest Radiographs: See Figures 21–3 and 21–4

Esophagograms: See Figures 21–5 and 21–6

Chest CT: See Figure 21–7

Laboratory Evaluation

ABGs (on room air): pH 7.38, $PaCO_2$ 48 mm Hg, PaO_2 60 mm Hg, HCO_3^- 28 mEq/liter, SaO_2 94 percent

Electrolytes (see Appendix for normal values): Na^+ 144 mEq/L, K^+ 3.7mEq/L, Cl^- 108 mEq/L, total CO_2 29 mEq/L, blood urea nitrogen (BUN) 20 mg/dL, creatinine 0.9 mg/dL

CBC (see Appendix for normal values):

White blood cells (WBCs) 16,500/mm³

Granulocytes 64 percent

Bands 14 percent

Lymphocytes 12 percent

Monocytes 4 percent

Eosinophils 2 percent

Basophils 1 percent

Hemoglobin (Hb) 12.1 g/dL

Platelets 415,000/mm³

Ca^{++} 12.5 mg/dL (range 8.5 to 10.5 mg/dL)

Liver function tests normal

LDH 240 IU/liter (range 100 to 190 IU/liter)

Total protein 5.2 g/dL (range 6 to 8 g/dL), albumin 3.0 (3.5 to 5.5 g/dL)

Sputum Gram Stain for Culture and Sensitivities:

4+ polymorphonuclear neutrophils (pus)

3+ gram-negative rods

1+ budding yeast with hyphae

Epithelial cells less than 3 to 5 per high-power field

Spirometric Studies (2 months before this visit):

Prebronchodilator

Forced vital capacity (FVC) 3.4 liters (68 percent predicted)
FEV_1 1.7 liters (55 percent predicted)
FEV_1/FVC 50 percent

Postbronchodilator

FVC 3.6 liters (72 percent)
FEV_1 1.9 liters (60 percent)
FEV_1/FVC 53 percent

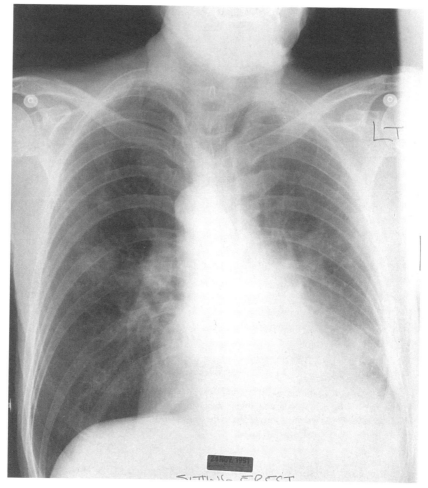

FIGURE 21-3   Chest radiograph taken two days earlier in an emergency room visit shows right lower lobe pneumonia with patchy infiltrate in the left lower lobe.

QUESTIONS

10. How would you interpret the ABG values?

11. What does the chest radiograph tell you about this patient's pulmonary condition?

12. What did the CT scan and esophagogram add to the information provided by the chest radiograph?

13. What pulmonary abnormality is suggested by the patient's pulmonary function data?

14. What is the significance of the elevated serum calcium?

15. What evidence indicates pneumonia in this case?

16. What diagnostic procedure would be most appropriate at this time?

17. Should the patient be hospitalized?

ANSWERS

10. The ABG is consistent with mild hypoxemia on room air. The acid-base status indicates compensated respiratory acidosis.

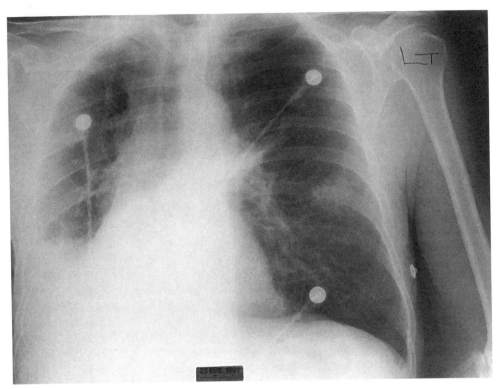

FIGURE 21–4   Chest radiograph (frontal view) of CS taken on day of admission demonstrates considerable atelectasis of the right middle and lower lobes with right pleural effusion due to obstruction of right bronchus intermedius. Evidence of bilateral metastatic disease most likely represents bronchogenic carcinoma.

11. Comparison of the admission chest radiograph to that taken the day before reveals a right bronchus intermedius obstruction, likely from tumor. There is also evidence of a cavitating metastasis to the left lung.

12. The CT scan of the chest demonstrates a mass in the right middle lobe and probable mediastinal and left lung metastases. On the esophagogram, tumor appears to have involved the esophagus (Figs. 21–5 and 21–6), causing high-grade obstruction to food passage. Overall stage of cancer appears to be more advanced.

13. The pulmonary function data indicate moderate obstructive pulmonary disease. The mild decrease in lung volumes may be due to air trapping or tumor. The patient demonstrates minimal improvement with bronchodilator therapy.

14. The elevated serum calcium may be responsible for the patient's confusion and lethargy. Of the various tumor types, squamous cell carcinomas have the highest association with hypercalcemia.

15. Indicators of pneumonia in this patient are the elevated WBC count with increased band cells (left shift to earlier WBC forms produced in response to significant infection), fever, pulmonary opacification on chest radiograph, and a sputum Gram stain positive for pus cells with predominance of gram-negative rod organisms.

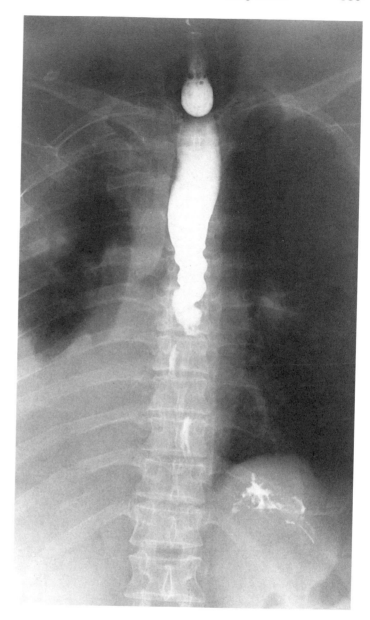

FIGURE 21-5 Frontal view of an esophagogram reveals high-grade obstruction of midesophagus, likely due to extensive mediastinal adenopathy or tumor invasion.

16. Bronchoscopy would quickly distinguish between common pneumonia and a cancer partially obstructing a bronchus, causing a postobstruction pneumonia. Not every patient with pneumonia needs bronchoscopy. In this patient, who has evidence of an obstructive lesion, weight loss, and a monophonic right lower lobe wheeze, bronchoscopy should have a high diagnostic yield for malignancy.

Sputum cytology is much less invasive than bronchoscopy, but it provides a specific tumor diagnosis in central airway lesions only up to 40 to 50 percent of the time.[14] It also provides little information about the extent of tumor.

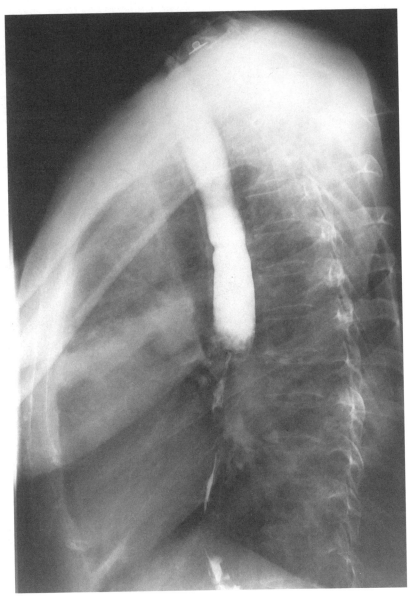

FIGURE 21-6   Lateral view of Figure 12-5.

17. The patient should be hospitalized for pneumonia and hypercalcemia and for symptoms suggestive of lung cancer. The lung cancer alone would not require hospital admission, but the combination of pneumonia and hypercalcemia requires intravenous (IV) drug therapy and close observation. For the pneumonia, antibiotics should be given; for the severe hypercalcemia, a course of IV saline and furosemide (Lasix), a diuretic to assist in urinary dumping of calcium, should be initiated. Cancer staging is necessary at this point, as is an assessment of the patency of the right bronchial airways.

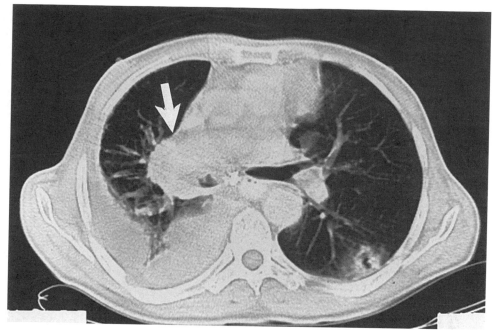

FIGURE 21-7 Computerized tomography of the chest shows a right hilar mass greater than 5 cm (*arrow*). A cavitary metastatic lesion is seen in the posterior left lung. There is evidence of pretracheal lymph-adenopathy with 2.5- to 3-cm lymph nodes. A moderate right pleural effusion is also visualized.

CASE STUDY—continued

CS was given IV antibiotics for the pneumonia and IV saline plus furosemide for the hypercalcemia. Flexible fiberoptic bronchoscopy was performed after 2 days of therapy. Bronchoscopy showed tumor totally obstructing the right bronchus intermedius with mucosal spread to within 2 cm of the carina. Analysis of tumor specimens revealed squamous cell carcinoma.

QUESTIONS

17. What is the TNM classification of this lung cancer, and what is its stage? (See Tables 21-3, 21-4, 21-5, and 21-6 for the classification systems.)

18. Is this patient a surgical candidate?

ANSWERS

17. The TNM classification is T4 (tumor greater than 3 cm in diameter indicated by chest CT, within 2 cm of carina, and involving the esophagus); N2 (2 cm mediastinal lymphadenopathy); M1 (evidence of metastasis to contralateral lung). A T4N2M1 classification is equivalent to cancer stage IIIB.

18. Surgical resection is not an option for stage IIIB lung cancer. Palliative therapy with radiation to shrink the tumor and reduce the symptoms of local and distant spread can be offered.

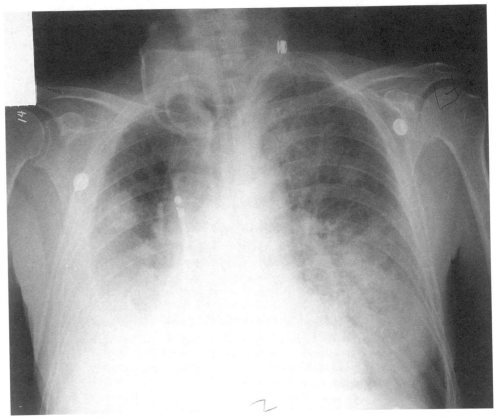

FIGURE 21-8   Chest radiograph (frontal view) shows pneumonia advanced to the lower left lobe with progressive postobstructive pneumonitis in the right lower and middle lobes.

CASE STUDY—continued

Two months after starting external-beam irradiation therapy to the thorax and mediastinum, CS returned to the emergency room for a sudden onset of massive hemoptysis. The patient coughed up about 800 mL of bright red blood over a 30-minute period. He was taken to the operating room for emergency rigid bronchoscopy. The airway was cleared of blood, a large clot was removed from the right mainstem bronchus, and tamponade with packing was successful. The packing was removed after about 15 minutes, and there was no further bleeding. After recovery from bronchoscopy, he was sedated with morphine to prevent coughing and transferred to the intensive care unit for observation. The patient enrolled in an outpatient hospice program. Six weeks later, the patient acquired postobstruction pneumonia (Fig. 21–8), was treated with oral antibiotics, and kept comfortable with supplemental oxygen and narcotics. He later died at home of respiratory failure.

REFERENCES

1. Parker, SL, et al: Cancer statistics, 1996. CA Cancer J Clin 65:5-27, 1996.
2. Khouri, NF, et al: The solitary pulmonary nodule: Assessment, diagnosis and management. Chest 91:128-133, 1987.
3. Silverberg, E, and Lubera, JA: Cancer statistics. Cancer 39:3-20, 1989.
4. Filderman, AE, et al: Bronchogenic carcinoma. In Brandstetter, RD (ed): Pulmonary Medicine. Medical Economics, Oradell, NJ, 1989, pp 525-549.

5. Wynder, EL: The etiology, epidemiology and prevention of lung cancer. Semin Respir Med 3:135–139, 1982.

6. Hirayama, T: Passive smoking and lung cancer: Consistency of association. Lancet 2:1425, 1983.

7. Weiss, ST: Passive smoking and lung cancer: What is the risk? (editorial) Am Rev Respir Dis 133:1–3, 1986.

8. Warnock, M, and Churg, A: Association of asbestos and bronchogenic carcinoma in a population with low asbestos exposure. Cancer 35:1236, 1975.

9. Hammond, EC, et al: Asbestos exposure, cigarette smoking, and death rates. Ann NY Acad Sci 330:473–490, 1979.

10. Samet, JM, et al: Personal and family history of respiratory disease and lung cancer risk. Am Rev Respir Dis 134:466–470, 1986.

11. Brincker, H, and Wilbek, E: The incidence of malignant tumors in patients with sarcoidosis. Br J Cancer 29:247, 1974.

12. Buzaid, AC, and Murren, JR: A progress report: Treating lung cancer. Contemp Int Med 9:78–90, 1990.

13. Muggia, FM, et al: Cell kinetic studies in patients with small-cell carcinoma of the lung. Cancer 34:1683, 1974.

14. Frost, JK, et al: Early lung cancer detection: Results of the initial (prevalence) radiologic and cytologic screening in the Johns Hopkins study. Am Rev Respir Dis 130:549, 1984.

15. Martini, N, et al: Early diagnosis of carcinoma of the lung. In Roth, JA, et al (eds): Thoracic Oncology. WB Saunders, Philadelphia, 1989.

16. Wang, KP, and Terry, PB: Transbronchial needle aspiration in the diagnosis and staging of bronchogenic carcinoma. Am Rev Respir Dis 127:344, 1983.

17. Chaffey, MH: The role of percutaneous lung biopsy in the work up of a solitary pulmonary nodule. West J Med 148:176–181, 1988.

18. Menzies, R, and Charbonneau, M: Thoracoscopy for the diagnosis of pleural disease. Ann Intern Med 114:271–276, 1991.

19. Bruderman, I: Bronchogenic carcinoma. In Baum, GL, and Wolinsky, E (eds): Textbook of Pulmonary Diseases, ed 4. Little, Brown & Co, Boston, 1989.

20. Carr, DT, and Holoye, PY: Bronchogenic carcinoma. In Murray, JF, and Nadel, JA (eds): Textbook of Respiratory Medicine. WB Saunders, Philadelphia, 1988.

21. Fletcher, EC, and Levin, DC: Flexible fiberoptic bronchoscopy and fluoroscopically guided transbronchial biopsy in the management of solitary pulmonary nodules. West J Med 136:477, 1982.

22. Menzies, R., and Charbonneau, M: Thoracoscopy for the diagnosis of pleural disease. Ann Int Med 114:271, 1991.

23. Bruderman, I: Bronchogenic carcinoma. In Baum, GL, and Wolinsky, E (eds): Textbook of Pulmonary Diseases, ed 4. Little, Brown, Boston, 1989, pp 1197–1237.

24. Carr, DT, and Holoye, PY: Bronchogenic carcinoma. In Murray, JF, and Nadel, JA (eds). Textbook of Respiratory Medicine. WB Saunders, Philadelphia, 1988, pp 1174–1250.

25. Faber, LP: Lung Cancer. In Holleb, AI, Fink, DJ, and Murphy, GP (eds). American Cancer Society Textbook of Clinical Oncology. American Cancer Society, Atlanta, 1991, p 194.

26. Morice, RC, et al: Exercise testing in the evaluation of patients at high risk for complications from lung resection. Chest 101:356, 1992.

27. Olsen, GN: Preoperative physiology and lung resection: Scan? Exercise? Both? (editorial) Chest 101:300, 1992.

28. Cummings, SR, Lillington, GA, and Richard, RJ: Estimating the probability of malignancy in solitary pulmonary nodules. Am Rev Respir Dis 134:449, 1986.

CHAPTER **22**

Sleep Apnea

Enrique Gil, MD, FCCP

Key Terms

central sleep apnea
continuous positive airway
   pressure (CPAP)
epoch
excessive daytime
   sleepiness
macroglossia
micrognathia
mixed apnea
narcolepsy

non–rapid eye movement
   (NREM) sleep
obstructive sleep apnea
   (OSA)
polysomnogram
rapid eye movement
   (REM) sleep
respiratory disturbance
   index
sleep apnea

sleep hypopnea
upper airway resistance
   syndrome
uvulopalatopharyngo-
   plasty (UPPP)

Introduction

Sleep apnea is not a trivial problem. Approximately 4 percent of women and 9 percent of men have significant **obstructive sleep apnea (OSA)**.[1] The implications from the medical and social standpoint are very important: Hypertension and stroke, among other disorders, are more commonly found in these patients, and daytime sleepiness is the cause of many accidents. Timely diagnosis and treatment of these patients may prevent serious medical complications.

Definitions

Sleep apnea is defined as a temporary pause in breathing lasting at least 10 seconds during sleep.[2] **Sleep hypopnea** is a period of hypoventilation or decreased airflow defined as a 50 percent reduction in thoracoabdominal movement lasting at least 10 seconds during sleep.[3] OSA/hypopnea is present when the respiratory drive is intact but the upper airway intermittently becomes obstructed during sleep. The **respiratory disturbance index** (also called the apnea/hypopnea index) is obtained by dividing the total number of events throughout the entire night by the total sleep time in hours. An index greater than 5 is abnormal, although it probably does not become clinically significant until it reaches 20.[4] The **upper airway resistance syndrome** is a form of obstructive sleep hypopnea in which the narrowing of the pharyngeal airway partially limits the airflow leading to an arousal during sleep. Usual measurements of airflow, effort, and oximetry fail to detect these events, which may be identified only by more sensitive means, such as measurement of intraesophageal pressures. These patients, however, may have significant daytime sleepiness and may respond to conventional treatment of sleep apnea.[5] **Central sleep apnea** is the cessation of airflow due to temporary loss of breathing effort during sleep.[2] **Mixed apnea** is the absence of ventilatory effort at the beginning of the event (*central component*) followed by effort with no airflow (*obstructive component*) with eventual resumption of breathing during sleep. An **epoch** is an arbitrary 30-second period used for staging sleep in the interpretation of a sleep study.

Sleep and Breathing

An understanding of sleep physiology is necessary in order to appreciate sleep disorders. Sleep is divided into two states: **rapid eye movement (REM) sleep** and **non–rapid eye movement (NREM) sleep**. NREM sleep is further divided into four stages. Normal sleep begins with stage 1, which is characterized by relatively low-voltage, mixed-frequency activity, with slow eye movements usually preceding sleep onset (Fig. 22–1). K complexes and sleep spindles with a similar background to that of stage 1 are characteristic of stage 2 (Fig. 22–2). Stages 3 and 4 (slow-wave sleep) are characterized by the presence of high-voltage slow waves in 20 to 50 percent of the epoch in stage 3 and in more then 50 percent in stage 4 (Figs. 22–3 and 22–4). REM sleep is characterized by rapid eye movements and absence of electromyographic activity (Fig. 22–5). The normal adult sleeper alternates between NREM sleep and REM sleep approximately every 90 minutes throughout the night.

REM and NREM sleep states both cause changes in breathing, even in healthy individuals. Typically, during the lighter stages of NREM sleep (stages 1 and 2) the breathing pattern is irregular because of the decrease in respiratory drive associated with the stimulatory effect of wakefulness and decreased metabolic rate associated

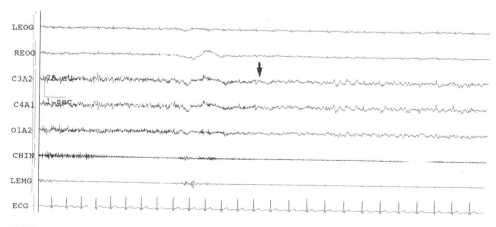

FIGURE 22–1   Polysomnogram demonstrating progression from being awake to stage 1 sleep. Note the low-voltage activity seen in the EEG leads (C3A2 & C4A1) characteristic of stage 1 sleep (*arrow*).

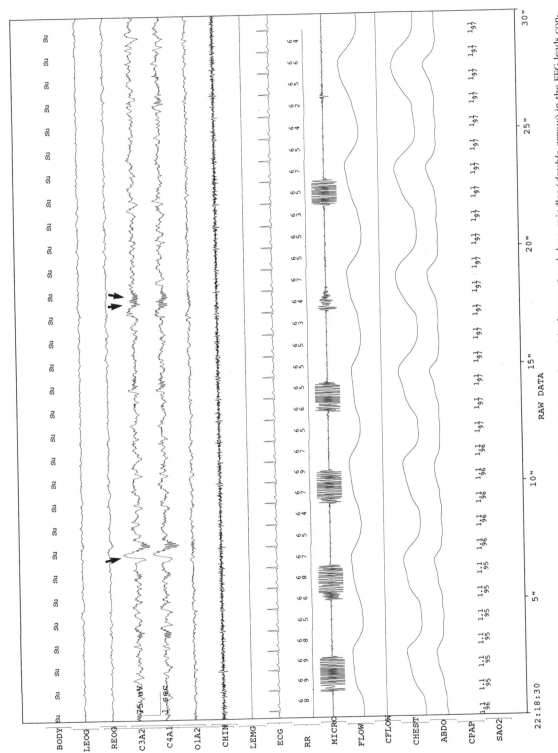

FIGURE 22-2 Polysomnogram demonstrating stage 2 sleep. Note the K complexes (*single arrow*) and sleep spindles (*double arrow*) in the EEG leads consistent with stage 2 sleep.

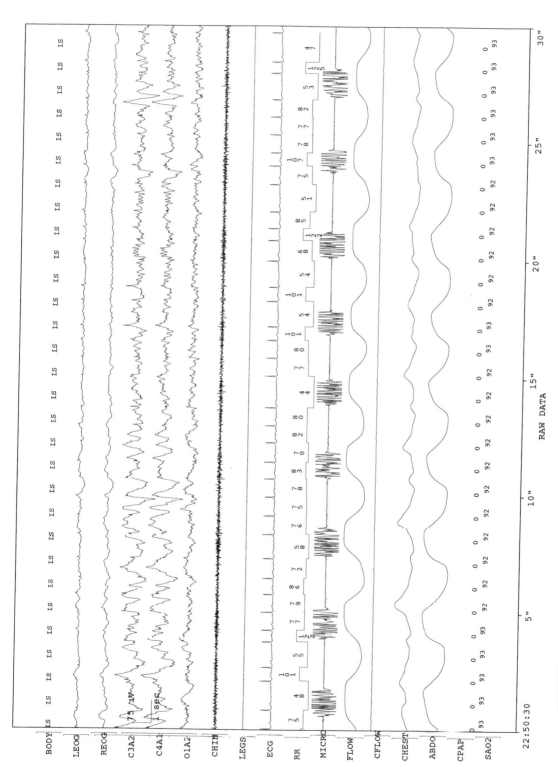

FIGURE 22-3 Polysomnogram demonstrating stage 3 sleep. Note the high-voltage slow waves seen in the EEG leads (C3A2, C4A1, O1A2).

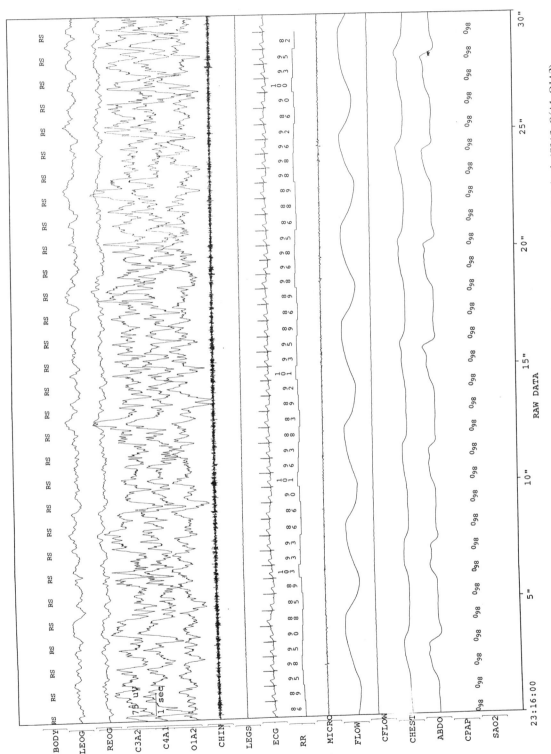

FIGURE 22–4 Polysomnogram demonstrating stage 4 sleep. Note the high-voltage slow waves seen in the EEG leads (C3A2, C4A1, O1A2).

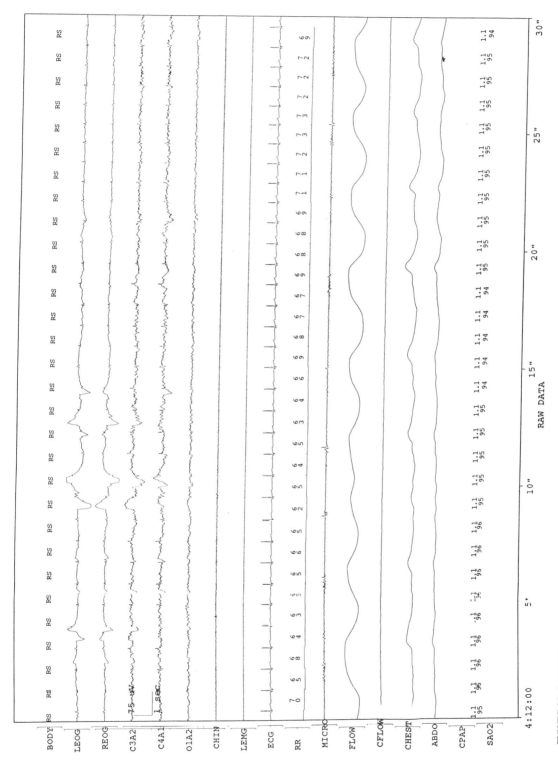

FIGURE 22–5   Polysomnogram demonstrating REM sleep. Note the large eye movements detected in the left and right eye oculogram tracings (LEOG and REOG) and the absence of EMG activity in the chin lead.

with sleep. In the deeper stages of NREM sleep, breathing is typically very regular; however, overall ventilation is reduced compared to that during wakefulness. During REM sleep, the respiratory drive is irregular because of the transient decrease in ventilatory response to chemical and mechanical stimuli. The influence of sleep on the upper airway is similar to its effects on other skeletal muscles, resulting in a general loss of muscle tone, and a reduction in tidal volume and minute ventilation.

Pathophysiology

Obesity, by narrowing the airway, is the most common cause of OSA. Structural abnormalities such as **micrognathia** (small mandible), **macroglossia** (enlarged tongue), or enlarged tonsils or adenoids can be contributing factors. OSA may be present in nonobese patients as a result of inherited or acquired anatomic narrowing of the upper airway. In the patient with OSA, whose airway is already compromised, the normal relaxation of the oropharyngeal muscles that occurs during sleep allows the airway to collapse even if the respiratory effort is normal or increased (Fig. 22-6). The resultant hy-

A

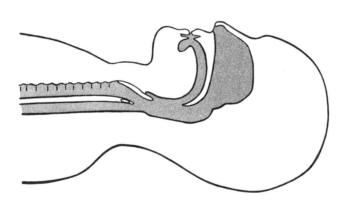

B

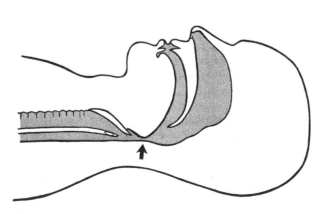

FIGURE 22-6 *(A)* Normal upper airway with patency; *(B)* obstructed upper airway typical for the patient with OSA *(arrow)*

poxemia and hypercapnia leads to an arousal that, by increasing muscle tone, terminates the obstruction. Repeated arousals lead to sleep fragmentation and daytime sleepiness.

The repeated episodes of hypoxemia during sleep result in adverse changes in the patient's hemodynamic system. Vagally mediated bradycardia may occur with the onset of hypoxemia. Tachycardia follows once breathing resumes. Systemic and pulmonary arterial blood pressures tend to rise during apneic episodes. The magnitude of the hypertension appears to be related to the degree of oxyhemoglobin desaturation. These pressures usually return to baseline once ventilation resumes; however, sustained pulmonary hypertension and cor pulmonale may develop in some patients. The incidence of systemic hypertension is higher in OSA patients than in the general population, especially in young, morbidly obese OSA patients.

Patients with central sleep apnea may have a decreased respiratory drive and therefore may have CO_2 retention and hypoventilation. The obesity hypoventilation syndrome fits this pattern. Most commonly in central sleep apnea, however, the respiratory drive is increased, and patients typically have hypocapnia. During sleep, the low CO_2 periodically inhibits the respiratory drive, resulting in an apneic event. This presentation is seen in patients with congestive heart failure who have Cheyne-Stokes breathing and at high altitude when hypoxemia leads to hyperventilation.

Clinical Features

The main features of OSA are **excessive daytime sleepiness** and loud snoring. Reports of apneic events by the bed partner are also common. Often the patient is seen by medical personnel at the insistence of the spouse, who either cannot tolerate the loud snoring or is concerned about the apneic events. Excessive daytime sleepiness interferes with many activities, such as driving an automobile, reading, and watching television. It can lead to accidents, interfere with family and social life, and cause loss of employment. Excessive daytime sleepiness is caused by sleep fragmentation stemming from frequent arousals necessary to relieve obstructive events during the night. Other symptoms related to OSA include poor memory, mood changes, morning headache, dry mouth, and impotence.

The OSA patient is typically an obese man with a short, thick neck. The OSA patient who is not obese may have anatomic defects of the upper airway, such as micrognathia, nasal obstruction, or a large tongue. These patients may have a narrow posterior pharynx and a large uvula. They may be hypertensive and present with signs of cor pulmonale, including lower extremity edema and venous distention. If obesity hypoventilation syndrome is present, arterial blood gases (ABGs) will reveal hypoxemia and hypercapnia during the awake hours. Otherwise, the daytime ABG is normal in OSA patients.

Sleep Studies

The definitive test for sleep apnea is the **polysomnogram**. Performed in a sleep center, this all-night recording of the patient's sleep is the "gold standard" for identifying the presence, type, and severity of sleep apnea. Using a multichannel recorder (polysomnograph), eye movements, airflow, respiratory movements, leg movements, electroencephalographic (EEG) readings, pulse oximetry, electrocardiographic (ECG) readings, and snoring are recorded. Recently, multichannel devices that record a limited number of parameters (e.g., respiratory movements, airflow, snoring, pulse oximetry, ECG) have been introduced for home studies, which may be comparable to a full polysomnogram. In patients with OSA, the polysomnogram demonstrates frequent episodes of apnea with corresponding periods of desaturation as demonstrated by pulse oximetry. The effort to breathe remains during the periods of OSA, as evidenced by the movement of the lower chest and abdomen.

If the polysomnogram is negative for OSA in the patient with significant daytime sleepiness, a multiple sleep latency test (MSLT) should be performed in a sleep center to rule out **narcolepsy**. The MSLT is performed the day after the polysomnogram, with the patient instructed not to take any medications such as sedatives and certain antidepressants for 2 weeks before the test. The patient is allowed to take four or five 15- to 20-minute naps 2 hours apart. Healthy subjects have a sleep latency of 10 to 20 minutes in the MSLT. A test is considered consistent with excessive daytime sleepiness if sleep onset occurs within 5 minutes. The presence of two sleep-onset REM episodes in the appropriate clinical setting is diagnostic of narcolepsy.

Treatment

For most patients with mild OSA, a combination of weight loss and avoidance of alcohol and sedatives is adequate treatment. More aggressive treatment is indicated if the respiratory disturbance index is higher than 20, or if the patient has excessive daytime sleepiness. It is important to remember, however, that patients with upper airway resistance syndrome may have a nondiagnostic polysomnogram. Therefore, a normal polysomnogram does not necessarily rule out OSA.

If the patient cannot lose weight, appetite suppressants such as phentermine and fenfluramine may be helpful; however, these drugs have been associated with pulmonary hypertension. Many OSA patients may already have a component of pulmonary hypertension, so the use of these appetite suppressants could potentially worsen it. No data are available regarding the use of appetite suppressants in the treatment of OSA; however their potential usefulness in a disease with significant morbidity and mortality is appealing. Our brief experience with their use suggests an improvement in symptoms in certain patients (unpublished observations).

Patients with moderate to severe OSA are treated with nasal **continuous positive airway pressure (CPAP),** which creates a "pneumatic splint" within the upper airway, preventing airway collapse and obstruction. The level of pressure needed to prevent obstruction (apnea and snoring) varies from patient to patient and must be determined by titration of the CPAP. Several nasal devices are available, including nasal mask and nasal "pillows." Both are effective, and their use depends on the patient's comfort and preference. The CPAP unit has some adjustable parameters, including pressure and a "ramp time" for slow increase of the CPAP up to the prescribed level in order to minimize patient discomfort and intolerance. Recently available units have two potentially very useful features:

1. The ability to record actual time of CPAP use under pressure. This feature may allow clinicians to evaluate patient compliance more efficiently, since it is impossible to distinguish between compliant and noncompliant patients on the basis of self-reports.[6] If compliance is poor, then a different treatment should be tried after every effort has been made to address any potential problems and side effects from CPAP use.

2. Ability to automatically titrate the CPAP needed during the night, providing optimal pressure at all times. This feature may minimize side effects and improve compliance.[7]

These devices may also allow home titration of nasal CPAP in those patients diagnosed as having OSA by multichannel home studies. One of the downsides of these units is their high cost.

Suboptimal patient compliance with CPAP remains a problem and an indication of our lack of a better treatment modality. Reported rates vary between 68 percent to 80 percent.[6,8,9] Reported side effects include nocturnal awakenings and nasal dryness, congestion and discharge, and sneezing.[10,11] The nasal congestion may be corrected with the addition of a humidifier in line with the CPAP unit, although not all patients find it helpful.[10] Recently, a heated humidifier has become available, which is probably better than the nonheated units; however, the cost of adding a humidifier is significant, and many insurance companies do not cover the added cost. Other simple measures that may be useful include the use of normal saline nasal spray and nasal corticosteroids. Other side effects include air leakage, causing ocular dryness and irritation; bruising of the bridge of the nose or gums; and facial irritation. Contraindications to the use of CPAP include acute severe sinusitis and nasal cerebrospinal fluid leak.

Of paramount importance in the treatment of OSA with nasal CPAP is regular follow-up to ensure compliance and address any potential side effects. The participation of an otolaryngologist/maxillofacial surgeon in the evaluation and management of patients with sleep apnea can be very important. Surgical approaches for the treatment of OSA bypass the site of obstruction or increase the size of the airway. Tracheostomy is very effective but not frequently used, and it is reserved for patients with severe, life-threatening disease or when other treatments have failed and the patient has severe OSA. In pediatric patients, removal of enlarged tonsils and adenoids removes the obstruction and is frequently effective.

Uvulopalatopharyngoplasty (UPPP) has a reported success rate of approximately 50 percent. Success rates of up to 66 to 78 percent have been reported when patients were evaluated with fiberoptic pharyngoscopy using the Müller maneuver or cephalometric studies to determine who would benefit from the procedure.[12,13] UPPP is useful in selected patients who fail to respond to nasal CPAP.[14] Laser UPPP may be useful, but there are few data in the medical literature regarding its benefits.[15] Laser UPPP may be useful in the treatment of snoring. Maxillofacial surgery should be considered in patients with craniofacial abnormalities. Dental appliances that relieve obstruction by repositioning of the tongue or advancing the mandible can be effective in selected patients.[16,17] Several surgical approaches directed toward weight loss have been tried, including gastric stapling.[18]

Patients with OSA have a higher risk of automobile accidents and should be informed regarding the risk of driving.[19] The legal implications for the patient and the treating physician can be significant.

CASE STUDY

History

Mr. L is a 47-year-old white man employed as a high school principal. Mr. L was seen in the outpatient clinic by his primary care physician because of excessive daytime sleepiness. He has had increasing problems over the past 6 months with daytime sleepiness, poor memory, and inability to concentrate. He often falls asleep while reading reports at work and while watching television at home. Within the past month he has been falling asleep while eating and during committee meetings. Two weeks ago, Mr. L was involved in a minor automobile accident in which he fell asleep while driving and ran off the road.

Mr. L's past medical history is noncontributory except for a tonsillectomy at age 6. He has no history of lung disease and denies having problems with coughing, sputum, shortness of breath, orthopnea, or hemoptysis. Mr. L reports using alcohol two to three times per week and has smoked two packs of cigarettes per day for the past 25 years.

QUESTIONS

1. What could be causing the symptoms of daytime sleepiness, memory loss, and lack of concentration?

2. What other symptom should the physician explore during the initial interview?

3. What signs should the physician identify during the physical examination?

4. Is there a connection between Mr. L's use of alcohol and tobacco and his symptoms? If so, what is the connection, and what should Mr. L be advised to do?

5. What simple techniques could the primary care physician suggest to Mr. L that might reduce his symptoms?

6. Does Mr. L require referral for objective evaluation of his condition?

ANSWERS

1. Both clinical depression and OSA are common causes of symptoms of daytime sleepiness, lack of concentration, and memory loss. The most common medical problem associated with excessive daytime sleepiness is OSA.[16]

2. The physician should ask Mr. L and his wife whether he snores. If he does snore, Mr. L's wife would probably be the best source for information regarding the intensity of his snoring, as well as the presence of pauses or snorts in breathing during sleep.

3. The physician should examine Mr. L for factors that may be contributing to upper airway obstruction (e.g., nasal polyps, obesity, neck size, large tongue) and for signs of heart failure. Evidence of heart failure in conjunction with OSA would suggest a more severe problem. The physical examination should also identify whether evidence of chronic lung disease is present in view of the patient's smoking history.

4. There probably is a connection between Mr. L's use of alcohol and his symptoms. Alcohol is known to worsen OSA symptoms. There is no evidence that the use of tobacco increases the severity of OSA symptoms, but patients with chronic lung disease who also have OSA are prone to more severe hypoxemia during periods of apnea. The more severe hypoxemia relates to the fact that these patients have some hypoxemia before apnea occurs, and once breathing stops, profound hypoxemia occurs more rapidly.

5. The primary care physician could recommend that Mr. L stop the consumption of alcohol, lose weight (if he is obese), sleep on his side or

prone, and avoid the using of sleeping pills. Although these suggestions may not completely relieve Mr. L's symptoms, they may markedly improve his condition.

6. Mr. L's attending physician should refer him to a sleep center, where a polysomnogram could be done to monitor his breathing during sleep.

Physical Examination

General: Patient alert and oriented, but apparently fatigued and sleepy; not in apparent distress; height 5 feet, 11 inches; weight 225 lb

Vital Signs: Body temperature 36.9°C (98.5°F); heart rate at rest 84/minute; respiratory rate 20/minute; blood pressure 138/85 mm Hg

HEENT: No evidence of nasal obstruction; narrow posterior pharynx with large uvula; pupils equal, round, and reactive to light and accommodation (PERRLA)

Neck: Supple, short, 19 inches in diameter; trachea midline; no stridor; carotid pulses ++ bilaterally with no bruits; no evidence of lymphadenopathy or thyroidomegaly; mild jugular venous distention (JVD) noted with the head of the bed elevated to 20°; no use of accessory muscles noted with breathing

Chest: Normal anteroposterior diameter with no use of accessory muscles at rest; no evidence of retractions or bulging with breathing

Lungs: Breath sounds slightly diminished bilaterally, with no adventitious lung sounds; no abnormalities noted with percussion over the lungs

Heart: Regular rhythm, with no evidence of murmurs or rubs; no heaves or abnormal pulsations over the precordium

Abdomen: Soft, nontender, markedly obese; normal bowel sounds; no organomegaly

Extremities: No clubbing or cyanosis; capillary refill normal; mild ankle edema

---

QUESTIONS

7. What is the most significant finding identified during the physical examination that may be contributing to Mr. L's problem?

8. Does the physical examination provide any evidence regarding the presence of lung disease?

9. What could explain the presence of mild JVD?

10. If OSA is causing Mr. L's problems, should the physical examination be more remarkable?

ANSWERS

7. The most significant findings of the physical examination are the presence of obesity, a narrow posterior pharynx, and a short, thick neck. Obesity appears to be the most common contributing factor to OSA.

8. The diminished breath sounds bilaterally may be the result of chronic obstructive pulmonary disease (COPD). It is also possible that obesity is making it more difficult to hear the breath sounds. Since Mr. L is a smoker, it would be prudent to order pulmonary function testing and a chest radiograph as a follow-up to the examination.

9. In some patients with OSA, JVD develops as a result of the frequent episodes of hypoxemia that occur during sleep. The pulmonary hypertension causes the right ventricle to fail and leads to a backup of blood into the venous system, which is seen as JVD. Since Mr. L is a smoker, it is also possible that he has developed COPD with hypoxemia. This could lead to chronic right heart failure and JVD. The presence of ankle edema also suggests the possibility of right heart failure.

10. It is not uncommon for OSA patients to have unremarkable findings during the physical examination. Only in very severe cases will complications such as heart failure cause significant findings during the examination.

CASE STUDY—continued

At the conclusion of the physical examination, the primary care physician referred Mr. L to a sleep laboratory for a polysomnogram. Fortunately for Mr. L, a nearby university hospital maintains a center for sleep disorders.

At the sleep center, a pulmonologist interviewed and examined the patient. The pulmonologist agreed with the primary care physician's tentative diagnosis of sleep apnea and arranged for an all-night sleep study. During the interview, Mr. L's wife indicated that he has been a habitual snorer for many years. She stated that his snoring had worsened recently and that she often sleeps in another room. She also has noticed pauses in her husband's breathing, but has never timed the pauses. She believes the pauses have lasted for no more than 1 minute.

At the conclusion of the interview, Mr. L and his wife were instructed regarding the purpose and procedures for the sleep study. They were given a brief tour of the facilities and advised to return later that evening for the sleep study. Mr. L returned to the sleep lab at 2110 hours and was put to bed at around 2300 hours. Mr. L had no trouble falling asleep in the laboratory and slept until 0530 the next day. The results of the sleep study follow.

Laboratory Evaluation

Sleep Latency: 8 minutes

Total Time in Bed: 381 minutes

Sleep Efficiency: 85 percent

Sleep Continuity: 23 awakenings, 56 minutes of wake time, and 261 EEG arousals (arousal index = 49)

Sleep Distribution: stage 1, 9 percent; stage 2, 69 percent; slow-wave sleep, 2 percent; REM sleep, 5 percent; REM latency, 213.5 minutes

Apnea Indexes: Apnea plus hypopnea index = 40; obstructive apnea index = 20; central apnea index = 1

Oxygen Parameters: Baseline SaO_2 levels, 90 percent; minimal SaO_2 during test, 69 percent; SpO_2 below 85 percent during 33 sleep periods

Leg Movements: 148 leg movements, 83 percent of which resulted in EEG arousals; leg movement index = 28

Cardiovascular Parameters: 114 cardiac rhythm abnormalities recorded, including unifocal premature ventricular contractions (PVCs)

Additional Findings: Loud snoring throughout the night

QUESTIONS

11. How would you interpret the following test results?

    a. Sleep latency?

    b. Sleep efficiency?

    c. Sleep distribution?

    d. Apnea indexes?

    e. Oxygen parameters?

    f. Leg movements?

    g. Cardiovascular parameters?

12. What is the probable cause of Mr. L's symptoms?

13. What treatment recommendations should be offered to Mr. L?

ANSWERS

11. The test results may been interpreted as follows:

    a. The sleep latency is in the normal range. Normal values for night-time sleep latency is less than 30 minutes.

    b. Sleep efficiency is abnormally low. Normal is greater than 90 percent.

    c. Sleep distribution is abnormal in this case. Normally stage 2 sleep represents 50 percent of sleep and slow-wave sleep 5 to 10 percent. REM latency is normally around 90 minutes. In this case, the REM latency of 213.5 minutes represents a significant delay in the onset of REM sleep. This abnormal distribution of sleep is consistent with someone who has numerous interruptions in sleep during the night.

    d. The apnea plus hypopnea index of 40 indicates that the patient averages 40 episodes per hour of abnormal ventilation during sleep. The obstructive apnea index of 20 suggests that approximately 20 of the 40 abnormal ventilation episodes each hour are due to obstructive apnea. (Figure 22–7 demonstrates a polysomnogram typical of an OSA patient.) The remaining 20 abnormal ventilatory periods each hour represent inadequate ventilation that may or may not be the result of upper airway obstruction. The central apnea index of 1 suggests that occasionally Mr. L experiences apnea as a result of a lack of ventilatory drive. This is not uncommon in normal sleepers, but is often found in the presence of OSA.

    e. The baseline Sao_2 of 90 percent represents a mild reduction in oxygenation while awake. The minimal Sao_2 value of 69 percent suggests that the patient experiences significant hypoxemia during sleep. An Sao_2 of 69 percent would correspond to a Pao_2 of less than 40 mm Hg. The patient had 33 episodes of hypoxemia throughout the night.

    f. The patient had an average of 28 leg jerks per hour and a total of 148 throughout the night. The majority (83 percent) of the leg jerks resulted in an EEG arousal. This suggests that the leg jerks are contributing to Mr. L's sleep fragmentation and daytime sleepiness; however, they may also improve with treatment of his sleep apnea, particularly if the movements are related to the apneic events.

    g. The numerous episodes of hypoxemia are causing abnormal cardiac function during sleep. Changes in heart rate and unifocal PVCs are common when the patient is hypoxic.

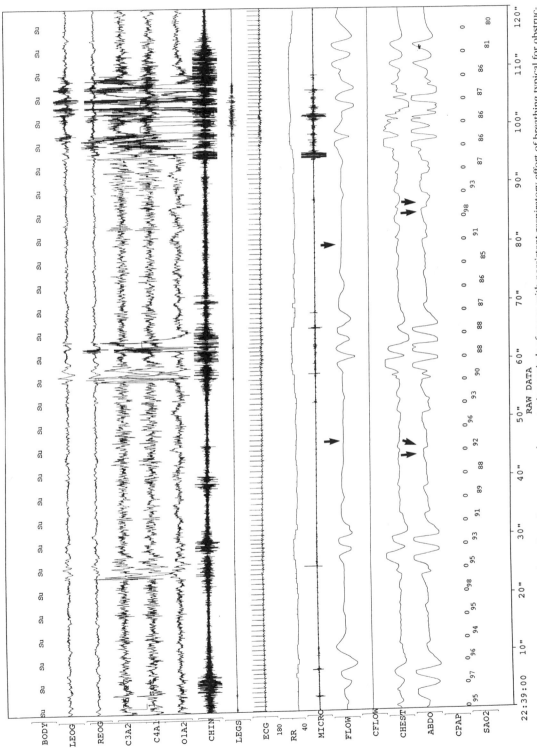

FIGURE 22–7   Compressed recording of a polysomnogram demonstrating periods of apnea with persistent respiratory effort of breathing typical for obstructive sleep apnea. Note the periodic lack of flow (*arrow*) in spite of breathing efforts, as seen by movement in the chest and abdomen leads (*double arrows*). EEG and chin leads show arousals terminating the obstruction. Note the desaturations (seen in the SaO_2 lead) associated with the obstructive events.

12. Mr. L's symptoms of excessive daytime sleepiness are probably the result of sleep fragmentation. The sleep fragmentation in this case is the result of OSA and leg jerks.

13. Treatment should include techniques for resolving the OSA and, if necessary, the leg jerks. Mr. L should be started on CPAP. He was advised to give up alcohol, since this can contribute to the problem, and to start a diet to lose weight.

CASE STUDY—continued

Follow-up

A diet plan was arranged for Mr. L. Nasal CPAP at 7 cm H_2O was successful in preventing the number of episodes of apnea and hypopnea. Mr. L tolerated the nasal CPAP well, and arrangements were made for home use. When Mr. L visited his attending physician 1 month after the initiation of treatment, his symptoms had improved, but he continued to have some daytime sleepiness. Compliance with treatment was confirmed. Leg jerks causing arousals were assumed to be the cause of Mr. L's continued daytime sleepiness. Periodic limb movement disorder is an entity of unknown etiology characterized by leg jerks that cause arousals and sleep fragmentation. This disorder often responds well to treatment with carbidopa-levodopa (Sinemet; a medication also used in the treatment of Parkinson's disease). Mr. L was started on Sinemet, and on a follow-up appointment his symptoms were reported to have significantly improved.

REFERENCES

1. Young, T, et al: The occurrence of sleep disordered breathing among middle aged adults. N Engl J Med 328:1230–1235, 1993.
2. Guilleminault, C, and Dement, W (eds): Sleep Apnea Syndromes. Alan R. Liss, New York, 1978, pp 1–12.
3. Gould, GA, et al: The sleep hypopnea syndrome. Am Rev Respir Dis 137:895–898, 1988.
4. He, J, et al: Mortality and apnea index in obstructive sleep apnea: Experience in 385 male patients. Chest 94:9–14, 1988.
5. Guilleminault, C, et al: A cause of excessive daytime sleepiness: The upper airway resistance syndrome. Chest 104:781, 1993
6. Rauscher, H, et al: Self reported vs measured compliance with nasal CPAP. Chest 103(6):1675–1680, 1993.
7. Meurice, JC. Efficacy of auto-CPAP in the treatment of the obstructive sleep apnea/hypopnea syndrome. Am J Respir Crit Care Med 153(2):794–798, 1996.
8. Reeves-Hoche, MK: Nasal CPAP: An objective evaluation of patient compliance. Am J Respir Crit Care Med 149:149–154, 1994
9. Meurice, JC: Predictive factors of long term compliance with nasal CPAP treatment in sleep apnea syndrome. Chest 105:429–433, 1994.
10. Hoffstein, V, et al: Treatment of OSA with nasal CPAP: Patient compliance, perception of benefits and side effects. Am Rev Respir Dis 145 (4 pt 1):841–845, 1992.
11. Pepin, JL: Side effects of nasal CPAP in sleep apnea syndrome. Chest 107(2):375–381, 1995.
12. Shepard, JW: Uvulopalatopharyngoplasty for treatment of obstructive sleep apnea. Mayo Clin Proc 65:1260–1267, 1990.
13. Aboussouan, LS: Dynamic pharyngoscopy in predicting outcome of UPPP for moderate and severe OSA. Chest 107(4):946–951, 1995.
14. Riley, RW, et al: Obstructive sleep apnea: Trends in therapy. West J Med 162(2):143–148, 1995.
15. Penek, J: Laser assisted uvulopalatoplasty: The cart before the horse (editorial). Chest 107(1):1–3, 1995.
16. Schmidt-Nowara, WW: Treatment of snoring and obstructive sleep apnea with a dental orthosis. Chest 99(6):1378–1385, 1991.
17. Eveloff, SE, et al: Efficacy of a Herbst advancement device in obstructive sleep apnea. Am J Respir Crit Care 149(4 pt 1):905–909, 1994.
18. NIH Conference: Gastrointestinal surgery for severe obesity: Consensus Development Conference Panel. Ann Intern Med 115 (12):956–961, 1991.
19. The official statement of the American Thoracic Society: Sleep apnea, sleepiness, and driving risk. Am J Respir Crit Care Med 150:1463–1473, 1994.

CHAPTER **23**

Croup and Epiglottitis

Robert L. Wilkins, PhD, RRT
James R. Dexter, MD, FCCP

Key Terms

croup
  (laryngotracheobron-
  chitis)

dysphagia
epiglottitis (supraglottitis)
intubation

retractions
stridor

Introduction

The upper airway, which consists of the nose, sinuses, pharynx, larynx, and trachea, is frequently exposed to a variety of irritants and infectious agents. It is not uncommon for these agents to cause inflammation and swelling of a portion of the upper airway. The inflammation may lead to significant narrowing of the airway and an increase in the work of breathing. Respiratory failure can occur if the patient fatigues. Additionally, complete obstruction is possible if the airway inflammation affects a particularly vulnerable portion of the upper airway (e.g., epiglottis). As a result, diseases of the upper airway represent a potentially life-threatening medical problem that clinicians must recognize and treat promptly.

A large number of medical problems are associated with diseases of the upper airway, but this chapter focuses on croup and epiglottitis. **Croup** is a viral infection of the larynx, trachea, bronchi, or a combination of these structures. It primarily affects infants and small children between 6 months and 3 years of age (Table 23–1). **Epiglottitis,** also called **supraglottitis,** is a bacterial infection of the epiglottis. It most often affects children between the ages of 1 and 5 years but occasionally occurs in infants and adults.

Croup

Etiology

Croup is almost always caused by viruses, the most common of which are parainfluenza viruses 1 and 3, influenza viruses A and B, respiratory syncytial virus (RSV), and adenovirus. Croup mostly occurs during the winter months.

TABLE 23-1   **Comparison Between Croup and Epiglottitis**

Parameter	Croup	Epiglottitis
Microorganism	Viral	Bacterial
Onset	Gradual	Acute
Most common age	6 months to 3 years	1 to 5 years
Site of disease	Below the glottis	Above the glottis
CBC	Often normal	Leukocytosis
Fever	Mild	Moderate to severe
Admission criteria	I & E stridor at rest	Admit all patients
Treatment	Cool mist, oxygen, racemic epinephrine	Endotracheal tube, antibiotics

CBC = complete blood count; I & E = inspiratory and expiratory

Pathology/Pathophysiology

Croup (laryngotracheobronchitis) causes inflammation and swelling of subglottic structures, such as the larynx, trachea, and larger bronchi. Croup can result in intrathoracic airway involvement, which leads to ventilation-perfusion ($\dot{V}/\dot{Q}$) mismatching and hypoxemia. Because croup can affect both upper and lower airways, the patient is at risk for ventilatory and oxygenation failure (see Chapter 3). If the upper airway obstruction becomes severe enough to jeopardize ventilation, the patient's respiratory muscles will eventually tire and the $Paco_2$ will rise.

Clinical Features

Croup frequently has a slow, insidious onset and commonly develops after 1 to 2 days of fever, nasal congestion, and coughing. The onset of croup is recognized by an increasingly severe cough that begins to take on a brassy or barking quality. Hoarseness is common and indicates inflammation of the vocal cords and larynx. Symptoms of respiratory distress develop when the trachea and bronchi become inflamed and narrowed. The symptoms associated with croup typically worsen at night, perhaps because of the drop in absolute humidity at night, which adds to the airway irritation.

Examination results of the croupy child may vary from nearly normal to markedly abnormal; the degree of tachycardia and tachypnea indicates the severity. A diminished sensorium should alert bedside clinicians to the onset of respiratory failure.

Inspiratory **stridor** is common and may frequently be heard without the aid of a stethoscope in patients with croup. Stridor is more common on inhalation because narrowing of the upper (extrathoracic) airway is increased momentarily with each inspiratory effort. When the airway obstruction is severe, however, stridor may occur on both inhalation and exhalation. **Retractions** are seen when the inspiratory effort is severe enough to cause a large drop in pleural pressure. This draws the skin surrounding the rib cage inward with each inspiratory effort and suggests a more severe problem. The retractions may be seen above or below the clavicles, as well as in the intercostal spaces.

Treatment

The majority of patients with croup respond to cool mist and do not need hospitalization. Keeping the child calm reduces stress on the respiratory system and may help minimize symptoms. Allowing the child to be held by a parent during examination and treatment may also be helpful.

Children with croup who present with inspiratory and expiratory stridor at rest, severe retractions, and tachypnea usually need to be hospitalized. Respiratory care practitioners administer cool mist and oxygen either by tent or face mask. Some infants and children do not tolerate a face mask and are more comfortable in a mist tent. A disadvantage of mist tents is that they make it difficult for clinicians to observe the patient and detect the onset of respiratory failure.

The use of racemic epinephrine may decrease airway edema and obstruction. Racemic epinephrine probably does not alter the overall course of illness, but it appears to offer temporary relief from upper airway edema and obstruction. The typical dose for racemic epinephrine is 0.25 mL of a 2.25 percent solution for children less than 6 months of age and 0.50 mL for older children. The racemic epinephrine is placed in 3 to 4 mL of saline and given by medication nebulizer or intermittent positive pressure breathing (IPPB) for 10 to 20 minutes. Repeat treatment may be needed in 1 to 2 hours. Tachyphylaxis is a common problem with racemic epinephrine and makes subsequent treatments less effective in some patients. Frequent use of racemic epinephrine may also lead to a "rebound" response that results in worsening of the airway obstruction.

In hospitalized patients with severe croup, corticosteroids have been shown to reduce the severity and duration of illness.[1] They are given if the patient appears severely ill or does not respond significantly to initial therapy of cool mist and racemic epinephrine. A single dose of dexamethasone (0.3 to 0.6 mg/kg) or an equivalent dose of prednisone is frequently adequate. Use of corticosteroids in the outpatient treatment of croup is controversial. A single intramuscular injection of dexamethasone (0.6 mg/kg) is associated with a reduction in symptoms within 24 hours of the visit to the emergency department in patients with moderate croup who are not hospitalized.[2]

The majority of croupy children respond favorably to treatment, but it is very important to monitor the patient closely in order to identify unexpected respiratory distress. Respiratory muscle fatigue proceeding to respiratory failure sometimes develops in croupy children. In such cases, the patient's sensorium, color, and arterial blood gases (ABGs) will deteriorate and endotracheal **intubation** is needed. In most cases, the child can be extubated in 2 to 3 days after airway inflammation has subsided. Criteria for extubation are lack of fever, minimal secretions upon suctioning, and presence of a small leak around the endotracheal tube.[3]

Epiglottitis

Etiology

Epiglottitis is most often caused by type B *Haemophilus influenzae,* although a small number of cases are caused by *Staphylococcus aureus*. It occurs year round and may follow a mild viral infection of the upper airway. Recent evidence suggests that the incidence of epiglottitis is decreasing, perhaps in response to the use of recently developed vaccines.[4]

Pathology and Pathophysiology

Epiglottitis causes inflammation and swelling of the epiglottis, aryepiglottic folds, and arytenoids (Fig. 23-1). The epiglottis often turns a bright, cherry-red color at the on-

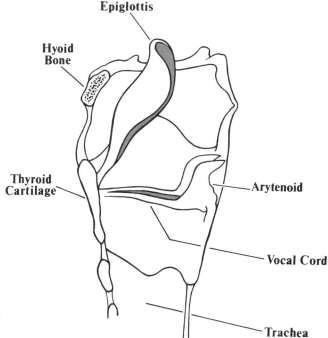

FIGURE 23-1   Cross-sectional view of the larynx.

set of the infection. The structures below the glottis are usually not involved. Supraglottic inflammation leads to difficulty swallowing (**dysphagia**) and airway narrowing, which is more pronounced during inspiratory efforts.

Patients with mild epiglottitis have normal ventilation and gas exchange as long as the upper airway remains patent. Ventilation is impaired, however, when the obstruction is severe, and death from ventilatory failure and asphyxia can occur if clinicians do not initiate proper treatment.

Clinical Features

Patients with epiglottitis typically have an abrupt onset of symptoms and appear more acutely ill compared to patients with croup. Patients with epiglottitis often complain of fever, sore throat, and difficulty swallowing. Drooling is common as a result of the patient's difficulty in swallowing.

The patient with epiglottitis appears toxic and prefers sitting upright. Sitting upright and leaning forward may make it easier for the patient to maintain a patent airway, since this position can help keep the swollen epiglottitis "out of the way." Inspiratory stridor and retractions are often present. Stridor varies with the position of the patient, level of activity, and degree of obstruction. Respiratory decompensation is associated with a diminished level of consciousness, and asphyxia may occur if treatment is not immediately implemented.

Although direct examination of the throat by depression of the tongue may reveal a bright red epiglottis and confirm the diagnosis, the procedure can also result in a sudden complete obstruction of the upper airway. Therefore, clinicians should perform the procedure *only* when equipment and personnel are available for intubation and tracheostomy.

Laboratory studies of the patient with epiglottitis reveals an elevated white blood cell (WBC) count with a left shift. A lateral neck x-ray demonstrates a swollen epiglottis and a normal subglottis. A chest x-ray reveals a complicating pneumonia in about 25 percent of epiglottitis patients.[5]

Treatment

All patients with the diagnosis of epiglottitis should be hospitalized because **intubation** or tracheostomy may be needed.[6] The risks associated with intubation or tracheostomy in patients with acute epiglottitis usually indicate placement of an artificial airway in the operating room. Initial airway management in the operating room is especially important because the upper airway occasionally obstructs completely in response to attempts at intubation, or even during simple inspection of the epiglottis. The physician and respiratory care personnel should stay with the patient at all times before successful placement of an artificial airway. If paralysis and mechanical ventilation are not employed, restraints may be needed in some cases to prevent accidental extubation.

Sedation and mechanical ventilation are not routinely needed in uncomplicated cases of epiglottitis because the problem is upper airway patency and the lungs are normal.[7] Humidity therapy applied to the endotracheal tube may prevent further airway irritation and mobilize respiratory secretions. A small condenser humidifier attached to the endotracheal tube does not need tubing and may reduce the risk of accidental extubation.[7] Oxygen therapy is not typically needed after intubation unless a complicating pneumonia is present.

Cultures of the epiglottis should be obtained after the airway is in place. The physician should order empirical intravenous (IV) antibiotic therapy to cover the most common organisms that cause acute epiglottitis (ampicillin 200 to 400 mg/kg per day, and chloramphenicol 100 mg/kg per day in divided doses every 4 to 6 hours for 7 to 10 days). The chloramphenicol can be discontinued if the culture results demonstrate that the *H. influenzae* strain is sensitive to ampicillin.

Extubation is often successful after 24 to 48 hours of treatment. The following are among the signs that the patient is ready for extubation: no fever within the past 12 hours, leak around the tube (which provides evidence that the inflammation has subsided), and improved general appearance of the patient. Daily direct visualization of the supraglottis is also an effective way to determine when extubation is acceptable. Extubation should be done with equipment and personnel available to replace the endotracheal tube should there be a sudden recurrence of partial airway obstruction.

CASE STUDY NO. 1

History

SR is a 6-year-old white girl brought to the emergency room by her parents at 3 A.M. The parents state that SR was healthy until the afternoon of the previous day. At that time she began complaining of sore throat, difficulty swallowing, and fever. Her mother obtained an oral temperature of 39.2°C (102.5°F) and gave her acetaminophen (Tylenol). Later that evening she became hoarse, her temperature increased to 39.4°C (103°F), and her breathing became rapid and labored. SR refused solid foods but was able to swallow small sips of juice. At 3 A.M. her parents decided to take her to the emergency room.

QUESTIONS

1. What medical problems do the symptoms in this case suggest?
2. What is the significance of SR's age?
3. What is the significance of SR's rapid onset of symptoms?
4. What physical examination techniques are useful in this case, and what purpose do they serve?

ANSWERS

1. The medial history suggests croup, epiglottitis, tonsillitis, strep throat, or pneumonia.
2. SR's age suggests that croup is not likely, since it occurs most often in children 6 months to 3 years of age.
3. The rapid onset of symptoms suggests epiglottitis.
4. The initial examination should focus on the vital signs and sensorium. This will help determine the severity of the illness. Auscultation of the chest and neck will be useful to identify adventitious lung or airway sounds that might suggest the location and severity of respiratory abnormalities. Inspection of the patient's breathing pattern to identify the presence of retractions and use of accessory muscles will assist in evaluating the severity of the problem.

Physical Examination

General: Alert and oriented; sitting upright and leaning forward, drooling, and apparently anxious

Vital Signs: Pulse 150/minute, respiratory rate 26/minute, temperature 39.4°C (103°F), blood pressure 110/75 mm Hg

HEENT: Unremarkable; throat not visualized at this time

Neck: Tracheal position normal; no lymphadenopathy; moderate use of accessory muscles with each inspiratory effort; inspiratory stridor noted on auscultation of the neck

Chest: Prolonged inspiratory time; clear breath sounds noted bilaterally; intercostal retractions

Heart: Tachycardia with a regular rhythm; no murmurs

Abdomen: Grossly normal; patient refused to lie down for abdominal examination

Extremities: No cyanosis or edema

QUESTIONS

5. Should the examination include direct visualization of the epiglottis to assist in making a correct diagnosis? Why or why not?
6. What do the vital signs and sensorium tell you about the patient's condition?
7. Why is the patient drooling?
8. What pathophysiology accounts for the retractions?
9. Why is the stridor heard only on inspiration? What would be indicated by stridor heard on inhalation and exhalation?

10. What is the most likely reason for the patient's refusal to lie down for the abdominal examination?
11. What laboratory tests would help make the correct diagnosis in this case? What are the anticipated results for each potential diagnosis?

ANSWERS

5. The attending physician should not attempt direct visualization of the patient's epiglottis until all the equipment and personnel are present to assist in emergency intubation and tracheostomy. This is important because the procedure of visualizing the back of the throat may initiate further inflammation of the epiglottis (if epiglottitis is the medical problem in this case), resulting in sudden, complete obstruction of the upper airway.

6. The rapid pulse and breathing rates suggest severe illness. The high fever is consistent with epiglottitis and is not common with croup. The normal sensorium indicates that the patient is probably not in respiratory failure.

7. The patient is drooling because of the painful swallowing. The pooling of secretions in the mouth and pharynx can cause aspiration.

8. The retractions are the result of changes in pleural pressure associated with strong contractions of the inspiratory muscles as the patient attempts to move air through a narrowed upper airway. This suggests that the patient's work of breathing is significantly increased.

9. Stridor is more common on inspiration because extrathoracic airways tend to narrow as the inspiratory muscles pull gas through the airway into the thorax. Inflammation of the upper airway causes narrowing that becomes more pronounced as the patient attempts to inhale. If the stridor were present on inspiration and exhalation, it would indicate a more severe case of upper airway obstruction.

10. Patients with a swollen epiglottis do not want to lie supine because this position makes breathing more difficult. The epiglottis is anterior to the tracheal opening, and leaning forward allows gravity to hold it away from the larynx. The swollen epiglottis is more likely to obstruct the larynx when the patient lays supine, which allows gravity to pull it back over the tracheal opening.

11. The complete blood count (CBC) helps to differentiate croup from epiglottitis. The WBC count, segmented neutrophils, and bands are usually elevated with epiglottitis. Lymphocytosis is more common with croup. A lateral neck film may show narrowing below the glottis with croup and an enlarged epiglottis with epiglottitis.

Laboratory Evaluation

CBC:

WBCs $15,500/mm^3$

Segmented neutrophils 74 percent

Bands 18 percent

Lymphocytes 4 percent

Hematocrit 39 percent

Lateral Neck Radiograph: Supraglottic narrowing consistent with epiglottitis (Fig. 23–2).

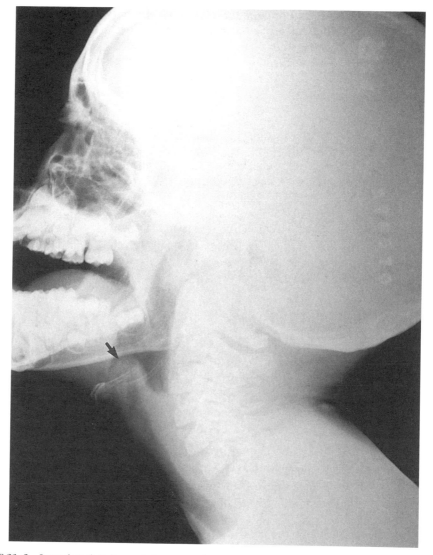

FIGURE 23-2   Lateral neck radiograph demonstrating an enlarged epiglottis (*arrow*). (Courtesy of Lionel Young, MD.)

QUESTIONS

12. Is an ABG important to obtain in this case? Why or why not?

13. Should the patient be hospitalized?

14. Should a throat culture be obtained?

15. What is the appropriate treatment?

ANSWERS

12. An ABG is not useful at this point. The procedure would probably add to the patient's anxiety and may worsen her condition.

13. All patients suspected of having epiglottitis should be hospitalized.

14. A throat culture should not be obtained until the integrity of the upper airway is assured. The procedure could lead to more swelling of the epiglottis.

15. The most urgent need for treatment is placement of a endotracheal tube. This would ensure a patent airway and prevent sudden obstruction of the upper airway should the epiglottis continue to enlarge. The procedure should be performed in the operating room, where an emergency tracheostomy can be performed if needed. IV antibiotics may be started as soon as an IV is placed.

CASE STUDY NO. 1—continued

SR was taken to the operating room, where an endotracheal tube was placed without complications. The tube was taped securely in place, and a cool mist with a fraction of inspired oxygen (FIO_2) of 0.35 was attached. SR was then taken to the pediatric intensive care unit (ICU) for further treatment. Her vital signs were as follows: pulse rate 128/minute, respiratory rate 24/minute, blood pressure 115/70 mm Hg, and temperature 39.2°C (102.5°F). Pulse oximetry demonstrated a saturation of 97 percent upon arrival at the ICU. A throat culture was obtained, and IV ampicillin and chloramphenicol were started.

QUESTIONS

16. What is the prognosis for this patient?
17. What is the most likely organism responsible for this infection?
18. When can the child be extubated?
19. How can accidental extubation be prevented?
20. Why is humidity therapy applied to the endotracheal tube?

ANSWERS

16. The prognosis for this patient is very good. A full recovery is expected.
17. The organism most likely responsible for this infection is *H. influenzae,* a small gram-negative bacillus. This organism may be resistant to ampicillin.
18. The patient can be extubated once the fever subsides for 12 hours and her general appearance has improved. This typically occurs 24 to 48 hours after intubation and the initiation of antibiotics.
19. Accidental extubation can be prevented by one or more of the following: close observation of the patient, careful explanation of the purpose of the tube to the child and parents, restraints, and sedation.
20. Humidity therapy is applied to the endotracheal tube to thin secretions and prevent obstruction of the tube with thick mucus. Since the upper airway is bypassed with an endotracheal tube the inhalation of dry gas directly into the trachea could be irritating to the mucosa. The application of humidity therapy may reduce airway inflammation.

CASE STUDY NO. 1—continued

After 36 hours, the patient's vital signs were normal and the patient was alert and oriented. At this point the patient was taken to the operating room, where she was extubated without complications. She was returned to the pediatric ICU for observation and continued IV antibiotics. Chloramphenicol was discontinued after the throat culture results demonstrated the presence of *H. influenzae* sensitive to ampicillin. After she was stable for 24 hours, the patient was discharged.

CASE STUDY NO. 2

History

RD is a 23-month-old white boy brought to the emergency room by his mother at 10 P.M. The patient's mother states that RD has had a cold over the past 2 days and developed a barking cough and respiratory distress earlier in the evening. The patient had been taking fluids poorly over the past 48 hours but refused to eat any solid food. He was given pediatric acetaminophen yesterday and today. The mother states that RD has "felt warm," but she did not actually take his temperature.

Earlier this evening shortly after the barking cough started, RD began to have labored breathing. At this point he was taken into the bathroom with the shower turned on for humidity. Although this seemed to provide some relief initially, RD began to have increased difficulty breathing at about 9:30 P.M. The patient's mother then brought him to the emergency room for treatment.

QUESTIONS

1. What are the possible medical problems suggested by this history?
2. What is the significance of RD's age and sex?
3. What physical examination techniques are useful in this case?
4. Was it a good idea for the patient's mother to take RD into the bathroom to breathe in a steamy environment? Why or why not?

ANSWERS

1. The differential diagnoses in this case include laryngotracheobronchitis (croup), epiglottitis, tonsillitis, and pneumonia.
2. The patient's age and sex are typical of croup, but they do not rule out epiglottitis, pneumonia, or tonsillitis.
3. Physical examination should identify the patient's general appearance, vital signs, level of alertness, breathing pattern, breath sounds over the chest and upper airway, skin color, and presence of retractions.
4. Yes, it was a good idea for RD's mother to take him into a steamy bathroom. The added moisture is often soothing to the irritated airways and may decrease respiratory distress.

Physical Examination

General: An alert child who is apparently anxious and working hard to breathe

Vital Signs: Pulse 144/minute, respiratory rate 36/minute, temperature 37.3°C (99.1°F), and blood pressure 150/P

HEENT: Normocephalic; eyes equally reactive to light; ears normal; dried nasal mucus discharge; nasal flaring on inspiration; throat apparently red upon brief inspection

Neck: Mild anterior cervical lymphadenopathy; loud inspiratory and expiratory stridor noted over neck

Chest: Severe intercostal and subcostal retractions; expiratory low-pitched wheezing noted over both sides of chest (loudest on the right)

Heart: Regular rate and rhythm without murmur; no heaves or lifts

Abdomen: Normal

Extremities: Skin warm and pink; normal pulses bilaterally in the upper and lower extremities

QUESTIONS

5. Based on the physical examination findings, would you consider this a mild, moderate, or severe case of upper airway obstruction? Upon what do you base this assessment?

6. What is indicated by the nasal flaring?

7. What is suggested by the low-pitched wheezing heard over the chest?

8. What laboratory tests would be useful, and what are the expected findings for each potential diagnosis?

ANSWERS

5. This appears to be a severe case of upper airway obstruction. This conclusion is based on the rapid pulse and respiratory rate, inspiratory and expiratory stridor, and severe retractions.

6. The nasal flaring suggests that the patient's work of breathing is increased.

7. The low-pitched expiratory wheezing heard over the chest suggests that the intrathoracic airways are involved in addition to the upper airway.

8. A CBC would be useful to differentiate croup from epiglottitis. Epiglottitis generally increases the WBC count, producing an increased percentage of segmented neutrophils and bands. The CBC may be normal with croup. If it is abnormal, there is usually only a slight elevation in the lymphocyte count. The CBC may be markedly abnormal with either croup or epiglottitis if a complicating pneumonia is present.

   A lateral neck film would be useful. Narrowing below the glottis is typical of croup; narrowing above the glottis is typical of epiglottitis. A chest film would be useful to evaluate the wheezing heard over the chest and to rule out pneumonia or atelectasis.

Laboratory Evaluation

CBC:

WBCs 12,800/mm^3

Segmented neutrophils 50 percent

Bands 3 percent

Lymphocytes 45 percent

Monocytes 2 percent

Radiography:

Lateral neck radiograph

    Subglottic narrowing (Fig. 23–3)

Chest radiograph

    Possible patchy infiltrate in the right middle lobe

QUESTIONS

  9. How would you interpret the CBC?

 10. Should an ABG be obtained?

 11. Should the patient be admitted to the hospital? Upon what information do you base your answer?

 12. What treatment is appropriate for this patient? State why each treatment modality is needed.

ANSWERS

  9. The CBC demonstrates a slight elevation in the WBC count. This appears to be primarily due to an elevation in the lymphocytes and is common with viral infections.

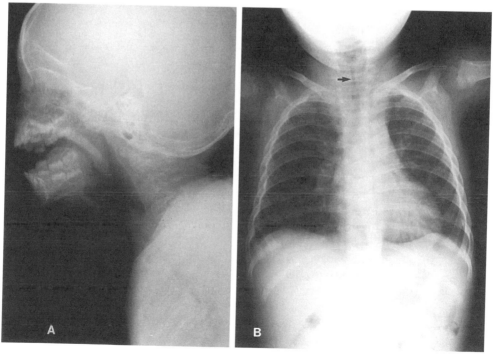

FIGURE 23–3   *(A)* Lateral neck and *(B)* AP radiographs demonstrating subglottic narrowing of the upper airway, typical for croup (*arrow*). (Courtesy of Lionel Young, MD.)

10. An ABG is not needed at this point. The procedure would be traumatic for the patient and would probably increase the severity of the symptoms.

11. The patient should be admitted. Severe cases of croup can lead to respiratory failure and asphyxia.

12. Initial treatment should include oxygen, cool mist, and racemic epinephrine. Oxygen is needed because the chest x-ray abnormality and wheezing suggest that intrathoracic airways are involved. $\dot{V}/\dot{Q}$ mismatching is likely and would result in hypoxemia. Cool mist should thin secretions and soothe the irritated airways. Racemic epinephrine may temporarily reduce swelling and inflammation of the upper airway and reduce the child's dyspnea. Corticosteroids should be used if the child responds poorly to this treatment.

CASE STUDY NO. 2—continued

In the emergency room, RD was given cool mist by mask with an FIO_2 of 0.40. Respiratory care administered racemic epinephrine by face mask via IPPB. The patient's mother was present throughout the treatment and was helpful in obtaining the child's cooperation. RD was admitted because of the severity of his symptoms and the abnormal chest film. He was taken to the pediatric ICU and placed in a mist tent with approximately 40 percent oxygen. A repeat treatment with racemic epinephrine was given 2 hours after the initial treatment. After the second treatment, the patient's vital signs were pulse 128/minute, respiratory rate 32/minute, and temperature 37.3°C (99.1°F). Pulse oximetry taken in the mist tent demonstrated an oxygen saturation of 95 percent. Stridor was present on inspiration, and low-pitched wheezing was still heard over the chest. The retractions were less noticeable.

QUESTIONS

13. What dangers are associated with the use of mist tents?
14. Should RD be given corticosteroids?
15. Should RD be given antibiotics?
16. What is a common problem associated with the use of racemic epinephrine?
17. Should the patient's mother be encouraged to remain at the bedside or to go home?

ANSWERS

13. Mist tents can make it more difficult to observe the patient. This may delay treatment if respiratory decompensation occurs. A pulse oximeter with an alarm is a useful monitoring tool for patients in a mist tent. Mist tents with oxygen represent a potential fire hazard and require appropriate posting of warning signs. The patient's mother should be advised of these concerns and should be told not to smoke or give the child any toys that may cause a spark.

14. Corticosteroids can be helpful in severe cases of croup. In this case the patient appears to be responding to more conservative treatment. Corticosteroids can be given if the patient does not continue to improve or if the upper airway obstruction worsens.

15. Antibiotics are not useful in the treatment of croup. This patient, however, has a suspicious infiltrate that may be pneumonia. A broad-spectrum antibiotic may be reasonable in this case while sputum specimens are obtained and analyzed.

16. Tachyphylaxis is a common problem with racemic epinephrine. This indicates that repeated treatments with racemic epinephrine may not be as effective as previous treatments. For this reason, the medication should not be given for mild cases of croup or on an outpatient basis for more severe cases to try and prevent hospitalization.

17. RD's mother should be encouraged to remain at the bedside. This may help reduce the child's anxiety and assist the hospital staff. Provisions should be made for the mother to sleep at the bedside.

CASE STUDY NO. 2—continued

The next morning, RD awoke in the mist tent with minimal symptoms. Mild inspiratory stridor was noted over the upper airway, and some coarse crackles were present over the chest. Vital signs were nearly normal, and RD was transferred to the basic care area. The racemic epinephrine treatments were stopped, but the mist tent continued. A repeat chest x-ray demonstrated improvement with partial resolution of the infiltrate. The patient continued to improve throughout the day and was discharged the following morning with normal vital signs and no symptoms.

QUESTIONS

17. Is the quick recovery in this case typical of most cases of croup?
18. Is this patient likely to have repeated episodes of croup?

ANSWERS

17. Yes, the quick recovery in this case is typical of croup.
18. Repeated episodes of croup are common in small children. As the child grows older, the episodes are likely to decrease in severity and frequency.

REFERENCES

1. Super, DM, et al: A prospective randomized double-blind study to evaluate the effect of dexamethasone in a acute laryngotracheitis. J Pediatr 115:323, 1989.
2. Cruz, MN, et al: Use of dexamethasone in the outpatient management of acute laryngotracheitis. Pediatrics 96:220-223, 1995.
3. Cressman, WR, and Myer, CM: Diagnosis and management of croup and epiglottitis. Pediatr Clin North Am 41:265-275, 1994.
4. Valdepena, JG, et al: Epiglottitis and *Haemophilus influenzae* immunization: The Pittsburgh experience—a five year review. Pediatrics 96:424-427, 1995.
5. Robotham, JL: Obstructive airways disease in infants and children. In Kirby, RR, and Taylor, RW (eds): Respiratory Failure. Year Book, Chicago, 1986.
6. Kimmons, HC, and Peterson, BM: Management of acute epiglottitis in pediatric patients. Crit Care Med 14:278-279, 1986.
7. Butt, W, et al: Acute epiglottitis: A different approach to management. Crit Care Med 16:43-47, 1988.

CHAPTER **24**

Respiratory Syncytial Virus

Victoria C. Sciacqua, BS, RRT

Key Terms

atelectasis
replication
respiratory syncytial virus
  (RSV)

ribavirin
small particle aerosol
  generator (SPAG)
teratogen

Introduction

Respiratory syncytial virus (RSV) was isolated in 1956 by Morris, Blount, and Savage,[1] and it remains a major cause of morbidity and mortality worldwide. It is recognized as the most frequent viral respiratory pathogen in infancy and early childhood. It is a leading cause of bronchiolitis and pneumonia in children and results in an estimated 90,000 hospitalizations and 4,500 deaths each year in the United States.[2]

Syncytium is defined as a "multinucleate mass of protoplasm produced by the merging of cells."[3(p1622)] At the level of the bronchioles, the virus causes neighboring cells to fuse together to form a syncytium, hence the name respiratory syncytial virus.

By the age of 2 years, nearly all children have been exposed to RSV. Although RSV infection can occur throughout a person's life, children less than 1 year of age tend to have the most severe disease. This appears to be due to their decreased immune response, smaller airway size, and lack of collateral ventilation. Because they are protected by maternal antibodies, it is very rare for infants 4 weeks old or younger to become infected with RSV.[4]

RSV outbreaks occur throughout the world every year and typically last 2 to 5 months. The virus is extremely common during the midwinter and early spring months. These epidemics tend to occur at regular, predictive intervals. During each epidemic there is a significant increase in the number of infants and small children admitted to hospitals with lower respiratory tract infections. Persons of all ages may have symptomatic RSV illness, as age does not play a role in immunity to the virus.

Etiology

The virus is usually introduced into the family by an older sibling or parent who is exhibiting coldlike symptoms. This infection poses a more serious threat to the younger siblings in the family.

The incubation period of RSV ranges from 2 to 8 days (average of 4 days).[5] The two most common modes of transmission are: (1) large particle aerosols that are transmitted during close personal contact; and (2) physical contact with contaminated secretions. The latter type of transmission can occur with hand-to-hand contact or touching of infected material. Infection usually occurs when the virus comes in contact with the victim's conjunctiva or mucous membranes via airborne particles or direct contact.[6] Although the virus is very labile, it remains infectious on cloth and paper for more than 30 minutes and is still contagious in nasal secretions after 6 hours.[7] Reinfections are common in both adults and children, but with each reinfection the severity of illness usually decreases.

Pathology and Pathophysiology

Once infection has occurred, the virus is spread along the respiratory tract by cell-to-cell transfer. Involvement of the lower respiratory tract may be a result of aspiration of secretions from the infected upper respiratory tract. **Replication** of the virus is limited to the respiratory tract mucosa but may involve the entire respiratory tract, thereby increasing the severity of illness.

The pathological findings associated with RSV infection include peribronchiolar mononuclear infiltration and necrosis of the epithelium of the small airways. Peribronchiolar mononuclear infiltration leads to edema of the bronchiole walls, submucosa, and adventitial tissue. Proliferation of the epithelium into the airway lumen due to necrosis leads to sloughing of the necrotic tissue into the airway. This sloughing, along with edema and the accumulation of mucus, leads to a decrease in airway lumen size. The airway may even become completely occluded. The virus causes an increase in mucus production, which enhances the severity of the airway plugging.

Once plugging of the airway occurs, areas of lung hyperinflation and **atelectasis** are likely to develop. Inspiration increases airway diameter and allows air to enter the lung around the mucus plugs. During expiration, the airways become narrower and inhibit the gas from escaping around the mucus plug, which results in air trapping. Atelectasis can occur in regions of the lung where mucus plugging is severe, resulting in minimal or no ventilation of the affected regions.

The combination of hyperinflation and atelectasis leads to abnormalities in ventilation-perfusion ($\dot{V}/\dot{Q}$) matching, resulting in hypoxemia. Reduced lung compliance and increased airway resistance result in increased work of breathing. The combination of hypoxemia and increased work of breathing may result in the patient's acute clinical deterioration.

Clinical Features

The clinical manifestations associated with RSV vary with both the age of the patient and the severity of the illness. Infants often present with evidence of severe disease.

Certain groups of children are also at an increased risk for severe RSV infection: children less than 3 months of age; children with congenital heart disease, bronchopulmonary dysplasia (see Chapter 26), cystic fibrosis (see Chapter 7), and immunodeficiencies (see Chapter 19); and premature infants (Table 24-1).

History of Present Illness

The infant who presents with RSV infection often has a history of being exposed to an older sibling or parent with coldlike symptoms; exposure to other children with RSV often occurs in day care centers. RSV infection may also occur as a result of nosocomial transmission during hospitalization. Often signs and symptoms of an upper respiratory tract infection (e.g., mild rhinorrhea, pharyngitis, cough, low-grade fever) precede the onset of more severe symptoms. The symptoms increase in severity as the disease progresses into the lower respiratory tract.

Physical Examination

The patient with RSV infection of the lower airways may exhibit several signs indicating an increased work of breathing. An increase in respiratory rate is typically present. Tachypnea is the best clinical sign correlating with hypoxemia.[6] The patient typically has intercostal or subcostal retractions, or both, and uses his or her accessory muscles to breathe. Other signs of increased work of breathing include nasal flaring, grunting, and the appearance of being "air hungry." Increased respiratory rate causes the patient to have a poor appetite; it also increases the patient's risk for aspiration if vomiting occurs.

Apneic episodes may occur during RSV infection and are a sign of severe illness. The cause of these episodes is uncertain; however, the immaturity of the central respiratory control mechanisms of very young children is thought to be a contributing factor.[8] As the disease becomes more severe, the frequency and severity of apneic episodes also increase. Infants of a young postnatal age, premature infants, and infants with a history of apnea are at highest risk for apneic episodes.[8]

Auscultation of breath sounds may help determine the severity of pulmonary involvement. Expiratory wheezing, diminished breath sounds, and crackles are the most common findings. Wheezing is a result of narrowed airways caused by inflammation and edema. Because the patient's lungs are often hyperexpanded, there is less airflow with each respiratory cycle and breath sounds are diminished. The cause of the crackles can be inferred from their pitch and timing during the respiratory cycle. Fine, late-inspiratory crackles are most likely the result of atelectasis due to mucus plugging of the airways. If the crackles are coarse and occur throughout the respiratory cycle, however, then pneumonia or retained bronchial secretions, or both, may be the cause. The extent to which the adventitious lung sounds occur over the chest

TABLE 24-1   **Risk Factors for Severe Infection in Infants
with Respiratory Syncytial Virus**

Congenital heart disease
Bronchopulmonary dysplasia
Prematurity
Immunodeficiency or immunosuppression
Chemotherapy treatment

indicates the amount of lung involved. Stridor may be heard over the upper airway if the trachea or larynx is affected.

Laboratory Data

In RSV infection, the complete blood count (CBC) is typically normal. An increase in white blood cell (WBC) count with a left shift (increase in the proportion of immature WBCs) may be seen when a superimposed bacterial infection is present.

Assessment of arterial blood gases (ABGs) will determine the degree of hypoxemia and the ventilatory status of the patient. The PaO_2 is usually decreased due to ventilation-perfusion ($\dot{V}/\dot{Q}$) mismatching. Hypoxemia due to RSV infection may last for weeks after acute recovery.[9] The $PaCO_2$ may be decreased because of hyperventilation. An increase in $PaCO_2$ indicates excessive dead space ventilation or fatigue of the respiratory muscles due to an increased work of breathing, or both. Progression to metabolic acidosis may occur if hypoxemia is severe and circulation compromised. Serial ABGs may help identify clinical deterioration in enough time to initiate appropriate treatment and avert a major crisis.

Chest radiographs commonly demonstrate at least one of the following findings: hyperinflation and interstitial pneumonitis.[6] Signs of hyperinflation and air trapping include flattened diaphragms, widened intercostal spaces, and an increase in anteroposterior diameter. If a lateral film is available, a prominent retrosternal airspace also will be noted when hyperinflation is present. Interstitial pneumonitis is commonly present in several lobes and is seen as areas of increased density. Atelectasis also may be seen on the chest radiograph.

Diagnosis

RSV should be suspected as the cause of illness based on the time of year, presence of a local outbreak, age of the patient, history of the illness, and the clinical picture. A definite diagnosis of RSV infection can be made by isolation of the virus or its antigens from the patient's respiratory secretions.[6] A good sputum specimen must be obtained and rapidly analyzed to ensure accurate results.

The bedside clinician can obtain a specimen with several different techniques. The more common techniques are nasal aspirate, nasal swabs, and nasal lavage. Although all techniques can be effective, some studies have shown that nasal washing is a more sensitive test than nasal swabs,[6] whereas others found nasal swabs to be nearly as effective.[10] The current gold standard of obtaining a specimen is *nasopharyngeal aspiration*. Complications associated with this method include local trauma, coughing spasms, vagal bradycardia, and transient hypoxemia.[11] This technique requires inserting a small catheter into the back of the oropharynx with subsequent aspiration of sputum into a mucus trap.

Nasal lavage appears to be a gentler method. A very small amount of saline is instilled into each nostril with simultaneous suctioning by a small catheter placed just inside the nose. Nasal lavage seems to be a superior method because it yields similar results and is free of the adverse effects of nasopharyngeal aspiration just mentioned.[11]

Once the specimen is obtained, rapid detection of the virus is found via *immunofluorescence,* which is defined as "any immunohistochemical method using antibody labeled with a fluorescent dye"[3(p823)] (e.g., enzyme-linked immunosorbent assay [ELISA]). Results of immunofluorescence tests usually can be obtained within 2 to 4 hours. Tests for rapid bedside diagnosis have been evaluated and have shown promising results.[12] It is very important to be able to diagnose the virus rapidly so that specific therapy can be initiated as soon as possible (see next section).

Treatment

The treatment of RSV, as with many other diseases, varies with the degree of severity. Most children require only supportive care for their illness. Some require supplemental oxygen to treat hypoxemia, especially if they have a lower respiratory tract infection. The patient with RSV should be hydrated adequately with intravenous (IV) fluids until normal feeding can resume. Pulse oximetry is useful to watch for hypoxemia, and ABGs help evaluate the degree of hypercapnia.

Bronchodilators may be helpful if the patient demonstrates wheezing or an increased work of breathing. Racemic epinephrine (Micronefrin or Vaponefrin) may be useful to decrease upper airway swelling when inflammation is severe enough to cause stridor. Mechanical ventilation may be necessary if the patient demonstrates increasing $PaCO_2$ with therapy, an excessive work of breathing, or episodes of apnea.

Since January 1986, **ribavirin** has been commonly used to treat patients who are extremely ill or at high risk for severe illness. Ribavirin is a virostatic agent whose exact mechanism of action is uncertain.[13,14] In some viruses, it prevents cap formation on the viral messenger RNA. This is thought to preclude translation of the virus. Another mechanism may be inhibition of viral nucleic acid polymerization and prevention of RNA replication. Ribavirin is different from most other antiviral drugs in both spectrum of activity and mode of administration.

Ribavirin is administered in aerosol form via a **small particle aerosol generator (SPAG)**. The SPAG-2 delivers particles in the range of 1.1 to 5.0 μm in diameter (Fig. 24–1). These small particles remain suspended in air until they reach the distal airways, where they are deposited. The drug is administered to the patient via hood, tent, or mechanical ventilation. Ribavirin (6 g/300 mL) is typically given for 12 to 18 hours/day for 3 to 7 days. Although this has been the standard regimen, studies have been done to evaluate the effects of using a high-dose, short-duration regimen. In one study regimen by Englund and colleagues,[15] the same ribavirin dose was used (6 g/300 mL), but the drug was administered for 2 hours three times a day. The therapeutic effects of this regimen were found to be similar to those of the standard regimen, but the study regimen resulted in a decreased release of ribavirin into the room. Therefore, use of this regimen would decrease health care workers' exposure to ribavirin and also allow greater access time to patients by health care workers and parents. Englund and colleagues observed that high-dose therapy regimens had no advantage in intubated patients, however, because environmental exposure to ribavirin is already limited, owing to the use of filters in the ventilator circuit.

The cost of 3 days of ribavirin treatment is approximately $2,100. Because of this high cost, ribavirin is usually given only after a sputum sample has been found to be positive for RSV in very sick infants. Exceptions to this include patients who have a high probability of having RSV and are severely ill. Initial studies looking at ribavirin use for RSV treatment found a more rapid clinical improvement with an increase in PaO_2 and SaO_2 and a decrease in hospital stay.[16] More recently, however, studies have not found it to be effective in clinical practice.[17] This has caused the American Acad-

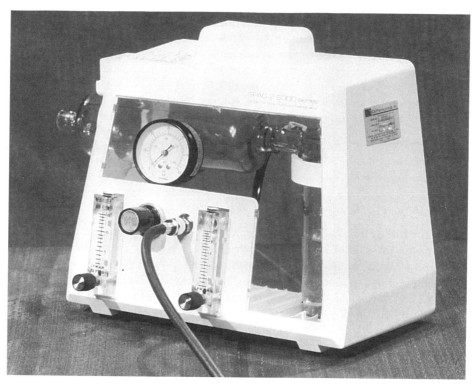

FIGURE 24-1   SPAG-2 unit used to administer ribavirin therapy.

emy of Pediatrics (AAP) to reconsider its recommendation in favor of the use of ribavirin. The Committee on Infectious Diseases of the AAP now states that ribavirin "may be considered" for use in certain infants at high risk for serious RSV disease (Table 24-2).[18] Infants with congenital heart disease, chronic lung disease, or underlying immunosuppressive disease, as well as infants who are severely ill with or without mechanical ventilation, are at high risk.[18]

TABLE 24-2   **Hospital Guidelines for Administration of Ribavirin Therapy**

I. Infants at high risk for severe or complicated infection with respiratory syncytial virus (RSV) because of the following concomitant conditions:
  A. Bronchopulmonary dysplasia or other chronic lung conditions
  B. Congenital heart disease
  C. Immunocompromising heart disease, or current administration of immunosuppressant therapy

II. Infants hospitalized with RSV who are severely ill, having the following findings:
  A. Oxygen desaturation: O_2 saturation < 93 percent by pulse oximetry
  B. Hypoxemia: Pao_2 < 65 mm Hg determined by arterial blood gas (ABG)
  C. Hypercapnia: Pco_2 > 40 mm Hg determined by ABG or CBG

III. Infants whose RSV disease is initially not severe, but who have the following risk factors for a more complicated course:
  A. Young age (<6 weeks)
  B. Multiple congenital anomalies
  C. Neurological or metabolic disease

Because ribavirin is very sticky, it may precipitate in either the ventilator circuit or the endotracheal tube. This precipitation can lead to malfunction of the expiratory valve in the circuit. The precipitation also may narrow the patient's endotracheal tube and increase expiratory resistance. This increase in resistance may cause inadvertent positive end-expiratory pressure (PEEP), also known as auto-PEEP, in the mechanically ventilated patient. The risks associated with ribavirin and mechanical ventilation may be reduced by: (1) frequent ventilator circuit changes (every 8 hours); (2) modifications to components of the circuit, such as filters and one-way valves; (3) frequent suctioning of the endotracheal tube; and (4) close and constant monitoring of the patient.[19,20]

Concern to Health Care Workers

The toxic effects of ribavirin in humans are unknown because safety reports are based primarily on animal studies. The drug has teratogenic effects in animals. A **teratogen** is "an agent or factor that causes the production of physical defects in the developing embryo of a pregnant woman."[4(p77)] Pregnant women and those who are trying to conceive should avoid exposure to ribavirin and should not provide care for people receiving ribavirin treatments.[21] This recommendation is based primarily on animal research, as no cases of human toxicity have been reported.[22] The most common human side effects have been rash, mild bronchospasm, and reversible skin irritation.[23] Health care workers also may complain of eye irritation and headache associated with ribavirin exposure.[23] Caregiver exposure can be limited by a tight-fitting mask that filters out particles with a mass median aerodynamic diameter of 0.5 μm. The use of a containment system has been shown to be effective in decreasing the level of exposure to ribavirin.[23,24]

Prevention of Nosocomial Infection

Since hospital-acquired RSV infection remains a major problem, many studies have evaluated techniques to decrease the spreading of the infection. One study showed that hand washing and isolating patients reduced the rate of nosocomial infection.[25] Another study showed that the use of gloves and gowns was beneficial.[26] Screening and isolating patients suspected of having RSV at the time of admission are also useful measures for decreasing nosocomial transmission.[27] The Centers for Disease Control recommends the following precautions: (1) use of masks if close to the patient; (2) use of gowns if soiling is likely; (3) use of gloves to prevent touching infected material; (4) use of disposable material or isolation of material before reprocessing; and (5) use of effective hand washing.[28] It is imperative that strategies be developed by health care workers to avoid unnecessary spread of the virus, especially to patients who are at highest risk.

What the Future Holds

Researchers have been trying to develop a vaccine against RSV for more than 20 years. Early vaccines not only have failed to protect infants, but have actually increased the severity of the disease.[29] Failure of early vaccines may have resulted from their inability to generate sufficient functional antibodies.[30] Efforts to develop an RSV vaccine continue.

CASE STUDY

History

NJ is a 2-month-old white female infant born to a 25-year-old woman, gravida 4, para 3 (four pregnancies, three live births), via a normal vaginal delivery. NJ was in her usual state of good health until February, when slight nasal congestion developed. The patient was seen by her primary physician and sent home on amoxicillin for symptoms associated with an upper respiratory tract infection.

Two days after the initial visit, the mother noticed that NJ had progressively worsening respiratory distress. She reported that NJ had increased congestion, decreased appetite, vomiting, and diarrhea and that the three older siblings had a history of upper respiratory tract infections. The patient was brought to the emergency room for repeat evaluation.

QUESTIONS

1. What risk factors indicate that RSV is the likely source of infection?

2. What suggests that this patient is at risk for a more severe case?

ANSWERS

1. A number of factors may point to RSV as the source of infection:

   a. The child's age puts her in a high-risk group.

   b. RSV is common in February. Most outbreaks appear to peak in January, February, or March.[8]

   c. The patient was treated a few days before admission for symptoms associated with an upper respiratory tract infection.

   d. The patient was exposed to older siblings with symptoms of upper respiratory tract infection. This is a very common clinical scenario for RSV infection.

2. The patient's age puts her at a greater risk for a severe RSV infection.

Physical Examination

NJ is awake, grunting, and in moderate to severe respiratory distress. She was placed on a pulse oximeter, which revealed oxygen saturations of 80 to 85 percent on room air. She experienced frequent coughing spells, during which her oxygen saturation fell into the 60s.

Measurements: Weight 4.3 kg (20th percentile); length 57 cm (50th percentile); head circumference 37 cm (10th percentile)

Vital Signs: Temperature 38.8°C (101.8°F), respiratory rate 50/minute, heart rate 180/minute, blood pressure 88/60 mm Hg (mean 63 mm Hg)

HEENT: Normal anterior fontanelle; pupils equal, round, and reactive to light and accommodation (PERRLA); tympanic membranes erythematous bilaterally; nasal flaring, with a small amount of yellow nasal discharge and crusting noted in the nostrils; throat clear

Neck: Trachea midline and mobile; inspiratory stridor noted

Chest: Costal and substernal retractions with each inspiration; chest hyperexpanded; diffuse inspiratory and expiratory coarse crackles and expiratory wheezes throughout all lung fields on chest auscultation

Heart: Regular rhythm at rate of 180/minute; no murmurs

Abdomen: Soft, nontender, and nondistended; normoactive bowel sounds

Skin: Pale, cool, and dry; no rashes; no evidence of cyanosis

Musculoskeletal: Examination significant for slightly decreased tone

Neurological: Deep tendon reflexes ++ and equal bilaterally; no ankle clonus; equivocal Babinski's sign

QUESTIONS

3. What effect does the elevated body temperature have on the patient's work of breathing?

4. What is the likely cause of the inspiratory stridor?

5. What are the likely causes of the crackles and wheezes heard on chest auscultation?

6. Why is the patient's chest hyperexpanded? How does this hyperexpansion affect the patient's work of breathing?

7. What clinical signs indicate that the patient's work of breathing is increased?

ANSWERS

3. Elevated body temperature increases metabolic rate and oxygen consumption. The patient's heart and respiratory rate will increase to accommodate the increased demand on the pulmonary and cardiovascular systems.

4. Stridor is a high-pitched, "crowing" sound heard on inspiration. It is usually caused by partial obstruction of the upper airway, which in this case is most likely due to inflammation from the viral infection.

5. Retained secretions are the most likely cause of the crackles because they are heard on inspiration and expiration and are coarse sounding. Viral infections often cause an increase in the production of mucus. The expiratory wheezing may be produced by edema, bronchospasm, or secretions in the airways.

6. The patient's chest is hyperexpanded because of the air trapping that results from intrathoracic airway obstruction. When the intrathoracic airways are obstructed, air enters the lung more easily than it exits. This is because airways enlarge during inspiration and narrow with exhalation. Air trapping causes hyperexpansion of the chest and increased functional residual capacity (FRC). As the FRC increases, the patient breathes at a higher lung volume. At high lung volumes, the elastic force of both the lung and the chest wall make chest expansion very difficult. To overcome these two forces, NJ must exert her respiratory accessory muscles to inhale.

7. NJ is exhibiting many signs of an increased work of breathing, including increased respiratory rate, retractions, expiratory grunting, and nasal flaring.

Laboratory Evaluation

Chest Radiograph: See Figure 24–2

ABGs (on room air):

	Observed	Normal
pH	7.37	7.35–7.45
$Paco_2$ (mm Hg)	48	35–45
Pao_2 (mm Hg)	52	85–100
HCO_3^- (mEq/liter)	25	22–26
Base excess (mEq/liter)	−1	(−2)–(+2)

CBC:

	Observed	Normal
WBCs/mm³	12,200	4,000–11,000
Red blood cells (RBCs)/mm³	3.9 million	4.1–5.5 million
Hemoglobin (g/dL)	11.1	11.5–15.5
Hematocrit (%)	37.2	30–40
Platelets	583,000	175,000–415,000

WBC Morphology:

	Observed (%)	Normal (%)
Segmented neutrophils	35	38–79
Bands	9	0–7
Lymphocytes	52	12–30
Monocytes	4	0–10

Chemistry: All within normal limits except for Na^+, which was slightly decreased at 132 mEq/liter.

QUESTIONS

8. What findings on the chest radiograph (Fig. 24–2) are consistent with the diagnosis of RSV? How do the findings on the chest film relate to the patient's symptoms?

9. How would you interpret the ABGs? What are the possible causes of the findings?

10. Interpret the CBC. What is the likely cause of the increase in the WBCs? Of what significance is the decreased hemoglobin?

11. What further diagnostic procedures should be done at this time?

12. What therapeutic interventions should be instituted in the emergency room?

13. Should this patient be mechanically ventilated?

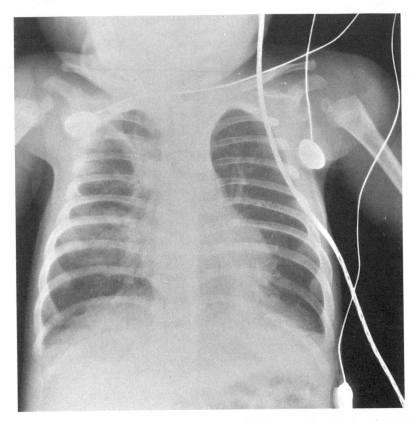

FIGURE 24-2   Chest radiograph demonstrating presence of diffuse opacities. (See text for complete description.)

ANSWERS

8. Hyperinflation and the presence of diffuse opacities are consistent with RSV infection. This chest film demonstrates both of these features. Flattened diaphragms, increased intercostal spaces, and increased radiolucency are consistent with hyperinflation.

Diffuse opacities are a common finding of RSV infection. Infiltrates are present in both the right middle lobe and right lower lobe, as shown by the increased opacity of the film in those areas. These densities are consistent with the diagnosis of RSV pneumonia.

The linear density seen in the right upper lobe is consistent with subsegmental atelectasis secondary to plugging of the airway.

The patient's symptoms correlate with the chest radiograph findings. Pulmonary hyperinflation leads to increased work of breathing as the infant is forced to breathe at a higher lung volume. Infection can cause air hunger, increased congestion, and elevated body temperature.

9. The ABG reveals mild respiratory acidosis. The decreased PaO_2 indicates moderate hypoxemia on room air. The increase in respiratory rate with an elevated $PaCO_2$ indicates that NJ has an impaired effective ventilation. Severe respiratory muscle fatigue is the most likely cause of the elevated $PaCO_2$. $\dot{V}/\dot{Q}$ mismatching and shunt due to excessive airway secretions and atelectasis are probable sources of the hypoxemia.

10. The CBC reveals a slightly elevated WBC count as well as a slightly reduced RBC count. The increase in WBC (leukocytosis) is most likely a response to the viral infection (lymphocytosis). WBCs are an integral part of the body's immune system and increase in number in response to the stress of infection. A decrease in hemoglobin reduces the oxygen-carrying capacity of the blood. This patient's oxygen content is low because of the decreased amount of circulating RBCs. This condition will stimulate cardiovascular compensation, but if the compensation is inadequate, it may result in decreased oxygen delivered to the tissues.

11. Appropriate diagnostic procedures at this time should include sputum analysis via immunofluorescence for the presence of RSV. Either a nasal swab or a nasal aspirate should be done to detect the virus or its antigens in NJ's nasal secretions.

12. Oxygen therapy is a mainstay in the treatment of RSV and should be instituted at this time to relieve NJ's hypoxemia. The amount of oxygen delivered should be titrated to maintain oxygen saturations between 90 to 95 percent. NJ's stridor requires immediate intervention since upper airway obstruction is potentially life threatening. The drug of choice to treat stridor is racemic epinephrine, which can be useful to reduce the amount of upper airway swelling. It should be continued if it is found to benefit the patient (decreased work of breathing and stridor) and discontinued if no relief is noted.

13. NJ's elevated Pa_{CO_2} (respiratory acidosis) dictates careful observation, but the condition is not yet life threatening. Mechanical ventilation will be needed if she does not respond to therapy or if the respiratory acidosis becomes more severe.

CASE STUDY—continued

NJ was admitted to the pediatric intensive care unit. The following were among the physician's orders:

1. Nothing by mouth (NPO)
2. IV dextrose 5% per normal saline (NS) 0.2% with 10 mEq KCl/liter at 15 mL/hour
3. Aminophylline 1:1 at 4.5 mL/hour
4. Theophylline level checked every morning (Qam)
5. Medication nebulizer: 0.25 mL Micronefrin every 3 hours as needed (prn) for stridor
6. Medication nebulizer: 0.3 mL albuterol in 2.5 mL NS every 3 hours
7. Chest physiotherapy every three hours after medication nebulizer
8. O_2 via hood to keep oxygen saturation at 90 to 95 percent
9. Continuous pulse oximeter and respiratory monitor

QUESTIONS

14. Why did the physician indicate that NJ should have NPO and start her on IV fluids?

15. What level of blood theophylline is considered therapeutic?

16. Are medication nebulizers and chest physiotherapy indicated in this patient?

17. Is ribavirin indicated in this case? If so, how should it be given, and what precautions should be taken by the respiratory care practitioner (RCP) to minimize his or her exposure to drug?

18. What precautions should be taken by all health care workers caring for this patient to prevent the spread of RSV?

19. What change in breathing pattern might occur in this patient that would indicate a more severe case of RSV infection?

ANSWERS

14. The physician ordered that NJ have NPO because she was experiencing moderate to severe respiratory distress. She not only was having difficulty eating, but was at risk for aspiration. IV fluids are necessary in this patient to maintain adequate hydration.

15. NJ's aminophylline drip should be titrated to a level of 10 to 20 μg/mL to ensure maximum benefits of bronchodilatation with minimum risk of toxicity.

16. Chest physiotherapy and medication nebulizer treatments are indicated for the treatment of bronchospasm. The presence of bronchospasm is suspected when wheezing is identified. Chest physiotherapy is indicated for patients who have difficulty bringing up secretions. Because of the child's age and condition, assistance with secretion removal is mandatory.

17. Ribavirin is indicated because NJ's illness is relatively severe. If ordered by the physician, the RCP should administer aerosolized ribavirin via a SPAG-2, which delivers particles of the appropriate diameter (range 1.0 to 5.0 μm) to reach the peripheral lung units.

    The RCP should wear a tight-fitting mask that will filter all particles with a mass median aerodynamic diameter of 0.5 μm. Whenever possible, a containment system (e.g., a vacuum system) should be used. This will minimize the RCP's exposure to the drug. Any RCP who may be pregnant should not administer ribavirin treatments.

18. All health care workers associated with this patient should wash their hands thoroughly before and after each patient contact. The use of gown and gloves with each contact is also important in preventing the spread of infection. The patient should be isolated from other patients who do not have RSV.

19. Apneic episodes, increased respiratory rate, and increased use of accessory muscles would indicate a more severe case of RSV infection.

CASE STUDY—continued

NJ was placed in isolation and started on 6 g ribavirin in 300 mL sterile water via mist hood. With the exception of an increased respiratory rate, vital signs remained stable throughout her hospitalization. The patient improved daily and was afebrile by day 3. On day 4, her medication nebulizers and chest physiotherapy were decreased to every 4 hours. They were decreased further as she improved until they were no longer required after day 6. Hypoxemia also decreased during that time, and her FIO$_2$ was titrated by pulse oximeter until, by day 7, room air oxygen saturations were 90 to 95 percent. The aminophylline drip was eventually discontinued, and she was started on oral aminophylline syrup (Somophyllin oral liquid) with the dose titrated to maintain a therapeutic level. At the time of discharge, NJ was feeding without difficulty, breath sounds were clear, and there were no signs of respiratory distress. NJ was discharged 8 days after admission and was sent home on oral theophylline syrup. NJ's mother was advised to bring her in 1 week later for a follow-up visit with her private physician.

REFERENCES

1. Morris, JA, et al: Recovery of cytopathogenic agent from chimpanzees with coryza. Proc Soc Exp Biol Med 92:544, 1956.
2. Morbitity and Mortality Weekly Report. Dec. 6, 1996, 45(48):1053–1054.
3. Dorland's Illustrated Medical Dictionary, ed 28. WB Saunders, Philadelphia, 1994.
4. Heierholzer, JC, and Tannock, GA: Respiratory syncytial virus: A review of the virus, its epidemiology, immune response and laboratory diagnosis. Austr Pediatr J 22:77, 1986.
5. McIntosh, K: Respiratory syncytial virus infections in infants and children. Pediatr Rev 9:191, 1987.
6. Hall, CB: Respiratory syncytial virus. In Fergin, RD, and Cherry, JD (eds): Textbook of Pediatric Infectious Diseases, ed 2. WB Saunders, Philadelphia, 1987.
7. Hall, CB, et al: Possible transmission by fomites of respiratory syncytial virus. J Infect Dis 141:98, 1980.
8. Hayden, FG, and Gwaltney, JM: Viral infections. In Murry, JF, and Nadel, JA (eds): Textbook of Respiratory Medicine. WB Saunders, Philadelphia, 1988.
9. Hall, CB, et al: Clinical and physiological manifestations of bronchiolitis and pneumonia. Am J Dis Child 133:798, 1979.
10. Barnes, SD, et al: Comparison of nasal brush and nasopharyngeal aspirate techniques in obtaining specimens for detection of respiratory syncytial viral antigen by immunofluorescence. Pediatr Infect Dis J 8:598, 1989.
11. Balfour, IM, et al: Diagnosing respiratory syncytial virus by nasal lavage. Arch Dis Child 72:58, 1995.
12. Krilov, LR, et al: Evaluation of a rapid diagnostic test for respiratory syncytial virus (RSV): Potential for bedside diagnosis. Pediatrics 93:903, 1994.
13. Boruchoff, SE, and Cheeseman, SH: Antiviral chemotherapy. In Kass, EH, and Platt, R (eds): Current Therapy in Infectious Disease, ed 3. BC Decker, Toronto, 1990.
14. Patterson, JL, and Fernandez-Larsson, R: Molecular mechanisms of action of ribavirin. Rev Infect Dis 12:1139, 1990.
15. Englund, JA, et al: High-dose, short-duration ribavirin aerosol therapy compared with standard ribavirin therapy in children with suspected respiratory syncytial virus infection. J Pediatr 125:635, 1994.
16. Rodriguez, WJ, et al: Aerosolized ribavirin in the treatment of patients with respiratory syncytial virus disease. Pediatr Infect Dis J 6:159, 1987.
17. Meert, KL, et al: Aerosolized ribavirin in mechanically ventilated children with RSV lower respiratory tract disease: A prospective double blind randomized trial. Crit Care Med 22:566–572, 1994.
18. Committee on Infectious Diseases: American Academy of Pediatrics: Reassessment of the indications for ribavirin therapy in respiratory syncytial virus infections. Pediatrics 97:137–139, 1996.
19. Adderley, RJ: Safety of ribavirin with mechanical ventilation. Pediatr Infect Dis J 9:5112, 1990.
20. Outwater, KM, et al: Ribavirin administration to infants receiving mechanical ventilation. Am J Dis Child 142:512, 1988.
21. Assessin, G: Exposures of health-care workers to aerosols of ribavirin—California. MMWR 37:560, 1988.
22. Torres, A, et al: Reduced environmental exposure to aerosolized ribavirin using a simple containment system. Pediatr Infect Dis J 10:217, 1991.
23. Janai, HK, et al: Ribavirin: Adverse drug reactions, 1986 to 1988. Pediatr Infect Dis J 9:209, 1990.
24. Bradley, J: Environmental exposure to ribavirin aerosol. Pediatr Infect Dis J 9:595, 1990.
25. Isaacs, D, et al: Handwashing and cohorting in prevention of hospital acquired infections with respiratory syncytial virus. Arch Dis Child 66:227, 1991.
26. LeClair, JM, et al: Prevention of nosocomial respiratory syncytial virus infections through compliance with glove and gown isolation precautions. N Engl J Med 317:329, 1987.
27. Krasinski, K, et al: Screening for respiratory syncytial virus and assignment to a cohort at admission to reduce nosocomial transmission. J Pediatr 116:894, 1990.
28. Peter, G (ed): Report of the Committee on Infectious Diseases, ed 21. American Academy of Pediatrics, Elk Grove village, IL, 1988.
29. Everard, ML: Bronchiolitis: Origins and optimal management. Drugs 49:885, 1995.
30. Toms, GL: Respiratory syncytial virus: How soon will we have a vaccine? Arch Dis Child 72:1, 1995.

CHAPTER 25

Respiratory Distress Syndrome in the Newborn

Patrice A. Johnson, BS, RRT
Cynthia Malinowski, MA, RRT

Key Terms

acrocyanosis
asphyxia
central cyanosis
exogenous surfactant
  therapy
grunting

hyaline membrane
  disease
nasal flaring
patent ductus arteriosus
  (PDA)

respiratory distress
  syndrome (RDS)
shunt
surfactant

Introduction

Respiratory distress syndrome (RDS) of the newborn occurs primarily in premature infants. It is characterized by a poor quantity and quality of surfactant and immature anatomy leading to progressive atelectasis and respiratory failure. Although many forms of respiratory failure can occur in the newborn, RDS is the most prevalent cause among premature infants. Advances in the prevention of premature delivery and treatment of RDS have reduced the number of deaths; however, RDS continues to be a significant cause of morbidity and mortality.[1] All neonatal intensive care unit clinicians should be able to recognize and treat this common cause of respiratory failure.

Etiology

The infant with RDS suffers from a **surfactant** deficiency. Surfactant must be produced in sufficient quantity and quality at birth to prevent collapse of the infant's alve-

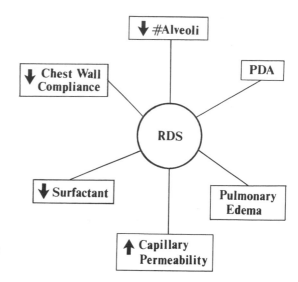

FIGURE 25-1   Diagram showing the abnormalities often associated with RDS.

oli at end exhalation. Functionally intact type II alveolar cells are responsible for producing this surface-active material so important for postnatal pulmonary function. The premature infant often does not have a sufficient amount of type II alveolar cells, or the cells that are present cannot produce an adequate quantity of surfactant. The incidence of RDS is therefore inversely related to gestational age, and any newborn delivered prematurely (less than 38 weeks' gestation) is at risk. RDS is most prevalent in newborns who are very premature (less than 29 weeks' gestational age) and who have a very low birth weight (less than 1500 g).[2]

The surfactant abnormality associated with RDS also consists of a qualitative alteration; that is, the surfactant often lacks all the components necessary for proper functioning.[3] The minor phospholipids are either not present or present only in small quantities.[4] The surfactant proteins (SP-A, SP-B, SP-C, and SP-D) have many important roles in the functioning of surfactant, including promoting adsorption of the phospholipids, enhancing immune properties, and promoting fluid clearance.[5] Because the preterm infant apparently has an immature metabolism of surfactant, these proteins are not metabolized properly.[6] The infant with RDS also has immature lung parenchyma with a decreased alveolar surface area for gas exchange, increased alveolar-capillary membrane thickness, a reduced lung defense system, an immature chest wall, and increased capillary permeability.[7,8] A left-to-right **shunt** through the **patent ductus arteriosus (PDA)** is often present with RDS. This shunting pattern leads to increased pulmonary blood flow and pulmonary edema (Fig. 25-1).

Any acute episode of perinatal **asphyxia** or reduction in pulmonary perfusion can interfere with appropriate surfactant production and contribute to the onset of RDS. Numerous maternal risk factors, such as diabetes, cesarean section without labor, and birth of an older sibling with RDS, increase the newborn's risk of RDS.[9,10]

Pathophysiology

Surfactant immaturity leads to alveolar collapse and irregular distribution of ventilation. As more and more alveoli collapse, the newborn must generate greater negative intrapleural pressures during inspiration in order to ventilate. The compliant chest

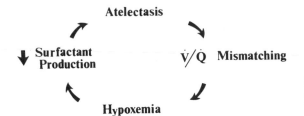

FIGURE 25-2   The vicious circle contributing to the deteriorating clinical condition of the infant with RDS.

wall of the newborn is an advantage during delivery, when the fetus must pass through the birth canal. This chest wall compliance can be a disadvantage, however, when the infant with RDS inhales and attempts to expand noncompliant lungs. As the infant generates greater negative intrapleural pressures in an attempt to expand the stiff lungs, the chest wall is pulled inward, thus limiting lung expansion. The progressive atelectasis causes a reduced functional residual volume which impairs gas exchange in the lungs.

Hyaline membranes, proteinaceous material caused by lung injury, are formed and further reduce the lung compliance. Thus, **hyaline membrane disease** is used as another term for RDS. Proteinaceous fluid, which leaks from areas of epithelial disruption into alveoli, further inactivates any surfactant that may be present.[11] This fluid and worsening hypoxemia due to large areas of intrapulmonary shunt lead to further inhibition of surfactant function. A vicious circle is produced by the continuing pattern of atelectasis, decreased compliance, ventilation-perfusion ($\dot{V}/\dot{Q}$) mismatching, and hypoxemia. Surfactant production decreases further, and atelectasis worsens (Fig. 25-2).

Maternal History

It is necessary to obtain a thorough maternal history in order to rule out other causes of respiratory distress, such as sepsis or congenital cardiac defects. β-Streptococcal pneumonia, transmitted in utero, can mimic RDS.[12] The clinician should suspect sepsis if there is a maternal history of prolonged rupture of the membranes or fever. A maternal history that includes alcohol ingestion, exposure to rubella virus, diabetes, or birth of an older sibling with a congenital cardiac defect should prompt the clinician to look for a cardiac defect in the neonate.[13]

Maternal history also helps to confirm the diagnosis of RDS if risk factors are present, including diabetes, history of RDS in siblings, second born twin, cesarean section without labor, and perinatal asphyxia.[1,14]

Clinical Features

The newborn with RDS has signs of distress soon after delivery.[4,14] Retractions are evident early in the disease. **Grunting,** the sound of expiration against a closed glottis, is a mechanism used by the newborn to increase functional residual capacity (FRC). Tachypnea is a common early finding; bradypnea and periods of apnea are late signs of respiratory failure. **Nasal flaring** and **central cyanosis** with the patient on room air are also typically present.[15] Chest auscultation may reveal fine inspiratory crackles, which are caused by abrupt opening of the distal lung units; or diminished breath sounds, which are due to shallow tidal volumes.[16]

The chest radiograph shows bilaterally decreased lung volumes, alveolar consolidation, and a ground-glass appearance with air bronchograms. Increased pulmonary vascularity will also be seen if there is a left-to-right shunt through the PDA (Fig. 25-3).

Pulmonary function testing shows moderate to severe reductions in lung compliance and FRC; however, these tests are not done regularly in unstable, critically ill infants with RDS. Newborns with RDS who also have elevated airway resistance are at increased risk for bronchopulmonary dysplasia (see Chapter 26).[17]

The most common abnormality detected by arterial blood gas (ABG) analysis in the infant with RDS is hypoxemia. Respiratory acidosis is also common in newborns with moderate to severe disease when the increased work of breathing leads to fatigue.[7,10] If a left-to-right shunt through the PDA is a complicating factor, metabolic acidosis may occur as a result of decreased perfusion to the lower body.

The clinical course of the newborn with RDS usually follows a predictable sequence of events. Unless **exogenous surfactant therapy** is given shortly after birth, symptoms typically worsen from delivery through the second or third day of life.[18] If exogenous surfactant therapy is administered promptly, the patient may improve dramatically. Another dose of surfactant is necessary if the patient deterio-

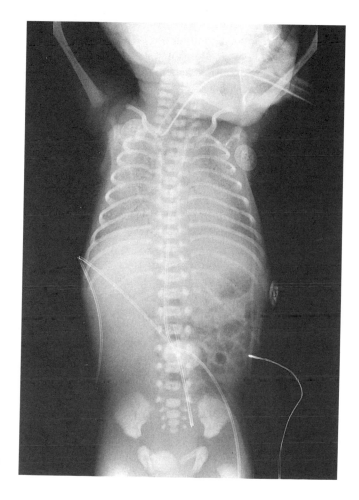

FIGURE 25-3   Chest radiograph showing RDS.

rates. Respiratory function then generally improves within 72 hours, when type II alveolar cell regeneration occurs and surfactant production reappears. If there are no complications, the newborn will recover within 5 to 7 days. The severely ill infant, who is usually of very low birth weight, often does not respond as quickly to treatment and frequently needs some type of ventilatory assistance.

Treatment

RDS can be prevented or its severity reduced through the administration of prenatal corticosteroids, delivered to the mother by an intravenous route. When given for preterm labor at 24 to 34 weeks' gestation, corticosteroids can reduce the mortality and morbidity of RDS.[19]

The initial resuscitation of the newborn suspected of having RDS includes careful thermoregulation to avoid increased oxygen consumption and metabolic acidosis.[20] Oxygen therapy is instituted to treat hypoxemia and monitored continuously with the use of a noninvasive device such as a transcutaneous monitor or pulse oximeter.

During the resuscitation process or shortly after delivery, exogenous surfactant therapy is initiated. The newborn is intubated, and artificial or modified natural surfactant is lavaged into the airway. Improvements in lung compliance and ABGs are likely to occur after the administration of artificial surfactant.[3] Prophylaxis, early treatment, and rescue are among the criteria for instillation of surfactant. The disadvantage of using a prophylactic approach, in which any newborn of a certain age or weight category would be automatically treated, is that some newborns would receive surfactant unnecessarily. If a prophylactic approach is not used, surfactant should be instilled at the earliest time possible after stabilization of the patient and confirmation of the presence of RDS.[21] The criteria for early surfactant delivery are (1) confirmation of RDS by radiographic findings and (2) administration of a fraction of inspired oxygen (FIO_2) of greater than 0.30. During the procedure, the dosage of surfactant may be given in two half-doses or four quarter-doses, with the newborn positioned to allow optimal distribution. Because of the large amount of fluid lavaged into the airway, the procedure may be complicated by one or more of the following: decreased oxygen saturation (SaO_2), change of color, and decreased heart rate. The clinician should treat these complications by temporarily increasing FIO_2 and peak inspiratory pressure (PIP). Multiple doses of surfactant may be needed, typically up to three, between 6 and 12 hours apart.[22]

In the newborn who does not receive surfactant, other forms of therapy can be instituted. If the infant requires an FIO_2 of greater than 0.60 to achieve adequate oxygenation and can continue to ventilate adequately, continuous positive airway pressure (CPAP) is needed. CPAP greatly improves outcome for newborns with RDS who are of a larger birth weight and older gestational age.[23] The obvious advantage of CPAP in RDS is that it increases FRC and keeps alveoli open throughout exhalation. This increases lung compliance and decreases the work of breathing, leading to improved arterial oxygenation at lower FIO_2 levels. CPAP is applied with nasal prongs or a face mask. The use of an endotracheal tube to apply CPAP has the disadvantage of increasing airway resistance, potentially making spontaneous breathing more difficult.

Currently, a predominant number of patients treated for RDS have a very low birth weight (less than 1500 g). CPAP has not been widely accepted as a treatment modality in these smaller, more immature newborns. Rather, they appear to benefit more from early intubation and mechanical ventilation.[24]

Continuous mechanical ventilation is needed when the infant fatigues and cannot maintain adequate ventilation, as evidenced by a $Paco_2$ that exceeds 60 to 70 mm Hg or by sustained apneic episodes. If mechanical ventilation is required, high PIPs and positive end-expiratory pressures (PEEPs) may be necessary initially because of poor lung compliance.[25] Mechanical respiratory rates of up to 60/minute may be needed. The general goals of mechanical ventilation in the infant with RDS are to keep the Pao_2 in the range of 60 to 70 mm Hg, $Paco_2$ less than 50 to 60 mm Hg, and pH between 7.3 and 7.4 while minimizing PIPs and Fio_2 levels. Minimizing PIPs and Fio_2 may reduce the risk of oxygen toxicity, barotrauma, cardiovascular compromise, and bronchopulmonary dysplasia (see Chapter 26).

As mentioned earlier, many premature newborns with RDS have a PDA with a left-to-right shunt, and this complicates their clinical course. Left-to-right shunting through the PDA causes blood to be shunted from the aorta into the pulmonary artery. This leads to "flooding" of the pulmonary circulation with blood, increases pulmonary capillary hydrostatic pressure, and causes leakage of fluid into the alveolar space. The shunting also leads to a decreased perfusion to the descending aorta, which may cause a metabolic acidosis. Clinicians should rapidly identify the presence of a PDA and employ pharmacological or surgical interventions to close the ductus arteriosus. Indomethacin, a prostaglandin inhibitor, often is given to help close the PDA.

CASE STUDY

Maternal History

A 24-year-old white woman, gravida 2, para 1, approximately 28 weeks pregnant, was admitted with a complaint of lower back pain. She had received prenatal care with regular visits. No medications were taken during her pregnancy except for prenatal vitamins. She stated that she was in a car accident 2 weeks ago, was seen by her obstetrician after the accident, and had no difficulty until an hour before admission. Upon arrival at the hospital, she was determined to be in premature labor and had spontaneous rupture of membranes. The amniotic fluid was clear. Delivery occurred 8 hours after the onset of labor via normal vaginal delivery.

Delivery History

A male infant, with an estimated gestational age of 28 weeks, was delivered weighing 1250 g (appropriate weight for gestational age). The Apgar scores were 5 and 7 at 1 and 5 minutes, respectively. The mother received no meperidine (Demerol) before the delivery. The infant had a cephalic presentation, and forceps were required to aid the delivery. The delivery team did not document any complications.

QUESTIONS

1. What does gravida 2, para 1 indicate?
2. Why is it important to know the color of the amniotic fluid?
3. Does the fact that there was a normal vaginal delivery have any bearing on the respiratory status of the infant?
4. Why is it significant to know that the mother did not receive meperidine before the infant's delivery?
5. What is the risk of development of RDS in an infant of this gestational age?

ANSWERS

1. Gravida refers to a woman's total number of pregnancies, including the current one. Para refers to the number of live births, *not* including the current one. Therefore, the gravida number will always be higher than the para number. A woman's pregnancy history also includes the number of abortions, which are divided into two categories: *spontaneous abortion* (often referred to as a miscarriage) and *therapeutic (medically induced) abortion*.

2. The amniotic fluid is typically clear. Yellow or green amniotic fluid, or green particles in the fluid, usually indicates that *meconium* (the newborn's initial stool) was released. This occurs for different reasons. Most often, meconium is released in association with periods of asphyxia. The resulting hypoxia, vasoconstriction, peristalsis, and ultimately anal sphincter relaxation causes meconium to be emitted into the amniotic fluid.[26] Meconium can cause airway obstruction and lung damage if drawn into the lungs before or during delivery. Red-tinged amniotic fluid indicates the presence of blood in the fluid. Other discolorations can be caused by infection that may develop when there has been a prolonged rupture of the membranes.

3. Yes, the type of delivery can influence the respiratory status of the infant. A vaginal delivery assists with the "squeeze" of the thoracic cavity, which helps to expel amniotic fluid from the lungs. When the chest has not been squeezed, as in the case of a cesarean section, the infant is prone to transient tachypnea.[27]

4. Meperidine can cross the placental barrier and affect the infant. If a mother receives meperidine within a few hours of delivery, the infant can become lethargic and apneic, requiring more advanced resuscitation.[28] The resuscitation may include administration of naloxone (Narcan) to reverse the effects of the meperidine and stimulate breathing.[20]

5. The incidence of RDS is inversely related to gestational age: As gestational age decreases, the risk of RDS development increases. RDS occurs in greater than 70 percent of newborns at 28 to 30 weeks' gestation.

Physical Examination

Vital Signs: Heart rate 168/minute, respiratory rate 64/minute, temperature 36.8°C (98.2°F), blood pressure 48/30 mm Hg, mean arterial pressure 39 mm Hg, and oxygen saturation (SpO_2) 93 percent determined by pulse oximeter

Measurements: Weight 1250 g (near 50th percentile); head circumference 27 cm (50th percentile); length 40 cm (greater than 50th percentile)

HEENT: Head round with some mild molding and mild bruising; anterior fontanelle flat and soft; sutures overlapping; external auditory canals patent; pupils equal, round, and reactive to light and accommodation (PERRLA); nares grossly patent

Lungs: Subcostal and intercostal retractions; breathing irregular; fine inspiratory crackles (rales) auscultated in both lungs

Heart: Regular rate and rhythm, with no murmur auscultated; pulses equal, but diminished bilaterally, brachially, and femorally

Skin: Acrocyanosis noted; multiple bruising on the extremities; initial capillary refill 3 seconds

Extremities: Creases on hands and feet; fingers and toes intact bilaterally

Neurological: Good muscle tone and activity

Abdomen: Soft, with no bowel sounds heard; no distention; liver down 1.5 cm; umbilical cord noted to have three vessels

Genitalia: Normal male; voided once; loose, meconium stool

QUESTIONS

6. How would you interpret the vital signs?
7. What is indicated by the retractions and inspiratory crackles?
8. What are the differential diagnoses in this case, and what is the most likely diagnosis?
9. What other diagnostic tests can be helpful in confirming the diagnosis?

ANSWERS

6. The infant has tachycardia and tachypnea. The normal heart rate for a newborn is 120 to 160/minute and the normal respiratory rate between 35 and 60/minute.[20] The infant should be observed closely because these signs could indicate hypoxemia. The blood pressure is within normal range.

7. Retractions indicate a significant increase in the work of breathing. Infants have a very compliant thoracic cage in contrast to adults. Retractions occur when the infant generates greater negative intrathoracic pressures in an attempt to overcome low lung compliance. Since the lungs of the infant with RDS are often less compliant than the chest wall, the forces of negative intrathoracic pressure collapse the chest wall inward instead of expanding the lungs. The fine inspiratory crackles indicate either fluid or atelectasis and are consistent with RDS.

8. The differential diagnoses include sepsis, pneumonia, and RDS. There is no history of prolonged rupture of the membranes or any maternal fever or infection, so sepsis is not the most likely diagnosis. RDS or pneumonia is the likely diagnosis, and further analysis is necessary to determine the diagnosis.

9. A CBC with a white blood cell count and differential may help identify the presence of infection. A chest x-ray could help confirm the diagnosis of RDS or pneumonia.

CASE STUDY—continued

The patient's clinical status began to deteriorate over the next hour with substernal (xiphoid) retractions in addition to the subcostal and intercostal retractions that were observed initially. A chest radiograph was obtained (Fig. 25–4). The infant exhibited nasal flaring and was grunting. The SpO_2 was 86 percent with the patient on room air. The infant became cyanotic and required an FIO_2 of 0.40 delivered via oxygen hood for improvement of his color.

The infant's current vital signs were as follows: heart rate 160/minute, respiratory rate 72/minute, and blood pressure 52/29 mm Hg with a mean arterial pressure of 40 mm Hg. Blood was drawn for ABG analysis after an umbilical artery catheter was placed. The results were as follows: pH 7.31, $PaCO_2$ 37 mm Hg, PaO_2 47 mm Hg, HCO_3^- 18 mEq/liter, and base excess −7 mEq/liter on an FIO_2 of 0.40.

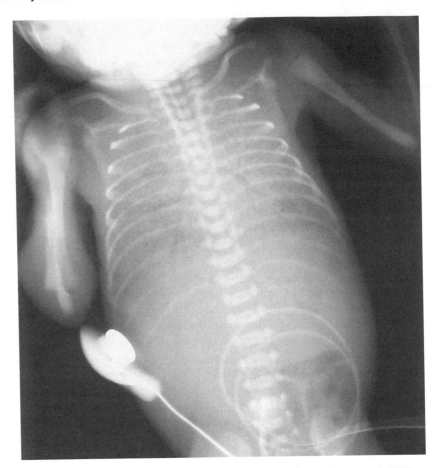

FIGURE 25-4   Chest radiograph obtained in the neonatal intensive care unit (ICU).

QUESTIONS

10. What is your interpretation of the chest radiograph?

11. What is the cause of the nasal flaring and grunting?

12. How would you interpret the ABG?

13. Is this patient a candidate for exogenous surfactant therapy?

ANSWERS

10. The chest radiograph reveals findings consistent with RDS: consolidation throughout both lungs, with decreased lung volumes and bilateral air bronchograms.

11. Nasal flaring is an infant's response to an increase in the work of breathing. In an attempt to decrease resistance to airflow into the lungs, the infant increases the diameter of the nostrils upon inspiration. Grunting occurs during exhalation, when the exhaled volume is pushed through a partially closed glottis. An infant may be able to increase FRC with this maneuver.

12. The ABG results reveal an uncompensated metabolic acidosis with hypoxemia. The $Paco_2$ is higher than expected, given the presence of metabolic acidosis, and represents early respiratory acidosis.

13. Because of this patient's young gestational age, his need for greater than 30 percent oxygen, and a chest radiograph indicating findings consistent with RDS, he is a candidate for exogenous surfactant therapy.

CASE STUDY—continued

The infant's oxygen requirements continued to increase. The SpO_2 of 88 percent was obtained while the patient was breathing an FIO_2 of 0.60 via oxygen hood. The ABG results were as follows: pH 7.26, $PaCO_2$ 50 mm Hg, and PaO_2 40 mm Hg

The physician intubated the infant with a 3.0-mm-diameter endotracheal tube. Auscultation of the chest and abdomen suggested proper placement of the tube. The infant was manually ventilated with 80 percent oxygen to determine the optimal pressures for chest expansion. His vital signs at that point were as follows: heart rate 150/minute, respiratory rate 60/minute, and SpO_2 94 percent, determined by pulse oximeter. The mechanical ventilator was set at a PIP of 22 cm H_2O, a PEEP of 4 cm H_2O, an intermittent mandatory ventilation (IMV) rate of 40/minute, and an FIO_2 of 0.80.

A modified natural surfactant (4 mL/kg) was administered via a 5-French feeding catheter, which had been inserted in the endotracheal tube to a point slightly beyond the tip of the endotracheal tube. The first quarter-dose was administered with the infant on his right side and his head and body turned to the right and in a downward slope. During the second quarter-dose administration, when the infant was positioned on his left side and in a downward slope, his heart rate dropped to 100/minute and his SpO_2 reading dropped to 80 percent saturation. He recovered with a temporary increase in the IMV rate to 60/minute and FIO_2 to 1.0. He was positioned with his head and body in an upward slope and turned to the right and then the left for the third and fourth quarter-doses, respectively. The ABG results after surfactant administration were as follows: pH 7.36, $PaCO_2$ 37 mm Hg, PaO_2 78 mm Hg on an FIO_2 of 0.80.

QUESTIONS

14. Why did this patient receive endotracheal intubation and mechanical ventilation?

15. Why did the patient's physiological parameters deteriorate during surfactant administration?

16. How would you interpret the most recent ABG, and what is the likely cause of the improvement?

17. What would be an alternative therapy for this patient?

ANSWERS

14. The need for intubation and mechanical ventilation was indicated by the persistent hypoxemia on a FIO_2 of 0.60 via oxygen hood and the infant's demonstration of fatigue with the increase in $PaCO_2$. The infant also met the criteria for surfactant administration, which would require endotracheal intubation.

15. The infant's deterioration during the surfactant administration—noted by decreasing heart rate, color, and oxygen saturation—is common and should be anticipated by clinicians. The large volume of surfactant (4 mL/kg) being lavaged into the airway can (1) lead to a vagal response and a slowing of the

heart rate; and (2) act as a blockage, causing a temporary decrease in oxygenation. This leads to decreased oxygen saturation and cyanosis. The infant should be allowed to stabilize for a minimum of 30 seconds between quarter-doses.

16. Improvement in ABGs is most likely due to the effect of surfactant in reducing alveolar surface area tension, thus improving the atelectasis and FRC. Lung compliance and oxygenation also show improvement, and the work of breathing is reduced.

17. An alternative to surfactant therapy at this time would be to place the patient on nasal CPAP, which could improve his FRC and thus his oxygenation. Because of the young gestational age of this infant, however, it is likely that he will tire more quickly as a result of his level of increased work of breathing, and therefore intubation with surfactant therapy is the preferred treatment.

CASE STUDY—continued

During the 8 hours after surfactant therapy, weaning from mechanical ventilation was started. The mechanical ventilator was set at a PIP of 18 cm H_2O, a PEEP of 4 cm H_2O, an IMV rate of 30/minute, and an FIO_2 of 0.35. The infant has been pink and has shown increased activity. His vital signs are as follows: heart rate 145 to 158/minute, respiratory rate 45 to 50/minute, mean arterial pressure 46 to 48 mm Hg, oxygen saturation 95 to 98 percent determined by pulse oximeter, and skin temperature 37.2°C (99.0°F).

Over the next 2 hours, the oxygen saturations began to decrease and a higher FIO_2 was required. Examination of the patient revealed diminished bilateral breath sounds, a heart rate of 168/minute, a pulse oximeter reading of 88 percent on 0.60 FIO_2, and apparent agitation. The infant was suctioned and placed back on the ventilator at an FIO_2 of 0.80. Blood for ABG analysis was drawn several minutes later, and ABG results were as follows: pH 7.25, $PaCO_2$ 53 mm Hg, PaO_2 47 mm Hg, HCO_3^- 22 mEq/liter, and base excess −5 mEq/liter.

QUESTIONS

18. How would you interpret the most recent ABG results?

19. What are the possible causes of the patient's deterioration?

20. What is the suggested treatment for this patient?

ANSWERS

18. The most recent ABG results reveal respiratory and metabolic acidosis with hypoxemia.

19. The causes for the inadequate ventilation and oxygenation could include a plugged endotracheal tube, a displaced endotracheal tube, air leak syndrome, progressive atelectasis, or worsening RDS.

    Had the endotracheal tube been plugged, the patient would have desaturated over a period of minutes instead of hours and would have responded positively to suctioning. Had the tube been displaced out of the trachea, the infant would have deteriorated dramatically immediately after the displacement. Tube displacement into the mainstem bronchus would have revealed unilateral breath sounds. In this case, a chest radiograph would be an appropriate diagnostic tool for determining whether the patient is experiencing air leak syndrome, worsening atelectasis, or RDS.

20. This patient is a candidate for another dose of surfactant therapy. In the very immature newborn, surfactant therapy may initially improve physiological parameters. However, while the exogenous surfactant has been used and is in the process of being catabolized and reutilized, the patient's endogenous surfactant may not be available or may not yet be mature enough to function properly, therefore requiring redosing with exogenous surfactant. An immediate treatment for this patient would be an increase in the PIP to 20 cm H_2O. This would increase the Pao_2 and decrease the $Paco_2$.

CASE STUDY—continued

The patient improved and by day 7 was extubated and placed on an Fio_2 of 0.30 via oxygen hood. By the end of day 7, the Fio_2 was increased to 0.40 because of low Spo_2 values. Physical examination revealed mild intercostal retractions and an increase in respiratory rate from 40/minute to 52/minute. Chest auscultation revealed bilateral inspiratory crackles and a systolic murmur. The patient also had bounding pulses and an active precordium. The chest x-ray revealed pulmonary edema and cardiomegaly. Umbilical line ABG measurements were as follows: pH 7.30, $Paco_2$ 37 mm Hg, Pao_2 52 mm Hg, HCO_3^- 18 mEq/liter, and base excess −8 mEq/liter on an Fio_2 of 0.40.

QUESTIONS

21. What is the most likely cause of this patient's respiratory distress?
22. Would the absence of a murmur change the suspected diagnosis?
23. What is the most likely cause of the metabolic acidosis as seen by the ABG?
24. What is the suggested treatment for this patient?

ANSWERS

21. The ductus arteriosus is the fetal vascular connection between the pulmonary artery and aorta. This patient is exhibiting symptoms of a PDA, which is associated with respiratory disease in newborn infants.[29] During the acute stages of respiratory disease, pulmonary vascular resistance can remain high. If the ductus arteriosus remains patent, a small amount of shunting will occur, but not enough to be clinically significant. When the pulmonary vascular resistance drops, with improved respiratory function, a PDA will allow a large amount of blood to shunt from the aorta through the ductus arteriosus into the pulmonary artery (left-to-right shunt). The increase in pulmonary blood flow leads to pulmonary edema and symptoms of respiratory distress.[27] Symptoms of a PDA include bounding pulses, murmur, active precordium, and respiratory distress, including retractions, tachypnea, and crackles. The incidence of PDA is highest in low-birth-weight infants.[30]

22. Even in the presence of a large PDA, a murmur may not be heard. In the absence of a murmur, findings of bounding pulses, active precordium, pulmonary edema, and cardiomegaly are indicative of a PDA.[31]

23. The metabolic acidosis is caused by decreased blood flow to the descending aorta and lower extremities. Blood flow shunts into the pulmonary artery, resulting in diminished flow through the descending aorta; this leads to the build-up of lactic acid and metabolic acidosis.

24. A PDA can be treated with indomethacin, a prostaglandin synthase inhibitor. The ductus arteriosus is stimulated to stay open by prostaglandins. Reducing the production of prostaglandins with indomethacin may lead to closure of the ductus arteriosus. A second method of closing the ductus arteriosus is surgical ligation.

CASE STUDY—continued

After administration of indomethacin, the systolic murmur and pulmonary edema resolved. The patient was weaned to room air within 24 hours. He remained hospitalized for 6 more weeks until he gained an appropriate weight for discharge. He had no other respiratory complications and was discharged at a weight of 1980 g.

REFERENCES

1. Bryan, H, et al: Perinatal factors associated with the respiratory distress syndrome. Am J Obstet Gynecol 162:476, 1990.
2. Robertson, B: Background to neonatal respiratory distress syndrome and treatment with exogenous surfactant. Dev Pharmacol Ther 13:159, 1989.
3. Morton, N: Pulmonary surfactant: Physiology, pharmacology and clinical uses. Br J Hosp Med 42:52, 1989.
4. Hallman, M: Fetal development of surfactant: Considerations of phosphatidylcholine, phosphatidylinositol, and phosphatidylglycerol formation. Prog Respir Res 15:27, 1981.
5. Poulain, F, and Clements, J: Pulmonary surfactant therapy. West J Med 162:43–50, 1995.
6. Moya, F, et al: Surfactant protein A and saturated phosphatidylcholine in respiratory distress syndrome. Am J Respir Crit Care Med 150:1672–1677, 1994.
7. Hallman, M, and Gluck, L: Respiratory distress syndrome: Update 1982. Pediatr Clin North Am 29:1057, 1982.
8. O'Brodovich, H, and Mellins, R: Bronchopulmonary dysplasia: Unresolved neonatal acute lung injury. Am Rev Respir Dis 132:694, 1985.
9. Samcon, L: Infants of diabetic mothers: Current perspectives. J Perinat Neonatal Nurs 6(1):61–70, 1992.
10. Hodson, W: Hyaline membrane disease: Remaining challenges. Semin Respir Med 6:111, 1984.
11. Ikegami, M, et al: A protein from airways of premature lambs that inhibits surfactant function. J Appl Physiol 57:1134, 1984.
12. Ablow, R, and Driscoll, S: A comparison of early-onset group B streptococcal neonatal infection and the respiratory distress syndrome of the newborn. N Engl J Med 294:65, 1976.
13. Streeter, N: High Risk Neonatal Care. Aspen Publishers, Rockville, MD, 1986.
14. Lapido, M: Respiratory distress revisited. Neonat Network 8:9, 1989.
15. Walti, H, et al: Neonatal diagnosis of respiratory distress syndrome. Eur Respir J Suppl 3:22S, 1989.
16. Downes, J: Respiratory distress syndrome of newborn infants: New clinical scoring system (RDS score) with acid-base and blood-gas correlations. Clin Pediatr 9:325, 1970.
17. Kraybill, E, et al: Risk factors for chronic lung disease in infants with birth weights of 751 to 1,000 grams. J Pediatr 115:115, 1989.
18. Chatburn, R: Similarities and difference in the management of acute lung injury in neonates (IRDS) and in adults (ARDS). Respir Care 33:539, 1988.
19. NIH Consensus Conference: Effect of corticosteroids for fetal maturation on perinatal outcomes. JAMA 273:413–418, 1995.
20. Bloom, R, et al: Textbook of Neonatal Resuscitation. American Heart Association, American Academy of Pediatrics, Elk Grove, Illinois, 1994.
21. OSIRIS Collaborative Group: Early versus delayed neonatal administration of synthetic surfactant: The judgment of OSIRIS. Lancet 340:1363–1369, 1992.
22. Hoekstra, R, et al: Improved neonatal survival following multiple doses of bovine surfactant in very premature neonates at risk for respiratory distress syndrome. Pediatrics 88:10–18, 1991.

23. Gregory, G, et al: Treatment of the idiopathic respiratory-distress syndrome with continuous positive airway pressure. N Engl J Med 284:1333, 1971.

24. Drew, J: Immediate intubation at birth of the very-low birthweight infant. J Dis Child 136:207, 1982.

25. Goldsmith, J, and Karotkin, E: Assisted Ventilation of the Neonate, ed 2. WB Saunders, Philadelphia, 1988.

26. Rossi, EM, et al: Meconium aspiration syndrome: Intrapartum and neonatal attributes. Am J Obstet Gynecol 161:1106, 1989.

27. Avery, G: Neonatology, ed 3. JB Lippincott, Philadelphia, 1987.

28. Yeh, TF: Neonatal Therapeutics, ed 2. Mosby–Year Book, St. Louis, 1991.

29. Fanaroff, A, and Martin, R. Neonatal-Perinatal Medicine: Diseases of the Fetus and Infant, ed 5, Vol 2. Mosby–Year Book, St. Louis, 1992, p 810

30. Hubbard, C: Ligation of the patent ductus arteriosus in newborn respiratory failure. J Pediatr Surg 21:3, 1986.

31. Cunningham, M, et al: Perinatal risk assessment for patent ductus arteriosus in premature infants. Obstet Gynecol 68:41, 1986.

CHAPTER **26**

Bronchopulmonary Dysplasia

Cynthia Malinowski, MA, RRT

Key Terms

atelectasis
bronchopulmonary
   dysplasia (BPD)
nasal flaring

necrosis
respiratory distress
   syndrome (RDS)
retractions

tracheal tugging

Introduction

Bronchopulmonary dysplasia (BPD), a chronic lung disease characterized by bronchiolar metaplasia and interstitial fibrosis, occurs primarily in premature infants who have received mechanical ventilation. Although all premature newborns receiving mechanical ventilation are at risk for BPD, the ones at highest risk are those who are ventilated at high peak inspiratory pressures (PIPs) or at an increased fraction of inspired oxygen (FIO_2), or both.[1] There are rare reports of BPD occurring in full-term newborns who have also received mechanical ventilation.[2] Because there is no standardized definition of BPD, there is a wide range in the reported incidence (2.4 to 68 percent).[3] Despite the discrepancies in the definition, it is clear that the occurrence of BPD is inversely related to gestational age. The disease develops in as many as 85 percent of newborns weighing 500 to 699 g; however, the rate drops to as low as 5 percent in newborns weighing more than 1500 g.[4]

There is little agreement on the criteria for the diagnosis of BPD. Suggestions range from an inclusive set of criteria, which would include all infants with respiratory sequelae who required supplemental oxygen beyond the age of 28 days, to more specific criteria involving radiographic and clinical findings.[5] An infant can be diagnosed with BPD if it received mechanical ventilation for more than 7 days, has persistent respiratory distress, requires an FIO_2 higher than room air after 28 days of age, and has a compatible chest radiograph.[6] These criteria are valid only if other causes of continued respiratory distress (e.g., pneumonia, pulmonary edema, apnea of prematurity) are ruled out.

Infants who are treated for BPD range in age from 3 weeks to a few years. The 3-week-old premature neonate presents different challenges in management than the 2-year-old child, who may need home care and frequent hospitalizations.

Etiology

BPD is caused by trauma to the lungs from the combined insults of mechanical ventilation and oxygen therapy.[7,8] The high incidence found in the lower gestational age and lower birth weight categories is due to the increased risk of this population to lung injury.[9] The development of the disease is facilitated by a complex interrelationship of factors, including pulmonary inflammatory autoinjury, an immature antioxidant system, and the presence of sepsis and pulmonary edema.[5] Many risk factors have been associated with the development of BPD (Table 26-1). The majority of infants with BPD have initially been diagnosed with **respiratory distress syndrome (RDS)** and often require high inflating pressures and oxygen concentrations because of the poor lung compliance associated with their initial disease process.[10] The fragile, immature lung may not tolerate the stretching forces likely to be produced by mechanical ventilation. Efforts have been made to identify the single factor associated with mechanical ventilation that causes the most harm. For example, is it high PIPs or high mean airway pressures? The evidence is inconclusive as to the exact factor, but most clinicians agree that the use of minimal PIPs may lessen the risk.[11,12]

In addition to having delicate airways and alveoli, the premature newborn has an immature antioxidant system. In the absence of a mature antioxidant system to neutralize oxygen radicals, even low FIO_2 levels (0.25 to 0.50) can predispose the lung to damage.[13] An abnormal inflammatory response may be part of the etiology of BPD. The infant with BPD has an increased number of inflammatory cells in its airway. The abnormal inflammatory response may favor an imbalance of protective versus destructive cells.[14] This promotes hydrolysis of the connective tissue matrix, leading to a propensity for injury. The presence of an endotracheal tube or infection, or both, may also play a role in the development of BPD.[15]

Many infants with BPD have had a patent ductus arteriosus (PDA) at some point in their clinical course. In premature newborns, a PDA usually results in left-to-right

---

TABLE 26-1   **Risk Factors for the Development of Bronchopulmonary Dysplasia**

- Prematurity
- Higher severity of respiratory distress syndrome
- Exposure to oxygen
- Barotrauma
- High inspiratory pressures
- Patent ductus arteriosus associated with pulmonary edema
- Fluid overload
- Male gender
- Nonblack race
- History of infection
- Perinatal asphyxia
- Family history of asthma

shunting of blood from the aorta into the pulmonary artery, which causes flooding of the pulmonary vasculature.[16,17] The premature newborn has a more permeable alveolar-capillary membrane, facilitating the movement of capillary fluid into the lungs. The resulting pulmonary edema may contribute to the lung injury in several ways:

1. Pulmonary edema results in greater oxygen requirements, which may worsen the oxygen toxicity problem.
2. The proteins found in the alveoli in the presence of pulmonary edema can in-activate surfactant, resulting in atelectasis, decreased lung compliance, and the need for higher ventilator pressures.[18]
3. The destruction of the alveolar-capillary membrane caused by mechanical ventilation further predisposes the infant with BPD to pulmonary edema, thus worsening the surfactant problem and leading to a vicious circle of **atelectasis,** higher ventilator pressures, continued alveolar-capillary damage, pulmonary edema, and inactivation of surfactant.

A high association between a family history of asthma or reactive airway disease and an increased risk for BPD has been identified, suggesting a familial link in the etiology of BPD.[5] The etiology of BPD, however, more likely involves a combination of factors, rather than one single mechanism (Fig. 26–1). Although mechanical ventilation plays a large part in the development of BPD, the unique characteristics of the premature lung are key factors in the etiology of this disease.

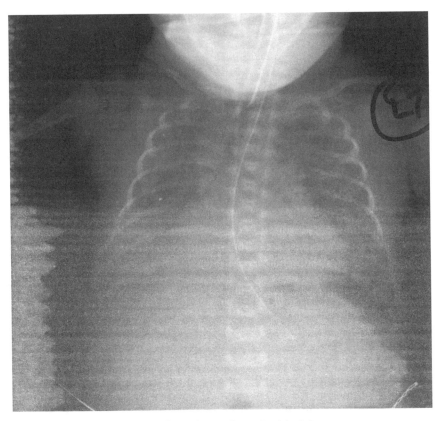

FIGURE 26–1   Chest radiograph of the infant.

Pathophysiology

In 1967, Northway, Rosan, and Porter were the first to describe BPD as a disease that occurs in stages associated with specific radiographic changes.[8] Since that time, other clinical investigators, including Northway, have reported that many patients with BPD do not manifest these specific chest radiographic stages.[19] It is helpful, however, to review the pathological changes in the lung associated with the radiographic stages as described by Northway and colleagues.

Stage 1 is characterized by the presence of hyaline membranes and is often indistinguishable from RDS. Atelectasis is present, and necrosis of bronchiolar mucosa has begun. Radiographic findings are similar to those of RDS (see Chapter 25).[20]

In *stage 2,* there is repair of bronchiolar and alveolar epithelium, but also areas of widespread **necrosis.** Areas of emphysema become evident, and cellular debris may obstruct airways. Atelectatic areas remain a problem, and the radiographic findings may show opacification.[6,21]

Stage 3 is associated with transition to the classic chronic findings in the lungs of the newborn with severe BPD. There is extensive bronchial and bronchiolar metaplasia and hyperplasia, as well as thickening of basement membranes. The alveolar emphysema that has been developing now leads to larger, spherically circumscribed groups of alveoli surrounded by atelectatic areas. Increased mucus secretion and interstitial edema are also present.[22]

Stage 4 is characterized by fibrosis. Smooth muscle hypertrophy is present. Progressive destruction of alveoli, airways, and vasculature can be seen. Lymphatic and mucus glands are deformed.[6,21]

These pathological changes in the lungs cause ventilation-perfusion ($\dot{V}/\dot{Q}$) defects: Areas of atelectasis have less ventilation than perfusion (low $\dot{V}/\dot{Q}$), and areas of emphysema have more ventilation than perfusion (high $\dot{V}/\dot{Q}$). The overall $\dot{V}/\dot{Q}$ mismatching results in hypoxemia.[10] Thickening membranes and pulmonary edema lead to diffusion defects and decreased gas exchange. Air trapping from alveolar destruction causes elevated Pa_{CO_2}. The infant with severe BPD (stage 4) has an increased functional residual capacity because of the air trapping.[2] The airways lose their structural integrity and become floppy, leading to scattered expiratory wheezing.

Mechanical characteristics of the lungs of newborns with BPD include decreased lung compliance and increased airway resistance. Increased airway resistance, possibly due to bronchospasm, also may contribute to the development of BPD. Infants with BPD generally have an elevated airway resistance on the first day of life, as compared to newborns of similar age and weight who do not have the disease.[23] The infant with BPD also may have an increased amount of thick secretions, which contributes to the elevated airway resistance.

Clinical Features

The clinical feature first noticed in the infant with BPD may be an inability to wean from mechanical ventilation. Later, the infant may manifest such a sensitivity to changes in F_{IO_2} that there may be large drops in oxygen saturation with small decreases in F_{IO_2}.

The infant's general appearance will demonstrate an increased work of breathing, including **tracheal tugging,** chest wall **retractions,** and tachypnea.[2] The infant in respiratory failure or impending respiratory failure will often remain pink even in the presence of moderate hypoxemia. This is because the presence of fetal hemoglobin shifts the oxygen-hemoglobin dissociation curve to the left, allowing a higher saturation of hemoglobin at a lower PaO_2. A lack of cyanosis cannot be interpreted as an indication of adequate oxygenation in premature infants.

Chest auscultation reveals diffuse, fine inspiratory crackles and expiratory wheezes. The crackles are due to the presence of pulmonary edema, which is associated with BPD or the opening of atelectatic areas on inspiration that have closed during expiration. Wheezes are present as a result of bronchospasm, anatomic narrowing of airways, or narrowing due to secretions.

The chest radiograph may not be definitive of BPD until later in the disease, when various degrees of irregular densities (from atelectasis and the formation of fibrosis) and hyperlucent areas can be seen.[24] The overexpansion is caused by air trapping, similar to that seen in adults with chronic obstructive pulmonary disease (COPD). The radiographic pattern in advanced BPD is often described as "bubbly" or cystic in appearance.[25] The complications of pulmonary edema or pneumonia may obscure the radiographic changes of BPD.

Pulmonary function studies typically reveal elevated total airway resistance, decreased lung compliance, and an increased work of breathing.[26] In most cases, pulmonary function testing is not done.

Arterial blood gas (ABG) measurements are similar to those seen in adults with COPD. Hypoxemia and a compensated to partially compensated respiratory acidosis are common findings. The hypoxemia usually responds to oxygen therapy.

An important part of assessing the newborn suspected of having BPD is to rule out other causes of continuing respiratory compromise, such as sepsis, aspiration, seizure disorders, apnea, immature chest wall, PDA, or intraventricular hemorrhage (IVH). In the newborn with respiratory distress and oxygen dependency lasting more than 28 days, a complete blood count (CBC), blood cultures, and ultrasound tests for PDA and IVH may be needed to rule out other causes for the respiratory compromise, especially in the absence of typical radiographic findings.

Treatment

The prevention of BPD is an important goal in management of the premature newborn. Strategies that lessen the incidence or severity of RDS and thus the need for mechanical ventilation and oxygen therapy have a preventative effect. The two treatment modalities that have the best preventative possibilities are the use of prenatal corticosteroids and exogenous surfactant therapy.[27,28]

Treatment of the infant with BPD is supportive in nature, emphasizing adequate nutrition and oxygenation to provide an environment for healthy lung growth. Although areas of lung damage may be permanent, the newborn has the ability to continue generating alveolar tissue. If the ratio of healthy alveoli to damaged alveoli improves, the newborn has a better chance of being successfully weaned from the mechanical ventilator, thus reducing his or her exposure to its damaging effects.

Pharmacological agents used in the treatment of BPD include bronchodilators, diuretics, and steroids.[29] Bronchodilators decrease the high airway resistance that is often seen in these infants.[30] Treatment with bronchodilators is warranted if wheezing, retractions, or gas trapping are noted. Isoproterenol, terbutaline, metaproterenol, albuterol, and isoetharine are the bronchodilators most commonly used in the treatment of BPD.[31] None of these bronchodilators appears to be superior to the others. Theophylline may be beneficial in reducing airway resistance and improving lung compliance in infants who are difficult to wean from mechanical ventilation.[9,31,32]

Diuretics are often necessary in infants with increased oxygenation requirements associated with pulmonary edema. Long-term diuretic therapy can lead to improved pulmonary function in infants with BPD.[33] Excessive weight gain due to fluid retention may precede pulmonary edema and identify the patient in whom diuretics may be necessary. Fluid management is monitored carefully to avoid fluid overload, which has been related to PDA development.

Steroid administration leads to short-term improvements in pulmonary function and more rapid weaning from mechanical ventilation in infants with BPD.[34] There is no clear evidence, however, that the use of steroids leads to a decrease in hospital stay, duration of oxygen therapy, or mortality rate. The best timing of steroid administration (i.e., early or later in the course of BPD), as well as the most effective dosage, is also unclear.[35] Steroids are associated with side effects such as immunosuppression, electrolyte imbalance, infection, hyperglycemia, and hypertension.[35] Even with the potential hazards and lack of evidence of long-term efficacy, steroids may be of benefit in the infant with BPD who has become ventilator-dependent and difficult to wean.

The spontaneously breathing newborn suspected of having BPD may require intubation and mechanical ventilation. ABG criteria for respiratory failure in the newborn vary, but generally include a pH less than 7.25, $Paco_2$ greater than 60 mm Hg, and Pao_2 less than 50 mm Hg on an Fio_2 greater than 0.60 to 0.80.[20,36]

Mechanical ventilation may be necessary for weeks or even months in some infants with BPD. Although there is no conclusive evidence that one strategy for mechanical ventilation is superior to another in these infants, it is generally agreed that the lowest PIP and Fio_2 necessary to achieve acceptable ABGs should be employed.[5,12] Inspiratory times should be long enough to provide even distribution of gases, but short enough to allow adequate expiratory times in order to ensure emptying of the lung and prevention of gas trapping. Low levels of positive end-expiratory pressure (PEEP, 2 to 4 cm H_2O) are helpful in preventing atelectasis. Higher levels may be necessary in the presence of a complicating pulmonary edema, but because the infant with BPD is prone to air trapping and overexpansion, higher PEEP levels should be used with caution.

Ideal ABG values are often different for infants with BPD than for those of similar gestational age who do not have the disease. For example, it is permissible for the newborn with BPD to have a $Paco_2$ within the range of 50 to 70 mm Hg as long as the pH remains above 7.28. Lowering the $Paco_2$ to 40 mm Hg may require significantly higher ventilator pressures and is far more detrimental to the infant than a mild to moderate increase in $Paco_2$. Adequate oxygenation appears beneficial for growth of the newborn.[37] Hypoxemia also has a detrimental effect on the pulmonary vasculature. Hypoxemia leads to pulmonary vasoconstriction and pulmonary hypertension in infants with BPD.[38] A Pao_2 range of 55 to 65 mm Hg is acceptable in these patients.[12]

If mechanical ventilation is an important etiological factor, then weaning the newborn from mechanical ventilator support may reduce lung damage. Aggressive weaning from the ventilator in the newborn not yet diagnosed with BPD, or showing very mild symptoms of BPD, can prevent the development of a severe case of BPD. The practice of "waiting" until the patient has perfect ABG values before weaning is less acceptable in the premature newborn at risk for BPD. Aiming for an "acceptable" range of pH, $Paco_2$, and Pao_2, which may be out of normal ranges, is an appropriate option for reducing lung damage and beginning the weaning process. For example, decreases in ventilator parameters may be attempted in the stable patient with a pH of 7.30, a $Paco_2$ of 52 mm Hg, and a Pao_2 of 55 mm Hg. The early use of continuous positive airway pressure (CPAP) in premature newborns with respiratory distress has been advocated to avoid the need for mechanical ventilation, also possibly preventing BPD.[39] The use of intravenous aminophylline can facilitate weaning from mechanical ventilation. Aminophylline improves respiratory function by improving diaphragmatic function, increasing chemoreceptor sensitivity to CO_2, and reducing pulmonary artery pressure.[35]

Monitoring of the infant during mechanical ventilation usually includes the use of a pulse oximeter. Transcutaneous monitoring has been less popular than oximetry in these infants because their transcutaneous Po_2 and Pco_2 values do not correlate well with arterial values.[40]

Nutritional management is an important treatment component for the infant with BPD. Weaning from mechanical ventilation can be difficult without adequate nutrition. The malnourished patient may not have the ability to grow new, healthy alveoli that would otherwise contribute to the healing process.[41]

Because of the evidence regarding the role of oxygen radicals in the development of BPD, investigations into the use of vitamins A and E to reduce oxygen-induced lung damage and promote normal lung healing have been initiated. The results have been mixed, and further controlled trials will be necessary before final conclusions can be made regarding their use.[42,43]

The infant with BPD needing long-term mechanical ventilation may benefit from a tracheostomy.[44] A tracheostomy can allow greater movement of the infant's head and improvement in feeding, both contributing to better overall development. However, the morbidity and mortality rates associated with tracheostomies is higher in pediatric patients compared to adults. Because of this, many clinicians leave the infant with chronic lung disease intubated for long periods of time, even several months, before considering tracheostomy.[45]

The infant may be discharged while still receiving oxygen therapy. Many infants with stable BPD who continue to need respiratory care will require home care. The home care of infants and children requiring respiratory therapy is evolving into a subspecialty that requires special education. Home care allows the infant with BPD the benefit of continued respiratory care at a much lower cost.

Outcome

Mortality rates of infants with BPD have been reported to be between 11 and 40 percent.[35,46] Of infants with BPD, cerebral palsy has been reported in 13 percent and neurological deficit in 27 percent.[47] Improved neurodevelopment has been reported in the presence of proper attention to nutrition and a favorable home environment.[4]

There is frequently an increased incidence of infections and repeated hospitalizations in this population of infants. Pulmonary function studies may remain abnormal, demonstrating reactive airway disease. The infant with BPD may become a child with chronic respiratory problems, such as wheezing, increased airway resistance, and airway obstruction.[32]

CASE STUDY

History

Baby Boy M is a 33-day-old prematurely born male who weighs 1420 g. At birth his estimated gestational age was 28 weeks. His initial diagnosis was RDS with PDA. He received exogenous surfactant therapy within 1 hour of birth and 12 hours later. He was on mechanical ventilation for 3 weeks with a PIP recorded as high as 38 cm H_2O on FIO_2 levels of 0.60 to 0.80 for more than 1 week. Initial radiographic findings were low lung volumes, a ground-glass appearance, and air bronchograms. At 1 week of age, the patient received indomethacin therapy to close his PDA. He was extubated, and is currently on a 35 percent oxygen hood. An examination revealed a respiratory rate of 78/minute; moderate substernal, subcostal, and intercostal chest wall retractions; and crackles bilaterally. ABG findings were as follows: pH 7.28, $PaCO_2$ 62 mm Hg, PaO_2 40 mm Hg, base excess (BE) +4, and HCO_3^- 30 mEq/liter.

QUESTIONS

1. What are the indications that Baby Boy M is in respiratory distress, and what further information should be gathered?

2. What diseases should be included in the differential diagnosis of this patient, and what is the most likely diagnosis?

3. What is your interpretation of the ABG, and what is the most likely cause of the decreased PaO_2?

ANSWERS

1. The indications of respiratory distress include tachypnea (respiratory rate 78/minute) and chest wall retractions. Additionally, an ABG analysis reveals hypoxemia on an FIO_2 of 0.35. Average respiratory rates for newborns are between 30 and 60/minute; rates in the higher range are typical of infants of this patient's age group. More important, the infant's current respiratory rate should be compared with rates counted in the past 48 hours to see if there has been an increase. Further information to gather would be a chest radiograph and CBC.

2. Diseases in the differential diagnosis include sepsis, aspiration, pulmonary edema due to fluid overload, and BPD. There is not enough evidence at this point to identify which of these potential problems is causing the respiratory distress. The history of mechanical ventilation strongly suggests BPD. In sepsis, findings of apnea and bradycardia are common,[47] but are not part of this patient's clinical findings. Blood cultures and a CBC would be important to rule out sepsis as a cause of the infant's respiratory distress. If the patient had aspirated, the clinical findings would likely be more acute.

3. The ABG reveals partially compensated respiratory acidosis with moderate hypoxemia. The decreased PaO_2 is caused by $\dot{V}/\dot{Q}$ mismatching and alveolar hypoventilation. The hypoxemia also could be caused by pulmonary edema, occurring as a result of injury to the alveolar-capillary membranes.

Physical Examination

General: Patient alert and agitated, under an oxygen hood; patient pink, but apparently in moderate respiratory distress

Vital Signs: Temperature 36.3°C (97.3°F), respiratory rate 78/minute, heart rate 166/minute, blood pressure 64/48 mm Hg

HEENT: Patient normocephalic; anterior fontanelle 2 × 2 cm, soft, and normotensive; pupils equally round and reactive to light and accommodation (PERRLA); nasal flaring present; throat clear

Neck: Supple without lymphadenopathy, but slightly increased tracheal tugging noted; no stridor

Chest: Normal anteroposterior diameter with symmetrical expansion; moderate substernal, subcostal, and intercostal retractions

Lungs: Rapid respiratory rate with fine inspiratory crackles throughout anterior lung fields bilaterally; wheezes heard on expiration

Heart: Regular rate and rhythm without murmur

Abdomen: Soft, nontender, nondistended with active bowel sounds and no hepatosplenomegaly

Extremities: Strong pulses in the upper and lower extremities bilaterally; no evidence of clubbing, cyanosis, or edema

QUESTIONS

4. What is the cause of the chest wall retractions?
5. Does the absence of a fever indicate that there is no infection?
6. Does the infant's pink color indicate adequate oxygenation? Why or why not?
7. What does tracheal tugging indicate, and what causes it?
8. What causes expiratory wheezes?
9. What is the significance of the presence of crackles?

ANSWERS

4. Chest wall retractions are present because of a high chest wall compliance and low lung compliance. When a large intrapleural subatmospheric pressure is generated by the diaphragm, the compliant chest wall collapses inward at the points of least resistance. As the infant's lung compliance worsens and greater diaphragmatic contractions are generated, the retractions worsen.

5. The absence of a fever does not necessarily indicate that the patient is free of infection. Sepsis can be associated with transient temperature imbalances that include hyperthermia or hypothermia.[5] An additional complicating factor with regard to assessment of body temperature is that the premature newborn's body temperature is often regulated by an incubator. In interpreting changes in body temperature, the incubator temperature must be assessed as well as the infant's body temperature.[48] For example, if the newborn has a normal core temperature but the incubator temperature has been increased several degrees to maintain the core temperature, thermal instability may be present.

6. The term newborn has only 25 percent adult hemoglobin, and the premature

newborn may have 0 percent adult hemoglobin.[49] Pink color in an infant does not indicate adequate oxygenation because fetal hemoglobin shifts the oxygen-hemoglobin dissociation curve to the left. The left-shifted curve means that the infant has a higher hemoglobin saturation at any Pao_2. The higher hemoglobin saturation makes it difficult to detect cyanosis. The newborn may remain pink until the Pao_2 drops very low—as low as 40 mm Hg—or until the arterial oxygen saturation (Sao_2) drops to 60 percent or less in some premature newborns.[6,49]

Fetal hemoglobin can be present in infants until 6 months of age. Although Baby Boy M is 33 days old, it is likely that he has significant amounts of fetal hemoglobin. The amount may vary as a result of the amount and frequency of transfusions of adult hemoglobin. Therefore adequate oxygenation cannot be assumed based on the patient's pink color.

7. Tracheal tugging is an indication of hyperinflation and respiratory distress. The infant with BPD has a low, flat diaphragm, similar to that of an adult with emphysema. When this low, flat diaphragm moves downward, the central diaphragmatic tendon pulls the trachea downward, causing tracheal tugging.[50]

8. Wheezing can be caused by narrowing of the airways, viscous airway secretions, and floppy airway walls. Bronchospasm with increased airway resistance is associated with BPD.

9. Crackles are often present in infants with BPD complicated by pulmonary edema. Pulmonary edema can be present in BPD owing to increased capillary permeability, fluid overload, or a PDA. Left-to-right shunting through the PDA causes blood to be shunted away from the aorta and into the pulmonary vasculature, leading to high hydrostatic pressure and leaking of fluid into the lung. This patient is 33 days old, and the presence of a PDA is usually diagnosed earlier in the clinical course.

Laboratory Evaluation

Chest Radiograph: See Figure 26–1

ABGs: pH 7.30, $Paco_2$ 71 mm Hg, Pao_2 49 mm Hg, BE +6, HCO_3^- 35 mEq/liter, oxygen hood at Fio_2 0.60

CBC (see Appendix for normal values):

White blood cells (WBCs) 13,000/mm³

Red blood cells (RBCs) 3.7 million/mm³

Segmented neutrophils 58 percent

Bands 1 percent

Lymphocytes 37 percent

Monocytes 1 percent

Eosinophils 1 percent

Hemoglobin 12.9 g/100 mL

Hematocrit 38 percent

During the time of this laboratory evaluation, the Fio_2 was increased to 0.70 based on pulse oximetry oxygen saturation values of less than 88 percent. The respiratory rate increased to 82/minute, and chest wall retractions became severe.

QUESTIONS

10. How would you interpret the ABG results?

11. What abnormalities are present on the chest radiograph, and what pathophysiology is causing these radiographic results?

12. What is significant about the CBC results?

13. What therapy would you suggest for this patient?

14. At what point would you consider intubation?

15. What is the optimal PaO_2 range?

ANSWERS

10. These ABGs reflect a partially compensated respiratory acidosis and hypoxemia. The pH is lower than normally acceptable. However, because of a decreased ability for renal retention of HCO_3^-, infants with BPD may not have the ability to compensate for a respiratory acidosis completely.[41] In order to make decisions in caring for this patient, the ABGs are best interpreted by examining any trends. If the acid-base status is typical for this patient, therapy may be different than if this is a significant change in his ABG status. Interpreted alone, this ABG represents typical values for infants with BPD. Except for the hypoxemia, the ABG results may be considered acceptable, even with a very high $PaCO_2$.[20]

11. The chest radiograph shows hyperexpanded lungs with irregular, streaky densities bilaterally in the perihilar region. The hyperinflation is typical of infants with BPD. Grossly, the lungs of infants with BPD have been described as having areas of emphysematous alveoli caused by cystic dilation of distal airways interspersed with dense, fibrotic areas.[51] The air trapping from the emphysematous component leads to the hyperinflation, and the fibrotic areas are represented by the irregular, streaky densities.

12. The significance of the CBC results is the absence of findings consistent with sepsis. There is a normal WBC count and no left shift. An abnormal WBC (increased or decreased) can occur during an active infection.[48] A WBC of 13,000/mm^3 is considered normal for an infant of this age.

13. The presence of wheezing is an indication for bronchodilator therapy. Aerosolized sympathomimetic agents such as metaproterenol, terbutaline, or isoetharine may provide relief of bronchoconstriction. The use of theophylline in infants with BPD has appeared beneficial in some cases, but because of potential relaxation of the cardiac-esophageal junction allowing reflux, it is used with caution. Additional therapy for this patient would include an increase in the FIO_2 to alleviate the hypoxemia.

14. There are two factors to consider in a decision to intubate this patient: (1) the work of breathing and (2) the evidence of respiratory failure by ABGs. This patient does not meet the ABG criteria for respiratory failure because the pH is greater than 7.28; however, impending respiratory failure is evidenced by an increase in respiratory rate, respiratory retractions, and FIO_2 requirements. This may be cause for intubation, even before the stated ABG criteria are met.

15. The PaO_2 should be maintained in the range of 55 to 65 mm Hg. If values greater than 55 mm Hg can be achieved, it is better to use the lowest FIO_2 necessary to be within the stated range. It is important to understand that

these desired Pao_2 values are ABG values and not those obtained from the heel (capillary ABG values). Heel-stick Pao_2 values do not reflect arterial values. Because of the difficulty in acquiring accurate Pao_2 values in the chronically ill newborn, pulse oximetry is used to monitor oxygenation. Values in the 90 to 95 percent oxygen saturation range are commonly the goal of oxygen therapy. It is necessary to maintain adequate Pao_2 levels in BPD patients because their growth rate and right ventricular function improve when chronic hypoxemia is avoided.[37]

CASE STUDY—continued

Baby Boy M's Fio_2 was increased to 0.80 over the course of 1 hour while he was monitored with a pulse oximeter to keep the saturation between 90 percent and 95 percent. He continued to have evidence of respiratory distress with retractions and tachypnea. Aerosolized medication treatments were ordered with terbutaline 0.25 mL in 2.75 mL saline. The patient's wheezing decreased after treatment. Oxygen requirement fluctuated but were eventually reduced to 0.45. Two days later it was noted that a weight gain in excess of 60 g/day (normal weight gain should be less than 50 g/day in a newborn this size) had been measured for 2 consecutive days. Crackles continued to be heard bilaterally, and a repeat chest x-ray revealed pulmonary edema superimposed on changes consistent with BPD. Respiratory rate increased to 90/minute, and heart rate was 150/minute. ABG results on a 1 liter/minute nasal cannula were as follows: pH 7.27, $Paco_2$ 85 mm Hg, Pao_2 40 mm Hg, HCO_3^- 37 mEq/liter, and BE +8. Because there was evidence of impending respiratory failure, the patient was intubated and given pressure-limited ventilation.

QUESTIONS

16. What is the cause of this patient's pulmonary edema?
17. Should any changes in bronchodilator therapy be made?
18. Can the low Pao_2 be treated with a higher Fio_2, instead of intubation and mechanical ventilation?
19. What is the Fio_2 for this patient on 1 liter/minute?
20. What additional pharmacological therapy could be used in this patient?
21. What initial ventilator settings would you suggest for this patient?

ANSWERS

16. This patient had a previous history of PDA, which was treated with indomethacin. It is unlikely that at the age of 33 days the ductus arteriosus would reopen and cause pulmonary edema. Because a PDA seems unlikely, the probable cause of pulmonary edema is the combination of increased capillary permeability due to injury and high pulmonary vascular pressures. Since pulmonary edema can be caused by fluid overload, the intake and output on this patient needs to be examined.
17. The findings do not indicate that the cause of his increasing respiratory distress is due to bronchoconstriction. As there is no evidence that any one bronchodilator agent is superior in the treatment of BPD, changing the medication probably will not have an effect on the patient's course.

18. Even though the patient shows evidence of continuing compensation for the respiratory acidosis, other signs indicate that he is in impending respiratory failure. His continued low PaO_2, increase in respiratory rate, increase in heart rate, crackles, and weight gain indicate a clinical picture of decompensation. Increasing the FIO_2 may improve his PaO_2 and is indicated as an immediate step; however, it probably will be only a temporary solution to the continued hypoxemia.

19. The FIO_2 of an infant on a 1 liter/minute cannula is not known. As is the case in adults, the FIO_2 is variable and influenced by the patient's ventilatory pattern. It is more likely that the infant will have high FIO_2 levels associated with low flows because of his small peak inspiratory flows and shallow breathing patterns. The FIO_2 may be as high as 0.60 with the infant on 1 liter/minute nasal cannula. In this case, it can be deceptive to consider the patient stable because he is only on a 1 liter/minute cannula.

20. Because the infant has had excessive weight gain, crackles, and a chest radiograph indicative of pulmonary edema, diuretics should be considered. Conservative management of this patient may include the use of diuretics before intubation to see if there is improvement in his respiratory distress. It still may be considered appropriate to intubate him before or during the administration of diuretics because of his continued deterioration and hypoxemia.

21. To determine ventilator settings, an assessment can be made after the patient is intubated and being ventilated manually. Chest excursion is observed, and a PIP that causes chest movement is chosen. The lowest PIP possible should be used to avoid further lung damage. PEEP levels of 2 to 4 cm H_2O should be applied to all newborns on mechanical ventilation.[52] A typical starting respiratory rate is 40 to 50/minute. Inspiratory to expiratory (I:E) ratios should favor longer expiratory times to avoid air trapping. For an infant with this diagnosis, commonly ordered settings are as follows: intermittent mandatory ventilation (IMV) 40/minute, PIP 24 cm H_2O, PEEP 2 cm H_2O, FIO_2 0.60, I:E ratio 1.0:2.5. As a guideline for choosing current parameters, it is also helpful to review the ventilator settings that the patient was on before extubation.

CASE STUDY—continued

Over the next 3 weeks, Baby Boy M was extubated twice and reintubated twice for respiratory failure. In each instance of extubation, he required an increased FIO_2 and demonstrated worsening respiratory distress. He has had one more episode of pulmonary edema, which was treated with diuretics. His ventilator settings were as follows: PIP 20 to 30 cm H_2O, IMV 40 to 50/minute, PEEP 2 to 5 cm H_2O, and FIO_2 0.50 to 0.80. The patient became very sensitive to small changes in FIO_2 and PIP.

QUESTIONS

22. What are the possibilities for treatment of this patient at this point?

23. What is the prognosis for this patient based on his current course?

ANSWERS

22. A trial of aminophylline may decrease airway resistance, improve diaphragmatic function, and allow the infant to be weaned from mechanical ventilation.

    The use of steroids could be considered at this point and may improve pulmonary function and facilitate weaning from the ventilator.

    If the patient continues to be ventilator dependent, tracheostomy may be considered. Advantages of tracheostomy in this patient would include better opportunities for environmental stimulation, range of motion, and more normal feeding habits.

23. Mortality rates of 11 to 40 percent have been reported for BPD. It is impossible to predict whether this patient will survive at this time.[35,46] The patients who die of BPD often have histories that include weeks of mechanical ventilation, difficulty weaning, and high FIO_2 requirements. If this patient does survive the chronic lung disease, his future outcome may involve ongoing health problems, neurological developmental problems, abnormalities of language development, and hearing difficulties.[53]

CASE STUDY—continued

The hospital course of this patient included another 3 months in the neonatal intensive care unit, repeated attempts at extubation, pneumonia, and nutritional difficulties. He was eventually extubated 6 months after admission and went home on oxygen therapy. Three months later, he was weaned from oxygen therapy. He was followed and treated for reactive airways, which required home use of bronchodilator therapy.

REFERENCES

1. Palta, M, et al: Development and validation of an index for scoring baseline respiratory disease in the very low birth weight neonate. Pediatrics 86:714, 1990.
2. O'Brodovich, H: Bronchopulmonary dysplasia: Unsolved neonatal acute lung injury. Am Rev Respir Dis 132:694, 1985.
3. Ehrenkranz, R, and Mercurio, M: Bronchopulmonary dysplasia. In Sinclair, J, and Bracken, M (eds): Effective Care of the Newborn Infant. Oxford University Press, New York, 1992, pp 399–424.
4. Parker, R, et al: Improved survival accounts for most but not all of the increase in BPD. Pediatrics 90:663–668, 1992.
5. Taeusch, H, et al: Schaffer and Avery's Diseases of the Newborn, ed 6. WB Saunders, Philadelphia, 1991.
6. Zimmerman, J, and Farrell, P: Advances and issues in bronchopulmonary dysplasia. Curr Probl Pediatr 24.159–170, 1994.
7. Barnhart, S, and Czervinske, P: Perinatal and Pediatric Respiratory Care. WB Saunders, Philadelphia, 1995, p 468.
8. Northway, WH, et al: Pulmonary disease following respirator therapy of hyaline membrane disease: Bronchopulmonary dysplasia. N Engl J Med 276:357, 1967.
9. Murphy, J: The human lung at 24 to 26 weeks gestation: Watershed of survival. Semin Respir Med 6:103, 1984.
10. Jackson, J: Bronchopulmonary dysplasia: Challenges for research. Semin Respir Med 6:119, 1984.
11. Kraybill, E, and Runyan, D: Risk factors for chronic lung disease in infants with birth weights of 751 to 1000 grams. J Pediatr 115:115, 1989.
12. Goldberg, R, and Bancalari, E: Therapeutic approaches to the infant with bronchopulmonary dysplasia. Respir Care 36:613, 1991.
13. Kelly, F: Free radical disorders of preterm infants. Br Med Bull 49(3):558–578, 1993.
14. Sluis, K, et al: Proteinase-antiproteinase balance in tracheal aspirates from neonates. Eur Respir J 7:251–259, 1994.
15. Stern, L, et al: Negative pressure artificial respiration: Use and treatment of respiratory failure of the newborn. Can Med Assoc J 102.595, 1970.
16. Dudell, GG, and Gersony, WM: Patent ductus arteriosus in neonates with severe respiratory disease. J Pediatr 104:915, 1984.
17. Brown, ER, et al: Bronchopulmonary dysplasia: Possible relationship to pulmonary edema. J Pediatr 92:982, 1978.

18. Kobayashi, T, et al: Inactivation of exogenous surfactant by pulmonary edema fluid. Pediatr Res 29: 353, 1991.

19. Bancalari, E, et al: Bronchopulmonary dysplasia: Clinical presentation. J Pediatr 95:819, 1979.

20. Thibeault, D, and Gregory, G: Neonatal pulmonary care, ed 2. Appleton-Century-Crofts, East Norwalk, 1986.

21. Kirkpatrick, B, and Mueller, D: Bronchopulmonary dysplasia. In Kendig, E (ed): Disorders of the Respiratory Tract in Children, ed 2. WB Saunders, Philadelphia, 1972, p 819.

22. Taghizadeh, A, and Reynolds, E: Pathogenesis of bronchopulmonary dysplasia following hyaline membrane disease. Am J Pathol 82:241, 1976.

23. Oliphant, M, et al: Pulmonary parenchymal patterns at one month as a prognostic indicator in neonatal chronic lung disease. Perinatol Neonatol Sept/Oct:21, 1987.

24. Fitzgerald, P, et al: Bronchopulmonary dysplasia: A radiographic and clinical review of 20 patients. Br J Radiol 63:444, 1990.

25. Greenough, A: Bronchopulmonary dysplasia: Early diagnosis, prophylaxis, and treatment. Arch Dis Child 65:1082, 1990.

26. Gerhardt, T, et al: Serial determination of pulmonary function in infants with chronic disease. J Pediatr 110:448, 1987.

27. NIH Consensus: Effect of corticosteroids for fetal maturation on perinatal outcomes. JAMA 273:413–418, 1995.

28. Kendig, J, et al: Surfactant replacement therapy at birth: Final analysis of a clinical trial and comparisons with similar trials. Pediatrics 82(5): 756–762, 1988.

29. Rozycki, H, and Kirkpatrick, B: New developments in bronchopulmonary dysplasia. Pediatr Ann 22(9):532–538, 1993.

30. Kao, L, et al: Effect of isoproterenol inhalation on airway resistance in chronic bronchopulmonary dysplasia. Pediatrics 73:509, 1984.

31. Davis, J, et al: Drug therapy for bronchopulmonary dysplasia. Pediatr Pulmonol 8:117, 1990.

32. Northway, W: Bronchopulmonary dysplasia: Then and now. Arch Dis Child 65:1076, 1990.

33. Kao, L, et al: Randomized trial of long-term diuretic therapy for infants with oxygen-dependent bronchopulmonary dysplasia. J Pediatr 124(5 pt 1):772–781, 1994.

34. Knoppert, D, and Mackanjee, H: Current strategies in the management of bronchopulmonary dysplasia: The role of corticosteroids. Neonatal Network 13(3): 53–60, 1994.

35. Abman, S, and Groothius, J: Pathophysiology and treatment of bronchopulmonary dysplasia: Current issues. Pediatr Clin North Am 41:277–315, 1994.

36. Koff, P, et al: Neonatal and Pediatric Respiratory Care, ed 2. Mosby–Year Book, St. Louis, 1993, p 326.

37. Cox, M, et al: Improved growth in infants with bronchopulmonary dysplasia treated with nasal cannula oxygen (abstract). Pediatr Res 13:492, 1979.

38. Southall, DP, et al: Recurrent cyanotic episodes with severe arterial hypoxaemia and intrapulmonary shunting: A mechanism for sudden death. Arch Dis Child 65:953, 1990.

39. Avery, ME, et al: Is chronic lung disease in low birth weight infants preventable? A survey of 8 centres. Pediatrics 79:26, 1987.

40. Hamilton, PA, et al: Underestimation of arterial oxygen tension by transcutaneous electrode with increasing age in infants. Arch Dis Child 60:1162, 1985.

41. Farnaroff, A, and Martin, R: Neonatal-Perinatal Medicine: Diseases of the Fetus and Infant, ed 5. CV Mosby, St. Louis, 1992, pp 871, 1296.

42. Watts, J, et al: Failure of supplementation with vitamin E to prevent bronchopulmonary dysplasia in infants <1500 g birthweight. Eur Respir J 4:188–190, 1991.

43. Chytil, F: The lungs and vitamin A. Am J Physiol 262:L517–L527, 1992.

44. Carlo, W, and Chatburn, R: Neonatal Respiratory Care, ed 2. Yearbook, Chicago, 1988.

45. Handler, S: Pediatric tracheostomy: Experience during the past decade. Ann Otol Rhinol Laryngol 91:628, 1982.

46. Yip, Y, and Tan, K: Bronchopulmonary dysplasia in very low birthweight infants. J Paediatr Child Health 27:34, 1991.

47. Koops, B, et al: Outpatient management and follow-up of infants with BPD. Clin Perinatol 11:101–122, 1984.

48. Streeter, N: High Risk Neonatal Care. Aspen, Rockville, MD, 1986.

49. Bancalari, E, and Flynn, J: Respiratory physiology, oxygen therapy, and monitoring. Birth Defects 24:41, 1988.

50. Glauser, F: Signs and symptoms in pulmonary medicine. JB Lippincott, Philadelphia, 1983.

51. Taghizadeh, A, and Reynolds, E: Pathogenesis of bronchopulmonary dysplasia following hyaline membrane disease. Am J Pathol 82:241, 1976.

52. Carlo, W, and Martin, R: Principles of neonatal assisted ventilation. Pediatr Clin North Am 33:221, 1986.

53. Markestad, T, and Fitzharding, P: Growth and development in children recovering from BPD. J Pediatr 98:597, 1981.

CHAPTER **27**

Persistent Pulmonary Hypertension of the Newborn

Cynthia Malinowski, MA, RRT

Key Terms

ductus arteriosus
extracorporeal membrane
   oxygenation (ECMO)

foramen ovale
maladaptation
nitric oxide (NO)

persistent pulmonary
   hypertension of the
   newborn (PPHN)

Introduction

The lungs do not participate in gas exchange before birth, as this is the function of the placenta. The lack of oxygen in the lungs causes the pulmonary vasculature to constrict, resulting in a marked elevation of the pulmonary vascular resistance (PVR). The elevated PVR inhibits blood flow through the lungs and causes blood to bypass the lungs by way of two normal fetal circulatory shunts: the **ductus arteriosus** and the **foramen ovale.** The ductus arteriosus is a connection between the pulmonary artery and the aorta. The foramen ovale is an opening between the right and left atria (Fig. 27-1). Blood flow through these two fetal shunts allows most of the oxygenated blood returning from the placenta to bypass the fetal lungs by shunting from the right side to the left side into the fetal systemic circulation.

    After birth, the pulmonary vasculature dilates as oxygen enters the lungs. The associated drop in PVR and simultaneous increase in systemic blood pressure facilitates closure of the fetal shunts. The foramen ovale closes in response to an increased volume of blood returning from the lung into the left atrium. This increased blood volume physically pushes against a flap valve lying in the left atrium and shuts it so that blood no longer has a pathway from the right to the left atrium. The ductus arteriosus constricts in response to the increases in oxygen tension. If the PVR does not decrease after birth, the fetal shunts will remain patent and blood flow to the lung will remain low. This syndrome, which consists of a high PVR, low pulmonary blood flow,

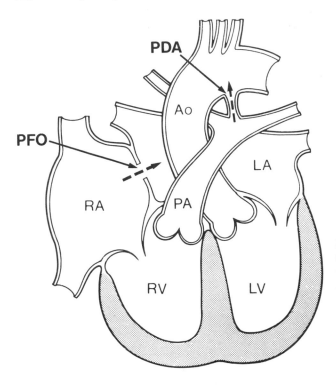

FIGURE 27-1 Fetal circulation is illustrated, showing right-to-left shunting (*dashed arrows*) through patent ductus arteriosius (PDA), pulmonary artery (PA) to aorta (Ao), and patent foramen ovale (PFO), right atrium (RA) to left atrium (LA). RV = right ventricle; LV = left ventricle. (Modified from Graves E, et al: Persistent pulmonary hypertension in the neonate. Chest 93:638, 1988, with permission.)

and a fetal state of circulation, is known as **persistent pulmonary hypertension of the newborn (PPHN).**[1] Although this condition may be treatable, the newborn with PPHN has a high mortality risk.[2]

Etiology

PPHN is a syndrome with a variety of clinical causes. Any pulmonary or cardiac disease that causes reactive pulmonary capillary constriction, an increase in pulmonary arterial musculature, or hypoplasia of the pulmonary vascular bed (with decreased total vascular area) may cause PPHN (Table 27-1).[1,3-5]

Interference with normal postdelivery reduction in PVR can be caused by prenatal anatomical changes. Chronic fetal hypoxemia can cause excessive muscularization of the pulmonary vessels and lead to PPHN.[6]

Infants with a normally structured arterial bed can have interference with the decrease in PVR and closing of fetal circulatory shunts that should occur at birth. This **maladaptation** to extrauterine existence can be caused by any initiating factor, such as acute perinatal stress, or by a disease that results in acidosis and hypoxemia. The low pH and hypoxemia leads to a continuation of the fetal PVR state after delivery, instead of the normal reduction of PVR.

Local endogenous mediators that affect PVR at birth are postulated to play a role in the maladaptation response. Mediators such as prostaglandins, leukotrienes, thromboxanes, and endothelin-1 have an effect on PVR through their vasoconstrictive or vasodilative properties. An imbalance of these mediators can lead to an elevated PVR after delivery.[7]

TABLE 27-1   **Causes of Persistent Pulmonary Hypertension of the Newborn (PPHN)**

Reactive pulmonary vasoconstriction
   Hypoxia/acidosis
      Pneumonia
      Atelectasis
      Meconium aspiration
      Hypoventilation
Increased pulmonary vascular musculature
   Chronic fetal hypoxia
   Prenatal pulmonary hypertension
Decreased cross-sectional area of pulmonary vasculature
   Hypoplasia of the lung
   Space-occupying lesions
      Diaphragmatic hernia
      Lung cysts

SOURCE: Adapted from Rudolph, AM: High pulmonary resistance after birth. Clin Pediatr 19:588, 1980.

Pathophysiology

Diminished pulmonary blood flow associated with PPHN results in areas of the lung where there is a high ventilation-perfusion ($\dot{V}/\dot{Q}$) ratio. Although the blood returning to the heart from the lung is well oxygenated (unless respiratory disease is the cause of the PPHN), a significant portion of the venous return is shunted through the ductus arteriosus and foramen ovale into the arterial system. As a result, the arterial blood is a mixture of desaturated venous blood and oxygenated arterial blood. Tissue oxygenation is often inadequate, and lactic acidosis occurs as tissue hypoxia develops. The combination of acidosis and hypoxemia results in a more profound increase in PVR and promotion of a vicious circle that leads to respiratory failure and death if not reversed.[4]

Clinical Features

Most infants with PPHN are term or post-term. The infant with PPHN may not exhibit signs of respiratory distress at birth, especially if respiratory disease is not the cause of the PPHN. Hypoxemia is often severe, associated with cyanosis, and poorly responsive to oxygen therapy.[8] A prominent right ventricular heave is visible or easily palpable during examination of the precordium. A loud second heart sound (S_2) or narrowly split S_2 with a loud pulmonic component (P_2) is often found during auscultation of the heart. A murmur is usually present as blood squirts through the ductus arteriosus or foramen ovale.[2,9] The lack of a murmur does not rule out PPHN because a large opening through the foramen ovale or ductus arteriosus may not result in turbulent blood flow. Examination of the respiratory system may reveal retractions and nasal flaring if lung disease is the cause of the PPHN. Otherwise, the lung examination is normal.

    The infant with PPHN may demonstrate signs and symptoms of neurological impairment when intrauterine asphyxia has occurred. Neurological impairment may be seen as seizures and abnormalities in level of consciousness, muscle tone, posture, reflexes, and pattern of breathing (e.g., periods of apnea).[10] Neurological impairment is an important finding, as it often determines the ultimate outcome.[11]

The chest radiograph will reveal clear lung fields and reduced pulmonary blood flow in the absence of lung disease. Although the chest radiograph is not diagnostic of PPHN, it is useful to assess sudden clinical deterioration caused by pneumothorax, bronchial intubation, or pneumonia.

Arterial blood gas (ABG) findings vary according to the severity of the shunting, the presence of underlying lung disease (e.g., meconium aspiration), and the site at which the arterial sample is drawn. Postductal arterial blood (blood in the arterial system that represents a mixture of shunted and nonshunted blood) will demonstrate severe hypoxemia. Preductal arterial blood (blood from the aorta before the opening of the ductus arteriosus) will often have good oxygenation because it contains blood that has passed through the lung. (This issue is explained later in greater detail, under Diagnosis.) The $Paco_2$ value of postductal blood is often found to be normal or elevated and is typically higher than expected for the level of ventilation. This is related to the large amount of dead space ventilation occurring while the lungs are adequately perfused.

Diagnosis

Neonates with PPHN may appear clinically similar to those with a cyanotic heart defect or any number of respiratory disorders. Bedside diagnostic tests, such as the hyperoxia test, comparison of preductal to postductal arterial Po_2, and the hyperoxia-hyperventilation test are often useful in the differential diagnosis.

The hyperoxia test identifies whether the patient's Pao_2 is responsive to the administration of oxygen. The newborn with a Pao_2 of 100 mm Hg or greater while breathing a fraction of inspired oxygen (Fio_2) of 1.0 probably has a $\dot{V}/\dot{Q}$ problem with an intrapulmonary origin (e.g., meconium aspiration), rather than a fixed right-to-left cardiac shunt, as in PPHN.[2] If the patient's Pao_2 remains less than 100 mm Hg while breathing an Fio_2 of 1.0, it is assumed that the hypoxemia is due to true shunting.[12] In such cases, PPHN or a cardiac lesion is the more likely diagnosis.

Comparing preductal to postductal arterial Pao_2 can reveal a right-to-left shunt through the ductus arteriosus (patent ductus arteriosus [PDA]). Blood that enters the root of the aorta from the left ventricle is considered *preductal arterial blood* because it has not reached the point at which the ductus arteriosus empties into the aorta. Preductal blood is oxygenated blood that has returned from the lung to the left side of the heart and exits the left ventricle into the aorta according to normal mechanisms. *Postductal arterial blood* is blood that is distal to the ductus arteriosus in the arch of the aorta. It is a mixture of venous blood that shunted through the ductus arteriosus and oxygenated blood from the left ventricle (Fig. 27–2).

Preductal and postductal blood can be assessed through ABGs and transcutaneous monitors. When ABGs are used to obtain preductal blood, the blood is most commonly drawn from the right radial artery. Preductal blood is drawn from this site because the right subclavian artery, which feeds blood into the right arm, branches from the brachiocephalic trunk of the aorta before the site at which the ductus arteriosus empties venous blood into the arch of the aorta (Fig. 27–2). The left radial is avoided because of the anatomical proximity of the left subclavian artery to the ductus arteriosus.

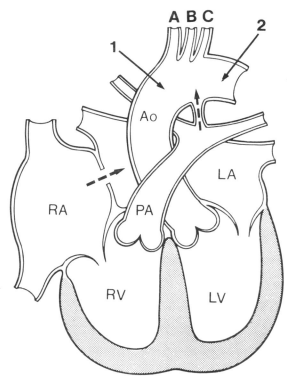

FIGURE 27–2   Preductal and postductal blood illustrated. 1 = preductal blood in the ascending aorta; 2 = postductal blood in the arch of the aorta; A = brachiocephalic trunk; B = left common carotid artery; C = left subclavian artery. (Modified from Graves, E, et al: Persistent pulmonary hypertension in the neonate. Chest 93:638, 1988.) Abbreviations as in Figure 27–1.

Postductal blood can be obtained from the umbilical artery. Transcutaneous (Tc) monitors can be used on the right upper body for preductal $TcPO_2$ and on the lower body for postductal $TcPO_2$. Simultaneous sampling revealing a difference of more than 15 mm Hg indicates a possible right-to-left shunt through the ductus arteriosus. A negative test result, however, does not rule out PPHN because shunting through the foramen ovale could be occurring and would not cause a significant difference between preductal and postductal PaO_2.[1,2]

The hyperoxia-hyperventilation test is accomplished by giving the newborn a high oxygen concentration (FIO_2 greater than 0.70) while a ventilator or manual resuscitator hyperventilates the patient. If the hypoxemia is due to PPHN, the respiratory alkalosis should decrease PVR, lessen the right-to-left shunting pattern, and improve oxygenation. A newborn with a fixed congenital heart lesion usually will not improve with this test.

Echocardiography can also confirm the presence of a PDA. This noninvasive procedure represents little risk to the patient.

Treatment

Treatment for PPHN focuses on lowering PVR or increasing systemic vascular resistance, or both. This should result in a reduction in right-to-left shunting and an increase in pulmonary blood flow.

Some infants may respond favorably to supplemental oxygen, but most will require assisted ventilation. The principal goal of mechanical ventilation in the treatment of PPHN is respiratory alkalosis. Respiratory alkalosis from hyperventilation should cause pulmonary vascular dilatation when the pH exceeds 7.50.[13] Hydrogen ion concentration, rather than $PaCO_2$, appears to be the mediating factor in the reduction of PVR.[14,15] Respiratory or metabolic alkalosis can induce vasodilation of the pulmonary vascular bed. Sodium bicarbonate or tromethamine (THAM) can be administered in order to produce a metabolic alkalosis to reduce PVR.[16]

Hyperventilation as a treatment for PPHN has been associated with various complications, including air leaks, bronchopulmonary dysplasia, neurodevelopmental abnormalities, and hearing loss.[17-20] Because of these potential complications, a more conservative ventilator management approach, including limiting ventilator pressures and tolerating higher $PaCO_2$ levels (50 to 60 mm Hg), has been attempted; outcomes have been successful.[21,22]

A newborn who is agitated and breathing out of synchrony with the ventilator may have periods of hypoxemia that may worsen the right-to-left shunting pattern. In such cases, paralysis and sedation can be used.

Pharmacological treatment of PPHN may include tolazoline (Priscoline) because of its potential ability to cause pulmonary vasodilation. Tolazoline is an α-adrenergic blockade with histamine-like action that has direct vasodilating effects. Unfortunately, the results of tolazoline use in infants with PPHN have been mixed.[4,13] Tolazoline is not a selective pulmonary vasodilator and can lower both systemic and pulmonary vascular pressures. If systemic pressures are lowered more than pulmonary pressures, the right-to-left shunting can increase. The use of tolazoline is also limited by complications, which include hypotension and gastrointestinal bleeding.[23] It may cause the patient to have a flushed appearance as systemic vasodilation occurs.

Severe systemic hypotension must be treated promptly because it increases the pressure gradient between the pulmonary artery and the aorta, leading to increased blood flow through the ductus arteriosus. Pharmacological agents such as dopamine may be needed to correct hypotension when it occurs.

Extracorporeal membrane oxygenation (ECMO) is an important option in the treatment of PPHN when conventional methods fail.[24] Arteriovenous ECMO is a method in which the infant's blood is withdrawn through a venous catheter and then perfuses a membrane oxygenator. After the blood is oxygenated, it is warmed and replaced into the infant's arterial system. This may be a lifesaving technique in severe PPHN because it allows adequate oxygenation and a reduction of the PVR. ECMO may be of value in patients with poor prognostic signs, such as an alveolar-arterial oxygen gradient (P[A − a]O_2) of greater than 600 mm Hg lasting for 12 hours.

High-frequency ventilation has been used to treat PPHN. It is most commonly used for newborns with a pulmonary air leak problem resulting in pulmonary interstitial emphysema. The role of high-frequency ventilation in the treatment of PPHN has not been clearly identified.

Nitric oxide (NO) is a pulmonary vasodilator, the effects of which appear to be identical to those of the endogenous vasodilator known as endothelium-derived relaxing factor. Low levels of inhaled NO have been associated with the reversal of hypoxemia in PPHN in both animals and human newborns.[25-27] The optimal concentration of NO has not been determined. There is evidence, however, that NO may have some toxic side effects, and the potential dangers of inhaled NO are currently being investigated.[28]

CASE STUDY

History

Baby Girl C is a term newborn who weighs 3250 g. She was the product of an uncomplicated pregnancy and was delivered to a 34-year-old mother with two healthy children at home. One hour before delivery, late fetal heart rate decelerations were noted. At delivery, meconium was seen in the amniotic fluid. After delivery, the patient's airway was suctioned to remove any meconium that may have been present in the trachea. The patient had Apgar scores of 7 at 1 minute (owing to poor color and respiratory effort) and 8 at 5 minutes (the patient had a more vigorous spontaneous respiratory effort). It was noted that the patient's color was cyanotic immediately after delivery, and she did not respond to an F_{IO_2} of 0.40 by oxygen hood. Examination revealed a respiratory rate of 40/minute, a heart rate of 130/minute, clear breath sounds, and absence of grunting or respiratory retractions. The F_{IO_2} was increased to 0.50, with no change in the patient's color. The infant was intubated and placed on a time-cycled, pressure-limited, continuous-flow infant ventilator.

QUESTIONS

1. What are the pertinent factors in the delivery history of this patient?
2. What diseases should be considered in the differential diagnosis of this patient, and what is the most likely diagnosis?
3. What diagnostic tests would you suggest be performed for further assessment of this patient?
4. What could explain why the cyanosis did not respond to oxygen therapy?

ANSWERS

1. One of the pertinent factors related to this patient's delivery history is the presence of meconium in the amniotic fluid. This finding indicates that the patient may have had an episode of asphyxia in utero or during delivery. The most common cause of in utero asphyxia is a reduction in placental blood flow, which impairs the transfer of oxygen from the mother to the fetus.[29] Symptoms of respiratory distress shortly after the delivery of a newborn through meconium-stained amniotic fluid is typically due to inhalation of meconium particles, which can cause pneumonitis, atelectasis, or pulmonary hyperinflation resulting from airway plugging.

   An additional factor of importance in the patient's history was the presence of late fetal heart rate decelerations. Normal fetal heart rates are between 120/minute and 160/minute. When bradycardia occurs, this is referred to as a deceleration. A common cause of heart rate decelerations in the fetus is asphyxia. The fetal heart rate is compared to the uterine contraction to see whether the deceleration occurred early or late in the uterine contraction. A heart rate deceleration occurring early in the uterine contraction cycle may be caused by a vagal response to the head's being compressed. A heart rate deceleration occurring late in the uterine contraction may be caused by uteroplacental insufficiency, which can lead to fetal asphyxia. A history of perinatal asphyxia can be an important finding in establishing the differential diagnosis.

2. The differential diagnosis should include meconium aspiration syndrome (MAS), PPHN, and congenital heart disease. It is necessary to have additional information before choosing the most likely cause of this patient's cyanosis. This infant has no retractions or grunting, signs that would be present if the cause of hypoxemia were due to lung pathology related to MAS. Because an increase in FIO_2 did not improve the patient's color, true shunting is likely to be the cause of hypoxemia.

3. Diagnostic tests that would further identify the cause of the infant's cyanosis are ABG analysis, chest radiograph and echocardiography. Bedside tests, such as a preductal and postductal PaO_2 comparison, may also be helpful.

4. Shunting of blood past the lungs, which is common in congenital heart disease and PPHN, may have caused the cyanosis.

Physical Examination

General: Patient alert and active, intubated with a 3.5-mm endotracheal tube, and receiving mechanical ventilation

Vital Signs: Temperature 36.5°C (97.7°F), respiratory rate 50/minute by mechanical ventilator and 20/minute spontaneously, heart rate 140/minute, blood pressure 60/45 mm Hg (mean arterial pressure 50 mm Hg)

HEENT: Normocephalic, with soft anterior fontanelle; eye motion normal; pupils equally round and reactive to light and accommodation (PERRLA); nasal shape normal with no flaring; pinnae well formed; throat examination precluded because of intubation

Neck: No masses, glands, or redundant tissue folds

Chest: Symmetrical, with no retractions

Heart: Regular rate and rhythm, without murmur or gallops

Lungs: Inspiratory crackles bilaterally

Abdomen: Nondistended; no masses or organomegaly on palpation; no bowel sounds heard on auscultation; umbilical cord with clean stump; umbilical arterial line and umbilical venous catheter lines in place

Extremities: Strong pulses in upper and lower extremities bilaterally; no evidence of edema; normal muscle tone demonstrated; cyanosis noted

---

QUESTIONS

5. Why are both a mechanical respiratory rate and a spontaneous respiratory rate given?

6. What is the significance of the patient's active alert state, reactive pupils, and normal muscle tone?

7. What does the finding of clear, equal breath sounds indicate?

8. Does the lack of murmur rule out the presence of a PDA in this patient?

9. Why would it be important to monitor the blood pressure or mean arterial pressure in this patient?

10. Is it significant that no chest wall retractions are present in this patient? If so, what is the significance?

ANSWERS

5. The patient is reported to be receiving mechanical ventilation at a respiratory rate of 50/minute, with a spontaneous rate of 20/minute. It is important to document both spontaneous and mechanical respiratory rates to identify whether the patient is exhibiting any spontaneous effort and how much of the total minute ventilation the infant is providing. The presence of spontaneous respirations is a positive neurological sign.

6. A normal sensorium, reactive pupils, and normal muscle tone represent significant positive findings in a patient with this kind of history (perinatal asphyxia and meconium-stained amniotic fluid) and indicate an intact neurological system. Meconium in the amniotic fluid can be considered a risk factor for the presence of an asphyxial episode in utero.[30] Although the normal neurological findings do not completely rule out future neurological abnormalities, it is unlikely that this infant has suffered more than minimal asphyxia.[31] If the patient were suspected of having sustained a moderate-to-severe brain injury, preparation would have to be made for the treatment of apneic episodes and seizures.

7. The findings of equal breath sounds could be important in ruling out pneumothorax or right mainstem intubation. A newborn with a history of meconium in the trachea is at risk for MAS, which is associated with a higher-than-normal incidence of pneumothorax. The presence of clear breath sounds does not rule out a lung parenchymal disease, although it may make it less likely.

8. The absence of a murmur does not rule out PDA. A newborn with PDA may not have a murmur if the opening is wide and blood flow through the ductus arteriosus is not turbulent.[1]

9. Patients with suspected PPHN syndrome should have their blood pressure monitored because changes in blood pressure can lead to changes in right-to-left shunting. The amount of blood bypassing the lungs and emptying directly into the aorta depends on both systemic and pulmonary pressures in addition to the size of the shunt. Systemic hypotension can facilitate a greater pressure gradient between the pulmonary artery and aorta and more shunting of blood from the pulmonary artery into the aorta, through the PDA, worsening the right-to-left shunt.

10. The absence of chest wall retractions is significant because it is a pertinent negative sign to be considered in distinguishing between a lung parenchymal problem and a right-to-left shunt, such as occurs with PPHN. Chest wall retractions are usually associated with the reduced lung compliance typical of lung parenchymal diseases. The presence of chest wall retractions is possible with lung disease or PPHN, but the absence of retractions would be more common in PPHN than with lung disease.

Laboratory Evaluation

Chest Radiograph:

Right lung somewhat hyperexpanded

Irregular, streaky densities bilaterally in the perihilar region

An endotracheal tube terminating approximately 1 cm above the carina (Fig. 27–3)

ABGs:

pH 7.26

$Paco_2$ 44 mm Hg

Pao_2 46 mm Hg

Base excess (BE) − 10 mEq/liter

HCO_3^- 18 mEq/liter

Fio_2 0.50

Intermittent mandatory ventilation (IMV) 50/minute

Peak inspiratory pressure (PIP) 20 cm H_2O

Positive end-expiratory pressure (PEEP) 4 cm H_2O

CBC:

White blood cells 13,000/mm^3

Segmented neutrophils 52 percent

Bands 8 percent

Lymphocytes 27 percent

Monocytes 6 percent

Eosinophils 2 percent

Hemoglobin (Hb) 18.2 g/dL

Pulse Oximeter (Left Foot): Arterial oxygen saturation (SpO_2) 85 percent

QUESTIONS

11. What is the pathophysiology causing the chest radiographic results?

12. Are these radiographic findings typical of PPHN?

13. How would you interpret the ABG results?

14. What are the possible causes of the hypoxemia?

15. What are the desired ABG values?

16. What is the significance of the anatomical location from which the pulse oximeter reading was taken?

17. What is the significance of the CBC findings?

18. What other diagnostic tests could be performed on this patient to confirm the presence of a right-to-left shunt through the PDA or foramen ovale?

ANSWERS

11. The radiographic findings are consistent with MAS, which is supported by the patient's history of meconium in the amniotic fluid.[32] Aspiration of meconium causes pneumonitis and can lead to atelectasis. Particulate meconium particles can lead to plugging of the airways and a pattern of hyperinflation, diffuse infiltrates, and areas of atelectasis. It is not clear whether this patient's ABG abnormalities are caused by the meconium aspiration or by PPHN.

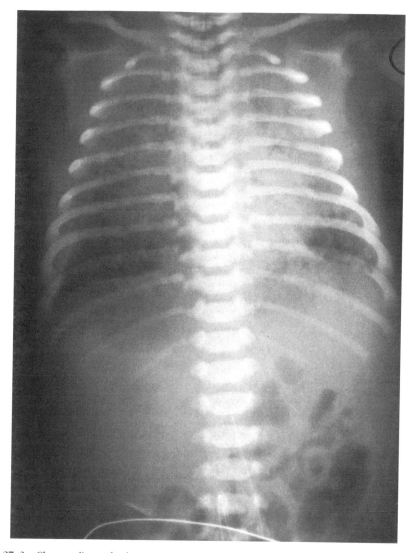

FIGURE 27-3   Chest radiograph showing irregular bilateral densities. Endotracheal tube is in good position.

12. The radiographic findings are not unusual in a patient with suspected PPHN caused by MAS. The radiographic findings suggest only that the meconium found in the amniotic fluid has been inhaled. They do not confirm or rule out PPHN and a right-to-left shunt as the cause of cyanosis.

13. These ABGs show an uncompensated metabolic acidosis and moderate hypoxemia on 50 percent oxygen. The cause of the metabolic acidosis could be the in utero asphyxia the patient may have suffered, reduced perfusion due to hypoxic systemic vasoconstriction, or severe hypoxemia due to PPHN.

14. The cause of this patient's hypoxemia could be atelectasis, small airway obstruction leading to $\dot{V}/\dot{Q}$ abnormalities, or a PDA.

15. The therapeutic range for ABG values in this patient would depend on the diagnosis. If the patient has PPHN, a pH of greater than 7.50, $Paco_2$ of 20 to

30 mm Hg, and a PaO_2 of greater than 100 mm Hg may lead to a lowering of PVR.[8,9,13] The patient with MAS without PPHN may be managed more conservatively, with lower ventilator rates and a lower FIO_2.[33]

16. The pulse oximeter reading should be interpreted as a postductal (left foot) sample. To help confirm the presence of a PDA, both preductal and postductal samples of blood should be obtained (described earlier in this chapter).

17. This is a normal CBC for a newborn. PPHN can be caused by sepsis, which is why a normal CBC is helpful in ruling out sepsis as the etiology of the persistent hypertension.

18. A diagnostic test that could confirm the presence of a PDA is echocardiography.

CASE STUDY—continued

Echocardiography confirmed the presence of a PDA and the absence of any other structural heart disease. With the patient receiving 100 percent oxygen, the PaO_2 remained in the high 40s. On an IMV of 60/minute, PIP of 20 cm H_2O, PEEP of 4 cm H_2O, and FIO_2 of 1.0, the umbilical artery blood gas results were as follows: pH 7.29, $PaCO_2$ 48 mm Hg, PaO_2 40 mm Hg, BE −8, and HCO_3^- 19 mEq/liter. Baby Girl C had episodes of decreased SaO_2 by pulse oximeter during suctioning or other procedures. During these procedures, she became agitated, respiratory efforts became uncoordinated with the ventilator, and saturation readings from the pulse oximeter dropped to as low as 70 percent.

QUESTIONS

19. Would you suggest any ventilator parameter changes for this patient?

20. What probably happens to this patient's delivered tidal volumes (VTs) when her respiratory efforts are not coordinated with the ventilator?

21. What approach is needed to decrease the patient's episodes of low SaO_2 values?

ANSWERS

19. This patient is hypoventilating and may benefit from hyperventilation in order to improve her PaO_2 and pH, which should decrease PVR. Increasing the IMV rate to between 60 and 80/minute may result in a higher pH and a lower $PaCO_2$. These ABG changes may facilitate a decrease in right-to-left shunting and improve the PaO_2. A PaO_2 of 70 to 80 mm Hg is a reasonable goal. Keeping the PaO_2 on the high side may help lessen the pulmonary vasoconstriction. This patient's PaO_2, however, is well below that goal. An alternative may be to increase the PIP, which will also have the effect of decreasing $PaCO_2$ and increasing pH. The disadvantage of using an increased peak pressure to achieve a higher pH is that excessive pressures can lead to barotrauma.[8,22,34]

20. The newborn receiving pressure-limited, time-cycled, continuous-flow **ventilation** may have a reduction in volume delivered into the lung when

fighting the ventilator. If the patient exhales during an inspiratory phase of the ventilator (active exhalation), the expiratory effort results in an increased resistance to the gas entering the lung through the ventilator. This increased resistance will cause a build-up of pressure in the circuit until the pressure limit of the ventilator is reached and no more gas enters the lung. On any given breath, it is difficult to determine how much volume actually reached the lungs of a patient who is not breathing in synchrony with the ventilator. Because the pressure developed in the lungs with pressure-limited ventilation determines the V_T, breathing out of synchrony with the ventilator is associated with a reduced V_T and minute ventilation. Decreases in minute ventilation can cause an increased $Paco_2$ and decreased pH, worsening the PVR and decreasing pulmonary blood flow in patients with PPHN.

21. Most clinicians would agree with the use of minimal stimulation, including a quiet environment, infrequent suctioning, and restrictions on handling the patient to reduce the patient's episodes of low Sao_2. Paralysis of the patient with PPHN is controversial and is usually reserved for patients such as Baby Girl C, in whom breathing out of synchrony with the ventilator is leading to impairment of oxygenation. Sedation can be attempted; if the patient improves, paralysis may not be necessary. This patient may also be a candidate for synchronized IMV (SIMV), now available with many infant ventilators.

CASE STUDY—continued

Baby Girl C was managed with hyperventilation (PIP increased to 30, IMV rate of 60/minute) and responded with an increase in Pao_2 to 60 mm Hg. She remained unstable with several episodes of cyanosis despite sedation. These episodes became longer and lasted up to 3 minutes. Her blood pressure was unstable (hypotensive). She showed no evidence of sepsis and had improved breath sounds. Her chest radiograph demonstrated improvement with reduced pulmonary vascular markings. At 36 hours of age, the following two ABG values were recorded, a half an hour apart:

ABG No. 1: pH 7.23, $Paco_2$ 19 mm Hg, Pao_2 15 mm Hg, BE −8 mEq/liter, HCO_3^- 20 mEq/liter

ABG No. 2: pH 7.12, $Paco_2$ 68 mm Hg, Pao_2 40 mm Hg, BE −9 mEq/liter, HCO_3^- 22 mEq/liter

These blood gases were obtained while the patient was receiving an IMV rate of 65/minute, a PIP of 35 cm H_2O, a PEEP of 4 cm H_2O, and an FIO_2 of 1.0.

QUESTIONS

22. What physical assessment information would you gather at this point?

23. What is the effect of the hypotension on the pathophysiology of PPHN in this patient?

24. Is this patient a candidate for ECMO?

ANSWERS

22. The physical assessment of this patient should include chest auscultation to

determine whether the breath sounds are bilateral. There has been a deterioration in the patient's ABG values, and two abnormalities that should be considered are pneumothorax and a right mainstem bronchus intubation. If breath sounds and chest radiograph confirm the absence of pneumothorax or right mainstem intubation, these ABG values could be considered indicative of intractable respiratory failure, which can occur in the course of PPHN.

23. Systemic hypotension associated with PPHN can increase the right-to-left shunt through the PDA. Hypotension often leads to lower systemic vascular pressures but not lower pulmonary vascular pressures and increases blood flow across the PDA.

24. Several criteria that have been suggested for ECMO are based on historical mortality predictions.[35] A $P(A - a)O_2$ greater than 600 mm Hg lasting 12 hours is a poor prognostic sign and means that ECMO may be warranted. In this patient, the first ABG (assuming 760 mm Hg barometric pressure) revealed a $P(A - a)O_2$ of 607 mm Hg and the second a $P(A - a)O_2$ of 588 mm Hg. Another criterion is acute deterioration associated with (1) PaO_2 less than 40 mm Hg lasting 2 hours or pH less than 7.15 lasting 2 hours; (2) PaO_2 less than 55 mm Hg and pH less than 7.40 lasting 3 hours; or (3) evidence of barotrauma, defined as the presence of four of the following seven: (a) pulmonary interstitial emphysema, (b) pneumothorax or pneumomediastinum, (c) pneumoperitoneum, (d) pneumopericardium, (e) subcutaneous emphysema, (f) persistent air leak lasting more than 24 hours, and (g) mean airway pressure greater than 15 cm H_2O.[36] Even though this patient is showing signs of acute deterioration, many physicians would manage her with conventional therapy (e.g., by stabilizing blood pressure, increasing ventilator settings) and continue to monitor her to see whether she continues to be unstable. If signs of intractable hypoxemia were to persist, she would be considered a candidate for ECMO.

CASE STUDY—continued

Baby Girl C's hospital course included a few more hours of instability, during which dopamine was used to control her blood pressure and neuromuscular blockers and sedation were administered in an attempt to reduce her cyanotic episodes. Her pH, $PaCO_2$, and PaO_2 all improved, and after another 24 hours of hyperventilation, she was gradually weaned from mechanical ventilation. She was discharged from the hospital 10 days later in good health.

REFERENCES

1. Fanaroff, A, and Martin, R: Neonatal-Perinatal Medicine: Diseases of the Fetus and Infant, ed 5. Mosby–Year Book, St. Louis, 1992, p 897.
2. Paul, V, et al: Persistent pulmonary hypertension in the neonate. Indian Pediatr 27:841–847, 1990.
3. Haworth, S, and Reid, L: Persistent fetal circulation: Newly recognized structural features. J Pediatr 88:614, 1976.
4. Peckham, GJ, and Fox, WW: Physiologic fac-

tors affecting pulmonary artery pressure in infants with persistent pulmonary hypertension. J Pediatr 93:1005, 1978.
5. Geggel, R, and Redi, L: The structural basis of PPHN. Clin Perinatol 11:525–549, 1984.
6. Griffin, P: Persistent pulmonary hypertension of the newborn: An update. VA Med Q 121:232–234, 1994.
7. Fineman, J, et al: The role of pulmonary vascular endothelium in perinatal pulmonary circu-

lation regulation. Semin Perinatol 15:58–62, 1991

8. Graves, E, et al: Persistent pulmonary hypertension in the neonate. Chest 93:638–641, 1988.
9. Taeusch, H, et al: Schaffer and Avery's Diseases of the Newborn, 6th ed. WB Saunders, Philadelphia, 1991, p 508.
10. Brann, A: Hypoxic ischemic encephalopathy. Pediatr Clin North Am 33:451–463, 1986.
11. Sexson, et al: The multisystem involvement of the asphyxiated newborn. Pediatr Res 10:432–439, 1976.
12. West, J: Respiratory Physiology: The Essentials, ed 5. Williams & Wilkins, Baltimore, 1995, p 56.
13. Drummond, W, et al: The independent effects of hyperventilation, tolazoline, and dopamine on infants with persistent pulmonary hypertension. J Pediatr 98:603–611, 1981.
14. Morray, J, et al: Effect of pH and P_{CO_2} on pulmonary and systemic hemodynamics after surgery in children with congenital heart disease and pulmonary hypertension. J Pediatr 113:474–9, 1988.
15. Schreiber, M, et al: Increased arterial pH, not decreased Pa_{CO_2}, attenuates hypoxia-induced pulmonary vasoconstriction in newborn lambs. Pediatr Res 20:113–117, 1986.
16. Walsh-Sukys, M: Persistent pulmonary hypertension of the newborn: The black box revisited. Clin Perinatol 20:127–143, 1993
17. Hageman, J, et al: Outcome of persistent pulmonary hypertension in relation to severity of presentation. Am J Dis Child 138:293, 1988.
18. Bifano, E, and Pfannenstiel, A: Duration of hyperventilation and outcome in infants with persistent pulmonary hypertension. Pediatrics 141:852, 1988.
19. Roberts, J, and Shaul, P: Advances in the treatment of persistent pulmonary hypertension of the newborn. Pediatr Clin North Am 40:983, 1993.
20. Sell, E, et al: Persistent fetal circulation: Neurodevelopmental outcome. Am J Dis Child 139:25, 1985.
21. Hsieh, W, et al: Non-hyperventilation respiratory therapy of persistent pulmonary hypertension of the newborn. Acta Paediatr Sin 36(1):24, 1995.
22. Dworetz, A, et al: Survival of infants with PPHN without ECMO. Pediatrics 84:1–6, 1989.
23. Ward, R: Pharmacology of tolazoline. Clin Perinatol 11:703–713, 1984.
24. Beck, R, et al: Criteria for extracorporeal membrane oxygenation in a population of infants with persistent pulmonary hypertension of the newborn. J Pediatr Surg 21:297–302, 1986.
25. Kinsella, J, and Abman, S: Efficacy of inhalational nitric oxide therapy in the clinical management of persistent pulmonary hypertension of the newborn. Chest (suppl)105:92S–94S, 1994.
26. Roberts, J, et al: Inhaled nitric oxide in persistent pulmonary hypertension of the newborn. Lancet 340:818–820, 1992.
27. Zayek, M, et al: Treatment of persistent pulmonary hypertension in the newborn lamb by inhaled nitric oxide. J Pediatr 122:743–750, 1993.
28. Giacoia, G: Nitric oxide: A selective pulmonary vasodilator. South Med J 88(1):33–41, 1995.
29. Abramovici, H, et al: Meconium during delivery: A sign of compensated fetal distress. Am J Obstet Gynecol 118:251, 1974.
30. Jacobsa, M, and Phibbs, R: Prevention, recognition, and treatment of perinatal asphyxia. Clin Perinatol 16:785–803, 1989.
31. Amiel-Tison, C, and Ellison, P: Birth asphyxia in the full term newborn: Early assessment and outcome. Dev Med Child Neurol 28:671–682, 1986.
32. Yeh, T, et al: Roentgenographic findings in infants with meconium aspiration syndrome. JAMA 242:60–63, 1979.
33. Wung, J, et al: Management of infants with severe respiratory failure and persistence of the fetal circulation, without hyperventilation. Pediatrics 76:488–494, 1985.
34. Duara, S, and Gewitz, M: Use of mechanical ventilation for clinical management of persistent pulmonary hypertension of the newborn. Clin Perinatol 11:641–667, 1984.
35. Nading, J: Historical controls for extracorporeal membrane oxygenation in neonates. Crit Care Med 17:423, 1989.
36. Loe, W, et al: Extracorporeal membrane oxygenation in newborn respiratory failure. J Pediatr Surg 20:684, 1985.

Glossary

α_1-protease inhibitor: A protein substance produced by the liver that blocks the action of the enzyme elastase; lack of this substance leads to a breakdown of the lung parenchyma and results in emphysema

A_2: Aortic component of the second heart sound

abdominal paradox: Abnormal inward movement of the abdomen with inspiratory effort; occurs with diaphragm fatigue or paralysis

acidosis: An abnormal increase in the hydrogen ion concentration, which leads to a decrease in the measured pH

acquired immune deficiency syndrome (AIDS): An immune disorder caused by infection with the human immunodeficiency virus (HIV), which reduces the body's ability to fight infections

acrocyanosis: Cyanosis of the extremities

acute postinfectious polyneuropathy: Progressive ascending paralysis caused by inflammation of the myelin sheath around peripheral nerves; also known as Guillain-Barré syndrome

adult respiratory distress syndrome (ARDS): Acute onset of respiratory failure due to increased permeability of the alveolar-capillary membrane and diffuse pulmonary edema

adventitious lung sounds: Abnormal sounds, such as crackles and wheezes, superimposed on the breath sounds

aerobic: Able to live or metabolize only in the presence of oxygen

afterload: The resistance to blood flow out of the ventricle during ventricular contraction

air bronchogram: An abnormal finding on the chest film seen when air-filled bronchi are visible as a result of surrounding consolidation

alkalosis: An abnormal decrease in the hydrogen ion concentration leading to elevation of the serum pH

amniotic fluid: A liquid produced by the fetal membranes that surround the fetus throughout pregnancy

amyotrophic lateral sclerosis (ALS): A progressive, fatal neurologic disease due to loss of motor neurons in the anterior horn cell; also known as Lou Gehrig's disease

anabolic metabolism: The constructive process by which the body converts simple substances into more complex compounds

anaerobic: Able to live or metabolize in the absence of oxygen

anatomical shunt: Blood bypassing the lung through anatomical channels; such blood is poorly oxygenated

anemia: An abnormal reduction in the number of circulating red blood cells

angina: Severe chest pain associated with coronary artery disease

angiography: The visualization of coronary arteries by x-ray after injection of radiopaque contrast medium

anion gap: The mathematical difference between the positive and negative ions of the blood

anorexia: Loss of appetite

anticholinergics: Medications designed to inhibit activity of the parasympathetic nervous system

anticoagulation: The process of inhibiting blood from clotting

antigens: Uniquely shaped molecules that are recognized by the immune system and stimulate a specific immune response

aortic rupture: The sudden fracture of the aorta caused by trauma

Apgar score: An evaluation system used to assess the newborn immediately after birth; system is based on a scale of 1 to 10, with 10 indicating the best physical condition of the infant

apnea: Cessation of spontaneous breathing for more than 10 seconds

arrhythmia: An abnormal rhythm of the heartbeat

arterial blood gases (ABGs): Measurements of oxygen, carbon dioxide, and pH in the arterial blood sample

asbestosis: A condition of pulmonary fibrosis related to the chronic inhalation of asbestos fibers

ascites: The accumulation of serous fluid in the peritoneal cavity

Aspergillus: A fungal organism that may infect the immunosuppressed patient

asphyxia: Cessation of life due to lack of effective gas exchange in the lungs

aspiration: Drawing in or out by the application of suction. In respiratory care patients, the term aspiration is often used to indicate the inhalation of vomitus into the trachea

asthma: A pulmonary disease characterized by reversible obstruction of the airways

atelectasis: Collapsed or airless condition of the lung

atopy: A term used clinically to apply to a group of diseases of an allergic nature; they differ from most allergies in that (1) they are inherited; (2) the antibody produced, called atopic reagin or skin-sensitizing antibody, is deposited in cutaneous tissues and may enter the blood stream; and (3) the primary reaction is edema, as occurs in hay fever or rhinitis; principal atopic manifestations are bronchial asthma, vasomotor rhinitis, and chronic urticaria

atrophy: A reduction in the size of a body part due to disease

auto-PEEP: The inadvertent build-up of positive end-expiratory pressure (PEEP) in the lung during mechanical ventilation as a result of inadequate expiratory time

autoimmune disease: Disease of the immune system that attacks the host

autonomy: Ability to function independently

autosomal recessive: A genetic feature that is not dominant

bands: Immature neutrophils that are recognized by the lack of neutrophil segmentation

barrel chest: An abnormal condition in which the anteroposterior diameter is increased because of hyperinflation of the lungs; often seen with emphysema

beneficence: The "do good" principle of ethics that prescribes the actions of health care workers to be of benefit to others

bradycardia: Abnormally slow heart rate; less than 60/minute in the adult

bradypnea: Abnormally slow breathing rate

bronchial breath sounds: Abnormal breath sounds heard over consolidated lung; sounds have equal inspiratory and expiratory components and are louder than vesicular breath sounds

bronchial provocation: Testing of the patient's airway responsiveness; asthmatics are known to have increased bronchospasm when exposed to the stimulating agent

bronchiectasis: Permanent dilatation of a portion of a bronchus due to structural weakness in the wall of the airway after infection

bronchiolitis: Inflammation of the bronchioles; most often occurs in infants and children

bronchitis: Inflammation of the bronchi, usually due to infection

bronchodilators: Medication designed to cause the smooth muscles of the airways to relax

bronchopleural fistula: An abnormal opening between the lung and the pleura that leads to a continuous lead of air into the pleural space

bronchopneumonia: A type of bacterial pneumonia that has segmental distribution

bronchopulmonary dysplasia (BPD): A chronic lung disease associated with infants who have been exposed to mechanical ventilation for significant periods of time

bronchoscopy: The process of placing a scope into the tracheobronchial tree for the purpose of diagnosis or therapy

bronchospasm: An abnormal contraction of the smooth muscles lining the intrathoracic airways

bruit: An adventitious sound of venous or arterial origin heard on auscultation and produced by turbulent blood flow

cachexia: A state of ill health, malnutrition, and wasting; may occur in many chronic diseases (e.g., certain malignancies, advanced chronic pulmonary disease)

carbon monoxide poisoning: Significant contamination of the blood with carbon monoxide, leading to reduced oxygen content of the arterial blood and tissue hypoxia when severe

carboxyhemoglobin (Hbco): Hemoglobin bound with carbon monoxide

carcinogens: Agents known to produce cancer

cardiac contusion: Trauma to the myocardium leading to tissue damage

cardiac index: The cardiac output divided by the patient's body surface area in meters squared. Normal cardiac index is 2.5 to 4.0 liters/minute per m^2

cardiac output: The quantity of blood pumped out of the left ventricle per minute. Normal values in the adult are 4 to 8 liters/minute

cardiac tamponade: Compression of the heart due to a build-up of blood in the pericardium

cardiomegaly: Hypertrophy (enlargement) of the heart

cardiomyopathy: Disease of the heart muscle

catabolic metabolism: The destructive process by which the body breaks down more complex compounds into more simple substances

central cyanosis: Bluish discoloration of the oral cavity due to hypoxemia

central sleep apnea: Pauses in breathing during sleep due to an inadequate drive to breathe

central venous pressure (CVP): Blood pressure in the central veins

chemotherapy: The use of chemical agents to treat cancer

chest pain: Abnormal pain in the region of the chest; may be of pleuritic or cardiac origin

chest physical therapy: Therapeutic procedures designed to improve expectoration of mucus from the tracheobronchial tree

Cheyne-Stokes breathing: An abnormal pattern of breathing characterized by periods of apnea lasting 10 to 60 seconds, followed by gradually increasing depth and frequency of breathing

chronic obstructive pulmonary disease (COPD): A chronic lung disease characterized by the presence of airflow obstruction; most often associated with emphysema and chronic bronchitis

circulatory failure: Inability of the circulatory system to meet the metabolic needs of the body; *see* shock

clubbing: Abnormal enlargement of the distal phalanges

common morality: A society's shared moral values

competent: Performance of a task at a satisfactory level; mentally sound

complete blood count (CBC): A laboratory test in which the red blood cell and white blood cell counts in the circulatory blood are reported

congestive heart failure (CHF): A clinical syndrome associated with left ventricular failure and diffuse pulmonary edema due to increased hydrostatic pressure in the pulmonary capillaries

consolidation: The process of becoming denser; often used in reference to the lung tissue when pneumonia is present

continuous positive airway pressure (CPAP): The provision of supra-atmospheric end-expiratory pressure to the spontaneously breathing patient

contractility: The ability to contract or shorten

contusion: An injury to the body in which the skin is not broken; a bruise

copious: Large amounts

cor pulmonale: A condition of right ventricular failure due to chronic lung disease

corticosteroid: Medication designed to reduce inflammation; often given to the patient with reversible obstruction of the airways, such as the asthmatic during an acute attack

coryza: Profuse discharge from the mucous membranes of the nose

cough: A sudden, forceful expiratory effort designed to expel mucus or foreign material from the lung and airways

crackles: Discontinuous adventitious lung sounds produced by the sudden opening of collapsed airways or by the movement of excessive airway secretions of fluid

crepitus: A dry, crackling sound or sensation

cromolyn sodium: A medication that inhibits mast cells from releasing mediators that cause bronchospasm; primarily useful in the prevention of asthma attacks

croup: A viral infection of the upper airways; most often seen in small children and infants

cyanosis: Slightly bluish, grayish, slatelike, or dark-purple discoloration of the skin due to the presence of abnormal amounts of reduced hemoglobin in the blood; may not appear in patients with severe anemia, even though their blood is poorly oxygenated, because there is not enough reduced hemoglobin present to cause the blue color to be visible

cystic fibrosis: A chronic inherited disease that affects the exocrine glands of the body, including the pancreas, lungs, and sweat glands

cytology: The study of cells through the use of a microscope

defibrillation: The application of direct electric shock to the chest in an effort to return the heart rhythm to normal

delayed hypersensitivity: The reaction of the cell-mediated immune system to an antigen

diaphoresis: Profuse sweating

diplopia: Double vision

disseminated intravascular coagulation (DIC): The abnormal diffuse form of coagulation that consumes several clotting factors, leading to generalized bleeding

diuresis: The excretion of large amount of urine

diuretic: An agent that increases the excretion of urine

drowning: Suffocation resulting from submersion
  a. **near drowning:** Drowning involving successful resuscitation after submersion
  b. **dry drowning:** Drowning without aspiration
  c. **wet drowning:** Drowning with aspiration

drug-induced lung disease: Disease of the lung that occurs as a side effect of certain medications

ductus arteriosus: An opening between the pulmonary artery and the aorta in the fetus; normally closes after birth

dysphagia: Difficulty swallowing

dysphonia: Difficulty speaking; hoarseness

dyspnea: Air hunger resulting in labored or difficult breathing; sometimes accompanied by pain; normal when due to vigorous work or athletic activity

edema: Abnormal collection of fluid in the tissues

ejection fraction: The portion of the ventricular volume ejected during contraction of the ventricle (systole); normally approximately 70 percent

electrocardiogram (ECG): A recording of the electrical activity of the heart

emphysema: A chronic obstructive pulmonary disease associated with abnormal dilatation of the distal airspaces
   a. **panlobular:** all the airways distal to the terminal bronchioles are involved
   b. **centrilobular:** distal lung units are spared and only the more central airways are involved

empyema: The collection of pus in the pleural cavity

end-diastolic volume: The amount of blood in the ventricle at the end of the diastolic period; represents the amount of blood available for ejection during the subsequent contraction of the ventricles

endogenous: Produced within or caused by factors within the organism

enuresis: Involuntary urination

epiglottitis: A bacterial infection of the epiglottis

epoch: A portion of the polysomnogram representing a 30-second period of time

erythema: Redness of the skin due to congestion of the capillaries

escharotomy: The surgical removal of burned skin that has formed scabs or dry, crusted tissue

ethics: A system of principles that governs conduct

euthanasia: The act of ending the life of a terminally ill patient

excessive daytime sleepiness: Abnormal sleepiness during the day that leads to decreased ability to function

exercise-induced asthma: Asthma attacks caused by exertion

exocrinopathy: Disease of the exocrine glands

exogenous surfactant therapy: The application of artificial surfactant to the lungs of a premature infant

external respiration: Gas exchange between the lung and an inhaled gas

extracorporeal membrane oxygenation (ECMO): The process of oxygenating the patient's blood by exposing it to a membrane oxygenator

extrinsic asthma: Asthma due to allergic reactions

exudates: Accumulations of fluid in a cavity; matter that penetrates through vessel walls into adjoining tissue; or pus or serum

fasciculations: Involuntary contraction or twitching of muscle fibers

fetid: Foul smelling

fetus: An infant in utero from the third month until birth

fever: An abnormal elevation of body temperature due to disease

fibrosis: The formation of fibrous tissue

fistula: An abnormal tubelike passage from a normal cavity or tube to another cavity or tube

flail chest: A condition of the chest wall due to two or more fractures on each affected rib that result in a "free-floating" portion of the rib cage; affected region moves in a paradoxical fashion with breathing; *see* paradoxical respiration

flash over: A wall of fire extending down from the ceiling and billowing out of open doors or windows

foramen ovale: An opening between the two atria of the heart in the fetus; normally closes after birth

forced vital capacity (FVC): The volume of air that is exhaled after full inspiration, during a forceful expiratory maneuver

Frank-Starling response: Increases in the force of myocardial contraction following increases in the stretching of the myocardium

functional residual capacity (FRC): The amount of gas in the lungs at the end of a normal tidal volume exhalation; represents a combination of the residual volume and the expiratory reserve volume

gallop: An abnormal rhythm of the heart characterized by an extra sound heard during diastole; this extra sound, added to the normal first and second heart sounds, results in a rhythm that resembles the pattern produced by the hooves of a horse during a gallop

Ghon complex: The combination of the initial lung lesion and the affected lymph node in the patient with tuberculosis

Glasgow coma scale: A scoring system used to document the neurological condition of the patient

granuloma: A granular growth or tumor

gravida: A pregnant woman; gravida 1 refers to a woman's first pregnancy, gravida 2 the second pregnancy, and so on

Guillain-Barré syndrome: *See* acute postinfectious polyneuropathy

Hb: Hemoglobin

HbCN: Hemoglobin bound with cyanide

Heave: An abnormal pulsation on the chest as the result of ventricular hypertrophy

HEENT: Head, ears, eyes, nose, and throat

helper T lymphocytes: White blood cells that promote the development of antibodies; play a key role in cell-mediated immunity

hemolysis: The breakdown of red blood cells resulting in the release of hemoglobin into the plasma

hemoptysis: Expectoration of blood arising from hemorrhage of the larynx, trachea, bronchi, or lungs

hemothorax: An abnormal build-up of blood in the pleural space

heparin: A medication designed to reduce blood clotting

hepatojugular reflex: A physical examination finding of jugular venous distention occurring shortly after pressure is applied over the liver; this finding suggests that the liver is engorged

hepatomegaly: Enlargement of the liver

hilum: A depression in an organ in which nerves and blood vessels enter or exit the lung

history of present illness: The section of the medical history that describes the details about the patient's current medical problem; details such as when the symptom first started, its level of intensity, and its location are included

honeycomb lung: A radiographic finding seen in end-stage interstitial lung disease caused by the formation of cysts

Hoover's sign: An abnormal breathing pattern, seen in patients with severe emphysema, in which the lateral portions of the chest wall move inward with each inspiratory effort

Horner's syndrome: A clinical syndrome caused by tumor compression of the cervical nerves

hyaline membrane disease: *See* respiratory distress syndrome (RDS)

hypercapnia: An abnormal increase in carbon dioxide in the arterial blood ($Paco_2$ > 45 mm Hg)

hyperkalemia: An abnormal increase in the serum potassium level

hypernatremia: An abnormal increase in the serum sodium level

hyperpnea: Deep breathing

hypersensitivity pneumonitis: A form of interstitial lung disease due to inhalation of organic dusts

hypersomnolence: An abnormal degree of sleepiness; *see* excessive daytime sleepiness

hypertension: An abnormal increase in the systemic blood pressure

hypertrophy: Enlargement of an organ or a part of the organ

hypocapnia: Reduction of the $Paco_2$ level below 35 mm Hg

hypoglycemia: An abnormal decrease in blood glucose levels

hypokalemia: An abnormal decrease in the potassium level in plasma of the circulating blood

hyponatremia: An abnormal decrease in the level of sodium in the plasma of the circulating blood

hypoplasia: Underdevelopment of a tissue or organ

hypopnea: Shallow breathing

hypotension: An abnormal decrease in the systemic blood pressure

hypothermia: An abnormally low body temperature

hypoxemia: Insufficient oxygenation of the arterial blood

hypoxia: Insufficient oxygenation at the tissue level

ICU: Intensive care unit

idiopathic: Disease occurring without a known cause

ileus: An obstruction of the intestines

infarction: Formation of an infarct; an area of tissue in an organ or body part that undergoes necrosis after cessation of blood supply

inotropes: Medications or compounds that affect the contractility of the heart muscle

insomnia: The inability to sleep

intermittent mandatory ventilation (IMV): A mode of mechanical ventilation in which the patient can take spontaneous tidal volumes in between the machine-delivered breaths

intermittent positive-pressure ventilation (IPPV): The application of positive pressure to the airway during inspiration

internal respiration: Gas exchange between the blood and tissues

intrinsic asthma: Asthma that is unrelated to allergic disorders

intubation: The process of placing an endotracheal tube into the trachea

ischemia: Local and temporary anemia due to obstruction of the circulation to a body part

jugular venous distention (JVD): Abnormal filling of the veins of the neck due to heart failure

kyphoscoliosis: Abnormal deviation of the spine laterally and from anterior to posterior

kyphosis: Excessive posterior curvature of the spine; gives rise to a condition commonly known as humpback or hunchback

lactic acidosis: A disturbance in the lactic acid balance of the body

laryngotracheobronchitis: *See* croup

leukocyte: A white blood cell

leukocytopenia: An abnormal decrease in the number of white blood cells in the circulation

leukocytosis: A transient increase in the number of white blood cells in the blood

leukopenia: Abnormal decrease in the number of white blood corpuscles, usually below 5000/mm^3

loud P$_2$: Refers to an abnormally loud second heart sound that occurs as the result of an abnormally forceful closure of the pulmonic valve; often the result of pulmonary hypertension

Lou Gehrig's disease: *See* amyotrophic lateral sclerosis

lung contusion: An injury to the lung that is the result of a blunt trauma, causing pathological changes; similar to a bruise

lymphadenopathy: Disease of the lymph nodes

lymphocytosis: An excess of normal white blood cells in the blood or an effusion

macroglossia: An enlarged tongue

macrognathia: Abnormal size of jaw

maladaptation: The lack of appropriate physiologic changes to extrauterine life

maximum inspiratory pressure (MIP): A test typically used to determine the strength of the patient's inspiratory muscles and their potential ability to wean from mechanical ventilation

mechanical ventilation: The application of positive-pressure breathing to a patient's lungs to maintain adequate gas exchange

meconium: A material that collects in the intestines of the fetus and forms the first stool of a newborn

metaplasia: The change in body cells from normal to abnormal for that type of tissue

metastatic malignancy: A tumor that is the result of a malignancy that has spread beyond the primary site

metered-dose inhaler (MDI): A device designed to deliver a specific dose of an aerosolized medication for inhalation

microemboli: Very small blood clots

micrognathia: Abnormal smallness of the jaws, especially the lower jaw

miliary tuberculosis: A uniquely disseminated form of tuberculosis that involves both lungs; *see* tuberculosis

mixed apnea: When both central and obstructive apnea are present in the same patient

mixed venous Po$_2$ (P$\bar{v}$o$_2$): The partial pressure of oxygen in the plasma of the venous blood in the right atrium, right ventricle, or pulmonary artery

morbidity: The condition of being diseased or unhealthy

mortality: The condition of being subject to death; often used to refer the death rate of a specific illness

mucoid: Clear, thick mucus from the tracheobronchial tree

mucus: Secretions from the tracheobronchial tree

murmur: A soft blowing or rasping sound heard on auscultation of the heart

myasthenia gravis: A neuromuscular disease associated with abnormal conduction of the nerve impulse through the neuromuscular junction

Mycobacterium: A genus of acid-fast organisms responsible for the lung infection known as tuberculosis

myocardium: The muscle making up the walls of the heart

myopathy: Disease of the muscles

narcolepsy: A chronic ailment consisting of recurrent attacks of drowsiness and sleep

nasal flaring: Flaring outward of the external nares with each inspiratory effort; usually indicates an increase in the work of breathing

nasal polyps: An abnormal growth protruding from the mucous membranes of the nasal passages

necrosis: The death of areas of tissue surrounded by healthy tissue

necrotizing: Causing death of areas of tissue or bone surrounded by healthy parts; *see* infarction

neoplasm: An abnormal growth of new tissue; can be benign or malignant

night sweats: Excessive sweating during sleep that often soaks the patient's pillow and pajamas and is the result of rapid decreases in body temperature following a fever

nitric oxide (NO): A pharmacological gas that causes pulmonary vasodilatation in low doses

nocturnal dyspnea: Shortness of breath that occurs during sleep; most often associated with congestive heart failure

nonmaleficence: The no-harm principle of ethics

non–rapid eye movement (NREM) sleep: Sleep not involving rapid eye movements, having four stages and making up the majority of sleep time in healthy people

normocephalic: Normal configuration of the head

nosocomial: Pertaining to or originating in a hospital; usually used in reference to an infection acquired by a patient while in a hospital

obstructive sleep apnea: The cessation of breathing for more than 10 seconds due to obstruction of the upper airway

obtunded: A condition of reduced response to stimuli

occupational asthma: Asthma attacks associated with a stimulant in the work place

oliguria: Diminished amount of urine formation

opportunistic infection: Infection caused by an organism that does not infect persons with a healthy immune system

optimal PEEP: The level of positive end-expiratory pressure (PEEP) that causes adequate oxygenation of the arterial blood without impeding cardiac output

oral thrush: Fungus infection of mouth or throat, especially in infants and young children, characterized by formation of white patches and ulcers, frequently fever and gastrointestinal inflammation

organomegaly: Abnormal enlargement of an organ in the body

orthopnea: Shortness of breath that occurs in the reclining position

oxygenation failure: Inability of the lungs to maintain adequate oxygenation of the arterial blood despite the use of supplemental oxygen

oxyhemoglobin: Hemoglobin bound with oxygen

P_2: Pulmonic component of the second heart sound. A loud P_2 is suggestive of pulmonary hypertension

para: A woman who has produced one or more viable offspring; often used along with the term gravida to indicate the number of pregnancies and resulting viable offspring; for example, gravida 2, para 1 refers to a woman who has been pregnant twice but has produced only one viable child

paradoxical pulse: Pulse that is abnormally suppressed during each inspiration

paradoxical respiration: Most often used to describe a condition seen with diaphragm fatigue or paralysis in which the diaphragm ascends with inspiration; seen as an inward sinking motion of the abdominal wall with each inspiratory effort by the patient; can also be used to describe a traumatized portion of the chest wall that sinks inward with inspiration in the patient with a flail chest; *see* flail chest

parenchyma: The essential parts of an organ that are concerned with its function; lung parenchyma refers to the distal portions of the lung involved with gas exchange

paresthesia: Sensation of numbness, prickling, or tingling often in the extremities

paroxysmal nocturnal respiration (PNR): A sudden onset of difficulty breathing that typically occurs during sleep; associated with congestive heart failure

patent ductus arteriosus (PDA): An opening between the pulmonary artery and the aorta of the fetus, which normally closes after birth

pectus carinatum: Abnormal protrusion of the sternum

pectus excavatum: Abnormal concavity of the sternum

pedal edema: Abnormal collection of fluid in the soft tissues around the ankles; often due to heart failure

perfusion: Passing of a fluid through spaces

pericardial tamponade: Compression of the heart due to a build-up of blood in the pericardial sac around the heart

pericarditis: Inflammation of pericardium (the double membrane sac enclosing the heart and the origins of the great blood vessels)

perihilar: Pertaining to the tissues around the hilum of the lung; the hilum is the opening that gives entrance to the pulmonary artery and veins for each lung

peristalsis: The rhythmic, coordinated contraction of smooth muscle that moves a substance through a canal; for example, peristalsis of the bowel moves food through the intestinal tract

peritoneal: Concerning the peritoneum, which is a serous membrane lining the abdominal cavity

permissive hypercapnia: The process of allowing the $PaCO_2$ to increase above normal by reducing the volume of the delivered tidal volume from the ventilator or by reducing the number of breaths per minute; done to reduce the negative impact of elevated mean intrathoracic pressure associated with mechanical ventilation

PERRLA: A mnemonic for *p*upils *e*qual, *r*ound, and *r*eactive to *l*ight and *a*ccommodation; part of the neurological component of the physical examination of the patient

persistent pulmonary hypertension of the newborn (PPHN): A clinical syndrome seen in infants, associated with increased pulmonary vascular resistance and decreased pulmonary blood flow

phagocytosis: The engulfing and destruction of foreign organisms by macrophages

pharyngitis: Inflammation of the pharynx

physiological shunt: Blood flow through the lung that passes by unventilated alveoli

plasmapheresis: The removal of plasma from withdrawn blood and replacement of the formed elements back into the patient

platypnea: Difficulty breathing in the upright position

pneumoconiosis: Disease of the lung caused by the chronic inhalation of dust, often of occupational origin

pneumonia: Inflammation of the pulmonary parenchyma

> a. **lobar pneumonia:** A form of bacterial pneumonia that affects a specific lobe as seen on the chest radiograph
> b. *Pneumocystis carinii* **pneumonia:** A pneumonia often seen in AIDS patients

pneumoplasty: A surgical procedure done to remove abnormal, hyperinflated lung tissue; also known as lung volume reduction surgery

pneumothorax: The presence of air in the pleural space

point of maximum impulse (PMI): Impulse generated by the contraction of the left ventricle

polycythemia: An excess of red blood cells; often due to chronic hypoxemia

polyphonic: A sound made up of multiple notes

polysomnogram: An all-night sleep study designed to help diagnose a patient's sleep problems

positive end-expiratory pressure (PEEP): The application and maintenance of positive pressure in the airways throughout the expiratory phase of mechanical ventilation

precordium: The surface of the chest wall overlying the heart

preload: The volume of blood filling the ventricle just before ventricular contraction

pressure-support ventilation: A method of ventilary support in which the patient's spontaneous breathing is assisted by the ventilator at a preset level of inspiratory pressure

primary hypoventilation: A disease caused by insufficient respiratory drive that leads to chronic elevation of the $Paco_2$

primary lung cancer: A lung tumor that originates in the lung

ptosis: Drooping of an organ such as the upper eyelid as a result of paralysis

pulmonary capillary wedge pressure (PCWP): The pressure used to evaluate left ventricular filling (preload)

pulmonary contusion: Trauma to the pulmonary tissue due to sudden impact

pulmonary fibrosis: A chronic lung disease associated with permanent fibrotic changes in the connective tissues of the lung following inflammation

pulmonary hypertension: Abnormal elevation of the pressure in the pulmonary artery

pulse pressure: The difference between the systolic and diastolic blood pressures

pulsus alternans: A pulse characterized by a regular alternation of weak and strong beats

pulsus paradoxus: An abnormal decrease in the systolic pressure during inspiration; associated with a significant increase in the patient's work of breathing

purified protein derivative (PPD): Used in the Mantoux skin test to diagnose tuberculosis

purulent: Containing pus; indicates the presence of bacterial infection

pyrogenic: Producing fever

radiolucency: Property of being partly or wholly permeable to radiant energy

radiopaque: Impenetrable to x-ray beams; for example, bones are usually impenetrable to x-ray beams and leave a white shadow on the radiograph

rales: A discontinuous type of adventitious lung sound heard on auscultation of the chest; *see* crackles

rapid eye movement (REM) sleep: sleep stage in which a person dreams and has rapid eye movements

refractory hypoxemia: Hypoxemia that does not respond adequately to significant increases in fraction of inspired oxygen

replication: To reproduce genetic material

respiratory alternans: An abnormal pattern of breathing where the patient alternates for short periods of time between breathing with accessory muscles and breathing with the diaphragm

respiratory distress syndrome (RDS): An acute failure of the lungs to provide gas exchange in the premature infant as a result of diffuse atelectasis and the formation of hyaline membranes

respiratory disturbance index: Obtained by dividing the total number of abnormal events during a night of sleep by the total sleep time in hours; indicates the severity of a patient's sleep disturbance

respiratory failure: Failure of the lungs to maintain adequate oxygenation with or without an elevated P_{CO_2}

respiratory syncytial virus: A common viral infection affecting infants and small children

retinopathy: Any noninflammatory disease of the retina

retractions: A visible sinking inward of the skin and soft tissues surrounding the bones of the thorax with each inspiratory effort; indicates that the work of breathing is significantly increased

rhinorrhea: Thin, watery discharge from the nose

rhonchus: A low-pitched, continuous type of adventitious lung sound heard during auscultation of the chest

ribavirin: A virostatic agent used to treat respiratory syncytial virus

S$_1$: First heart sound; produced by the closure of the mitral and tricuspid valves

S$_2$: Second heart sound; produced by the closure of the aortic and pulmonic valves

S$_3$: Third heart sound; may be normal in young persons, but usually indicates heart disease in adults

S$_3$ gallop: An abnormal third heart sound

S$_4$: Fourth heart sound; often heard in adult patients with heart disease

sarcoidosis: A disease of unknown etiology characterized by widespread granulomatous lesions that may affect any organ in the body, but more often the lungs

scoliosis: Abnormal lateral curvature of the spine

segmented neutrophils: Mature neutrophils, most of which are able to fight infection

sensorium: Portion of the brain that functions as a center of sensations

sepsis: Pathologic state, usually febrile, resulting from the presence of microorganisms or their poisonous products in the blood stream

shock: A clinical condition resulting from inadequate blood flow to the vital organs; often characterized by a reduced urine output, diminished level of consciousness, hypotension, peripheral cyanosis, and tachycardia
   a. **anaphylactic:** shock due to injection of a protein substance to which the patient is sensitized
   b. **hypovolemic:** shock due to inadequate blood volume
   c. **septic:** shock that occurs in septicemia, when endotoxins are released from certain bacteria in the blood stream; characterized by hypotension from a significant drop in systemic vascular resistance
   d. **toxic:** severe, acute shock brought on by infection with strains of *Staphylococcus aureus*

shunt: Blood that passes from the right side of the heart to the left side without coming into contact with gas exchange units of the lung

silicosis: Pulmonary fibrosis due to inhalation of silica dust

sleep apnea: Temporary pauses in breathing during sleep lasting at least 10 seconds

sleep hypopnea: A period of decreased airflow during sleep defined as a 50 percent or greater reduction in thoracoabdominal movement lasting at least 10 seconds

small particle aerosol generator (SPAG): Most often used to deliver ribavirin to patients with respiratory syncytial virus

sputum: An aggregation of secretions from the tracheobronchial tree and mouth

stable asthma: Asthma that has not caused an increase in symptoms over the past 4 weeks

static compliance: The lung compliance calculated by using the static pressure in the airways during an expiratory hold maneuver; results reflect the compliance of the lung and chest wall

status asthmaticus: Persistent and intractable asthma unresponsive to conventional treatment

stenotic: Abnormal narrowing of a body passage or opening

stridor: Harsh or high-pitched sound (like blowing of the wind) heard during respiration; due to obstruction of air passages

stroke volume: The amount of blood ejected by the left ventricle with each beat

subcutaneous emphysema: An abnormal accumulation of air in the subcutaneous tissues due to a leak from the lung

supraglottitis: *See* epiglottitis

surfactant: An agent that lowers surface tension; pulmonary surfactant is a phospholipid substance that helps prevent alveolar collapse

sweat chloride: The level of the chloride ion in the sweat of the patient; a sweat chloride test is done to assist the physician in the diagnosis of cystic fibrosis

sympathomimetic: Medications that stimulate the sympathetic nervous system; often given in an attempt to dilate the smooth muscle of the airways in patients with obstructive pulmonary disease

tachycardia: Abnormal increase in heart rate

tachyphylaxis: Rapid immunization against the effect of toxic doses of an extract by previous injection of small doses of it

tachypnea: Abnormal increase in the respiratory rate

tamponade: Pathological compression of a body part

teratogen: An agent that causes a physical defect in the developing embryo of a pregnant woman

tetany: A nervous system problem characterized by spasms of the muscles, typically in the extremities

theophylline: A xanthine type of bronchodilator

thromboembolism: A blood clot that has broken loose from its site of origin and is traveling in the vascular system; often lodges in the lung

thrombosis: The formation of a blood clot

thyromegaly: Enlargement of the thyroid gland

tracheal tugging: The physical examination finding in which the trachea is seen or felt to tug downward with each inspiratory effort; indicates an increase in the work of breathing

tram tracks: Abnormal findings on the chest film associated with hypertrophy of the bronchial walls; often seen in patients with cystic fibrosis

tuberculosis: Infection due to *Mycobacterium;* often involves the lungs, but can occur in most body tissues

universal precautions: The practice of treating all patients as though they were infected with a blood-borne infection; requires the use of precautionary measures, such as wearing latex gloves, a gown, and a mask whenever contact with a patient's blood or secretions could occur

unstable asthma: Asthma that has caused an increase in symptoms during the past 4 weeks

upper airway resistance syndrome: A form of obstructive sleep hypopnea in which narrowing of the upper airway partially limits airflow, leading to an arousal

uvulopalotopharyngoplasty (UPPP): A surgical procedure designed to remove redundant tissue from the upper airway and therefore reduce the likelihood of hypopneas or obstructive events during sleep

vasopressor: A medication given to increase peripheral vascular resistance in an attempt to elevate the blood pressure

ventilatory failure: Inadequate ventilation that causes an increase in $Paco_2$

ventricular hypertrophy: Abnormal enlargement of one or both of the ventricles of the heart

vesicular breath sounds: Normal breath sounds occurring over the lung; represent filtered bronchial breath sounds produced by turbulent airflow in the larger airways

viral pneumonia: Viral infection in the lung most often associated with inflammation of the interstitial tissues

virulent: Very poisonous

vital capacity (VC): The volume of air a person is able to exhale after a maximum inspiratory effort

weaning: The process of gradually discontinuing mechanical ventilation of a patient

wheeze: A high-pitched, continuous type of adventitious lung sound resulting from narrowing of the intrathoracic airways.
  a. **monophonic:** wheeze with a single tone
  b. **polyphonic:** wheeze with multiple notes occurring at the same time

REFERENCE

Taber's Cyclopedic Medical Dictionary, 18th Edition. F.A. Davis Company, Philadelphia, 1997.

APPENDIX

Normal Laboratory Values

Hoai N. Tran

ADULT

Arterial Blood Gases (ABGs)

pH	7.35–7.45
$Paco_2$	35–45 mm Hg
Pao_2	80–100 mm Hg
HCO_3^-	22–26 mEq/liter
Base excess (BE)	−2 to +2
Arterial saturation with oxygen (Sao_2)	>95 percent

Complete Blood Count (CBC)

Red blood cell (RBC) count	
Men	4.6–6.2 million/mm³
Women	4.2–5.4 million/mm³
Hemoglobin (Hb)	
Men	13.5–16.5 g/dL
Women	12.0–15.0 g/dL
Hematocrit (Hct)	
Men	40–54%
Women	38–47%
Erythrocyte index	
Mean cell volume (MCV)	80–96 μ³
Mean cell hemoglobin (MCH)	27–31 pg
Mean cell hemoglobin concentration (MCHC)	32–36%
White blood cell (WBC) count	4,500–10,000/mm³
Differential of WBCs	
Neutrophils	40–75%
Bands	0–6%
Eosinophils	0–6%
Basophils	0–1%
Lymphocytes	20–45%
Monocytes	2–10%
Platelet count	150,000–400,000/mm³

Chemistry

Na$^+$	137–147 mEq/liter
K$^+$	3.5–4.8 mEq/liter
Cl$^-$	98–105 mEq/liter
CO$_2$	25–33 mEq/liter
Blood urea nitrogen (BUN)	7–20 mg/dL
Creatine	0.7–1.3 mg/dL
Total protein	6.3–7.9 g/dL
Albumin	3.5–5.0 g/dL
Cholesterol	150–220 mg/dL
Glucose	70–105 mg/dL

Hemodynamic Values

Variable	Abbreviation	Normal
Cardiac output	Q̇T	4–8 liters/minute
Cardiac index	CI	2.5–4.0 liters/minute/m^2
Stroke volume	SV	60–130 mL
Ejection fraction	EF	65–75%
Central venous pressure	CVP	0–6 mm Hg
Pulmonary artery pressure	PAP	25/10 mm Hg
Pulmonary capillary wedge pressure	PCWP	6–12 mm Hg
Systemic vascular resistance	SVR	900–1400 dynes/second/cm^5
Pulmonary vascular resistance	PVR	110–250 dynes/second/cm^5

Pulmonary Function Tests

Variable	Abbreviation	Normal
Forced vital capacity	FVC	>80% of predicted
Slow vital capacity	SVC	80–120% of predicted
Forced expiratory volume in 1 second	FEV$_1$	>80% of predicted
Forced expiratory volume in 1 second/Forced vital capacity	FEV$_1$/FVC	>75%
Forced expiratory flow	FEF$_{25-75\%}$	>80% of predicted
Carbon monoxide diffusing capacity	D$_{LCO}$	25 mL CO/minute/mm Hg
Total lung capacity	TLC	6000 mL
Functional residual capacity	FRC	2400 mL
Residual volume	RV	1200 mL
Vital capacity	VC	4800 mL

Vital Signs	Normal Range
Temperature range	36.1–37.5°C
Heart rate	60–100/minute
Respiratory rate	12–20/minute
Blood pressure range	120/80 mm Hg Systolic 95–140 mm Hg Diastolic 60–90 mm Hg

CHILDREN (AGE 1 to 12 YEARS)

ABGs

Refer to adult values

CBC Tests

RBC count	3.8–5.5 million/mm³
Hb	11–16 g/dL
Hct	31–43%
Erythrocyte index (refer to adult values)	
WBC count (refer to adult values)	
Differential of WBCs (refer to adult values)	

Chemistry

Na⁺	135–145 mEq/liter
K⁺	3.5–5.0 mEq/liter
Cl⁻	100–106 mEq/liter
Ca⁺⁺	9.2–10.8 mg/dL
Mg⁺⁺	1.5–2.0 mEq/liter
Glucose	60–105 mg/dL

Hemodynamic Values

CI	3.5–4.5 liter/minute/m²
CVP	2–6 mm Hg
PAP	30/8 mm Hg
PCWP	4–8 mm Hg

NEWBORN

ABG

pH	7.25–7.35
Pa_{CO_2}	26–40 mm Hg
Pa_{O_2}	50–70 mm Hg
HCO_3^-	17–23 mEq/liter
BE	−10 to −2

CBC Count

RBC count	4.8–7.1 million/mm^3
Hb	14–24 g/dL
Hct	44–64%
Erythrocyte index	
MCV	96–108 μ^3
MCH	32–34 pg
MCHC	32–33%
WBC count	
Mean value	18,100/mm^3
Range	9,000–30,000/mm^3
Lymphocytes	
Mean value	5,500/mm^3
Range	2,000–11,000/mm^3

Chemistry

Na^+	133–149 mEq/liter
K^+	5.3–6.4 mEq/liter
Cl^-	87–114 mEq/liter
CO_2	19–22 mEq/liter
Total protein	4.8–8.5 g/dL
Albumin	2.9–5.5 g/dL
Glucose	30–110 mg/dL

Hemodynamic Values

Cardiac output	
Newborn	0.8–1.0 liter/minute
6 months old	1.0–1.3 liters/minute
1 year old	1.3–1.5 liters/minute
CI	2.5–4.5 liters/minute/m^2
SV	
Newborn	5 mL
6 months old	10 mL
1 year old	13 mL

Vital Signs

Temperature range	36.1–37.5°C
Heart rate	100–160 minute
Respiratory rate	30–60/minute
Blood pressure	75/50 mm Hg

Index